Physiotherapy is both an art and a science, drawing from knowledge of several sciences including anatomy, physiology, medicine, pathology, biomechanics and behavioural psychology. This scientifically and research based text, with extensive reference to the literature, is designed to provide a scientific basis from which clinical expertise is developed in neurological rehabilitation. This book is intended for undergraduate students and qualified physiotherapists who may find it a useful refresher. The post-graduate research student is also invited to seek thought provoking questions which require investigation.

Common themes throughout the chapters include: consideration of the theoretical basis of treatments and scientific evidence of their effectiveness; a non-prescriptive, multidisciplinary approach to patient management; involvement of the patient and carer in goal setting and decision making; use of outcome measures to evaluate the effects of treatment in everyday practice; and a problem solving approach to management (a model is described in Chapter 7).

SECTION 1: BASIC CONCEPTS IN NEUROLOGY

These chapters provide a basis for understanding subsequent sections and are referred to widely throughout the book. A degree of basic knowledge is assumed in Chapters 1 and 2, in which applied neuroanatomy and neurophysiology, and motor control are discussed. Assessment by the neurologist (Chapter 3) and physiotherapist (Chapter 4) are then outlined. This section ends with discussion of abnormalities of muscle tone and movement (Chapter 5), and the recovery mechanisms of neural and muscle tissue involved in plasticity (Chapter 6).

SECTION 2: NEUROLOGICAL AND NEUROMUSCULAR CONDITIONS

Each chapter in this section contains contributions from physiotherapists and medical practitioners. The neurological conditions in Chapters 7 to 13 are not presented in any particular order, but the neuromuscular conditions are organised from proximal to distal parts of the motor unit. Disorders of nerves are presented in two sections: I – motor neurone disease (Chapter 14) which involves the anterior horn cell (but also upper motor neurones) and II – polyneuropathies (Chapter 15) which involve the motor nerves. Disorders of muscle (Chapter 16) are then covered to include the neuromuscular junction (myasthenia gravis) and muscle fibres (muscular dystrophies). Muscle disorders of childhood onset are dealt with in Section 3 and mainly include muscular dystrophies and spinal muscular atrophy (the latter being a problem of the anterior horn cell, but so placed as the onset is in childhood).

Specific issues related to each disorder are discussed and, to avoid repetition of aspects common to all disorders, reference is made to chapters on general topics such as assessment, treatment concepts and techniques, drugs etc. Case histories illustrate certain aspects of some conditions and a problem solving approach is used.

SECTION 3: LIFETIME DISORDERS OF CHILDHOOD ONSET

This section is not simply termed paediatric conditions, since children with disorders such as muscular dystrophy and cerebral palsy are frequently surviving into adulthood. The introduction to paediatric neurology discusses some of the rarer conditions which physiotherapists may come across (Chapter 17). The continuation of care into adulthood is stressed throughout Chapters 17 to 21.

SECTION 4: TREATMENT APPROACHES TO NEUROLOGICAL REHABILITATION

This final section begins with a review of the theoretical basis of treatment concepts (Chapter 22). Adequate evaluation has not been performed although it is likely that no single approach has all the answers. Aspects from the different concepts can be selected for use in an individual patient. This eclectic approach is being applied in all areas of physiotherapy, as rigid adherence to one school or another is progressively thought not to be in the best interest of patients.

Two treatment concepts are introduced which were developed in orthopaedics and can be applied to neurology: adverse neural tension (Chapter 23.1) and muscle imbalance (Chapter 23.2). Specific treatment techniques and management of muscle tone are discussed in Chapters 24 and 25, explaining the types of treatments available, their proposed mode of action (if known) and situations in which they might be applied.

Pain (Chapter 26) and psychological issues (Chapter 27), which may influence physiotherapy treatment, are then discussed. The final chapter covers drug treatments used in neurology (Chapter 28) and provides a useful glossary with details of effects and side effects of drugs, some of which may influence physical management.

CURRENT ISSUES IN REHABILITATION

Certain areas which are relevant to neurological rehabilitation in general, some being controversial, are discussed briefly below.

Impairment, Disability and Handicap (IDH)

The international classification of impairment, disability and handicap (ICIDH) was first published by the World Health Organisation (WHO) in 1980 and is currently under revision by a Working Party. The two main outcomes of the classification system are definitions of IDH and a categorisation system for describing specific items.

Impairment is defined as loss or abnormality of body structure or appearance, organ or system function,

NEUROLOGICAL PHYSIOTHERAPY

PROFESSOR MARIA STOKES PhD, MCSP

Director of Research
Royal Hospital for Neuro-disability
London

Mosby
London Philadelphia St Louis Sydney Tokyo

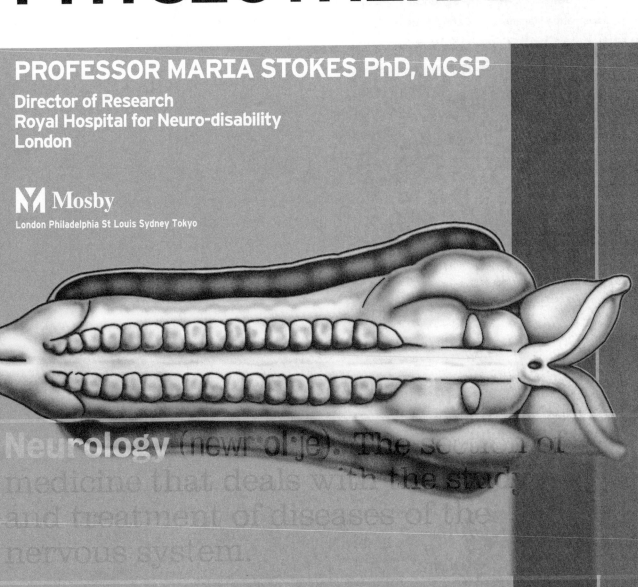

Neurology (newr·ol·je). The science or medicine that deals with the study and treatment of diseases of the nervous system.

Publisher	**Jill Northcott**
Development Editor	**Gillian Harris**
Project Manager	**Louise Patchett**
Design	**Greg Smith**
Layout	**Gisli Thor**
Cover Design	**Greg Smith**
Illustration Manager	**Danny Pyne**
Illustrators	**Deborah Gyan**
	Matthew McClements
	Marion Tasker
	Lynda Payne
Production	**Hamish Adamson**

resulting from any cause. Impairments thus represent disturbances at the organ level and may be of an anatomical, physiological or psychological nature.

Disability is the lack or restriction of ability, resulting from an impairment, in terms of functional performance and activity, representing disturbance at the level of the person.

Handicap is the disadvantage experienced by the individual, as a result of impairments or disabilities, which prevents them from fulfilling their normal role. Handicap thus reflects interaction with, and adaptation to, the individual's surroundings, and is influenced by their age, sex and social and cultural background.

An example of how the classification codes are used is shown in Table 1. The codes and specific items are listed in the relevant sections of the WHO (1980) manual.

Uses of the classification system include health care planning for management and prevention, policy making, epidemiology, and assessment in occupational health, employment and social security. The coding system is potentially useful for rehabilitation research but requires further refinement before it can be established as a reliable measurement system. A major part of rehabilitation research is currently concerned with developing methods for measuring impairments and disability.

For clinical purposes, it is useful to apply the definitions of impairment and disability when planning treatment, without necessarily using the coding system for specific items. There is some disagreement amongst clinicians as to which aspect of function treatment should be aimed at. It is argued by some that treatment should only involve functional tasks, thus focusing on disability. It is certainly true that the specificity of training is vital to the re-education of normal activities, and there is a growing body of evidence to support this (see Chapter 24). It is also true that unless a threshold level of muscle function is available, a functional task cannot be achieved and cannot therefore be practised.

If an example for this argument is taken from the information in Table 1, without a threshold level of strength in the quadriceps muscles (impairment), a patient is unable to stand up from sitting and go up and down the stairs (disability). In order for these activities to be practised, specific exercises to improve quadriceps' strength are required. When an appropriate level of strength is achieved, then standing up and stair walking need to be practised, as quadriceps exercises alone will not prepare the patient for these specific activities which involve skill and the co-ordination of other muscles. It is suggested that each situation needs to be assessed as to whether impairments require specific attention in order to help reduce disability.

The Multidisciplinary Team and Problem Solving
The medical model, in which the doctor made all the management decisions, is being replaced by the team approach as standard practice in rehabilitation. The disciplines share information and negotiate a set of priority goals for each patient. The balance of input from different team members is indicated in the chapters on the different conditions, but the role of the physiotherapist is elaborated due to the nature of this particular book.

Areas of overlap in roles exist between different disciplines and these very much depend on the individual hospital or institution. Examples of overlap between physiotherapists and occupational therapists appear in the book and, ideally, some tasks should be carried out jointly between the two disciplines.

Decisions on general management goals and planning are made by the team as a whole and involve the patient and carer/family as much as possible. The aims are to solve functional problems, rather than simply to treat specific impairments which form only part of the overall management (discussed above).

Importance or Otherwise of Diagnosis
The specific diagnosis may not always be important when analysing a patient's physical problems, or applying certain treatments, but overall management is undertaken with a background knowledge of diagnosis, prognosis and signs and symptoms of a condition. All these aspects are covered in this book.

	Impairment	Disability	Handicap
Examples of classification of impairment, disability and handicap according to World Health Organisation (1980)			
Problem	Muscle weakness of lower limbs	Inability to climb stairs	Mobility - social restriction of being confined to one level
Classification code	I 74.3	D 42	H 3 (scale 0-9)

Table 1 **Examples of classification of impairment, disability and handicap according to World Health Organisation (1980).**

Treatment goals differ for degenerative, terminal conditions (e.g. Huntington's disease and motor neurone disease), and those where a degree of recovery is expected and where rehabilitation aims to improve the patient's independence and quality of life (e.g. brain injury, stroke, spinal cord injury). Knowledge of prognosis is therefore important.

Knowledge of specific signs and symptoms is important so that strategies can be used to deal with them e.g. behavioural management of unilateral neglect in stroke patients and visual cueing to overcome 'freezing' in Parkinson's disease.

While knowledge about diagnosis is important for general management, it may not be directly relevant to the use of certain treatment approaches and techniques. For example, many of the treatment concepts in neurological rehabilitation have been developed for stroke patients but these could be applied to any condition where there is loss of motor ability and a capacity for learning. This is one reason why treatment approaches have not been presented in detail in chapters on specific conditions, and the physiotherapist can select an approach which seems appropriate for a particular patient, regardless of diagnosis.

Reference

World Health Organisation. *International classification of impairments, disabilities and handicaps (1994 reprinted version)*. Geneva: WHO; 1980.

ACKNOWLEDGEMENTS

Many people have been involved in producing this book, whether by writing chapters or providing support and encouragement. Firstly, my thanks go to the authors who have shared their knowledge, expertise and time as senior clinicians and academics. I am very grateful to Lilian Hughes for administrative assistance, with her invaluable attention to detail, sense of humour and kindness. I thank the Royal Hospital for Neuro-disability, the Living Again Trust and the team at Mosby for enabling me to undertake this project.

A special thank you to Professor Archie Young for giving me an excellent training and the confidence to pursue an academic career. I also thank the following friends and colleagues for their help: Sue Newsom and Mary Reaich BSc MSCP for assistance with literature searching, Dr Keith Andrews, Professor Di Newham, Gabrielle Rankin MSc MCSP and Marian Trelawny MCSP for useful feedback on parts of the text, Michael Ortmans for general support, Tony Peake (author and literary agent) for very helpful advice, and fellow ex-London Hospital physiotherapy students Ann Doherty, Jo Lawrence, Sharon Lloyd-Brown and Sue Nancollas for helpful after dinner discussions at Alfred's.

It is not possible to mention all those who were close at hand for their friendship and support, but I would particularly like to thank James Curran and his son Joseph, Margaret and Rosaleen Hegarty, Mary Chester-Klabis and family, Mark Comerford, Ann Conway and family, Helen Donoghue and family, Pat and Steve Falconer, Mary and John Gale, Dorothea and David Lee and Mary Daly, Eva, Chris and Theo Sykes, the Murphy family, the Murray family, the O'Hara family and, not least, my own family.

This book is dedicated in memory of

Dr Pam Edwards
(1963-1997)

For your friendship, and the warmth and joy you gave.

Maria Stokes
December 1997

Jane Armistead MCSP
Physiotherapist, Royal National Orthopaedic Hospital, Stanmore. Chapter 10

Dr Ann Ashburn PhD MPhil MCSP
MSc Course Co-ordinator, Lecturer in Rehabilitation Studies, University Rehabilitation Research Unit, University of Southampton. Chapter 4

Gillian Baer MSc MCSP
Lecturer, Department of Physiotherapy, Queen Margaret's College, Edinburgh. Chapter 7

Dr David Bates MA MB BChir FRCP
Consultant and Senior Lecturer, Department of Neurology, Royal Victoria Infirmary, Newcastle. Chapter 11

Professor J Graham Beaumont BA MPhil PhD CPsychol FBPsS
Head of Clinical Psychology, Royal Hospital for Neuro-disability, London. Chapter 27

Mr Rolfe Birch MChir FRCS
Consultant Orthopaedic Surgeon, Royal National Orthopaedic Hospital, Stanmore. Chapter 10

Dr Eva Bower PhD MCSP
Senior Research Fellow, University Rehabilitation Research Unit, University of Southampton. Chapter 4

Dr Tom Britton MA MD BChir MRCP
Consultant Neurologist, Kings College Hospital, London. Chapter 5

Dr Christine Collin FRCP
Consultant in Neurological Rehabilitation Medicine, Battle Hospital, Reading. Chapter 8

Barbara Cook MCSP
Superintendent Physiotherapist III, Royal Hospital for Neuro-disability, London. Chapter 13

Gaynor Daly MCSP
Consultant Physiotherapist, Princess Alice Hospice, Esher. Chapter 8

Dr Carlos deSousa BSc MD MRCP
Consultant Paediatric Neurologist, Great Ormond Street Hospital for Children, London. Chapter 17

Professor Lorraine DeSouza PhD FCSP
Director of Research, Department of Physiotherapy, Brunel University College, London. Chapter 11

Sally Durham MCSP
Senior Paediatric Physiotherapist, Queen Mary's Hospital, Roehampton. Chapter 19

Dr Brian Durward PhD MSc MCSP
Senior Lecturer, Department of Physiotherapy, Queen Margaret's College, Edinburgh. Chapter 7

Professor Richard HT Edwards PhD FRCP
University Department of Medicine, Royal Liverpool University Hospital. Chapters 16 & 21

Professor Peter Ellaway BSc PhD
Professor of Physiology, Division of Neurosciences, Imperial College School of Medicine, London. Chapter 1

Dr Ibrahim H Fahal MRCP
Consultant Physician, Havering Hospitals NHS Trust, Romford. Chapters 16 & 21

Helen Forde MCSP Grad Dip Phys
Senior I Physiotherapist, The London Spinal Injuries Unit, Royal National Orthopaedic Hospital Trust, Stanmore. Chapter 9

Dr Scott Glickman FRCS
Senior Lecturer in Medical Rehabilitation, Division of Neurosciences, Imperial College School of Medicine, London. Chapter 9

Dr RB Godwin-Austen MD FRCP
Consultant Neurologist, Queens Medical Centre, Nottingham. Chapter 12

Dr Elizabeth Green MD BA Hons DCH
Consultant Neuropaediatrician, Chailey Heritage Rehabilitation and Development Centre, Lewes. Chapters 18 & 19

Noreen Hare MCSP
Physiotherapist, The Hare Association, Nottingham. Chapter 19

Joanna Jackson BA MSc MCSP Cert Ed DipTP
Senior Lecturer in Physiotherapy, School of Health and Social Science, Coventry University. Chapter 24

Diana Jones MCSP
Research Physiotherapist, Institute of Health Sciences, University of Northumbria, Newcastle. Chapter 12

Professor Christopher Kennard PhD FRCP FRCOphth
Professor of Clinical Neurology, Division of Neurosciences, Imperial College School of Medicine, London. Chapter 3

Dr Madhu Khanderia PhD MR PharmS
Chief Pharmacist, Royal Hospital for Neuro-disability, London. Chapter 28

Cherry Kilbride MSc MCSP
Superintendent Physiotherapist, Neurosciences, Royal Free Hospital NHS Trust, London. Chapter 25

Dr Dawn Langdon MA MPhil PhD CClin Psychol
Clinical Neuropsychologist in Neurological Rehabilitation, Neuro-Rehabilitation Unit, National Hospital for Neurology and Neurosurgery, London. Chapter 26

Dr Margaret B Lowrie PhD BSc
Senior Lecturer, Department of Anatomy and Cell Biology, St Marys' Hospital Medical School, London. Chapter 6

Dr Gillian McCarthy FRCP DCH
Consultant Neuropaediatrician, Royal Alexander Hospital, Brighton. Chapter 20

Dr Frederick Middleton FRCP
Consultant in Rehabilitation Medicine, Spinal Unit, Royal National Orthopaedic Hospital, Stanmore. Chapter 9

Dr Gregory Moran MRCP
Senior Registrar, Department of Clinical Neurophysiology, Newcastle General Hospital. Chapter 11

Jane Nicklin MCSP
Clinical Specialist in Physiotherapy, National Hospital for Neurology and Neurosurgery, London. Chapter 15

Betty O'Gorman MCSP
Superintendent Physiotherapist, St Christopher's Hospice, London. Chapter 14

Dr David J Oliver BSc FRCGP
Medical Director, The Wisdom Hospice, Rochester. Chapter 14

Elia Panturin Med PT
Lecturer, Department of Physiotherapy, University of Tel Aviv, Israel. Chapter 23.1

Professor Rowena Plant PhD MCSP
Professor of Rehabilitation Therapy, University of Northumbria, Newcastle. Chapter 22

Teresa Pountney MA MCSP
Senior Paediatric Physiotherapist, Child Development Centre, Worthing. Chapter 20

Dr Oliver Quarrell BSc MD FRCP
Consultant in Clinical Genetics, Centre for Human Genetics, Sheffield. Chapter 13

Hillary Rattue MSc, MCSP Cert Ed
Senior Paediatric Physiotherapist, St George's Hospital, London. Chapter 17

Dr John Rothwell PhD
Head of Movement Disorder Section, MRC Human Movement and Balance Unit, Institute of Neurology, Queen Square, London. Chapter 2

Sue Rowley MCSP Grad Dip Phys
Superintendent III Physiotherapist, The London Spinal Injuries Unit, Royal National Orthopaedic Hospital, Stanmore. Chapter 9

Professor Maria Stokes PhD MCSP-Editor
Director of Research, Royal Hospital for Neuro-disability, London, and Visiting Professor, St George's Hospital Medical School, University of London. Chapter 23.2

Nicola Thompson MSc MCSP
Clinical Specialist in Gait Analysis, Oxford Gait Laboratory, Nuffield Orthopaedic Centre NHS Trust, Oxford. Chapters 16 & 21

Heather Thornton MCSP
Superintendent Physiotherapist and Paramedical Co-ordinator, Regional Rehabilitation Unit, Northwick Park and St Mark's NHS Trust, Harrow. Chapter 25

Dr John Wade MA MD FRCP
Consultant Neurologist, Wexham Park Hospital, Slough. Chapter 7

This section lists some national charities which help those with neurological disabilities and their carers. The list is not exhaustive, as other groups exist locally and there are also national groups for some of the rarer disorders. Some of these charities also fund medical research.

BRAIN DAMAGE
Headway
National Head Injuries Association, 7 King Edward Court, King Edward Street, Nottingham NG1 1EW

BASIC
Brain and Spinal Injuries Charity, Hope Hospital, Stott Lane, Salford, Manchester M6 8HD

CEREBRAL PALSY
SCOPE (formerly the Spastics Society)
12 Park Crescent, London W1N 4EQ

Hare Association
c/o Chartered Society of Physiotherapy (CSP)
14 Bedford Row, London WC1R 4ED

FRIEDREICH'S ATAXIA
Friedreich's Ataxia Group
The Stable, Wiggins Yard, Bridge Street, Godalming, Surrey GU7 1HW

GENERAL SUPPORT SERVICES
Association of Medical Research Charities (AMRC)
29-35 Farringdon Road, London EC1M 3JB

Disabled Living Foundation (DLF)
380-384 Harrow Road, London W9 2HU

Disability Action - Northern Ireland
2 Annadale Avenue, Belfast BT7 3JH

Physically Handicapped and Able Bodied (PHAB)
Summit House, Wandle Road, Croydon, London CR0 1DF

Royal Association for Disability and Rehabilitation (RADAR)
12 City Forum, 250 City Road, London EC1V 8AF

Scottish Council on Disability
Princes House, 5 Shandwick Place, Edinburgh EH2 3ND

Communications Aids
Glacier Building, Harrington Road, Brunswick Business Park, Liverpool L3 4DF

Care and Respite
Crossroads
Association Office, 10 Regent Place, Rugby, Warks CV21 2PN

Leonard Cheshire Foundation
26-29 Maunsel Street, London SW1P 2QN

Sport
British Wheelchair Sports Foundation
Ludwig Guttman Sports Centre for the Disabled, Harvey Road, Stoke Mandeville, Aylesbury, Bucks HP21 8PP

Riding for the Disabled Association
Avenue R, National Agricultural Centre, Kenilworth, Warks CV8 2LY

Sexual Counselling
SPOD
Association to Aid Sexual & Personal Relationships of People with a Disability, 286 Camden Road, London N7 0BJ

GUILLAINE BARRE SYNDROME (GBS)
GBS Support Group of the UK
Lincolnshire County Council Offices, Eastgate, Sleaford, Lincs NG34 7EB

HUNTINGTON'S DISEASE
Huntington's Disease Association
108 Battersea High Street, Battersea, London SW11 3HP

MOTOR NEURONE DISEASE (MND)
Motor Neurone Disease Association
PO Box 246, Northampton NN1 2PR

MULTIPLE SCLEROSIS
Multiple Sclerosis Society of Great Britain and Northern Ireland
25 Effie Road, Fulham, London SW6 1EE

Multiple Sclerosis Society in Scotland
27 Castle Street, Edinburgh EH2 3DN

NEUROCUTANEOUS DISORDERS
Dystrophic Epidermolysis Bullosa Research Association (DEBRA)
DEBRA House, 13 Wellington Business Park, Dukes Ride, Crowthorne, Berks RG45 6LS

NEUROMUSCULAR DISORDERS
Muscular Dystrophy Group
7-11 Prescott Place, London SW4 6BS

Myasthenia Gravis Association
Central Office, Keynes House, Chester Park, Alfreton Road, Derby DE21 4AS

Neuromuscular Centre (NMC)
Woodford Lane West, Winsford, Cheshire CW7 4EH

PARKINSON'S DISEASE
Parkinson's Disease Society,
22 Upper Woburn Place, London WC1H 0RA

SPINA BIFIDA
Association for Spina Bifida and Hydrocephalus (ASBAH)
ASBAH House, 42 Park Road, Peterborough, Cambs PE1 2UQ

Scottish Spina Bifida Association
190 Queensferry Road, Edinburgh EH4 2BW

SPINAL CORD INJURY
Association of Spinal Injury Research, Rehabilitation and Reintegration (ASPIRE)
Royal National Orthopaedic Hospital Trust, Brockley Hill, Stanmore, London HA7 4LP

Back Up
Room 102, The Business Village, Broomhill Road, London SW18 4JQ

Spinal Injuries Association
Newpoint House, 76 St. James' Lane, London N10 3DF

also see **BASIC** (under **BRAIN DAMAGE**)

STROKE
The Stroke Association
CHSA House, Whitecross Street, London EC1Y 8JJ

Chest, Heart and Stroke Association (Scotland)
65 North Castle Street, Edinburgh EH2 3LT

Northern Ireland Chest Heart and Stroke Association
21 Dublin Road, Belfast BT2 7FJ

also see **BASIC** (under **BRAIN DAMAGE**)

OTHER LOCAL SERVICES FOR THE DISABLED
Crossroads (Care Attendants Scheme Ltd)
Dial-a-ride
Meals on wheels
Stroke Clubs

PROFESSIONAL GROUPS FOR PHYSIOTHERAPISTS
These are all contactable via:

The Chartered Society of Physiotherapy
14 Bedford Row, London WC1R 4ED

AGILE - Chartered Physiotherapists Working with Older People

Association of Chartered Physiotherapists Interested in Neurology (ACPIN)

Association of Chartered Physiotherapists in Oncology & Palliative Care (ACPOPC)

Association of Community Physiotherapists

Association of Paediatric Chartered Physiotherapists for People with Learning Disabilities

Association of Chartered Physiotherapists in Mental Health Care

Association of Chartered Physiotherapists in Riding for the Disabled

Association of Chartered Physiotherapists in Women's Health

Association of Chartered Therapists Interested in Electrotherapy

British Association of Bobath Trained Therapists

British Association of Hand Therapists

Hydrotherapy Association of Chartered Physiotherapists

SECTION 1

BASIC CONCEPTS IN NEUROLOGY

Neurology (new-rol'je). The science or medicine that deals with the study and treatment of diseases of the nervous system.

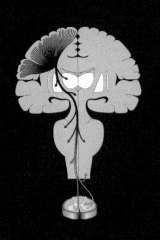

1

PH Ellaway

APPLIED NEUROANATOMY AND NEUROPHYSIOLOGY

CHAPTER OUTLINE

INTRODUCTION

The peripheral nervous system and central nervous system (CNS) consist of neurones that provide both lines of communication and a means of integrating information. They allow the body to move around and to interact with its environment in a meaningful and controlled manner. This chapter outlines the more functional aspects of the nervous system and is presented as a basis for understanding normal function and the clinical and pathological conditions presented later. The special senses and autonomic nervous system are not discussed. The reader should consult more comprehensive texts for detailed descriptions of the anatomy and physiology of all aspects of the nervous system (e.g. Schmidt, 1978, 1986; Carpenter, 1990; Nicholls *et al.*, 1992; Shepherd, 1994).

NEURAL TISSUES

The tissues of the nervous system consist of excitable neurones and nonexcitable neuroglial cells.

NEURONES

No neurone can be described as 'typical', but the cortico-spinal neurone shown in Figure 1.1 includes all the important features. The cell body, or soma, contains the cell nucleus and other organelles. Most of the cell processes arising from the soma are dendrites that extend several times the average width of the soma. The axon is a single process that may extend for a considerably greater distance, in this case from the cell body in the motor cortex of the brain down to the motoneurone pool in the spinal cord. The axon may become myelinated (see 'Schwann cells') shortly after it leaves the soma. Axons typically make contact with other neurones (or muscle fibres, or gland cells) at synapses. Most synapses involve transmission of a signal from an axon to a dendrite but there are also axo-axonic (Figure 1.1) and dendrodendritic synapses. Some dendrites are covered in specialised spines at the points of synaptic contact. Axon terminals are also specialised at synaptic junctions, often having a 'bouton' appearance. The presynaptic axonal terminals contain many vesicles, which are stored packets of neurotransmitter chemical.

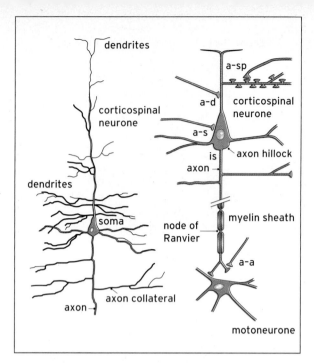

Figure 1.1 A corticospinal neurone.
Semidiagrammatic views of a corticospinal neurone and some synaptic connections. Abbreviations: is, initial segment of axon; a-a, axoaxonic synapse; a-d, axo-dendritic synapse; a-s, axo-somatic synapse; a-sp, axon to dendritic spine synapse. Note that for clarity dendritic spines are shown on only one dendrite.

Although only one axon leaves the soma, that axon usually branches many times. Thus, a neurone such as the corticospinal cell makes contact with many neurones along its route in addition to a target group of motoneurones in the spinal cord. A common feature of long neurones is the presence of recurrent axon collaterals. These warrant special attention in that the collaterals make contact with local neurones that tend to suppress (inhibit) further discharge of the output neurones. Such negative feedback is a common feature of neural control systems.

Axonal Transport
Neurones produce and transport a number of trophic factors that help to characterise undifferentiated targets during development. Other substances manufactured within neurones and transported along axons are neurotransmitters or hormones. Axonal transport of molecules can occur in either an anterograde (soma to axonal terminals) or retrograde (axonal terminals to soma) direction. In addition to the loss of electrical signalling following an injury that severs nerve axons, the disruption to axonal transport results in marked morphological and functional changes in both target cells and the parent cell body.

NEUROGLIA
Neurones in the CNS (brain and spinal cord) are outnumbered approximately 10:1 by neuroglial cells. The cells of the neuroglia are not excitable, i.e. they do not generate or transmit action potentials. However, they clearly interact with neurones and subserve several functions that are intimately linked with the successful operation of nerve cells.

Astrocytes
An astrocyte has a large nucleus and numerous protoplasmic processes radiating from the central cell body. Astrocytes are found principally in the grey matter of the CNS. Whilst closely applied to neurones, astrocytes appear to make more direct contact with the walls of blood capillaries. They probably have several functions amongst which is the exchange of specific substances with the bloodstream.

Oligodendrocytes
Oligodendrocytes predominate in the white matter of the CNS. They have less protoplasm surrounding the nucleus and fewer processes than astrocytes. The processes are long and made almost exclusively of myelin. They make contact with many neurones winding in tight spirals around axons.

Schwann Cells
Schwann cells are found in peripheral nerves and have a similar form to oligodendrocytes. Each Schwann cell is in contact with the axon of a single neurone. It provides a tight spiral of myelin broken at intervals of approximately 1 mm along the length of the axon by gaps (nodes of Ranvier) where the axon is in open contact with the extracellular space. Myelin is a fatty substance and provides a high degree of electrical resistance between axons and the extracellular space. This insulation is important in the transmission of nerve impulses (see below).

SIGNALLING IN THE NERVOUS SYSTEM

Neurones and muscle fibres are referred to as excitable cells because they generate and transmit action potentials.

RESTING POTENTIAL
A difference in electrical potential exists across the membrane of an excitable cell (Figure 1.2A) with the inside, say of a nerve axon, being at a potential of some −70 to −80 mV (up to −90 mV inside a muscle fibre). This is the resting potential of the cell and is the immediate result of a difference in permeability of the cell membrane to the major ionic constituents of the intracellular and extracellular fluids. Extracellular fluid has a high concentration of both sodium ions (Na$^+$:140 milliequivalents [meq] per litre) and chloride ions (Cl :105 meq/litre), whereas the predominant charged particles inside cells are potassium ions (K$^+$:150 meq/litre) and negatively charged organic molecules (anions). Under resting conditions the permeability of the cell membrane to K$^+$ (P_K) is much greater than that to Na$^+$ (P_{Na}). The cell membrane also has relatively high permeability to Cl (P_{Cl}) but is virtually impermeable to the large intracellular anions. The

concentration gradients that exist across the cell membrane mean that there will be diffusion of permeable ions down those gradients. Such diffusion of charged particles generates an electromotive force opposing diffusion. If we consider the situation for K^+ in isolation, the equilibrium potential for K^+ (E_K), i.e. the potential difference that would balance the diffusion of K^+ out of and into the cell, is given by the Nernst equation:

$$E_K = 61 \log_{10}[K^+]_O/[K^+]_I = -90 \text{ mV}$$

where $[K^+]_O$ and $[K^+]_I$ are the concentrations of K^+ outside (5 meq/litre) and inside (150 meq/litre) the cell, respectively. The factor 61 is determined by a number of constants and the temperature. In order to calculate the value of the actual resting membrane potential (V), all ions and their permeabilities have to be taken into consideration, using the Goldman derivative of the Nernst equation:

$$V = 61 \log_{10} (P_{Na+}[Na^+]_O + P_K[K^+]_O + P_{Cl}[Cl]_I \\ /(P_{Na+}[Na^+]_I + P_K[K^+]_I + P_{Cl}[Cl]_O = -70 \text{ mV}$$

Under resting conditions Na^+ ions continue to move into the cell since they are driven by both the concentration gradient (high outside) and the attraction of the negative intracellular potential. The resting membrane potential does not run down with time since the influx of Na^+ is balanced by active extrusion of Na^+ through a metabolically fuelled pump sited in the membrane (Figure 1.2A). The pump may be coupled to the active transport of K^+ in the opposite direction and, when the exchange is 3 Na^+ for 2 K^+, the pump is electrogenic and contributes directly to the genesis of the resting membrane potential.

ACTION POTENTIAL

The action potential is a transient reversal of the membrane potential that reaches approximately +30 mV (the inside of the cell is positive) and returns within 1 millisecond (ms) to the resting potential (Figure 1.2B). Action potentials are transmitted along the length of an axon or muscle fibre without decrement and constitute the signalling process of excitable cells. During an action potential, and for a short period (~1 ms) afterwards, the cell is refractory and cannot generate a second action potential. This places an upper limit on the frequency with which an axon can transmit such impulses.

If an axon is depolarised to a critical threshold, voltage-sensitive channels for Na^+ open in the membrane and the permeability suddenly becomes greater for Na^+ than for K^+ (Figure 1.2A). The membrane potential, as given by the Goldman equation, now reaches a value close to the equilibrium potential for Na^+ (+30 mV). Within 1 ms there is a transient increase in P_K, and a reduction in P_{Na}, resulting

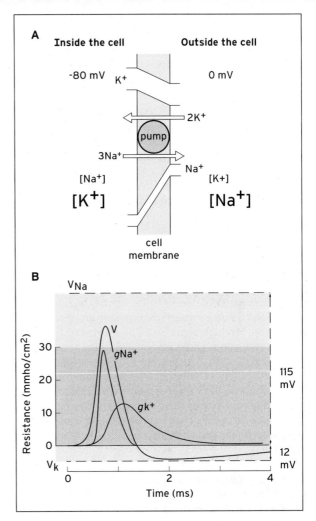

Figure 1.2 The action potential. (A) Genesis of the resting membrane potential in an excitable cell. Active and passive movement of the principal cations, sodium (Na^+) and potassium (K^+), across the cell membrane. The relative concentrations of the two ions inside and outside the cell are indicated by the size of the symbols in square brackets. Broad and narrow channels indicate high and low permeabilities; steep and shallow channels indicate high and low electrochemical gradients. The active pump is fuelled metabolically and is electrogenic, contributing to the negative resting membrane potential. (B) Theoretical calculations of the changes in conductance (g), or reciprocal of membrane resistance (mmho/cm²), of Na^+ and K^+ ions during an action potential and the resultant change in membrane potential (V). V_{Na} and V_K are the equilibrium potentials for Na^+ and K^+. (Redrawn from Hodgkin, 1958, with permission.)

in a swift return of the membrane potential to the resting conditions. The complete process constitutes the action potential. The transient depolarisation, in turn, generates an electric current that depolarises the membrane further along the cell and so the action potential becomes a transmitted impulse.

Myelinated axons conduct action potentials more quickly than do unmyelinated axons and muscle fibres. The myelin acts as an electrical insulator so that current can leave the cell membrane only at nodes of Ranvier. Current from an action potential at one node is able to depolarise the next node rather than be short-circuited by adjacent uninsulated regions (as occurs in unmyelinated axons). In effect, the action potential jumps from node to node, transmission known as saltatory conduction.

Factors Affecting Nerve Conduction

Conduction velocity decreases with a fall in tissue temperature and increases with a rise. Exposure to cold can result in a reversible nerve block, usually aggravated by vasoconstriction that reduces the warming process of blood circulation. Mechanical pressure and anoxia can also block nerve conduction. Large myelinated afferent axons are more susceptible to these processes than are smaller axons. Local anaesthetics can be used to block transmission by interfering with the voltage-sensitive Na+ channels. They are used in pain management since, in low concentrations, they block the smaller nociceptive afferent axons rather than large myelinated afferents. (See also 'Peripheral nerve function'.)

Electrical Recordings

The electrical activity of neurones and muscle fibres can be recorded. Electrodes placed on the skin record only a minute fraction of the current generated by action potentials, and the potential difference recorded between two electrodes reaches only a few microvolts. Nevertheless, useful signals can be recorded, particularly from nerves and active skeletal muscle (electromyography; EMG), the heart (electrocardiography; ECG) and the brain (electroencephalography; EEG). Details of electrophysiological tests can be found in Misulis (1993).

Sensory Evoked Potentials (SEP)

It is possible to look for neural events in the brain related to specific stimuli, such as flashes of light, sound tones or skin stimulation. To record these sensory evoked potentials, electrodes are placed on the scalp (EEG) specifically over the part of the cerebral cortex that is known to process that type of afferent (sensory) input, e.g. the occipital lobes for visual stimuli.

Motor Evoked Potentials (MEP)

These can be recorded using EMG. Stimulation of a nerve, the brain or the spinal cord may be achieved using electrical or magnetic pulses. Electrical stimulation applied through electrodes attached to the skin is used to test peripheral nerve conduction or reflex function (e.g. the H reflex). Stimulation excites the underlying neural tissue by depolarising neuroneal axons. It may often be painful if the axons or terminals of sensory axons involved in signalling noxious events are closer to the electrodes than the target nerve. This is particularly the case when electrically stimulating the brain or spinal cord, which is not tolerated well by subjects. The relatively new and painless technique of transcranial magnetic stimulation (TMS) is preferred for stimulation of the CNS (Barker et al., 1987). To stimulate the motor cortex, for example, an electrically insulated coil is placed over the cranium. A high current is discharged through the coil for a fraction of a millisecond. This generates a magnetic field which passes through the cranium, unattenuated by the skin and bone, and excites neurones in the brain. Twitches in arm, leg and even respiratory muscles can be evoked by such TMS and recorded by EMG.

Invasive techniques are employed less routinely to record muscular and neural activity. Needle electrodes applied percutaneously can be used selectively to record the activity of single motor units (see below). The shape of the action potential during voluntary effort or the timing relative to a stimulus can be used diagnostically for many disorders of muscle and neural function.

SYNAPTIC TRANSMISSION

Transmission of impulses across a synapse occurs by either a chemical or an electrical process.

Chemical Transmission

Chemical transmission occurs at synapses within the central and peripheral nervous systems. The time course of transmission varies from a few milliseconds to 100 ms or even seconds. The mechanism of transmission at the neuromuscular junction between a motoneurone axon and muscle fibres has many elements that are common to other chemically transmitting synapses. The arrival of an impulse in the presynaptic terminal increases the permeability of the presynaptic membrane to Ca^{2+}. Ca^{2+} enters the cell and causes a large increase in the rate at which small vesicles in the terminal coalesce with the cell membrane. As a result, the transmitter (in this case, acetylcholine) contained in the vesicles is liberated into the cleft and diffuses across to the postsynaptic membrane. The adjacent postsynaptic membrane has ion channels that are sensitive to acetylcholine. These open, resulting in an indiscriminate increase in the permeability of the postsynaptic membrane to Na^+, K^+ and Cl^-. As a result the membrane becomes depolarised, creating a local endplate potential. This quickly reaches a threshold at which voltage-sensitive Na^+ channels open, causing an action potential to be initiated. The action potential is propagated along the muscle fibre, in which it triggers the processes leading to muscle contraction.

The endplate potential is a transient event because the enzyme acetylcholine esterase, located in the postsynaptic membrane, quickly denatures acetylcholine, splitting it into choline and acetic acid. Much of the choline is taken up locally into the presynaptic terminal, recycled into acetylcholine and stored in the vesicles.

Fast Synaptic Transmission

Glutamate is an example of an excitatory neurotransmitter in the CNS that can have a fast synaptic action. Acetylcholine at nicotinic receptors located at the neuromuscular junction and in autonomic ganglia is also capable of fast transmission.

Excitatory Postsynaptic Potential (EPSP)

The electrical stimulation of a number of axons in an excitatory nerve depolarises the postsynaptic neurone by increasing the permeability of its membrane to cations (e.g. Na^+, K^+ and Ca^{++}). The resultant EPSP may now be several millivolts in amplitude (Figure 1.3).The total EPSP is the sum of a large number of small EPSPs evoked by the synchronous actions of the individual excitatory axons. The EPSP in a motoneurone has a rise time of about 1 ms and decays over 10–15 ms. Because of the long decay time there is opportunity for temporal summation with other synaptic events. If these are from different sources, this is referred to as spatial summation. If the summation is sufficient, the threshold for generation of an action potential will be reached at the initial segment of the axon at the axon hillock (the junction between soma and axon).

Inhibitory Postsynaptic Potential (IPSP)

Activation of fast inhibitory synapses between axons and the soma or dendrites of neurones may result in hyperpolarisation of the postsynaptic membrane. The IPSP has a similar time course to the EPSP. IPSPs are subject to temporal and spatial summation with other IPSPs and EPSPs. IPSPs result from an increase in permeability to Cl^- (or K^+) and tend to move the membrane potential away from the threshold, thus lessening the chance that an action potential will occur. If the membrane potential is already close to the equilibrium potential for Cl^-, the release of the inhibitory transmitter may not hyperpolarise the postsynaptic neurone. However, any coincident EPSP will be attenuated due to the increased Cl^- conductance (Figure 1.3). The simple amino acids glycine and gamma aminobutyric acid (GABA), are examples of inhibitory neurotransmitters acting on this time scale.

Slow Synaptic Transmission

Another broad category of chemically mediated synaptic transmission is less directly coupled with ion channels than is fast synaptic transmission and hence is slower in action. The transmitter molecule binds to a receptor that triggers a chain of reactions involving G-proteins and second messengers, terminating in the phosphorylation of components of ion channels. The opening or closure of those ion channels alters the permeability of the membrane to various ions, which tends to modulate the other synaptic actions on the cell. Monoamines (e.g. dopamine, 5-hydroxytryptamine) and neuropeptides (e.g. substance P) are neurotransmitters or neuromodulators that are involved in slow synaptic transmission. As an example, although excitatory amino acids act as transmitters (fast) in central pain pathways, substance P released from pain

afferent terminals in the dorsal horn of the spinal cord modulates that transmission.

Presynaptic Inhibition

Some inhibitory pathways have axons that act on other axons, rather than directly on the soma or dendrites of the target neurone. Axons of the inhibitory pathway depolarise the terminals of axons with an excitatory input to the target neurone. Any action potentials arriving in the excitatory axons when they are depolarised will be reduced in amplitude. Presynaptic inhibition is more selective than postsynaptic inhibition in that it acts on specific excitatory inputs rather than affecting all synaptic inputs to the target output neurone.

Electrical Transmission

Electrical transmission is encountered less frequently than chemical transmission. An example is the transmission of the action potential from one cardiac muscle cell to another across the closely approximated membranes that form an intercalated disc. In the nervous system the synaptic junctions associated with electrical transmission comprise tight membrane appositions called gap junctions. Gap junctions allow sufficient flow of electrical current from a presynaptic action potential to generate an action potential in the postsynaptic neurone and this occurs without the delay

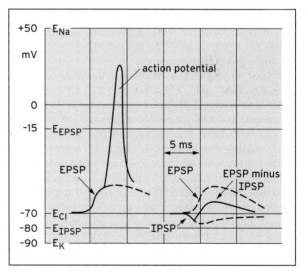

Figure 1.3 The effect of excitatory and inhibitory synaptic inputs on the membrane potential and generation of the action potential. Excitatory postsynaptic potential (EPSP) produced by stimulation of the homonymous muscle nerve. Inhibitory postsynaptic potential (IPSP) produced by stimulation of the antagonist muscle nerve. Equilibrium potentials for Na^+, K^+, Cl^-, the EPSP and IPSP are indicated on the y axis. Note that the temporal summation of an IPSP with the EPSP results in a failure of the membrane potential to reach the threshold for generation of an action potential. (Redrawn from Schmidt, 1978, with permission.)

associated with the release and diffusion of a neurotransmitter at a chemically transmitting synapse.

PERIPHERAL NERVE FUNCTION

Peripheral nerves are referred to as either sensory or mixed (motor and sensory) nerves. Mixed nerves innervate muscles and contain both myelinated and unmyelinated axons, innervating a wide range of sensory receptors, skeletal muscle fibres (α-motoneurone axons) and the intrafusal muscle fibres of muscle spindles (γ-motoneurone axons). The skin, joints, ligaments and interosseous membranes are innervated by sensory nerves also comprising both myelinated and unmyelinated afferent axons. In addition, both sensory and mixed nerves contain unmyelinated, efferent axons, the postganglionic fibres of the sympathetic nervous system, that innervate blood vessels (vasomotor) and, additionally in the case of cutaneous nerves, the sweat glands (sudomotor).

Classification of Nerve Fibres

There are two principal myelinated fibre groups in cutaneous nerves, a fast-conducting (30–80 m/s) A$\alpha\beta$ group and a slow-conducting (5–30 m/s) Aδ group. The unmyelinated afferents (C-fibres) give rise to very slowly conducting action potentials (<1–2 m/s). B-fibres are not found in peripheral nerves and refer to preganglionic sympathetic axons.

The sensory axons of a mixed (muscle) nerve fall into four groups. Group I (conducting at 70–120 m/s), group II (30–70 m/s) and group III (5–30 m/s) are all myelinated axons. The unmyelinated afferent axons in mixed nerves constitute group IV (<1–2 m/s).

Clearly there are some parallels in the two nomenclatures. Group IV and C-fibres both refer to unmyelinated axons. Group III and Aδ axons have similar diameters, as do group II and A$\alpha\beta$ axons. There are very few Aα axons in cutaneous nerves that equate in diameter to the large group I axons of muscle nerves. Articular nerves (innervating joints and ligaments), which are purely sensory in their myelinated complement of axons, have a unimodal spectrum of fibre diameters that is skewed towards the small diameter end. Just to add to the confusion in this nomenclature, the two subdivisions of motor axons in mixed nerves have been labelled α (skeletomotor) and γ (fusimotor). Matthews (1972) presented a comprehensive review of this nomenclature.

Nerve Conduction Velocity

The largest myelinated axons are found almost exclusively in the mixed nerves to muscle. These axons (12–20 µm in diameter) innervate the primary endings of muscle spindles and Golgi tendon organs, receptors important respectively in the regulation of position of the limbs and control of the force exerted by muscles (see below). The size of an axon relates to the speed at which it conducts nerve impulses (action potentials). The axon diameter (in µm) multiplied by 6 equals velocity (in m/s); this relation applies reasonably well for myelinated axons, indicating that the fastest afferent axons from muscle (diameter 20 µm) conduct nerve impulses at 120 m/s whereas those from the skin (12 µm) reach only 72 m/s.

The complement of afferent axons in peripheral nerves includes two thirds that are unmyelinated axons with non-differentiated nerve endings. The other third are myelinated axons, nearly all of which innervate sensory structures with some form of specialised receptor organ. The unmyelinated axons are all small (<1–2 µm diameter) and conduct at velocities of the order of 1 m/s or less. Despite having low conduction velocities, their high numbers and ubiquitous presence in peripheral nerves betokens important functions. They signal damage to tissues (nociceptors), the workload of a muscle (ergoreceptors), temperature (thermoreceptors), chemicals released within tissues and a range of non-noxious mechanical events. Some of these unmyelinated afferents are polymodal, in that they respond to a mix of noxious and non-noxious stimuli.

Electrical Stimulation Threshold

The threshold for excitation by an electrical stimulus is also related to axon size, with the largest axons having the lowest threshold. Since particular modalities of sensory receptor tend to be innervated by axons with a narrow range of axon diameter, it is possible to achieve a degree of selectivity when using externally applied electrical current to stimulate peripheral nerves. To date, this facility has been of more use to physiologists investigating the nervous system than to physiotherapists treating patients. Indeed, most commercial, therapeutic electrical stimulators, whether they are intended to produce muscular contraction or sensory excitation, are not at all selective in their action.

SOMATIC SENSORY RECEPTORS

Somatic sensory receptors are those receptors not included amongst the special senses. Comprehensive reviews may be found in Willis and Coggeshall (1978), Barlow & Mollon (1982) and Brown (1991).

STIMULUS TRANSDUCTION

Most receptors respond preferentially to one form of energy (e.g. mechanical, chemical, thermal). Receptor end organs are designed to convert a specific form of energy into electrical energy (nerve impulses). Transduction involves the production of a nonpropagated generator (or receptor) potential in the unmyelinated terminal part of the axon. This local, depolarising potential is graded and additive if two separate stimuli are presented in quick succession. Current from the generator potential flows along the axon, emerging at the first node of Ranvier in a myelinated axon, where it generates a propagated action potential. If the generator potential persists in response to a stimulus, then a train of action potentials will result.

Information transmitted along axons can be coded in two ways; the frequency of nerve impulses and the number of channels (axons). As a stimulus increases in intensity, the frequency of discharge in afferent axons increases in proportion to the logarithm (or some power) of the stimulus intensity. Such a relationship accords individual axons the ability to signal a very wide range of stimulus intensities.

Table 1.1 lists cutaneous, muscle and articular receptor afferents innervated by somatic and cranial nerves, the type of stimulus involved, and the classification of the afferent axons.

THE SKIN

Glabrous (non-hairy) skin has many receptor types responding to contact or to stretch of the skin during movement. Each receptor has a receptive field, i.e. a particular area of skin from which it is possible to excite that receptor. Receptive field size and the density of receptors vary according to location and determine the degree of discrimination. For touch, this can be tested using a pair of dividers (two point discrimination test) and asking the subject (blindfolded) to discriminate one or two points of contact. The fingertips are able to discriminate two points only 1 mm apart, whereas skin on the abdomen cannot discriminate points closer than 5–10 mm.

Some cutaneous receptors, such as the paciniform endings, are rapidly adapting and signal only a change in the stimulus, such as initial contact; they are particularly sensitive to vibration. Others, such as the Meissner's corpuscle and Merkel cells, adapt slowly to mechanical stimulation and continue to fire impulses while the stimulus persists.

In hairy skin, a further range of receptors exist that have their terminals intricately attached to hair follicles. They respond to movement of hairs, are rapidly adapting and can be exquisitely sensitive.

All these receptors in glabrous and hairy skin are innervated by myelinated axons. Other afferents innervated by myelinated axons (Aδ range) have no specialised receptor ending and respond only to intense stimuli that are potentially damaging ('noxious'). These are nociceptors and their stimulation gives rise to the sensation of sharp pricking or cutting pain. The skin also has afferents that are innervated by slow-conducting unmyelinated axons. These are receptors that respond to changes in temperature, both warmth and cold, and to noxious stimuli that cause dull, aching pain. There are also some polymodal, unmyelinated afferents that respond to both noxious and innocuous stimuli (see 'Pain').

The actual role of a particular cutaneous receptor is rarely restricted to the generation of sensation. Depending upon the destination of the afferent axon, the stimulus may produce a reflex change in skeletal muscle (e.g. the flexion reflex), contribute to the control of precise voluntary muscular activity such as a precision grip, cause local vascular responses (skin flare) or elicit widespread vascular and sudomotor (sweat) changes through the autonomic nervous system.

SKELETAL MUSCLE

The principal receptors in skeletal muscle innervated by myelinated axons are muscle spindles and tendon organs. They were reviewed in detail by Matthews (1972).

Muscle Spindles

Large numbers of muscle spindles are found in muscles engaged in posture and fine voluntary movements. The muscle spindle consists of about 6 or 7 thin intrafusal muscle fibres surrounded by a capsule in their central region. The central part of each intrafusal fibre is filled with nuclei and has no striations. There are one or two long bag fibres and shorter chain fibres, bag and chain referring to the characteristic distribution of nuclei. The nucleated part of both types of fibre supports spiral endings of a single, large myelinated afferent axon, the primary ending. To either side there are one or more secondary afferent endings but these tend to be restricted to the shorter chain intrafusal fibres. The intrafusal fibres are innervated by small myelinated axons of fusimotor neurones (γ-motoneurones). There is also some fusimotor innervation by branches of α-motoneurone axons, the so-called β-innervation of intrafusal muscle fibres.

The primary and secondary endings respond to stretching of the muscle by increasing their firing rate. The primary ending has a greater dynamic sensitivity than the secondary ending and gives a high-frequency burst of impulses during the lengthening of a muscle. The discharge adapts to a lower rate when the muscle is held at the longer length. The discharge of both primary and secondary endings tends to pause if the muscle contracts. These responses are consistent with the spindles lying in parallel with skeletal muscle fibres. However, it is important to realise that such responses are rather different when a muscle is under voluntary drive. The difference is due to the activity in the fusimotor neurones.

Fusimotor innervation produces contraction of intrafusal muscle fibre poles, stretching the central region bearing the afferent terminals and causing an increase in the discharge rate of spindle afferents. There are two types of fusimotor neurone. Static fusimotor neurones produce an increase in the overall discharge rate of primary and secondary afferents but reduce substantially the phasic, or dynamic, component of muscle stretching. Static fusimotor neurones innervate the chain fibres. In contrast, dynamic fusimotor neurones, as their name suggests, increase the dynamic response to stretch and this increase is proportionally greater than the concomitant increase in steady state discharge. Dynamic fusimotor neurones innervate the specialised 'dynamic bag' intrafusal muscle fibre in the spindle (Boyd, 1980).

Recordings in people (Vallbo et al., 1979) and freely moving animals have shown that the discharge of muscle spindle afferents is maintained, or may increase, during voluntary contraction of a muscle. During voluntary contraction, coactivation of skeletomotor and fusimotor neurones (α/γ-coactivation) ensures that the unloading to be expected from any shortening of the muscle is

Classification of sensory receptors in skin, muscle and joints

Tissue	Receptor		Afferent axons	Preferred stimulus	Response	
	Name	Type			Phasic	Tonic
Skin	Hair follicle endings	Mechanoreceptors	$A_{\alpha\beta}$ & A_{δ}	Hair/skin displacement	+++	?
	Merkel cell Type SA1	Mechanoreceptors	$A_{\alpha\beta}$	Skin displacement	+	+++
	Ruffini ending Type SA2	Mechanoreceptors	$A_{\alpha\beta}$	Skin displacement	?	+++
	Meissner's corpuscle	Mechanoreceptors	$A_{\alpha\beta}$	Indentation Low frequency	+++	?
	Pacinian corpuscle	Mechanoreceptors	$A_{\alpha\beta}$	Indentation High frequency	+++	?
	Free nerve endings	Nociceptors	A_{δ}	Damage (mechanical, thermal or chemical)	+	+++
	Free nerve endings	Nociceptors	C Polymodal	Damage (mechanical, thermal or chemical)	+	+++
	Free nerve endings	Thermoreceptor	A_{δ}	Cold (cooling)	+	+++
	Free nerve endings	Thermoreceptor	C	Warmth (warming)	+	+++
Muscle	Muscle spindle primary ending	Mechanoreceptor	Gp Ia	Muscle length	+++	++
	Muscle spindle secondary ending	Mechanoreceptor	Gp II	Muscle length	+	+++
	Golgi tendon organ	Mechanoreceptor	Gp Ib	Muscle contraction	+	+++
	Free nerve ending	Mechanoreceptor & ergoreceptor	Gp III	Various (mechanical)	?	++
	Free nerve ending	Nociceptor	Gp IV	Damage (mechanical, thermal or chemical)	?	++
Joint/ ligament	Ruffini ending	Mechanoreceptor	Gp II (& I?)	Joint movement	++	+++
	Paciniform ending	Mechanoreceptor	Gp II (& I?)	Joint movement	+++	?
	Tendon organ-like	Mechanoreceptor	Gp II (& I?)	Joint stress	+	++
	Pacinian corpuscle	Mechanoreceptor	Gp I (& II?)	Vibration/stress	+++	?

Table 1.1 Classification of sensory receptors in skin, muscle and joints.

counteracted by intrafusal contractions. The spindles are thus able to continue to signal any additional, imposed length change, whether it is a shortening or lengthening of the muscle.

Golgi Tendon Organs

These receptors have a rather simple histological structure and are found just at the point where muscle fibres insert into a tendon. Tendon organs are not found deep within the collagenous tendon. They are thus placed strategically to monitor the tension that develops as a muscle contracts and pulls on its tendons. Recordings from single tendon organ afferents show that they are capable of responding vigorously to the contraction of a single motor unit (see 'The motor unit') amongst the possible hundreds of units that make up a muscle. The role of tendon organs is to provide force feedback to the CNS (see the review by Jami, 1992).

Free Nerve Endings

Muscle contains large numbers of undifferentiated or free nerve endings connected to small-diameter, slow-conducting myelinated and unmyelinated axons. These endings respond to a wide range of stimuli, including pressure, contraction, stretch, chemicals and noxious events. Some are polymodal and respond to several types of stimulus. Little is known of the function of these free nerve endings but it would be wrong to think that they signal exclusively events that might damage muscle. Stimulation of these afferents causes adjustments in cardiovascular and respiratory function. Some may function therefore as ergoreceptors, signalling the work that muscles perform.

JOINTS AND LIGAMENTS

Several types of sensory end organs innervated by myelinated axons are found in joints and ligaments. The three main types are Ruffini endings, paciniform endings and endings resembling tendon organs. In addition, membranes between bones have Pacinian corpuscles. The paciniform types of ending respond phasically to joint movement or vibration and the tendon organ-like endings detect persistent distortion or stress. The receptor that signals joint movement is the Ruffini ending. More of these receptors discharge as the joint approaches one or other end of the range of movement. Like the muscle spindle primary ending, Ruffini endings signal both the steady position (tonic or static discharge) and movement (phasic or dynamic discharge).

SENSORY PATHWAYS

Somatic and visceral afferents enter the CNS through cranial nerves or spinal dorsal roots. Sensory axons in cranial nerves have their cell bodies within the brainstem; other sensory afferents have their cell bodies in ganglia associated with the dorsal roots.

DERMATOMES

Each spinal root innervates a well delineated area of skin known as a dermatome; these are illustrated in anatomy texts (e.g. Williams, 1995). Each dermatome overlaps slightly with the neighbouring dermatome. Dermatomes may be visualised in the condition of shingles (herpes zoster viral infection) which causes painful skin eruptions confined to particular portions of the skin. Sensation may be tested during clinical neurological examination, e.g. for a nerve root problem. Abnormality in a certain dermatome indicates which nerve root is the source of the problem.

DORSAL COLUMNS

There are several routes within the spinal cord by which sensory afferents project to the brain (Figure 1.4). The dorsal column pathway constitutes well defined white matter lying on the dorsal (posterior) aspect of the cord. It contains mainly the branches of large, myelinated primary afferent axons from a wide range of sensory receptors signalling innocuous events. These include skin receptors signalling vibration, touch (e.g. two point discrimination) and proprioceptors from muscles and joints (e.g. sense of position and movement). The axons ascend in the ipsilateral dorsal columns and synapse with second-order neurones in the dorsal column nuclei in the medulla oblongata (caudal brainstem). The gracile nucleus receives afferents from the lower body and legs. The cuneate nucleus receives afferents from the upper body and arms.

Second-order axons from the dorsal column nuclei decussate (cross over) and pass through the medial lemniscus to synapse with third-order cells in the contralateral thalamus. Typically, if this pathway is damaged there is a loss of fine touch (glove and stocking anaesthesia) and movements are unco-ordinated, reflecting the loss of positional sense.

SPINOTHALAMIC PATHWAY

This route ascends the spinal cord in the lateral and anterior (ventral) white matter. Spinothalamic axons belong to second- or third-order neurones that receive synaptic inputs from small myelinated and unmyelinated afferent axons innervating nociceptors and temperature-sensitive sense organs (also some touch-sensitive receptors). The primary axons enter the spinal cord and usually travel up a few segments in Lissauer's tract before synapsing with dorsal horn cells. The axons of those second-order neurones decussate and ascend in the contralateral spinothalamic tract to terminate in a nucleus of the thalamus separate from the terminations of dorsal column projections.

SOMATOPY

Both the dorsal column and the spinothalamic pathways show a degree of somatotopic organisation. That is, there is segregation of axons within each tract according to the part of the body in which they originate. However, of more relevance to clinical conditions is the difference in level at which each tract decussates. The fact that fibres conveying

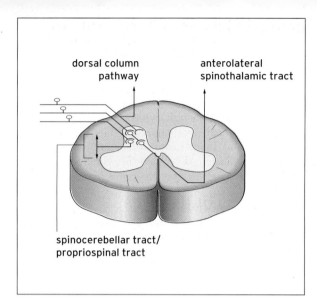

Figure 1.4 The major ascending sensory pathways in the spinal cord. The dorsal (or posterior) column pathway conveys afferent information from mechanoreceptors (skin) and proprioceptors (muscle and joints) destined for the somatosensory cortex. The spinothalamic tracts in the anterior (ventral) and lateral white matter convey information mainly from nociceptors and thermoreceptors to the thalamus, and on to the cortex. Spinocerebellar tracts in the lateral white matter route proprioceptive inputs to the cerebellum. Propriospinal tracts link the different segments of the spinal cord.

painful and thermal sensory inputs cross within the spinal cord, whereas those involved in more discrete skin sensation and positional sense cross in the medulla (lower brainstem), allows clinicians to estimate the location of spinal cord lesions. The classical example is the Brown-Séquard syndrome, in which damage to one side of the spinal cord disrupts thermal and pain sensation from the opposite side of the body and touch and kinaesthesia (positional sense) from the same side below the level of the lesion (see Chapter 9).

SPINOCEREBELLAR TRACTS

Two ascending spinal cord tracts ascend to the cerebellum. The dorsal spinocerebellar tract (DSCT) ascends in the most lateral and medial white matter. It consists of second-order neurones, the cell bodies of which are located in Clarke's column, a dorsally located nucleus in the spinal grey matter. The primary afferents that synapse with cells of Clarke's column are from muscle, tendon and joint receptors, and some types of skin receptors. The DSCT projects without decussation to the ipsilateral cerebellum. The ventral spino-cerebellar tract (VSCT) ascends in the white matter just ventral to the DSCT. The neurones of the VSCT are located diffusely in the medial grey matter. They receive inputs from peripheral receptors and interneurones, as well as from descending neurones that convey central commands to motoneurones. The VSCT pathway crosses and ascends contralaterally but most fibres recross in the pons to give an ipsilateral representation in the cerebellum. The net result is that the cerebellum receives both sensory and motor infor-mation related to activity of the ipsilateral musculature.

PROPRIOSPINAL NEURONES

In addition to the sensory pathways that project to supraspinal locations we should consider here the propriospinal neurones (Figure 1.4) that link different segments of the spinal cord, particularly the lumbar and cervical levels. Propriospinal neurones may transmit both

sensory and motor information between locations within the spinal cord.

SENSORY CORTEX

The representation of sensory modalities in the cerebral cortex is well defined. There are major areas devoted to the special senses, e.g. vision in the occipital lobes and hearing in the temporal lobes. Somatic sensation has a primary receiving area in the parietal cortex, posterior to the central sulcus (Rolandic fissure).

PRIMARY SOMATOSENSORY CORTEX

There is a somatotopic organisation of the primary sensory cortex (S1) representing the contralateral side of the body. The foot and leg occupy the most dorsal position on the postcentral gyrus, with the body mapped in an inverted manner through trunk, arms and face, progressing over the lateral and more ventral aspect of the gyrus. The dermatomal organisation of the periphery is replaced by a somatopy in the cortex that gives emphasis to acuity of sensation. Thus, each finger has a relatively large repre-sentation in the somatosensory cortex compared, say, with the trunk. Although the somatotopic map is well defined, the sensory cortex has the potential to become reorganised (plasticity, see Chapter 6) if sensory systems are disrupted in the periphery. If, for example, a finger is amputated, then the cortex originally dedicated to that area is taken over by afferents from adjacent fingers. This plasticity is thought to account for the increased sensitivity and acuity that results for the fingers that are preserved.

SECONDARY SOMATOSENSORY CORTEX

A second, smaller area of cortex also receives somatic afferent input and is located close to the ventral border of S1 almost within the lateral cerebral fissure (Sylvian fissure). Here there is a bilateral map of the body. Neurones

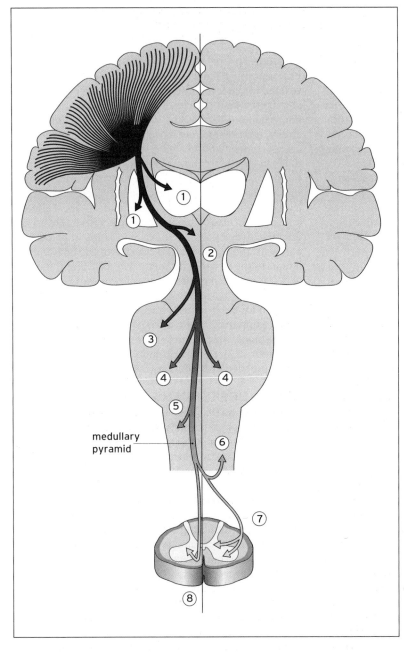

Figure 1.5 The pyramidal tract.
Diagrammatic representation of the pyramidal tract and its major connections through collateral branches.
1: corticostriatal and corticothalamic;
2: corticorubrospinal;
3: corticopontocerebellar;
4: corticorubrospinal;
5: cortico-olivocerebellar;
6: corticocuneate and corticogracile;
7: crossed corticospinal;
8: uncrossed corticospinal.
(Redrawn from Phillips & Porter, 1977, with permission.)

medullary pyramid

within this secondary somatosensory cortex (S2) have directional sensitivity. For example, a neurone in S2 may respond to brushing the left hand from palm to finger but not to brushing the left hand from finger to palm. Thus, S2 is involved in integrating sensory input that is relevant to actual behaviour.

ASSOCIATION AREAS

Another area of cortex that lies adjacent to S1 also receives somatic afferent input but does not have a clear somatotopic organisation. It is known as an association area and, using Brodmann's system for classifying those areas of the cerebral cortex that can be ascribed different functions,

constitutes areas 5 and 7, just posterior to S1 (areas 1, 2 and 3). Association areas of the cortex are thought to be involved in the perception of stimuli rather than the sensation.

MOTOR CORTEX

Areas of the motor cortex include the primary, premotor and supplementary cortices.

PRIMARY MOTOR CORTEX

The primary motor cortex is located on the precentral gyrus (see Figure 2.1). As with the primary sensory cortex, the neurones of the motor cortex constitute an inverted topographical map of the body. The leg and foot musculature is represented dorsally on the gyrus, the hand and arm laterally, and the face and tongue ventrally. Areas of motor cortex that subserve muscles involved in manipulative tasks and fine control are proportionally larger than any others. Plasticity is a property of the motor cortex. If areas of the motor cortex lose contact with their target muscles due, for example, to a spinal cord lesion or amputation, that cortical area becomes 'reassigned' to adjacent, intact muscles, particularly if those muscles are now used more frequently, to compensate for the loss of function (see Chapter 6). The primary motor cortex is a thin layer of grey matter spread over several gyri and often located deep in sulci. There are six distinguishable layers in the cortex, based on different cell types. Layer V contains large neurones known as Betz cells. Betz cells give rise to axons that pass into the pyramidal tract (see below).

PREMOTOR CORTEX AND SUPPLEMENTARY MOTOR CORTEX

Other motor cortical areas have been identified (see Figure 2.1). The premotor cortex (Brodmann's area 6) lies just anterior to the primary cortex; there is also a medially located area of cortex in the frontal lobes known as the supplementary motor cortex. These motor cortical areas are known to be involved more in the preplanning of movement rather than the synthesis of the final output signals to motoneurones. In addition, a frontal eye field (area 8) controls eye movements.

The functional anatomy of the brain is described in more detail in relation to motor control mechanisms in Chapter 2.

MOTOR PATHWAYS

Descending pathways include the corticospinal tract as well as other smaller tracts.

CORTICOSPINAL TRACT (PYRAMIDAL)

The principal route through which voluntary commands reach motoneurones in the spinal cord is the corticospinal (pyramidal) tract (Figure 1.5). It has its origin mainly in the primary motor cortex (Brodmann's area 4) of the precentral gyrus. Axons from the cortex pass through the internal capsule to the brainstem, where most decussate in the medullary pyramids (hence the name). A small proportion of axons remain uncrossed and descend in the ventromedial white matter before decussating at the level of the target motoneurones in the spinal cord.

Only a small proportion (~3%) of the pyramidal tract consists of large myelinated axons arising from Betz cells. The larger proportion of pyramidal tract axons are small in diameter and hence conduct impulses slowly. Corticospinal axons give off axon collateral branches throughout their length, beginning in the grey matter of the cortex, terminating finally on interneurones or motoneurones within the grey matter of the spinal cord (see Figure 1.1). Rather few make direct contact with motoneurones but these connections are important in that they engage muscles involved in precision tasks.

Damage to Corticospinal Transmission

Primate animals in which the pyramidal tracts have been severed at the level of the pyramids recover quickly and show few motor deficits. They can stand, balance, walk and reach out for objects. What they clearly lose is the ability to make intricate movements with the hand. They are no longer able to grasp effectively or to perform independent finger movements. People with stroke suffer far greater disability. Stroke affecting this area typically results from thrombotic obstruction of blood vessels at the level of the internal capsule in the brain. Cortical efferent and afferent axons are particularly vulnerable to the disrupted blood flow. There is a longlasting or permanent paralysis and numbness on the side of the body contralateral to the vascular accident. The fact that the motor deficit is so much greater than following surgical section of the pyramids shows that cortical efferents are not all destined for the pyramidal tract. Cortical efferents project to other important motor areas of the brain, including the basal ganglia, the red nucleus, cerebellum and brainstem (see Figure 2.3). Porter & Lemon (1993) reviewed corticospinal function and voluntary movement.

OTHER DESCENDING TRACTS

Other pathways that descend from the brain to influence motoneurones and interneurones in the spinal cord include the rubrospinal, tectospinal, vestibulospinal and reticulospinal tracts. In addition, the spinal cord contains propriospinal neurones (Figure 1.4) with long ascending and descending axons that co-ordinate muscular activity in the upper and lower limbs (see Chapter 2).

Vestibulospinal Tract

This tract mediates a number of reflexes that originate in the labyrinth sense organs (vestibular system). The labyrinths detect both linear acceleration due to gravity (the two otolith organs; the saccule and utricle) and rotational acceleration (semicircular canals) of the head during movement.

Reticulospinal Tracts

The reticular system consists of a complex set of brainstem nuclei. They regulate spinal cord reflex function by facilitating or inhibiting afferent input at a spinal segmental level. They also regulate afferent input related to transmission of nociceptive input (see 'Pain').

Tectospinal Tract

This pathway originates in the superior colliculus where visual information related to spatial awareness is processed. It descends only to cervical levels and controls the neck musculature and hence head position.

Rubrospinal Tract

This tract has its origin in the red nucleus. It communicates with the thalamus and cerebellum and exercises a less than well understood role in the co-ordination of movement. It may be vestigial in humans.

SEGMENTAL INNERVATION OF MUSCLES

In a similar way in which sensory innervation is segmental and can be mapped by dermatomes, the innervation of skeletal muscles is segmental. Most limb muscles are innervated from more than one spinal segment, e.g. quadriceps is innervated from the 3rd and 4th lumbar segments (L_3 and L_4). Injury to a nerve root will cause paralysis of the muscles innervated by it (see Chapter 10) and damage to the spinal cord will result in paralysis of all muscles innervated by egments below the level of injury (see Chapter 9).

THE MOTOR UNIT

A motor unit consists of a single motoneurone, its axon (and axon collaterals) and the muscle fibres that it innervates. During development, muscle fibres have multiple innervation from several motoneurones. In the adult, any muscle fibre is innervated by only one motoneurone. The number of muscle fibres innervated by a motoneurone varies from less than ten in the small extraocular muscles to many hundred in a large limb muscle.

MUSCLE FIBRE TYPES

The gross appearance of skeletal muscle reveals two distinct types, red and white muscle reflecting different amounts of the respiratory pigments haemoglobin and myoglobin. The twitch and tetanus contraction characteristics of the two muscle types are very different. Red muscle has a slow twitch contraction profile and generates a modest amount of force in an isometric contraction. The twitch of a predominantly white muscle has a faster time course and generates a higher force. Tetanic fusion occurs at lower stimulation rates for red than for white muscle. However, the force generated by a tetanic contraction is well maintained in red muscle whereas it declines rapidly over a period of a few minutes in white muscle.

If the histological appearance of a cross-section of muscle is examined, using a stain for the glycolytic enzyme adenosine triphosphatase (ATPase), three principal types of muscle fibre can be distinguished (Table 1.2). Large, dark staining fibres (type IIb) have few mitochondria and few accompanying blood capillaries (see Figure 21.2). Such fibres predominate in white muscle. Type IIb fibres have a basically anaerobic metabolism (glycolytic enzymes) and are characterised by fast twitch contractions. Other smaller fibres (type I) are lighter staining and have more mitochondria and capillaries. These are found predominantly in red muscle, have an aerobic metabolism and a slow twitch profile. A third, less frequently encountered, type of fibre (type IIa) is intermediate in size. Like type I fibres, type IIa fibres are rich in oxidative enzymes and surrounded by capillaries. However, in a twitch contraction, type IIa fibres can generate tension as quickly as can type IIb fibres.

Some muscles in animals can be exclusively of one fibre type but all human muscles have a mixture of fibres of varying proportions.

MOTOR UNIT TYPES

The muscle fibres of any one motor unit are of the same type. Burke (1980) classified motor units on the basis of the speed of contraction and susceptibility to fatigue. Three types can be distinguished. Fast fatiguable (FF) units comprise type IIb muscle fibres, have fast twitch contractions and fatigue rapidly (Table 1.2). Slow (S) motor units comprise type I fibres, have slow twitch profiles and are very resistant to fatigue. Less numerous are the fast fatigue-resistant (FR) motor units comprising type IIa fibres, having a fast twitch and more resistance to fatigue than FF units. Figure 1.6A summarises the characteristics of the three types of unit.

There are some motor units that have properties intermediate between FF and FR types. These can be influenced by training regimens (see Chapter 6, Plasticity). Regular training for explosive tasks requiring maximum effort, such as weightlifting, shift some motor units more towards the FF type. Endurance training, such as long distance running, results in a greater proportion of FR units in the relevant muscles. Interestingly, biopsy studies also show a greater proportion of FR units in the limb muscles of animals that migrate over long distances.

MOTOR UNIT RECRUITMENT

Voluntary contraction of skeletal muscle consists of an orderly recruitment of motor units based on the size principle of Henneman (1957). Small motor units are recruited during weak voluntary contraction. As a contraction increases in strength, larger motor units are recruited, with the largest being reserved for contractions approaching maximum voluntary force (Figure 1.6B). Repeated contractions recruit motor units in the same order with the general rule that S units are recruited first, followed by FR and then FF units. The reverse order is followed during derecruitment as a muscle relaxes. The same recruitment order appears to occur in reflexes such as the stretch reflex (see over).

Figure 1.6B indicates the range of muscle contraction over which any particular type of motor unit is used. Note the curvilinear relation between force and number of motor units used in a task. Motor tasks that generate weak forces (e.g. standing and walking) recruit a disproportionately large percentage of the motoneurone pool compared with activities (e.g. running and jumping) that generate much greater forces. The advantage of this strategy is that a finer degree of control can be exercised during weak contractions. Motor acts such as ballistic movements (e.g. jumping, hurling an object) require the generation of high forces but may not need so fine a degree of control (see Chapter 2).

TROPHIC INFLUENCE, REINNERVATION

Motoneurones exert a trophic influence on the muscle fibres that they innervate. If a nerve is cut, the axons distal to the cut die, leaving Schwann cells along the original path of the nerve. The motoneurone cell bodies survive and their axons have the potential to reinnervate muscle by growing out along the path of the Schwann cells. However, when the axons reach the muscle they branch and make synaptic contact with a number of muscle fibres, irrespective of

Classification of skeletal muscle fibres and motor units							
Muscle fibre type		Motor unit	Motoneurone	Twitch contraction		Fatigue resistance	Enzymes	
				Speed	Force		Oxidative	Glycolytic
Red	Type I or C	S	Small	Slow	Low	High	High	Low
Red	Type II a or B	FR	Medium	Fast	Medium	High	Very high	Moderate
White	Type II b or A	FF	Large	Fast	High	Low	Low	High

S = Slow	FR = Fast fatigue-resistant	FF = Fast fatiguable

Table 1.2 **Classification of skeletal muscle fibres and motor units.**

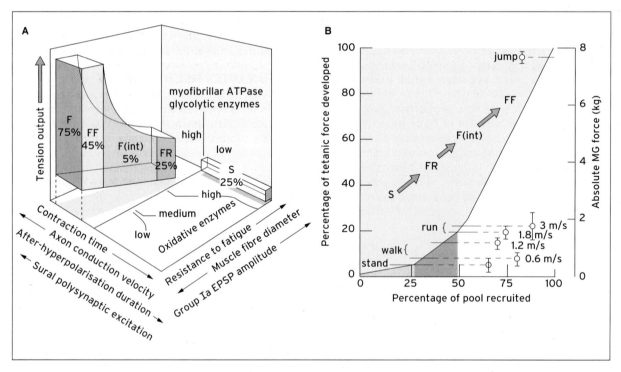

Figure 1.6 Properties of motor units and their recruitment during skeletal muscle activities in the cat. (A) Three-dimensional representation of a range of properties of individual motor units. The boxes represent clusters of motor units with rather similar properties. Abbreviations: F and FF: fast fatiguable; FR: fast fatigue-resistant; F(int): fast with intermediate fatigue resistance; S: slow; EPSP: excitatory postsynaptic potiential. (Redrawn from Burke *et al.*, 1973, with permission.) (B) Graph showing the range of muscle activity over which motor units with different properties are recruited. Note that muscle activity that recruits half the available motor unit pool generates only 20% of maximum force. (Redrawn from Walmsley *et al.*, 1978, with permission.)

muscle fibre type. Those muscle fibres will then change their histological and histochemical profile (type Ia, Ib or II) to those properties characteristic of the particular type of motoneurone (S, FR or FF) that has reinnervated them.

The frequency and pattern of motoneurone firing (discharge of action potentials) can also influence the physiological properties of motor units. If the nerve to a muscle is subjected to periodic electrical stimulation it is possible to change the profile of the motor units towards the S or FF types, according to the frequency of stimulation (see Chapter 24). The change is transient and motor units soon revert to their original type if the stimulation is discontinued.

SPINAL CORD REFLEXES

Movements are termed reflex if they are largely automatic responses to a specific stimulus, such as blinking. Reflexes are involuntary and do not have to be learnt. They tend to be invariant, although the extent of the reflex response will usually depend upon the magnitude of the stimulus. It is important, however, to realise that reflexes may be influenced by activity in other parts of the CNS and in some cases may be suppressed by willpower. Some types of automatic behaviour that involve complex or repetitive sequences of skeletal muscle contractions are referred to as motor reactions or motor programmes rather than reflexes. An example of a motor reaction is cough. This is a precise sequence of events: inhalation, closure of the glottis, contraction of expiratory and abdominal muscles, opening of the glottis, contraction of facial and buccal cavity muscles and, finally, expiration. Motor programmes include activities such as quiet breathing and locomotion.

Some reflexes seen during development of the nervous system in childhood are lost as the child matures (see Chapter 18).

STRETCH REFLEXES

There are three types of stretch reflex: phasic, tonic and long-latency.

Phasic Stretch Reflex

In the normal condition, tapping the tendon of muscles that have an antigravity role elicits a short-latency, brief contraction known as the (phasic) stretch reflex. The knee jerk is a typical example (Figure 1.7). Tapping the patellar tendon extends the quadriceps muscles (extensor, agonist) of the thigh. Muscle spindles in the quadriceps are excited and many of them discharge, causing a fairly synchronous afferent volley of impulses in group I afferents. These afferents make excitatory monosynaptic connections with α-motoneurones to the same (homonymous) muscle. A proportion of the motoneurones discharge and cause a twitch-like contraction in the muscle. The reflex thus acts to correct the displacement (lengthening) of the muscle. The stretch reflex is the only reflex arc that has a monosynaptic connection between afferent and efferent neurones. Other reflexes have one or more interneurones (intercalated neurones) in the reflex arc. The excitability of interneurones may be modulated by other segmental afferent inputs and by descending pathways from the brain. This allows a substantial amount of control to be exercised over reflex function.

Facilitation/Reinforcement of Reflexes

The phasic stretch reflex (the tendon jerk) is increased in amplitude by manoeuvres such as clenching the teeth or hands (Jendrassik's manoeuvre). The act of producing distant muscle activity activates descending, supraspinal pathways that facilitate the stretch reflex through two routes (Figure 1.7). One is direct facilitation of the α-motoneurones such that more of the motoneurone pool will discharge in response to the spindle afferent volley. The other route is

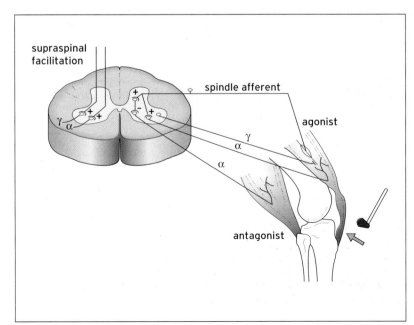

Figure 1.7 The stretch reflex pathway. Afferent axons from muscle spindles make excitatory monosynaptic connections with α-motoneurones to the agonist muscle. Branches of the spindle axons also innervate interneurones that inhibit α-motoneurones to the antagonist muscle at the same joint (reciprocal inhibition). On the left of the diagram (for clarity) are shown descending pathways from supraspinal sites that can facilitate the stretch reflex, either by direct excitatory connections with the α-motoneurones or indirectly through excitation of γ-motoneurones.

through facilitation of the γ-motoneurones to the muscle spindles of the agonist muscle. The γ-motoneurones cause contraction of intrafusal muscle fibres making the spindle endings more sensitive to the stretch. The result is that a larger number of spindles discharge in response to the stretch. Again, these descending pathways are likely to be involved in adjustments to reflex sensitivity during normal motor behaviour, involving postural stability.

Tonic Stretch Reflex
Supraspinal control is involved in the tonic stretch reflex, in which sustained stretch of a muscle elicits a persistent reflex contraction. The sense organ is, again, the muscle spindle, but transmission is through an oligosynaptic (several synapses) pathway. In a normal, relaxed person, the interneurones in that pathway are insufficiently excitable for the reflex to be elicited. However, supraspinal sites can raise the excitability of this pathway and enable the tonic stretch reflex to contribute to postural stability.

Long-latency Reflexes
There are other mechanisms contributing to posture that appear to have a pathway from spindle afferents through the brain and back down to motoneurones in the spinal cord. They are the so-called long-latency stretch reflexes and can be turned 'on' or 'off' by making the voluntary decision either to resist or to give way to an anticipated increase in the load imposed on a muscle that would displace a limb. The long-latency stretch reflex is augmented in sufferers of Parkinson's disease who typically have rigidity and uncontrollable resistance to imposed or willed movements.

RECIPROCAL INHIBITION
During the stretch reflex, motoneurones supplying the antagonist muscle operating at the same joint are inhibited (Figure 1.7). This reciprocal inhibition is effected through branches of the spindle afferent axons synapsing with inhibitory interneurones in the spinal cord. The function of this reflex is to prevent opposition by the antagonist muscle to the stretch reflex correction of position of the agonist muscle.

FLEXION OR WITHDRAWAL REFLEX
Many reflexes have a protective role. When a limb touches a hot or sharp object there is a reflex withdrawal of the limb away from the stimulus. This occurs before the subject is aware of the nature of the stimulus. The reflex is effected through an oligosynaptic spinal cord pathway. The receptors are several but mostly fit the category of nociceptor, i.e. receptors that are excited by stimuli that have the potential to damage tissues. The afferent limb of the reflex is through relatively slow-conducting, myelinated Aδ axons, which also signal sharp pain. The reflex is a well co-ordinated movement involving flexion at several joints. There may be a 'local sign' to the reflex, e.g. dorsiflexion at the ankle if the stimulus is to the heel, which ensures that there is an effective withdrawal from the potentially damaging source. The reflex is not invariable and, to some extent, can be suppressed by willpower. Also, the reflex is suppressed in the leg during the stance phase of locomotion whereas it is enhanced during the swing phase. These are meaningful adjustments that ensure effective progression. Clearly, collapsing on to the source of a painful stimulus if the other leg were off the ground would be counterproductive.

CROSSED EXTENSION REFLEX
The flexion reflex in one leg may be accompanied by extension of the opposite leg. This crossed extension reflex is mediated through branches of the same Aδ afferent axons. The axons synapse with interneurones, the axons of which decussate in the spinal cord to excite motoneurones of contralateral extensor motoneurones. The reflex adds a postural element to the protective nature of the ipsilateral flexion/withdrawal reflex. It strengthens the limb support on the side opposite to the limb that is withdrawn. In addition to the crossed extension there is a more subtle reflex adjustment of muscle tone in axial muscles of the trunk to ensure that the centre of gravity is shifted over the supporting leg.

AUTOGENETIC INHIBITION
Golgi tendon organ afferents make reflex connections with motoneurones of their own muscle through a disynaptic pathway involving inhibitory interneurones. Tendon organs detect the generation of force during active ontraction of muscle. The pathway provides fast feedback for the moment-by-moment control of muscle force from the weakest to the strongest contractions. It is not a protective reflex but, through negative feedback, assists in the precise regulation of muscle tension.

CLASP-KNIFE REFLEX
The clasp-knife reflex is the sudden relaxation and lengthening of a muscle that occurs during vigorous contraction when the muscle is suddenly stretched. It is a protective reflex, initiated by extreme tension, as occurs in eccentric (lengthening) contractions. The sense organs are free nerve endings in muscle and tendons, the axons of which synapse with interneurones that inhibit the homonymous muscle.

POSTURAL REFLEXES

Reflexes involved in posture are difficult to demonstrate in normally functioning people due to the overriding influence of voluntary actions. For that reason, the following accounts are based on observations from animal experiments. The decerebrated animal has no conscious experience but is reflexly active. Decerebration removes the cerebral cortices and other forebrain structures such as the thalamus and basal ganglia, but leaves the midbrain and brainstem in contact with the cerebellum and spinal cord. Decerebrate animals exhibit rigidity in antigravity muscles. The rigidity is supported by an overactive stretch reflex that disappears on cutting the dorsal roots to a limb.

MAGNET OR PLACING REACTION

If a firm surface is brought into contact with the feet of a decerebrated cat, suspended about its midriff, the limbs extend. Muscle tone is then adjusted reflexly to keep the feet in contact with the surface. The afferents involved in this magnet or placing reaction are pressure receptors in the skin of the foot and proprioceptors within joints and muscles of the toes. The function of the reflex is to stabilise the animal with respect to the surface and to support its weight.

HEAD-ON-NECK REFLEXES

Rotation of the head on the body elicits very specific patterns of muscle contraction in the limbs. For example, twisting the head upwards elicits a persistent reflex contraction of extensor muscles in both forelimbs and simultaneous flexion in the hindlimbs. This reflex adjustment makes sense behaviourally as the posture is appropriate for an animal anticipating a leap. Likewise, rotating the head over the right forelimb results in reflex extension of that limb and flexion of the left forelimb (the boxer's attitude to an opponent). Such an adjustment is a meaningful reaction to the anticipated transfer of weight as the animal moves off to the right. The reflexes are not influenced by destroying the labyrinths but are abolished by cutting the high cervical dorsal roots. The receptors involved are proprioceptors in neck muscles and vertebral joints. These reflexes are easily elicited in a child born anencephalic, that is, with a grossly underdeveloped forebrain. Despite the difficulty of demonstrating such reflexes in normal people, they clearly exist and have a role to play in orienting the limbs appropriately during both voluntary and involuntary head movements.

RIGHTING REFLEX

We are able to keep ourselves upright as a result of visual and gravitational influences. The righting reflex is a complex series of manoeuvres that can be observed in a decerebrated animal. First, the head rotates on the body so that it assumes the normal head-up orientation. Head misalignment is detected by vestibular (otolith) organs in the inner ear (labyrinths) which are sensitive to the earth's gravitational field. Secondly, the body twists under the head so that it too is aligned for a normal upright posture. This part of the reflex adjustment is effected by the head-on-neck reflexes described above. Reflex righting can be prevented in a decerebrated animal by putting pressure on the flank opposite that which is in contact with the ground. Clearly, receptors in the trunk exposed to uneven distribution of body weight also contribute to the reflex, since it can be blocked by such an opposing action. Finally, in the righting process, the placing (magnet) reactions and stretch reflexes described above contribute to balanced standing in an upright position. In intact animals and people, vision also plays a major role in the initiation of the righting reflex.

VESTIBULO-OCULAR REFLEXES

If the visual scene is moving, or if the body is rotating, the eyes make involuntary movements known as nystagmus. This consists of a series of alternating quick (saccadic) and slow eye movements, the two movements being in opposite directions. The fast movement, or saccade, establishes a new focus of attention for the eye. The eye then tracks this point in the field of vision (the slow movement). Although nystagmus may be triggered by visual inputs (optokinetic nystagmus) it also occurs in response to head or body rotation (vestibular nystagmus). If a blindfolded person is rotated in a chair, nystagmus is elicited with the fast and slow phases occurring in directions that would be appropriate if the subject could see. However, the eye movements stop after a few seconds of rotation only to appear again briefly, in the reverse direction, when rotation is stopped. Under these conditions, the nystagmus is triggered by stimulation of the semicircular canals in the labyrinths of the inner ear. The receptor organs in the semicircular canals respond to angular accelerations but cease responding (as the nystagmus ceases) once the head achieves a constant angular velocity. Nystagmus in the opposite direction is then triggered as the head decelerates.

In intact persons, visual and vestibular influences combine to elicit compensatory adjustments through vestibulo-ocular reflexes. During movement of the head, vestibulo-ocular reflexes execute eye movements to keep the field of view fixed on the same point on the retina. The central nervous pathways include the vestibular nuclei in the brainstem and the motor nuclei for the eye muscles in the midbrain. Other important elements of control over eye position, not discussed here, are the mechanisms achieving conjugate and vergence eye movements.

ABNORMAL REFLEXES

Clonus is a pathological sign that may be seen when attempting to elicit a stretch reflex. Instead of a single brisk response to stretch of a muscle, rhythmic repeated contractions of the muscle occur. Clonus is typically seen in hemiplegia (as after stroke) resulting from damage to the corticospinal tract as it passes through the internal capsule. Although clonus is a sign of pyramidal tract damage, cortical output to other parts of the brain may also have been affected.

Brisk stroking of the lateral border of the sole of the foot elicits a reflex plantaflexion of the toes in normal adults. In hemiplegia the response is dorsiflexion of the toes, the so-called Babinski response. The Babinski response is also an indication of damage to the corticospinal tract. However, it is quite normal to see the Babinski response in neonates and in infants up to the age of approximately 9 months. This is because the corticospinal tract is still developing in neonates and infants and the tract does not become fully myelinated until 9 months of age (see Chapter 18).

MUSCLE TONE

The level of muscle tone varies from person to person, as differences in the firmness of handshakes testify. Muscle tone is the active resistance of a muscle to gentle stretching. It should not be confused with stiffness of joints due to long-term physical damage. The neural mechanisms supporting muscle tone are the short- and long-latency stretch reflexes. However, muscle tone is clearly influenced by voluntary decisions to resist or submit to stretch. Such decisions can have a profound effect on the long-latency component of the stretch reflex, which is thought to have a transcortical component. Voluntary control cannot be exercised over the short-latency component, which is transmitted through the spinal cord. Muscle tone is discussed in detail in Chapter 5.

RIGIDITY

Decerebrate rigidity in animals has been described above. It is abolished by dorsal root section and is therefore reflex in nature. Clinical rigidity can occur in man after brain injury and is evident as an abnormally high level of muscle tone in flexor and extensor muscles, of both upper and lower limbs, to passive movement of joints.

Rigidity also occurs in extrapyramidal disorders such as Parkinson's disease and can be associated with a cog-wheel type of response to brisk stretch of a muscle. The long-latency stretch reflex is enhanced in patients with parkinsonian rigidity, implicating a supraspinal route for the reflex support of such pathological levels of muscle tone.

SPASTICITY

Spasticity differs from rigidity in that the abnormally high levels of tone are evident in the antigravity muscles, which are the extensor muscles of the lower limbs and the flexor muscles of the upper limbs. Stretch reflexes are enhanced in spasticity and contribute to the tone that is evident on passively moving a limb. The condition is commonly a result of corticospinal damage as occurs in cerebral palsy, stroke and head injury.

HYPOTONUS

In this condition there is a lack of muscle tone and an absence of stretch reflexes. On attempting to elicit a knee jerk, the response is a pendular motion of the leg, i.e. simply a passive swing following displacement. Hypotonus is characteristic of cerebellar disease, probably as a result of decreased supraspinal facilitation of α- and γ-motoneurones.

PAIN

The perception of pain depends very much on the psychological state of the person.

The management of pain in patients with neurological conditions is discussed in Chapter 26.

NOCICEPTORS

Sense organs (nociceptors) dedicated to the detection of stimuli likely to cause damage to tissues are found in most parts of the body except the nervous tissue of the brain. Nociceptors comprise free nerve endings and do not have elaborate, encapsulated receptor organs. They respond to noxious stimuli such as extremes of heat and cold, excessive mechanical stimulation and to certain chemicals (see Table 1.1). Some receptor endings respond to more than one type of noxious stimulus and are known as poly-modal nociceptors. In the viscera, nociceptors in the walls of hollow organs tend to respond to excessive distension. Sharp pricking or cutting pain of an acute nature is sensed by nociceptors elsewhere in the body that are supplied by slow-conducting (5–30 m/s) myelinated axons (Aδ in skin nerves and group III in muscle nerves). Dull, burning or nauseous pain, especially of a chronic nature, is signalled by receptors supplied by slowly conducting (1–2 m/s) unmyelinated axons (C-fibres in skin nerves and group IV in muscle nerves).

PAIN PATHWAY

The pain pathway ascends in the spinal cord to the brain as the anterolateral spinothalamic tract (see above). It is formed of axons from second- and third-order neurones lying in the dorsal horn on the opposite side of the spinal cord. These neurones receive synaptic inputs from first-order nociceptive afferents entering the spinal cord through dorsal roots and sympathetic rami. They also receive inputs from a number of other sources. It is clear that a considerable degree of integration is carried out at this early stage in the transmission of nociceptive information. The axons in the anterolateral spinothalamic tracts terminate in specific parts of the thalamus. Although thalamic neurones continue the transmission process on to the sensory cortex, the thalamus is very much involved in the generation of pain as a sensed experience. Thalotomy has been employed to relieve otherwise intractable pain but restricted lesions within the thalamus can produce paradoxically persistent (thalamic) pain.

HYPERALGESIA

It is a common experience that a prior painful event can result in a lowered threshold for experiencing pain at the same location. An area of skin around the original site of stimulation becomes tender, such that stimuli not normally giving rise to pain now do so. The mechanisms behind hyperalgesia include an increased sensitivity in nociceptive afferents, so that they discharge more impulses to repeated stimuli, and the release of local chemical agents which sensitise adjacent areas. In addition, transmission at the points of synaptic convergence in the CNS, particularly in the dorsal horn of the spinal cord, becomes modified. The changes include the up-regulation of various neurotransmitters and neuromodulators, such as the excitatory amino acids (glutamate and aspartate) and certain peptides (substance P and calcitonin gene-related peptide).

REFERRED PAIN

Pain associated with visceral disorder may be felt in some remote part of a limb or the trunk. For example, cardiac ischaemia is felt as pain in the left arm and gallstones as shoulder pain. The reason for this referred pain is that neurones lying in the dorsal horn of the spinal cord receive converging inputs from nociceptors in the limbs and from afferents coming from the viscera. The brain apparently interprets the activity in the projection pathway as coming from the somatic rather than the visceral source.

PAIN CONTROL

Melzack & Wall (1965) formulated the 'gate control' theory of pain transmission incorporating the complex convergence of segmental afferents and descending inputs on to centrally projecting neurones. The basis of the theory is that other non-noxious inputs can modulate activity in the nociceptive pathway through inhibitory interneurones. This theory can account for the known facility of rubbing the skin to ease the pain or itch arising nearby. The activity of the inhibitory interneurones can also be increased or decreased by descending pathways from the brain. Melzack and Wall likened this mechanism to a gate that can be open or shut to the traffic in the pain pathway.

There are several locations within the brain that produce endorphins and encephalins, peptides that have an endogenous action similar to that of administered opiates such as morphine. Endorphins are found in neurones of the hypothalamus where they may contribute to the autonomic and endocrine changes associated with pain states. In the brainstem, two important locations where encephalin- containing neurones are located are the peri-aqueductal grey matter and the raphe nuclei. These locations are involved in the modulation of pain transmission. Neurones in the raphe nuclei have axons that descend into the spinal cord and contact cells in the dorsal horn. The raphe neurones produce a monoamine neurotransmitter, 5-hydroxytryptamine.

Another system descending to the dorsal horn originates in the locus coeruleus, the neurones of which are noradrenergic. These descending fibres exercise control over pain transmission at the first synapses on the pain pathway. Finally, encephalins are again found in the spinal cord associated with dorsal horn cells. We do not fully understand the organisation of this complex set of interacting systems involved in modulating pain transmission. However, the existence of endogenous opiate-like neuromodulators, and the multitude of locations at which pain transmission is regulated, hold much promise for more effective intervention for pain relief.

REFERENCES

Barker AT, Freeston H, Jalinous R, Jarrett IA. Magnetic stimulation of the human brain and peripheral nervous system: an introduction and the initial results of a clinical evaluation. *Neurosurgery* 1987, **20**:100-109.

Barlow HB, Mollon JD. *The Senses*. Cambridge: Cambridge University Press; 1982. (Cambridge Texts in the Physiological Sciences; volume 3).

Boyd IA. The isolated mammalian muscle spindle. *Trends Neurosci* 1980, **3**:258-265.

Brown AG. *Nerve cells and nervous systems. An introduction to neuroscience*. London: Springer Verlag; 1991.

Burke RE. Motor unit types: functional specialisations in motor control. *Trends Neurosci* 1980, **3**:255-258.

Burke RE, Levine DN, Tsairis P, *et al.* Physiological types and histochemical profiles in motor units of the cat gastrocnemius. *J Physiol* 1973, **234**:723-748.

Carpenter RHS. *Neurophysiology*. London: Edward Arnold; 1990. (Physiological principles of medicine series).

Henneman E. Relation between size of neurones and their susceptibility to discharge. *Science* 1957, **126**:1345-1346.

Hodgkin AL. Ionic movements and electrical activity in giant nerve fibres. *Proc R Soc B* 1958, **148**:1:37.

Jami L. Golgi tendon organs in mammalian skeletal muscle: functional properties and central actions. *Physiol Rev* 1992, **72**:623-666.

Matthews PBC. *Mammalian muscle receptors and their central actions*. London: Edward Arnold; 1972. (Monographs of the Physiological Society, No. 23).

Melzack R, Wall PD. Pain mechanisms: a new theory. *Science* 1965, **150**:971-979.

Misulis KE. *Essentials of neurophysiology*. Boston: Butterworth Heinemann; 1993.

Nicholls JG, Martin AR, Wallace BG. *From neurone to brain*. Sunderland, Mass: Sinauer Associates; 1992.

Phillips CG, Porter R. *Corticospinal neurones*. London: Academic Press; 1977. (Monographs of the Physiological Society, No. 34).

Porter R, Lemon R. *Corticospinal function and voluntary movement*. Oxford: Clarendon Press; 1993.

Schmidt RF. *Fundamentals of neurophysiology*. New York: Springer Verlag; 1978.

Schmidt RF. *Fundamentals of sensory physiology*. Berlin: Springer Verlag; 1986.

Shepherd GM. *Neurobiology*. New York: Oxford University Press; 1994.

Walmsley B, Hodgson JA, Burke RE. Forces produced by medial gastrocnemius and soleus muscles during locomotion in freely moving cats. *J Neurophysiol* 1978, **41**:1203-1216.

Williams P. *Gray's anatomy, 38th edition*. Edinburgh: Churchill Livingstone; 1995.

Willis WD, Coggeshall RE. *Sensory mechanisms of the spinal cord*. New York & London: Plenum Press; 1978.

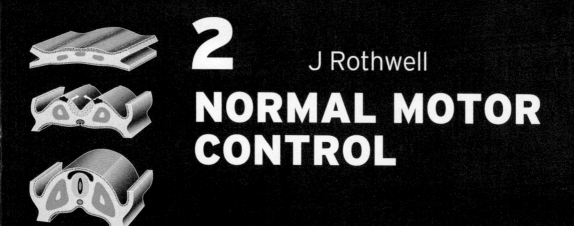

2

J Rothwell

NORMAL MOTOR CONTROL

CHAPTER OUTLINE

- Movement plans and programmes
- Descending motor pathways
- Areas of the cerebral cortex involved in control of movement
- Subcortical structures involved in control of movement
- Posture

INTRODUCTION

This chapter gives a brief summary of the basic principles used by the nervous system to control movement, together with the major central nervous structures involved.

MOVEMENT PLANS AND PROGRAMMES

A simple but fundamental observation about the control of movement can be made by anyone who has learned to write. A signature written small with a fine hard-tipped pencil on a sheet of paper will look virtually identical (if allowance is made for size) to the signature of the same person written using a blunt piece of chalk on a wall-mounted blackboard. Although the muscles used are different, ranging from the small muscles of the hand and forearm to the whole arm, shoulder and even legs when writing on the blackboard, the identity of the signature remains clear. The observation implies that within the motor system there is an idea of the signature and that this is transformed into the appropriate action irrespective of the precise combination of muscles and joints needed to achieve it. It is this transformation of an idea into a plan or programme of movement that is the fundamental task of the motor system.

APRAXIA

Apraxia is a condition in which this transformation is compromised (Geschwind & Damasio, 1985). It occurs after lesions in several parts of the brain, and is particularly common in patients with damage to the left hemisphere or with lesions of the anterior part of the corpus callosum. There are many varieties of apraxia. Ideo-motor apraxia refers to the inability of patients to produce a correct movement in response to a simple external command. For example, if a patient is asked to hold out the tongue, he or she may be unable to do so, or will make an inappropriate movement such as chomping the teeth. However, although unable to use the tongue on command, the same patient may be able to move it quite normally in automatic movements such as licking the lips or speaking. Careful testing shows that the patient understands what he or she should do, but simply cannot transform the command into an appropriate movement. Exactly where in the brain this transformation occurs is not clear. One idea is that apraxia can result from disconnection of areas of the brain which receive the instruction to move or which formulate the idea of the movement, from the final effector areas of the motor system.

DEAFFERENTATION

The production of any movement involves co-operation between plans or programmes of movements and feedback from sensory receptors in the periphery. Before discussing the role of the latter, it is useful to have some idea of the extent to which the central motor command system can store and replay sequences of movement without reference to sensory input. Studies of 'deafferented' patients have shown that the central command system can store and execute an extraordinarily wide range of movement commands. An example was seen in a patient with a severe peripheral sensory neuropathy affecting the hands and feet (Rothwell *et al.*, 1982). This patient had no sense of movement, touch, temperature or pin prick in his hands, although his motor power was virtually unaffected. Despite an almost total lack of sensation, he could move his thumb to touch each finger in turn with his eyes closed, even though he could not feel the touch of each finger to the thumb. He could repeat this movement for several cycles quite well, but over the course of half a minute or so the movement would deteriorate and finally ended up with the fingers missing the thumb. What appeared to happen was that small errors crept into the performance of each cycle of the movement. They went uncorrected and gradually built up to produce severe disruption of movement. The conclusion from such observations is that the central nervous system (CNS) can store a remarkably detailed set of movement commands which is quite sufficient in this example to orchestrate the timing and sequencing of the very many small muscles in the hand and forearm needed to produce finger and thumb movement.

ROLE OF SENSORY FEEDBACK
Sensory feedback may involve interaction with reflexes during motor activity or adaptation after the movement, to update later motor commands.

Reflexes
It is now believed that sensory feedback interacts in two ways with these preformed movement commands. The most familiar way is in the 'reflex' correction of movements (see Chapter 1). In the textbook example of a stretch reflex, if a subject holds a weight by flexing the biceps, then sudden increase in the weight will cause elbow extension and stretch the biceps to recruit a stretch reflex that opposes the applied disturbance. Engineers refer to this as 'on-line' correction of the central motor command. Under most circumstances, though, such reflex corrections are not very efficient. This is readily verified if we move from the textbook to the real world and note what happens to the angle of our elbow when someone unexpectedly places a heavy glass on to a light tray which we are holding in one hand. When the weight is added, the elbow extends and the tray moves downwards. Reflexes in the biceps may occur but they are insufficient to prevent movement of the tray and restore the angle of the elbow. In engineers' terms, the 'gain' of the reflex is low. In fact, the rule for many reflexes is that they are relatively inefficient as compensatory mechanisms when the disturbance to movement is large, such as in the example of the glass on the tray, but in other conditions, when the disturbance is small, they may act very powerfully indeed.

In the example of the biceps, careful experiments have shown that very small disturbances of movement, at around the perceptual threshold of the subject, are almost totally compensated by reflex mechanisms, even though the disturbance itself may remain undetected by the subject. Under many conditions, this makes some sense. If a large disturbance occurs, it might be inappropriate to recruit the full strength of a muscle like the biceps in a reflex manner. Instead, it is more likely that we would wish to consider voluntarily whether a completely different movement strategy would be more appropriate (Marsden *et al.*, 1983). Of course, this rule will not apply to all reflexes. Life-preserving or damage-limiting reflexes often operate at a very high gain in all conditions. Consider the enormous movements of the arms that we make if we begin to tip forward off balance when standing on the edge of a wall with the sea several metres below our feet. These arm movements are postural reflexes which try to force the body back to the safety of dry land (see below).

Adaptation
Sensory feedback is also used to update the instructions in the central motor command system so that subsequent movements are performed more accurately. The important distinction here is that the sensory correction is not 'on-line', but is used after the movement is complete to update the motor commands for the next time they are used. The information is used to adapt or improve an already formed set of movement commands. A good example of this way of using sensory feedback was noted during the study of the deafferented man referred to earlier. Despite the lack of sensation in his hands and feet, this man still drove a manual gear-change car. He considered himself to be safe, even though he could feel neither the gear stick nor the pedals. During the course of his illness, he bought a new car but found that he could not learn to drive it. Despite trying for several weeks, he ended up by selling the new car and buying back his old one. The interpretation was that without sensory feedback from his arms and legs, he was unable to update his centrally stored commands for car driving and adapt them to the subtleties of the new driving position.

Another example of sensory adaptation of motor commands can be demonstrated in most normal subjects using prism spectacles (Thach *et al.*, 1992). Such spectacles typically deviate gaze by, say, 30 degrees to the right, so that objects which appear to be straight ahead to the subject are actually 30 degrees to the left of the midline. If subjects are asked to point rapidly at objects in front of them, then their aim is to the right of the target. This effect is seen only on the first few trials after the spectacles are put on. Over the next 20 trials or so, subjects gradually become more accurate. Because the task is to point as fast as possible (the experiment works better if, rather than pointing, subjects throw an object at the target), it seems unlikely that visual feedback is used to correct the arm movement 'on-line'. That is, it is unlikely that subjects see that their arm is moving in the wrong direction and use that information immediately to correct the movement as it is taking place. It is more likely that visual feedback of the error from one movement is used to update subsequent commands for the next attempt. After 20 or so trials, the improvement in accuracy means that subjects have reorganised the commands for arm movements to take account of the displacement of the visual field. When a subject points at an object which appears to be straight ahead, the arm movement control system points the arm 30 degrees to the left of the midline.

We can show that this replanning occurs automatically by examining performance in the first few trials a subject makes after the spectacles are removed. In these trials a subject points to the left of the target as if the motor system was still 'assuming' that the visual world was shifted to the right. Subjects have to relearn the new relation between a normal visual world and their arm-pointing movements as their motor systems recalibrate. The results of a prism experiment featuring dart throwing in a normal subject contrasted with those of a patient with cerebellar disease (Thach et al., 1992). Whereas the normal subject showed the adaptations described above after putting on and removing the prism spectacles, the cerebellar patient was more inaccurate at the start of the experiment but, more importantly, did not show any adaptation to the prism spectacles or any after-effect on removing them. The implication is that cerebellar connections may be involved in this type of adaptation.

Finally, it is important to be aware that such adaptation is not an unusual phenomenon. For example, movement of a cursor on a computer screen rarely corresponds in distance to the amount by which the mouse is moved on the mouse-pad, but we can adjust quickly to the change in gain between mouse and cursor. Such adaptation is not the result of 'on-line' reflex correction of movement, but the result of adapting our commands for arm movements to the new displacement that we see before us.

DESCENDING MOTOR PATHWAYS

Many parts of the brain are involved in the control of movement, but before we examine them in detail, it is useful to review briefly the descending pathways which convey the motor commands. The detailed anatomy of these pathways is dealt with in Chapter 1 and by Rothwell (1994). In humans, the major motor pathways are the pyramidal tract, the reticulospinal tracts and the vestibulospinal tracts (see below). Other descending motor pathways also exist, but they are probably small compared with the three main systems. In particular, it should be noted that the rubrospinal tract, from the red nucleus to the spinal cord, is quite prominent in the cat; however, it is thought to be virtually non-existent in people.

PYRAMIDAL TRACT

The corticospinal or pyramidal tract carries information from the cerebral cortex to the spinal cord. Its projections are primarily contralateral and have a strong influence on the activity of groups of spinal motoneurones which innervate distal muscles of the hands and feet. Like most other descending systems, the axons of the corticospinal tract usually synapse on to interneurones in the spinal cord. These interneurones then contact the motoneurones which innervate a muscle. However, particularly in higher primates and man, the corticospinal system has developed many direct projections to motoneurones which omit the spinal interneurones. These monosynaptic connections are most prominent to motoneurones innervating distal muscles, and are termed the corticomotoneuronal component of the corticospinal tract.

RETICULOSPINAL TRACTS

The reticulospinal tracts arise in the pontine and medullary areas of the reticular formation. These pathways are predominantly bilateral and have the largest density of projections to axial and proximal muscles. The input to the reticulospinal tracts comes from many areas of the brain including the cerebral cortex. There are no direct terminations on spinal motoneurones.

VESTIBULOSPINAL TRACTS

The vestibulospinal tracts arise in the vestibular nuclei, which receive input from the balance organs of the ear. Their projections to the spinal cord are mostly bilateral and to proximal and axial muscles.

LESIONS OF DESCENDING MOTOR PATHWAYS

In the late 1960s Lawrence & Kuypers (1968) conducted a classic series of experiments in which they described the behavioural effects of lesions of various descending systems in monkeys. When the animals awoke from anaesthesia following bilateral section of the pyramidal tract, their behaviour looked virtually indistinguishable from normal. They ran around the cage, climbed up the bars and fought with other animals as usual. However, they were noted to have problems in picking up small pieces of food from the floor of the cage.

When the monkeys were tested in a special apparatus that involved retrieving food from small wells drilled into a wooden board, Lawrence & Kuypers noted that the most persistent deficit was an inability to produce what they termed 'fractionated' movements of the fingers. When intact monkeys retrieved food pieces from each well they did it by forming a precision grip between the forefinger and thumb, flexing the other three fingers out of the way into the palm of the hand. Following pyramidotomy, animals could no longer perform a precision grip. They tried to retrieve the food by using all four fingers and the thumb in concert. The result was that they were mostly unsuccessful. The conclusion from these experiments was that in the monkey the pyramidal tract is particularly important for fine, fractionated control of distal arm muscles. (It should be noted that pyramidotomy produces relatively little muscle weakness and no detectable increase in muscle tone.)

In a separate series of experiments, Lawrence & Kuypers also tried to evaluate the effect of transsecting the brainstem–spinal pathways. Their experiments involved two stages. In the first stage the animals were given a pyramidotomy and allowed to recover. Later the brainstem pathways were also cut. The reason for the double lesion was that if the brainstem pathways alone were damaged, then part of their function could be taken over by the pyramidal system. Although recovery was good after the initial pyramidal lesion, animals appeared to be very impaired after the second lesion involving the vestibulospinal and reticulospinal tracts. Even after some weeks' recovery, they had severe postural deficits and tended to slump forward when sitting. They had great difficulties in avoiding obstacles when walking, and an absence of righting reactions so that they could not readily stand up again if they fell. The conclusion was that these brainstem pathways are used chiefly in the control of gross postural movements. Although the pyramidal tract might also be involved to some extent in such movements, its most important role seems to be to superimpose upon them the ability to produce fractionated movements of the distal hand muscles.

AREAS OF THE CEREBRAL CORTEX INVOLVED IN CONTROL OF MOVEMENT

The motor areas of the cerebral cortex are defined as having: (1) a direct (corticospinal) projection to the spinal cord; and (2) cortico-cortical connections with the primary motor cortex. Three major areas are usually distinguished (Figure 2.1): the primary motor cortex itself, lying anterior to the central sulcus; the premotor cortex, which occupies an area in front of the primary motor cortex on the lateral surface of the brain; and the supplementary motor area, a region of the medial surface of the hemisphere anterior to the leg area of the primary motor cortex. The primary motor cortex corresponds anatomically to Brodmann's area 4; the premotor cortex to the lateral part of area 6; and the supplementary motor area to the medial part of area 6.

Some-times the premotor cortex is itself subdivided into a dorsal and a ventral portion. In addition, several other motor areas have recently been described that lie on the cingulate gyrus in the medial surface of the hemisphere. The function of these areas is still under investigation (He et al., 1995).

PRIMARY MOTOR CORTEX

The primary motor cortex is so called because it has the lowest threshold for production of movement after direct electrical stimulation of the cortex (see review by Porter & Lemon, 1994). Early mapping experiments in both primates and humans revealed the well known 'motor homunculus'. Stimulation of medial portions of the primary motor cortex produced movements of the legs, whilst stimulation of progressively more lateral regions produced movements of the trunk, arm, hand and then face on the opposite side of the body. Of all motor areas, the primary motor cortex has the largest number of corticospinal connections and it contributes some 40% of the total number of fibres in the pyramidal tract. This is one reason for its very low threshold to direct electrical stimulation or magnetic stimulation (see Chapter 1).

When a movement is made, the discharge of motoneurones in the spinal cord reflects the activity of all the inputs that they receive, both from local spinal circuits and from descending input in the corticospinal, vestibulospinal and reticulospinal pathways. Each input provides only part of the final motor command, and in different tasks the importance of each input may vary. In most voluntary movements, recording of single cell activity in the brains of conscious primates shows that primary motor cortex cells discharge in a manner very similar to that of spinal motoneurones. The cortical cells fire before the onset of movement often at a rate proportional to the force exerted in the task. In these circumstances, the primary motor cortex probably provides a large proportion of the input to spinal motoneurones. In less voluntary tasks, such as swinging the arms when walking, the motor cortical contribution may be smaller.

Because such a large proportion of the corticospinal

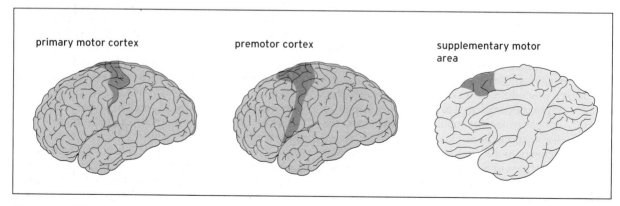

primary motor cortex

premotor cortex

supplementary motor area

Figure 2.1 The three main motor areas of the cerebral cortex of the human brain. These locations are only approximate since the detailed neuroanatomical and neurophysiological studies that have been performed in monkeys have not been performed in humans.

system originates in the primary motor cortex, lesions here can have very pronounced effects on movements. Such lesions also interrupt indirect output to the spinal cord via cortical projections to the reticular formation and the reticulospinal tracts. This explains why lesions of the motor cortex differ in their effects from the pure pyramidal lesions described above. Small lesions of the primary motor cortex result in weakness of a limited group of muscles on the contralateral side of the body. If the lesion is very small, recovery is good with little increase in muscle tone and little permanent deficit except in fine discrete movements (Hoffman & Strick, 1995). Larger lesions produce greater weakness in more muscles, and there is less recovery of function. After an initial period of flaccid paresis, muscle tone may be permanently increased. Lesions in the internal capsule tend to affect a large number of descending (corticospinal as well as corticoreticulospinal) fibres because they are bundled together in a small volume. Thus, capsular lesions usually result in widespread and permanent deficits. It is as if the effect of small lesions can be compensated to a large extent by activity in remaining structures, but if the lesion is large then compensation is less likely.

Reorganisation in the Primary Motor Cortex

Recently, there has been a good deal of interest in how motor cortical areas reorganise after injury (Donoghue & Sanes, 1994). The clearest effects are seen after injury to the peripheral motor system. Figure 2.2 shows an example of the changes which can occur. The upper part of the figure shows a map of the motor cortex of a rat indicating the forelimb area, the extraocular representation around the eyes, and a region in-between, stimulation of which produces movement of the vibrissa (whiskers). After mapping the cortex (Figure 2.2A), the experimenters cut the 7th cranial nerve which supplies the vibrissa, with the result that the rat could no longer move its whiskers. Figure 2.2B shows that preventing vibrissa movement leads to a substantial reorganisation of the cortex, such that when electrical stimuli are applied to what was previously the vibrissa area, they now produce movements of either the forelimb or of the extraocular muscles. It is as if the representation of these two muscle groups has expanded into the area previously occupied by the projection to the vibrissa.

These changes occur very quickly, and can be documented even in the space of 60 minutes or less. They appear to be due to changes in the activity of intrinsic cortical circuits rather than to reorganisation of the pattern of corticospinal projections. Figure 2.2C illustrates what is thought to happen. In the diagram, there are a number of cortico-cortical connections between the arm and the vibrissa area which are drawn as being excitatory. Under most conditions, the excitability of these connections is suppressed by the activity of local inhibitory interneurones. It is thought that these in turn are controlled by (amongst other things) sensory input from the periphery. When the nerve to the vibrissa is cut, sensory input from the whiskers is altered and this reduces the excitability of some of the inhibitory interneurones in the arm area. The effect is to 'open up' the excitatory connections from the vibrissa to the arm area so that when the vibrissa area is stimulated electrically, activity in the cortico-cortical connections to the arm area can excite pyramidal output neurones which project to the arm. This change in the excitability of corticocortical connections can occur very rapidly indeed and explains why the effects on the motor cortex map occur after such a short time interval. It is possible that after a longer period of time such changes may become permanent through growth of new synaptic connections.

Similar changes have been demonstrated in patients with limb amputation or spinal cord injury using the new technique of transcranial magnetic stimulation (TMS) of the motor cortex (Cohen et al., 1991). Unfortunately, such reorganisation of the cortex does not seem to occur so readily after damage to central structures. Perhaps one reason for this is the dependence of the reorganisation on sensory input from the periphery. If this is disrupted in any way, or if the circuitry of the cortex itself is damaged, then this type of reorganisation may be compromised. This process of re-organisation, plasticity, is discussed in Chapter 6.

PREMOTOR AND SUPPLEMENTARY MOTOR AREAS

The corticospinal projection from premotor and supplementary motor areas is smaller than that from primary motor cortex and the threshold for electrical stimulation is higher. These areas are thought to be more remote from the peripheral motor apparatus, and because of this they are often referred to as secondary motor areas. They receive input from separate parts of the brain. In particular, the basal ganglia project (via thalamus) more strongly to the supplementary motor area than to the premotor cortex whereas the situation is reversed for cerebellar projections.

When a movement is made, an appropriate plan or programme for the movement must be selected. It has been proposed that this selection occurs in one of two ways. In 'externally cued' movements the instructions are retrieved on the basis of external signals in the environment. For example, a red traffic light means retrieve the programme for leg extension to press the brake to stop the car. In 'internally cued' movements instructions are retrieved from memory without any external cues. It is thought that the supplementary motor area has a preferential role in internally cued movements, whereas the premotor cortex is preferentially involved in externally cued movements. Recent work suggests that this division of function is most prominent in the anterior parts of each area.

In the 1980s, Passingham in Oxford conducted several experiments which confirmed this idea (Passingham, 1995). 'Externally cued' and 'internally cued' tasks were used to train monkeys in which the premotor cortex or supplementary motor areas were removed bilaterally. The implication of the findings of these lesion studies is that the premotor cortex is concerned with the retrieval of movements made on the basis of information provided by external cues, whereas the supplementary motor area is concerned with retrieval of movement on the basis of information within the animal's motor memory.

This subdivision of movements into two types has some important practical implications. In patients with Parkinson's disease the degeneration of dopaminergic cells, in the substantia nigra pars compacta, compromises the output of the basal ganglia. Such patients often have particular difficulty in performing 'internally cued' movements, whereas their performance is often much better when external cues are provided. A typical example is the freezing which patients may experience when walking. Very often, walking can be improved if visual cues, such as lines or squares, are drawn on the floor indicating to the patient where to place his or

her feet next. Indeed, some patients who are particularly prone to freezing episodes may even go to the extent of always carrying an umbrella with them. If they experience a freezing episode, then they may be able to turn their umbrella upside down and place the handle in front of them so that they can use that as a visual cue to step over in order to initiate gait (see Chapter 12).

In the context of the theory outlined above, perhaps the disordered basal ganglia output in Parkinson's disease is primarily affecting the (internally cued) performance of a supplementary motor area, whilst externally cued movements mediated through the premotor system may be able to function relatively well.

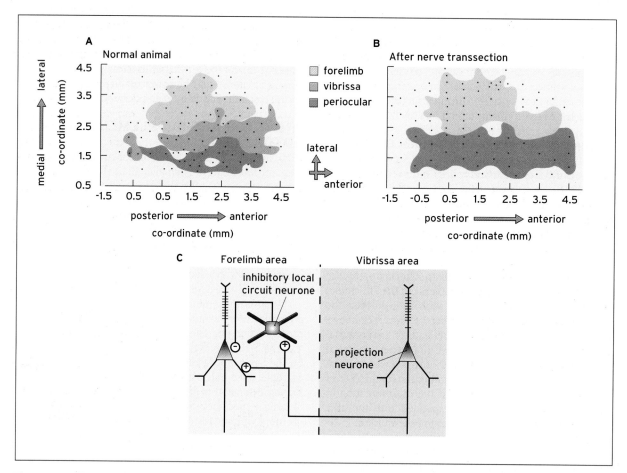

Figure 2.2 Reorganisation of motor map of the primary motor cortex. (A) Surface view of the motor cortex of a normal rat, illustrating the major functional regions. (B) Surface view of the motor cortex in a rat 123 days after transsection of the buccal and mandibular branches of the facial (7th cranial) nerve. Each dot indicates an electrode site at which movement occurred with small intracortical stimuli. Shading shows the periocular, vibrissa and forelimb areas of the cortex. Note that after nerve transsection, there is an apparent expansion of the forelimb and periocular sites into the vibrissa zone. (Redrawn from Sanes & Donoghue, 1991, with permission.)

(C) Hypothetical circuits to explain the reorganisation. Ordinarily, stimulation of the vibrissa area results only in vibrissa movement because spread of excitation (see branching axons from vibrissa output neurone to forelimb area) is limited by simultaneous activation of a local circuit inhibitory interneurone. It is thought that the activity of the inhibitory neurone is influenced by afferent input coming from the periphery. When the sensory input from the whiskers is altered by cutting the 7th cranial nerve, this reduces the excitability of some of the inhibitory interneurones in the forelimb area and opens up the excitatory connections from the vibrissa area.

SUBCORTICAL STRUCTURES INVOLVED IN CONTROL OF MOVEMENT

Anatomical and physiological features of these structures are discussed and clinical examples of dysfunction are given.

BASAL GANGLIA

The basal ganglia have no direct connections either to or from the spinal cord, so that in order to understand their role in movement it is important first to understand their connections with other parts of the motor system (see Rothwell, 1995, for review).

Anatomy

The basal ganglia consist of five main nuclei (Figure 2.3) that lie deep within the cerebral hemispheres between the cortex and thalamus. The caudate nucleus and the putamen are two large nuclei, separated by white matter in humans, but in other animals they form one structure which is known as the striatum. The globus pallidus is placed medial to the striatum. Its name comes from the pale colour of the nucleus in fresh sections of the brain. It is divided into two parts, the external or lateral nucleus (GPe) and the internal or medial (GPi) nucleus, by a thin lamina. Although both subdivisions look similar, they have very different functions. The final two structures of the basal ganglia are the subthalamic nucleus, which is a small lens-shaped nucleus underneath the thalamus, and the substantia nigra, which is readily visible in cut sections of the brain as a dark streak (due to the melanin pigment in the cells) in the midbrain. The substantia nigra is divided into two portions, the pars reticulata (SNpr) and the pars compacta (SNpc). As with the globus pallidus, the two subdivisions have very different functions.

The basal ganglia receive their main input from the cerebral cortex, and send the majority of their output back to the cortex via the thalamus. This circuit is known as a cortico, basal ganglia–thalamo-cortical loop. A small proportion of the output also goes directly to structures in the brainstem rather than the thalamus. Two important targets are the superior colliculus, an area involved in the control of eye movement, and the pedunculopontine nucleus, an area known in the cat to be important in the control of locomotion.

Cortical input projects mainly to the caudate nucleus and putamen, which together constitute the receiving nuclei of the basal ganglia. The main output structures are the GPi and the SNpr. Although the latter two regions are separated by some distance anatomically, they are thought to form part of the same structure which has been split in the course of evolution by fibres of the internal capsule. The flow of information through the basal ganglia from input to output is shown in Figure 2.4. There are basically two main pathways through the basal ganglia: the direct and indirect pathways. The direct pathway consists of direct projections from the striatum to the Gpi or SNpr. The indirect pathway comprises projections from the striatum to the GPe, and thence to the subthalamic nucleus (STN),

and finally to the GPi (or SNpr). It is now known which transmitters are released at each of the synapses in the pathway, and whether they are excitatory or inhibitory to the target cells.

The inhibitory and excitatory connections are shown in Figure 2.4; from tracing the two pathways it can be seen that the direct and indirect routes produce opposite effects on the final output nucleus. Activation of the direct pathway inhibits the output neuron, whereas activity in the indirect pathway produces final excitation of the output neurone. This opposite action is often likened to a neuronal brake and accelerator. It is not known whether the two pathways actually converge onto the same output cell, as shown in the diagram, or whether the two pathways project to two separate populations of output cells.

A final important piece to add to the anatomical jigsaw is the dopaminergic pathway, which arises from cells in the SNpc and has axons that terminate in the striatum where they release dopamine. Dopamine has opposite actions on the cells of the direct and indirect pathway, being excitatory to those involved in the direct pathway and inhibitory to those involved in the indirect pathway (see Figure 2.4).

It was once thought that the function of the basal ganglia was to integrate information from many cortical areas before relaying it back to the cortex for final use.

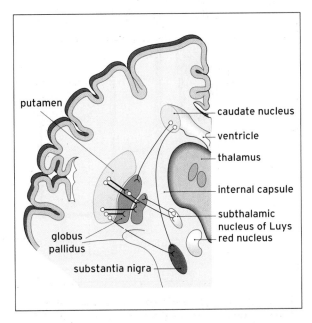

Figure 2.3 Location of the nuclei comprising the basal ganglia. This coronal section through the brain is slanted anterioposteriorly in order to show all the structures on one section. Note the two parts of the globus pallidus. The two subdivisions of the substantia nigra (pars reticulata and pars compacta) are not shown in this picture. The connections from the caudate nucleus and putamen to the substantia nigra are shown terminating in the pars reticulata. The dopaminergic connection from the pars compacta is not shown.

Anatomically, this appears to be what might happen, since the cross-sectional area of the receiving nuclei is much larger than that of the final output nuclei, giving ample opportunity for anatomical compression of the information to occur. This idea is now thought to be incorrect, however. Information from different cortical areas appears to remain separate in its passage through the basal ganglia and flows through many independent parallel channels. For example, in the motor circuit, information from the somatomotor areas of cortex converges onto the putamen, which then sends information via the direct/indirect pathways back to the same areas of the cortex. Similarly, prefrontal areas of the cortex project on to the caudate nucleus, which then projects to particular subareas of the globus pallidus and

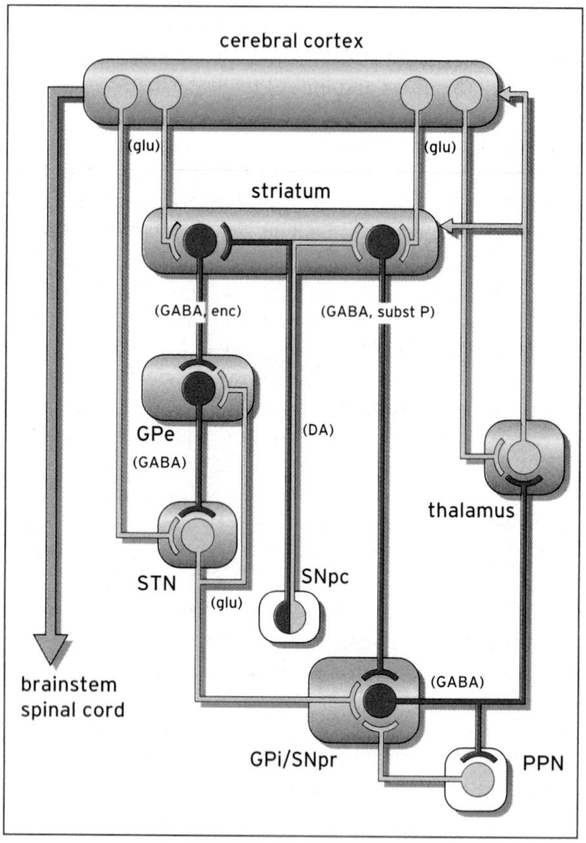

Figure 2.4 The main flow of information through the basal ganglia. The caudate nucleus and putamen are grouped together as the striatum in this diagram. The direct pathway from the striatum to the GPi is shown as the right-hand projection, whereas the indirect pathway is shown as the left-hand projection from the striatum. Filled neurones are inhibitory; pale connections are excitatory. Transmitters are shown in small type. (Abbreviations: DA, dopamine; enc, encephalin; glu, glutamate; GABA, gamma-aminobutyric acid; PPN, pedunculopontine nucleus. (Redrawn from Alexander & Crutcher, 1990, with permission.)

back to the cortex. The oculomotor loop is one loop which will be referred to later. This receives input from frontal areas of the cerebral cortex, including frontal eye fields and supplementary eye fields, and sends output mainly to the superior colliculus in the brainstem.

Theories of Basal Ganglia Function

There are many theories about the possible role of the basal ganglia in control of movement. Many make use of an unexpected property of the final output neurones in the GPi and SNpr. These neurones are GABAergic (i.e. they produce gamma aminobutyric acid) and are inhibitory to their target cells in the thalamus. In animals at rest, the firing rate of these cells is very high (50–200 Hz). The consequence is that even when no movement is occurring, a large amount of inhibitory output leaves the basal ganglia. The simplest interpretation of this is that the output acts as a brake on movement and that when it is removed movement may occur (the thalamocortical projection is excitatory, so that tonic inhibition of this projection would remove excitatory input to the cortex).

There is some evidence for this simple interpretation from studies of the eye movement control system. Just before the onset of a visually guided saccadic eye movement, cells in the SNpr that project to the superior colliculus reduce their firing rate. At about the same time, a burst of activity occurs in collicular neurones, which then starts the eyes moving. In the simple model it looks as if removal of the inhibitory output of the oculomotor loop of the basal ganglia 'allows' the eye movement to start. In fact, this interpretation is probably oversimplified. Removal of the tonic inhibitory output of the basal ganglia probably does not cause an obligatory eye movement. For the eyes to move, other, excitatory inputs must probably converge upon the superior colliculus and other output centres in the brainstem. Removal of the inhibitory output from the basal ganglia is therefore regarded as being a facilitatory influence on the final movement.

Staying with this simple interpretation, we can use the anatomy of the basal ganglia to explain many of the movement disorders caused by basal ganglia disease (Wichmann & DeLong, 1993). These are considered in the following paragraphs and also discussed in Chapter 5.

Hemiballism

Hemiballism is caused by a lesion of the subthalamic nucleus on one side of the brain. It is characterised by wild involuntary movements of the contralateral side of the body which may be so large as to prevent patients from feeding or dressing themselves. This is usually caused by a vascular lesion, and often resolves within a few weeks. In the diagram of the basal ganglia circuit (Figure 2.4), we see that removing the influence of the STN will reduce excitatory input to the GPi and SNpr. This will reduce the firing of the output nuclei, and therefore reduce inhibitory output to the thalamus. The final effect is similar to removing the brake of a car, and results in excessive motor output.

Huntington's disease

Huntington's disease is characterised by uncontrollable choreiform movements of the limbs and trunk, which often worsen with time (see Chapter 13). In the later stages of the disease the chorea may lessen and may be replaced by an akinetic–rigid state. Pathologically, Huntington's disease begins with preferential death of striatal neurones in the indirect pathway. Following the anatomy, we can see that reduction of inhibition from the striatum to the GPe will produce additional inhibitory activity in the pathway from the GPe to the STN (Figure 2.4). This extra inhibition of the STN can be compared to a lesion of the STN, since it results in less excitatory output to the Gpi and SNpr. The final result is less inhibitory input from the basal ganglia and an excess of movement.

Parkinson's disease

Parkinson's disease is due to a degeneration of the dopaminergic neurones in the midbrain, particularly those which project to the striatum. Following the model, we can see that this will result in overactivity in the indirect pathway and underactivity in the direct pathways through the basal ganglia (Bergman *et al.*, 1990). The final result is excess inhibitory output from the basal ganglia and hence a reduction in the amount of movement (Figure 2.5). Indeed, recent recordings taken from monkeys made parkinsonian by injection of the toxin MPTP (*N*-methyl-4-phenyl-1,2,3,6-tetrahydropyridine) show just this type of behaviour: neurones in GPi do indeed fire at a higher rate in parkinsonian monkeys than in normal monkeys. This has led to the idea that one way to treat Parkinson's disease may be to damage either the GPi (thereby decreasing the inhibi-tory output to the basal ganglia) or the STN (thereby removing some of the excitatory input to the output nuclei). Both approaches work very successfully in the monkey model, and are now being used in people.

Although the model of basal ganglia function is very successful in explaining many of the symptoms of basal ganglia disease, several questions are left unanswered. For example, the model predicts that lesions of the globus pallidus in normal subjects should produce a syndrome characterised by excess involuntary movement. In fact, bilateral lesions of the globus pallidus (as seen, for example, after carbon monoxide poisoning) actually produce a condition which resembles mild Parkinson's disease rather than chorea. Similarly, we would also predict that lesions of the thalamus might sometimes produce a parkinsonian state (by removing the excitatory input to cortex). In fact, this is never seen. Thalamic lesions in the areas which receive input from basal ganglia normally produce a dystonic syndrome rather than a parkinsonian syndrome.

There have been many attempts to improve this model of basal ganglia function. In particular, the spatial pattern of the output to different cortical areas is likely to be important. Thus, basal ganglia projections to areas of the cortex which are involved in a movement might decrease their firing rate (thereby removing inhibition), whilst those cortical areas which are uninvolved in the movement might receive an increased output from the basal ganglia. The effect would be that the pattern of basal ganglia output might help to focus excitation within the motor cortex.

CEREBELLUM

As with the basal ganglia, a great deal is known about the anatomy and synaptic connectivity of the cerebellum, but there is little consensus about its role in the control of movement (see Stein, 1995).

Anatomy

In man, the most conspicuous features of the cerebellum are the two lateral hemispheres which lie either side of a narrow ridge known as the vermis. Two main fissures divide the cerebellum transversely: the primary fissure divides the anterior from the posterior lobe, and the posterolateral fissure divides the much smaller flocculonodular lobe from the rest of the cerebellum (Figure 2.6A). These structures form the cerebellar cortex, which sends its output to the cerebellar nuclei deep within the cerebellum (Figure 2.6B).

Cerebellar cortex and nuclei

Three main longitudinal strips of cerebellar cortex project to the three main cerebellar nuclei. The medial zone (which is mainly equivalent to the vermis) projects to the fastigial nucleus; the intermediate zone projects to the interposed nuclei (globosus and embelliform nuclei in man); and the lateral zone of the cerebellar hemispheres projects to the dentate nucleus. The vestibular nuclei also receive some direct output from the flocculonodular nodule lobe and parts of the vermis. The vestibular nucleus has a direct output to the spinal cord. The fastigial nucleus projects both to the vestibular nuclei and to other nuclei in the brainstem. However, the main output of the cerebellum arises in the interposed and dentate nuclei. They have projections to the red nucleus and (via the thalamus) to motor areas of the cerebral cortex, as well as direct outputs to brainstem structures. The cerebellum therefore has no direct motor output.

All inputs to the cerebellum project both to the cerebellar nuclei and to the cerebellar cortex. Since the output of the cortex goes uniquely to the nuclei, it appears as if the cerebellar cortex is working as a 'side loop', modulating the main flow of information to the nuclei. However, the extent to which this is true physiologically is unknown.

Output neurones from the cerebellum

The Purkinje cells are the main, and largest, neurones of the cerebellar cortex (Figure 2.7). They are the only output cells and their axons are inhibitory to the target neurones within the nuclei. The Purkinje cell dendrites stretch up to the surface of the cerebellar cortex, and the dendritic trees lie in a flat plane parallel to the axis of each cerebellar folium. The dendritic trees of adjacent Purkinje cells appear to stack on top of each other like plates.

Input neurones to the cerebellum

The cerebellar cortex receives two types of input fibre: climbing fibres and mossy fibres. Both are excitatory.

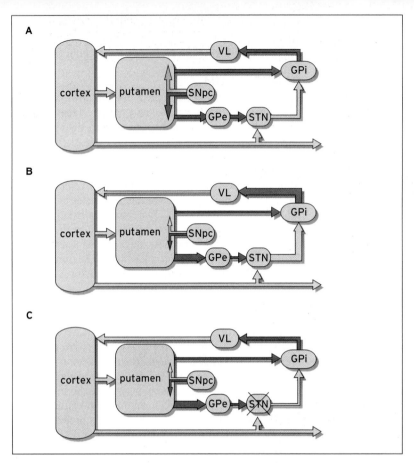

Figure 2.5 Basal ganglia circuitry changes in Parkinson's disease.
(A) Normal activity in basal ganglia circuits; (B) changes in Parkinson's disease; and (C) reversal of these changes after lesion of the subthalamic nucleus (STN). Parkinson's disease causes underactivity in the direct pathway from the putamen to the GPi and overactivity in the indirect pathway to the GPe. The result is excessive activity in the inhibitory output neurones of the GPi and a reduction in the final excitatory output from the thalamus to the cerebral cortex. This situation can be normalised by lesion of the STN. Less excitatory drive in the indirect pathway to the GPi leads to a reduction in the pallidal inhibition of the ventrolateral thalamus (VL).

Climbing fibres arise in the inferior olivary nucleus, and each forms 100–200 powerful synapses directly with one Purkinje cell. Mossy fibre input arises in cells of the pontine nuclei. The mossy fibre axons do not synapse directly with Purkinje cells. They synapse with granule cells within the cerebellar cortex which have long axons that run perpendicular to the dendritic trees of Purkinje cells for several millimetres along the length of the cerebellar cortex. Each parallel fibre contacts very many Purkinje cells, but since the synapses are at the tip of the Purkinje dendrites each synapse is not very powerful. Thus the parallel fibre input is very diverse and weak compared with the very strong and focal input from the climbing fibres. Sensory input from the spinal cord may enter the cerebellar cortex directly in the mossy fibres, or travel via the olive to the climbing fibres. A similar arrangement applies to the input from motor areas of the cerebral cortex.

A special feature of the cerebellar circuitry is the adaptable synapse between the parallel fibre and the Purkinje cells. If the Purkinje cell is activated simultaneously by both parallel fibre and mossy fibre input, then the effectiveness of the synapse from parallel fibres to the Purkinje cell is decreased. This effect might allow the cerebellum to 'learn' or 'unlearn' associations between different inputs. Since the cerebellum has no direct motor output, it influences movement via projections to both brainstem–spinal and corticospinal motor systems. It is thought that the projection to vestibular nuclei and the reticular formation is important in the control of axial and proximal muscles, whereas the projection to the cerebral motor cortex is involved in the control of limb movements.

The Role of the Cerebellum

There are three main theories concerning the nature of the cerebellar contribution to movement control: (1) timing; (2) learning; and (3) co-ordination (Thach *et al.*, 1992). All three are related to the symptoms of cerebellar disease.

Timing

Hypermetria (the tendency of cerebellar patients to over-reach a target to which they are pointing) is usually caused by inappropriate timing of muscle activity such that antagonist force arises too late to stop a movement at the appropriate end point. It has been proposed that the time taken for impulses to travel along the long parallel fibre system to a particular group of Purkinje cells might be used to calculate times of muscle activation.

Learning

A second deficit in cerebellar movement control is a failure to adapt motor commands to changes in the environment. An example of this in subjects wearing

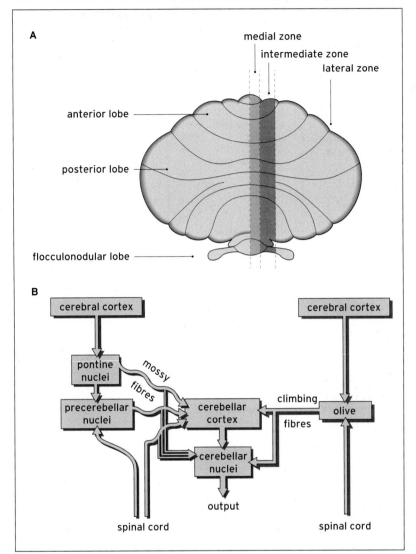

Figure 2.6 Subdivisions and connections of the cerebellum.
(A) The transverse and longitudinal subdivisions of the cerebellum. (B) A highly simplified diagram of the input and output connections of the cerebellum. Note that all inputs go both to the cerebellar cortex and to the cerebellar nuclei.

laterally deviating prism spectacles was given earlier. Experiments on animals have shown that such adaptation fails to occur if the cerebellar cortex is inactivated, and it has been suggested that changes in the effectiveness of the parallel fibre-to-Purkinje cell synapse might underlie this type of adjustment.

Co-ordination
The third function proposed for the cerebellum is that of co-ordination. Inco-ordination is one of the classical symptoms of cerebellar disease and is caused by both a deficit in timing of muscle activity and in the amount of activity in different joints.

POSTURE

The postural control system performs three main functions: (1) it supports the body, providing forces which bring form to the bony skeleton; (2) it stabilises supporting portions of the body when other parts are moved; and (3) it balances the body on its base of support. Like the rest of the movement control system, the postural system performs these functions in two different ways. It can act as an 'on-line' feedback correction system, in which disturbances of posture are noted and corrected immediately by reflex mechanisms. Alternatively, it may predict that a postural disturbance will occur and provide anticipatory forces that will minimise the expected postural disturbance. For example, if we rapidly elevate our arms, then postural contractions occur simultaneously in muscles at the back of the leg and trunk. These contractions tend to pull the trunk backwards and compensate for the expected forward displacement which would be produced by holding the arms out in front of the body. Such anticipatory responses are often known as 'feedforward' corrections.

It is not known in which centres of the CNS these various functions are performed. They are likely to be

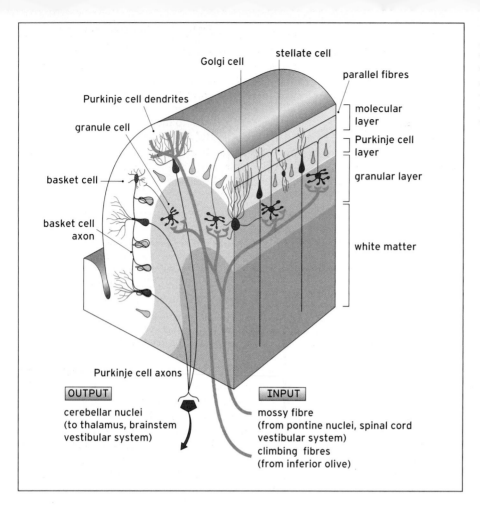

Figure 2.7 Three-dimensional diagram of the principal circuitry within the cerebellar cortex. Input enters via the mossy and climbing fibres; the only output is via Purkinje cell axons.

Golgi cell

stellate cell

parallel fibres

Purkinje cell dendrites

granule cell

molecular layer

Purkinje cell layer

granular layer

basket cell

basket cell axon

white matter

Purkinje cell axons

OUTPUT

cerebellar nuclei
(to thalamus, brainstem
vestibular system)

INPUT

mossy fibre
(from pontine nuclei, spinal cord
vestibular system)
climbing fibres
(from inferior olive)

distributed in many regions of the spinal cord, brainstem and even cerebral cortex (Horak & Wollacott, 1993).

Disturbances to posture are detected by three main sensory systems: the somatosensory system (including muscle and joint receptors providing information on the position of body parts, as well as pressure receptors that provide an indication of the distribution of forces at points of contact); the vestibular system (the semicircular canals and otolith organs); and the visual system. In many circumstances, the same disturbance is signalled by all three inputs. For example, if the body falls forward, visual input indicates approach of the visual scene as the head moves forwards, vestibular input indicates a shift in the angle of the head relative to gravity, and the somatosensory system signals rotation at the ankle and trunk as well as changes in the distribution of pressure on the soles of the feet.

All three of these inputs contribute to the corrective responses which may occur. However, in many cases things are not as simple as this, and discrepancies can arise between the different inputs. If we are standing upright in the cabin of a rocking boat, our bodies may sway together with the cabin. If the two movements are in phase, then there will be no apparent movement of the visual field, nor any change in angle of the ankle. Only the vestibular receptors will signal that the body is moving relative to gravity and this signal will conflict with the apparently stable signals coming through somatosensory and visual systems. One of the jobs of the postural system is to decide which inputs are providing the most useful information in different circumstances, so that if conflicts of information arise, more weight can be placed upon the most reliable input.

PLATFORM STUDIES

The fact that the postural system can 'grade' the importance of different sensory inputs means that at the limit, each type of input can on its own produce a postural response. This can be demonstrated in the following situation (see articles in Horak & Wollacott, 1993). Subjects stand on a special platform that can either rotate and tilt up and down (causing plantarflexion and dorsiflexion), or move backwards or forwards in the horizontal plane. The platform is placed within a special tent-like space which can, if necessary, sway backwards and forwards with the body so that the visual environment appears to be constant. In the situation when the platform is simply moved backwards, the subjects sway forwards, and all three channels of sensory input are activated: the visual field approaches, the ankle dorsiflexes, and vestibular input signals a change in the direction of the pull of gravity with respect to the body.

Given the design of the platform, it is possible to arrange that the dorsiflexion of the ankle produced by backwards translation is cancelled out by a simultaneous plantar flexion rotation of the platform around the ankles. In this situation, the subject is moved backwards, and the toes are rotated downwards, so that although the body tips forwards, the angle at the ankle remains constant. This therefore removes much of the somatosensory input to the postural system, but nevertheless postural responses are still generated by visual and vestibular input. It is also possible to remove the visual input, either by having subjects close their eyes, or by making the room around the subject move with the body. In this situation, vestibular input alone can generate corrective electromyographic responses in the leg and trunk. Although the pattern of response is very similar, the responses to different types of sensory inputs are not all the same. The latency of responses evoked by visual or vestibular input is longer than those produced when somatosensory inputs are available.

Moveable platforms can also be used to demonstrate how the postural system interacts with other local reflex circuits. If the platform is rotated toes up, then subjects tend to fall backwards. However, a dorsiflexion of the ankle stretches the gastrocnemius/soleus muscles and tends to evoke a local stretch reflex, which if uncorrected would tend to pull the body further backwards off balance. Under these conditions the postural system rapidly learns, after only one or two trials, to reduce the stretch reflex in the gastrocnemius/soleus and increase the size of the corrective response in the anterior tibial muscles.

Finally, it is also possible to show that the postural system can modify its responses according to the way in which the body is supported. For example, when a moveable platform is moved backwards or forwards, subjects correct their posture by exerting torque around the ankle to oppose body sway. For this to work, the platform must be stable, so that the foot can exert pressure on the platform and move the body. If, instead, subjects are balanced on a seesaw then it is no longer possible to exert torque at that joint to oppose movement of the body. Balance in this condition is controlled by movements of the arm and trunk (rescue reactions). A change of postural strategy is produced by making the ankle muscle irrelevant to balance. It is an example of the postural system achieving the same end by different means.

RESCUE REACTIONS

The reactions that help to restore balance once the centre of gravity has fallen outside the postural base are perhaps most familiar. These rescue reactions involve obvious, gross movements of the whole body and may be classified as stepping, sweeping and protective reactions (Roberts, 1979).

If a standing subject is given a large unexpected push from behind, this will cause him or her to step forwards in order to capture the forwards moving centre of gravity. Often, the postural system does not wait until the centre of gravity has actually fallen outside the postural base before initiating the step; it predicts whether or not an initial displacement is likely to cause such a movement to occur and initiates a step before the point of no return is passed.

Under some conditions, stepping reactions are inappropriate and can be suppressed. For example, if a swimmer begins to overbalance when standing on the edge of the pool, he or she will rapidly swing the arms forwards in an attempt to use the reaction forces of the arm movements on the trunk to push the body back into equilibrium. In some circumstances, such reactions may also locate stable objects in the environment onto which the subject can hold to maintain balance (sweeping reactions). Finally, if all else fails and balance is lost, powerful protective reactions occur which are designed to protect the head and body during falls. The arms are thrown out, and the trunk rotated to break the fall. These reactions are not easily suppressed. The arms will be thrown out through panes of glass or into fire in order to fulfil their protective role. These reactions are not dependent on vestibular function, they are all present in vestibular defective individuals. However, all rescue reactions are depressed in certain diseases of the basal ganglia.

REFERENCES

Alexander GE, Crutcher MD. Functional architecture of basal ganglia circuits: Neural substrates of parallel processing. *Trends Neurosci* 1990, **13**:266-271.

Bergman H, Wichmann T, DeLong MR. Reversal of experimental parkinsonism by lesions of the subthalamic nucleus. *Science* 1990, **249**:1436-1438.

Cohen LG, Bandinelli S, Findley TW, Hallett M. Motor reorganisation after upper limb amputation in man. *Brain* 1991, **114**:615-627.

Donoghue JP, Sanes JN. Motor areas of the cerebral cortex. *J Clin Neurophysiol* 1994, **11**:382-396.

Geschwind N, Damasio AR. Apraxia. In: Fredericks JAM, ed. *Handbook of Clinical Neurology*. Amsterdam: Elsevier; 1985: vol. 1, 43-432.

He SQ, Dum RP, Strick PL. Topographic organisation of cortico-spinal projections from the frontal lobe: motor areas on the medial surface of the hemisphere. *J Neurosci* 1995, **15**:3284-3306.

Hoffman DS, Strick PL. The effects of a primary motor cortex lesion on the step/tracking movements of the wrist. *J Neurophysiol* 1995, **73**:891-895.

Horak FB, Woollacott M. [Editorial] In: Special issue on 'Vestibular control of posture in gait.' *J Vestib Res* 1993, **3**:1-2.

Lawrence DG, Kuypers HGJM. The functional organisation of the motor system in the monkey, Parts 1 and 2. *Brain* 1968, **91**:1-14;15-36.

Marsden CD, Rothwell JC, Day BL. Long latency automatic responses to muscle stretch in man, their origins and their function. In: Desmedt JE, ed. *Advances in neurology*, vol. 39. New York: Raven Press; 1983:509-540.

Passingham RE. The status of the premotor areas: evidence from PET scanning. In: Ferrell WR, Proske U, eds. *Neural control of movement*. New York: Plenum Press; 1995:167-178.

Porter RR, Lemon RN. *Corticospinal function and voluntary movement*. Oxford: Oxford University Press; 1994.

Roberts TDN. *Neurophysiology of postural mechanisms*. London: Butterworth; 1979.

Rothwell J. *Control of human voluntary movement*. London: Chapman & Hall; 1994.

Rothwell JC. The basal ganglia. In: Cody FWJ, ed. *Neural control of skilled human movement*. London: Portland Press; 1995:13-30.

Rothwell JC, Traub MM, Day BL, *et al.* Manual motor performance in a deafferented man. *Brain* 1982, **105**:515-542.

Stein J. The posterior parietal cortex, the cerebellum and visual control of movement. In: Cody FWJ, ed. *Neural control of skilled human movement*. London: Portland Press; 1995:31-49.

Sanes JN, Donoghue JP. Organisation and adaptability of muscle representations in primary motor cortex. In: Caminiti P, Johnson PB, Burnod Y, eds. *Control of arm movement in space*. Berlin: Springer; 1991:103-127.

Thach WT, Goodkin HP, Keating JG. The cerebellum and the adaptive coordination of movement. *Ann Rev Neurosci* 1992, **15**:403-442.

Wichmann T, DeLong MR. Pathophysiology of parkinsonian motor abnormalities. *Adv Neurol* 1993, **60**:53-61

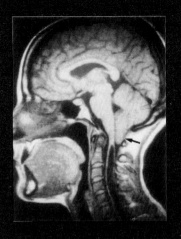

3

C Kennard

MEDICAL DIAGNOSIS OF NEUROLOGICAL CONDITIONS

CHAPTER OUTLINE

- **Taking a neurological case history**
- **The neurological examination**

- **Neurological investigations**

INTRODUCTION

The diagnosis of neurological conditions is often viewed as complex, demanding a vast knowledge of neuroanatomy, neurophysiology and the large number of neurological diseases. It should, however, be remembered that in everyday neurological practice a relatively limited number of conditions are encountered. With a knowledge of these conditions and the manner of their presentation, and by taking a systematic history and carrying out an appropriately oriented neurological examination, it is usually possible to arrive at a correct diagnosis.

TAKING A NEUROLOGICAL CASE HISTORY

For the clinical neurologist, taking the patient's history is often more important than the clinical examination, which is simply confirmatory. Indeed it is often claimed that about 80–90% of patients with neurological symptoms may be correctly diagnosed from the history alone. When taking a neurological history the examiner should always try to achieve two goals. The first is to try and localise along the neuraxis, from the cerebral hemispheres to the peripheral nerve and muscle, where the pathological process is taking place. For example, a patient complaining of weakness in both legs but none in the arms is most likely to have pathology in the peripheral nerves or muscles of the leg, or in the thoracic or lumbar spinal cord. The additional symptom of disturbed urinary function would strongly favour the spinal cord or cauda equina but not the peripheral nerves

and muscle. The second goal is to identify the nature of the disease process from the description of the onset, evolution and course of the illness. For bilateral weakness in the legs, a gradual progression would suggest a chronic disorder of the peripheral nerves or muscles, whereas an acute onset with rapid progression would suggest either an acute peripheral neuropathy, such as the Guillain–Barré syndrome, or an acute spinal cord lesion. The sudden onset of a hemiplegia is likely to be due to infarction or haemorrhage in the contralateral cerebral hemisphere, whereas a progressive development would suggest a cerebral tumour.

The commonest neurological symptoms are headache, dizziness and blackouts. Patients complaining of headaches are often fearful of having a brain tumour, but in fact this is a rare presentation. Most will have either muscle contraction (tension) or migraine headaches. Dizziness is a very vague symptom which may indicate a rotatory illusion of movement, called vertigo. However, more commonly the patient describes a vague lightheaded, or 'swimmy' sensation. Whereas vertigo usually indicates a disturbance in the vestibular apparatus or more centrally in the brainstem, other symptoms of dizziness may be very difficult to diagnose accurately.

Blackouts or 'funny turns' indicate an epileptic seizure or a syncopal episode (faint), and careful questioning of the patient, as well as an eye witness, about events preceding, during and following the episode is absolutely crucial. There are many other symptoms which have neurological significance, including disorders of memory and consciousness, visual disturbances, speech and swallowing abnormalities, localised pain, sensory and motor symptoms, abnormal involuntary movements, problems with bladder control, and walking difficulties. By elucidating the nature, location and timing of a particular symptom, and its association with other symptoms, it is often possible to reach either a single diagnosis or at least a reasonably limited set of differential diagnoses. These can then be further evaluated during the neurological examination and by appropriate investigations.

THE NEUROLOGICAL EXAMINATION

The neurological examination is primarily carried out to localise the site of the pathology in the neuraxis, and requires a knowledge of the course and innervation pattern of the cranial and peripheral nerves, and of the major fibre tracts in the brain and spinal cord. It commences as soon as the patient enters the consulting room, sits down and begins to relate the history of illness. Alertness, gait and speech may all provide important clues to the diagnosis. The manner in which the history is told may indicate impairments of judgement or memory, confusion, or difficulties with comprehension or expression of ideas. After the history has been taken, before the patient is taken to the examining couch, a few moments should be spent in evaluating the mental state and some aspects of cognitive function. This should include determining whether the patient is oriented in time and place. Tests of attention, memory and clarity of thought include the immediate repetition of a series of digits forwards and backwards, serial sub-traction of 7s from 100, and recall of an address or set of objects after an interval of 3 minutes. The ability of the patient to read, write, name objects, solve simple mathematical problems, copy diagrams, and draw a clock face (for evidence of spatial neglect) should be noted.

The neurological examination should now proceed with the patient lying comfortably on the examination couch in a well lit and warm room. It is preferable to examine the patient in undergarments. The examination should then proceed in a systematic manner, starting with the cranial nerves and then motor, reflex and sensory function in the trunk and limbs. Formal assessment of gait and balance should complete the examination.

The function of each cranial nerve is examined in turn: sense of smell (olfactory nerve); visual function including visual acuity, visual fields and examination of the optic fundi with an ophthalmoscope (optic nerve); examination of the pupils and eye movements (oculomotor, trochlear and abducens nerves); facial sensation, corneal sensation and reflex and jaw movement (trigeminal nerve); facial movement (facial nerve); hearing (auditory nerves); palatal sensation and movement, gag and cough reflex (glossopharyngeal and vagus nerves); movements of the sternomastoid and trapezius muscles (accessory nerve); and tongue movement (hypoglossal nerve) are all examined and any abnormalities noted.

Motor function should be examined next. This commences with observation of the patient's limbs and trunk looking for wasting or fasciculation of the muscles (suggestive of damage to the anterior horn motor neurones), abnormal posture and involuntary movements such as

tremor (usually indicating an extrapyramidal disorder). If the tremor is present only at rest then Parkinson's disease should be considered. If present only during maintained posture this may be physiological, due to stress or associated with thyrotoxicosis. The other likely diagnosis is of benign essential tremor, which may be hereditary. Tremors and other involuntary movements are discussed in Chapters 5 & 25.

The muscle tone in the limbs is then assessed. If increased, as in spasticity and rigidity, either an upper motor neurone (pyramidal tract) or an extrapyramidal disorder, respectively, is suggested. The strength and speed of movement in each muscle group is then systematically assessed, and any weakness should be graded according to the Medical Research Council (MRC) scale from 0 to 5 (0 = absent contraction, 5 = full strength). In addition, it is useful to observe the patient's ability, in prone and supine positions, to maintain against gravity his or her arms outstretched, and then both legs; the weak arm or leg usually tires first and then sags. The ability to sit up from the lying position and the strength of neck flexion and extension should also be assessed.

Motor co-ordination, usually an indicator of cerebellar function, is then assessed by finger–nose and heel–shin movements, and asking the patient to perform rapid alternating movements of the limbs. To complete the motor examination the reflexes are tested including the biceps, supinator, triceps, knee, ankle and cutaneous abdominal reflexes. Finally, the plantar responses (Babinski response) are assessed.

Testing sensory function is undoubtedly the most difficult part of the examination and should not be prolonged for more than a few minutes, since the patient will tire and the responses become inconsistent. All areas of the skin surface should be tested first for pain sensation with a pin, assessing whether there are differences between the two sides of the body, a level below which sensation is impaired, or an area where sensation has been lost completely. Testing of other sensory modalities including light touch (cotton wool), joint position sense (by small movements of a finger or toe), vibration (tuning fork) and temperature is performed only if indicated by the history or other aspects of the examination which has been carried out earlier.

Finally, the patient should be asked to stand with eyes open and then closed (Rhomberg's test), and any unsteadiness noted. The patient's gait should then be tested, noting particularly posture, step amplitude, and ability to turn. For further information on taking a neurological examination the reader is referred to Fuller (1993).

NEUROLOGICAL INVESTIGATIONS

After taking the history and completing the neurological examination, it should be possible to determine to what extent additional investigations are needed either to confirm a diagnosis or to differentiate between a range of possible diagnoses. However, it should always be remembered that neurological dysfunction may result from disease in another part of the body. It is also important to plan investigations which are going to provide the maximal amount of information about the patient's illness but which will result in the least possible discomfort and risk. The principal investigations for diagnosing brain and spinal cord disease are computerised tomography (CT) scanning, magnetic resonance (MR) imaging, evoked potentials (EP) and electroencephalography (EEG), and for peripheral nerve and muscle disease electromyography (EMG) and nerve conduction studies.

NEUROIMAGING

The imaging technique used will depend on the quality of image required and the availability of the technique.

Plain Radiology of the Skull and Spinal Column

Following the introduction of CT scanning, the use of X-rays has declined. However, routine lateral and antero-posterior radiographs of the skull are still of use in the initial assesment of patients with head injuries, particularly those in whom there has been any alteration in the level of consciousness, when evidence of a skull fracture is an indication for hospital admission for observation. X-ray images of the skull also provide information about the integrity of the pituitary fossa, the presence or absence of intracranial calcification, and whether the frontal, maxillary and sphenoidal paranasal sinuses show opacification suggestive of infection or neoplasia.

Radiographs of the spine are taken to identify changes in the vertebrae themselves, the intervertebral discs and the intervertebral foramina. However, it should be appreciated that the intervertebral disc is not radiopaque, and a radiograph of the lumbosacral spine taken in a patient with a presumed acute disc prolapse is likely to be normal. It is only after a disc protrusion has been present for months or years that the margins of the prolapsed disc start to calcify, producing posterior osteophyte formation of the borders of the upper and lower vertebrae. Collapse of the vertebrae revealed by plain radiography may occur due to osteomyelitis, Paget's disease, fracture, and neoplasia, either benign or malignant, which may result in cord compression.

CT Scanning

This is a technique in which the transmission of photons across the head, through the brain, is recorded using crystals. The tissue density of the brain is measured across several tomographic horizontal levels, and computers construct images of slices of the brain (Latchaw, 1984). The differing densities of the grey and white matter, cerebrospinal fluid (CSF), blood and bone can be distinguished, as can abnormal tissue such as haemorrhage, tumour, oedema and abscess (Figure 3.1A). Enhancement of the images, produced by the intravenous injection of a contrast medium, may add precision to diagnosis. Because of artefact from the surrounding bone, CT scanning is not ideal for examination of the posterior fossa and the spinal cord.

CT scanning is widely available, not only for the diagnosis and identification of focal cerebral lesions, but also to assess the presence or absence of ventricular dilation in cases of possible hydrocephalus (Figure 3.1B), or of cortical atrophy resulting from ageing.

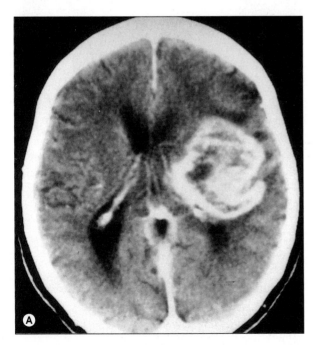
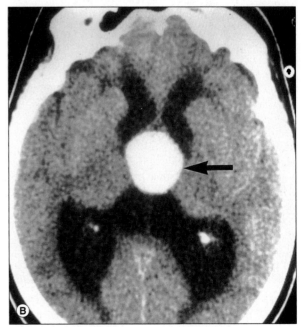

Figure 3.1 CT scans of the brain. (A) A malignant glioma in the right hemisphere. (B) Ventricular dilation (hydrocephalus) due to a colloid cyst (arrow) in the IIIrd ventricle, causing obstruction of CSF flow from the IIIrd to the IVth ventricle through the aqueduct of Sylvius.

MR Imaging

This relatively new technique produces, in a similar manner to CT scanning, 'slice' images of the brain in any plane, and has the great advantage of using non-ionising radiation (Moseley, 1988). The patient's head is placed in a powerful magnetic field that produces temporary physical changes in the atoms of the brain. This results in the production of radio-frequency energy, subjected to computer analysis, from which an image is constructed. This technique provides excellent visualisation of anatomical detail, particularly the difference between grey and white matter. Abnormalities in the white matter, as in multiple sclerosis (Figure 3.2A), and the spinal cord with its cervical (Figure 3.2B) and lumbar roots are clearly defined. As this technique becomes more available it is superceding CT scanning.

Angiography

In this technique a contrast medium opaque to X-rays is injected into the blood vessels leading to the brain to outline their intracranial course. It is extremely useful for the diagnosis of cerebral aneurysms (Figure 3.3A,B), vascular malformations and occluded or stenosed arteries (Figure 3.3C) and veins. Recent developments in MR angiography, which is non-invasive, suggest that it will eventually take over from X-ray angiography as the technique of choice (Sellar, 1995).

Positron Emission Tomography (PET)

Just as the transmission of X-rays through the head (transmission tomography) can be used to generate CT scans, so similar pictures can be obtained using positron-emitting radioisotopes (emission tomography; Sawle, 1995). These isotopes are produced in a cyclotron and are used to label various naturally occurring products, e.g. water and carbon dioxide are labelled with ^{15}O and glucose with ^{18}F. A variety of such ligands can be generated and delivered to the subject by inhalation or by injection. The isotopes produce positrons that, after a very short distance, collide with electrons, resulting in annihilation and the release of photons. Multiple arrays of detectors are used to detect the photons and CT techniques allow maps of regional cerebral blood flow to be produced. In addition, cerebral blood volume and cerebral glucose uptake can be measured simultaneously, allowing the oxygen extraction ratio and cerebral metabolic rate for oxygen to be calculated. The density of neurotransmitter receptors can also be studied using appropriately labelled ligands, as can activation of the brain during specific neurobehavioural tasks. This technique is extremely costly and is available in relatively few centres throughout the world.

ELECTRODIAGNOSTIC TESTS

These tests involve the amplification and recording of the electrical activity of the brain and peripheral nerves, which may be either spontaneous or induced by appropriate stimulation. Details of these tests can be found in textbooks such as Misulis (1993).

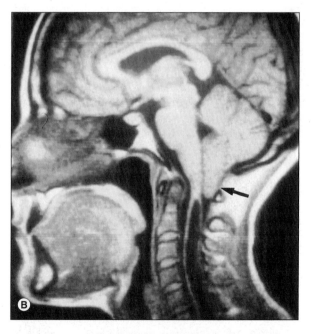

Figure 3.2 MR scans of the brain. (A) Axial section (T2 weighted) through the brain of a patient with multiple sclerosis. The plaques of demyelination appear as areas of high signal attenuation in the white matter (arrowed). (B) A sagittal section (T1 weighted) through the brain of a patient with cerebellar ectopia (Arnold-Chiari type 2 malformation) and syringomyelia. Note that the cerebellar vermis (arrowed) descends into the cervical canal well below a line drawn between the first cervical vertebra and the posterior margin of the foramen magnum. The spinal cord is expanded by the fluid-filled syrinx, which appears as a black core in the centre of the cord.

Electroencephalography (EEG)

EEG is a method of recording spontaneous cerebral electrical activity through the intact skull. A set of electrodes is attached to the scalp and the electrical activity is amplified to provide 16 or more channels of activity, usually displayed on a chart recorder. It is of use in the diagnosis of different types of epilepsy, in certain forms of encephalitis and in some cases of coma.

Evoked Potentials (EP)

Sensory EPs are the time-locked electrical activations of specific parts of the brain in response to a stimulus that may be visual (flashed light or pattern such as an alternating checkerboard), auditory (click or tone) or somatosensory (electrical pulse) stimulus. The latency (the delay between the onset of the stimulus and the onset of the response) is measured and provides a measure of conduction along the sensory pathway, e.g. the optic nerve. These techniques have been used particularly to identify clinically silent lesions in sensory pathways due to multiple sclerosis and are of value in the differential diagnosis of a variety of cerebral metabolic disorders in infants and children.

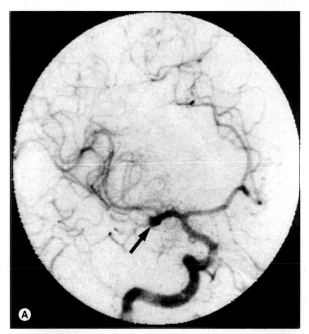

(A)

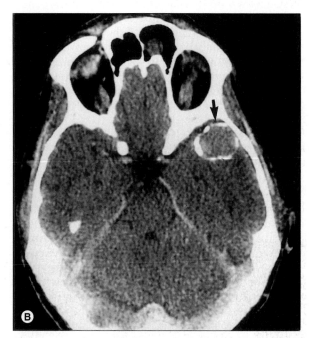

(B)

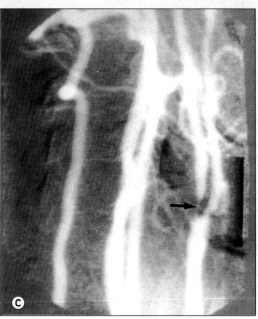

(C)

Figure 3.3 Imaging aneurysms and stenosis.
(A) Cerebral angiogram showing a small aneurysm arising from the right middle cerebral artery (arrowed).
(B) A contrast-enhanced CT scan of the same patient shows that the aneurysm (arrowed) located at the tip of the temporal lobe has a calcified wall and is in fact much larger than was shown on the angiogram. This indicates that the majority of the aneurysm is thrombosed.
(C) A cerebral angiogram showing a tight stenosis of the right internal carotid artery (arrowed) at its origin from the common carotid artery. The patient presented with recurrent episodes of amaurosis fugax (monocular blindness) of the right eye.

Nerve Conduction Velocity

Conduction along the sensory or motor component of a peripheral nerve can be measured by recording the sensory or motor response downstream from a site of electrical stimulation. The time taken for the action potential to travel along a defined segment of nerve allows the conduction velocity to be calculated. This technique is used in the diagnosis of entrapment syndromes, such as the carpal tunnel syndrome due to compression of the median nerve at the wrist, and in diagnosing peripheral neuropathies that may be axonal or demyelinating.

EMG

EMG involves the insertion of recording electrodes into a variety of muscles in different parts of the body and recording spontaneous (at rest) and induced (by contraction of the muscle) electrical muscle activity. It can be used to differentiate between primary muscle disease and denervation of muscle due to lower motor neurone dysfunction. It is therefore useful in the diagnosis of neuromuscular diseases such as motor neurone disease, muscular dystrophies and polymyositis.

LUMBAR PUNCTURE AND EXAMINATION OF THE CEREBROSPINAL FLUID

Examination of CSF is sometimes of great importance in the diagnosis of neurological disease, particularly in patients suspected of having meningitis, subarachnoid haemorrhage and suspected inflammatory brain disease (Thompson, 1995). Lumbar puncture carries a risk of tonsillar herniation, however, and possible death if the intracranial pressure is raised; if this is a possibility, a CT scan is required beforehand to exclude a mass lesion. A lumbar puncture is performed under sterile conditions; a local anaesthetic is given and then a fine-bore needle is inserted into the L3–L4 interspace until it enters the subarachnoid space and CSF is obtained. As well as obtaining CSF for analysis of its cellular, chemical and bacteriological constituents, the CSF pressure may be measured.

MUSCLE BIOPSY

Muscle biopsy can be extremely valuable in the diagnosis of neuromuscular diseases, particularly intrinsic pathology of the muscle as in inflammatory disorders such as polymyositis, or degenerative disorders such as the muscular dystrophies (Dubowitz & Brooke, 1973). The biopsy is taken from an affected muscle and then processed for light and electron microscopy. Special staining techniques are used to identify the different muscle fibre types and abnormalities in specific enzyme pathways. Recently, the introduction of immunocytochemical and immunohistochemical techniques has allowed the localisation of specific proteins. The interpretation of a muscle biopsy usually includes the description of a constellation of changes and then the association of these changes with a specific diagnosis (see Chapters 16 & 21).

OTHER TESTS

Routine haematological, biochemical and serological analysis of blood may sometimes assist neurological diagnosis. In addition to analysis of red and white cells, haematological testing should include the platelet count in patients with cerebrovascular disease. Erythrocyte sedimentation rate (ESR) should be measured, especially in patients over the age of 50 years presenting with headache, to exclude temporal arteritis. In addition to the routine biochemical assessment of renal, liver and calcium function, measurement of creatine phosphokinase (CPK) is useful in the evaluation of neuromuscular disease, since raised levels indicate muscle damage. Patients with movement disorders should have the levels of serum copper and plasma caeruloplasmin (a copper transporter protein) checked to exclude Wilson's disease, which is treatable with chelating agents (Marsden, 1987).

Serological testing should include tests for syphilis and the human immunodeficiency virus (HIV) if the patient has specific risk factors. Tests for HIV can be performed only after the patient has received appropriate counselling.

Conclusions

This chapter has provided a brief overview of the clinical examination and investigative techniques which a neurological patient may undergo before being referred to the physiotherapist. Further details may be obtained from the recommended texts detailed below. Aspects of the medical examinations that are performed during the physiotherapy assessment are discussed in Chapter 4.

REFERENCES

Dubowitz V, Brooke MH. *Muscle biopsy.* London: WB Saunders; 1973.

Fuller G. *Neurological examination made easy.* Edinburgh: Churchill Livingstone; 1993.

Latchaw RE. *Computed tomography of the head, neck and spine.* Chicago: Mosby Year Book; 1984.

Marsden CD. Wilson's disease. *Q J Med* 1987, **65**:959-967.

Misulis KE. *Essentials of clinical neurology.* London: Butterworth Heinemann; 1993.

Moseley I. *Magnetic resonance imaging in diseases of the nervous system.* Oxford: Blackwell Scientific Publications; 1988.

Sawle GV. Imaging the head: functional imaging. *J Neurol Neurosurg Psychiat* 1995, **58**:132-144.

Sellar RJ. Imaging blood vessels of the head and neck. *J Neurol Neurosurg Psychiat* 1995, **59**:225-237.

Thompson EJ. Cerebrospinal fluid. *J Neurol Neurosurg Psychiat* 1995, **59**:349-357.

GENERAL READING

Walton J. *Brain's diseases of the nervous system, 10th edition.* Oxford: Oxford University Press; 1993.

Warlow C. *Handbook of neurology.* Oxford: Blackwell Scientific Publications; 1991.

Wilkinson IMS. *Essential neurology, 2nd edition.* Oxford: Blackwell Scientific Publications; 1993.

4

E Bower & A Ashburn

PRINCIPLES OF PHYSIOTHERAPY ASSESSMENT AND OUTCOME MEASURES

CHAPTER OUTLINE

- The principles of evaluation
- Characteristics of measurements
- Procedures for using measurement tools
- Importance of evaluation

INTRODUCTION

Although physiotherapy practice has evolved over the years, the pressure for change has increased in recent times. The demand for evidence-based treatment and cost-effectiveness has challenged many traditional practices and has brought pressures on therapists to change attitudes and develop skills. Physiotherapists have been forced to be aware of the greater need for accountability, particularly if they are to remain professional practitioners and not become technicians in the healthcare system (Rothstein, 1989). There is a requirement to justify treatment plans, monitor client responses, predict outcome, and defend length, frequency and content of treatment programmes.

The role of physiotherapy within the broader sense of rehabilitation, which aims to protect or restore the personal and social identity of clients (Ward & McIntosh, 1993), is reported to be key, but still there is a paucity of evidence of effectiveness (Anonymous, 1992). Management of disordered movement and function forms the focus of the profession and has been described by Edwards (1996) and Ward & McIntosh (1993) as problem-solving, goal-directed and reliant on the accurate measurement and analysis of movement, posture and function. However, the use of quantitative measures to record movement does not form a part of routine practice of many physiotherapists. In a systematic descriptive study of four centres (Bower & McLellan, 1994a) none of the physiotherapists at any of the centres routinely used established assessment scales. All the physiotherapists set aims or goals for treatment, but at three of the four centres therapists were not very systematic and their aims or goals often did not lend themselves to precise measurement.

It is possible that therapists actively resist the use of appropriately developed and validated measures. The following concerns have been suggested: (1) formal assessments could take up too much treatment time; (2) measures may not provide an accurate reflection of the movement or function under treatment; (3) the assessment process could identify an individual physiotherapist as just 'muddling through' rather than giving therapy in a structured and logical way; (4) the accurate measures add nothing to the treatment process; (5) the specific treatment given may not be as successful as the physiotherapists had hoped; and (6) on-going measurements could show that an individual physiotherapist was not as successful at delivering a treatment as assumed. Two other reasons could be that therapists are often unaware of the different measures available and that they often do not know which measures to choose for which purpose. Any resistance to documenting responses in order to practice objectively in a climate of evidence-based therapy needs to be overcome or adequately justified.

The aim of this chapter is to raise an awareness of the importance of quantifying. A description of assessment, measurement and outcome from physiotherapy is provided in the section on principles of evaluation. Paediatric neurology appears to have more established scales than have been developed for adults, and this is reflected in the greater use of examples of paediatric measurement in this chapter. The final section challenges the poor use of quantitative measures in current practice and proposes that future developments within the profession are dependent on the accurate analysis of the effect of treatment.

BACKGROUND

Physiotherapy is rarely provided in isolation and so interventions need to be considered in the wider context of rehabilitation or habilitation. The World Health Organisation (WHO, 1980) defined rehabilitation as a set of influences, procedures and resources to be applied both to the disabled person and to the environment. It involves the recovery or improvement of function as well as prevention of disability and the maintenance of social role (McLellan, 1997), which implies that, while a focus is placed on disability, the aim is to reduce handicap (Wade, 1992).

DEFINING THE PROBLEM

The WHO model of illness provides a useful framework for understanding rehabilitation; the consequence of illness is identified at three key levels (see 'Preface'; Wade, 1992; McLellan, 1997):
- Impairment is the lack of body part or function as a direct consequence of pathological damage; loss of movement, vision, hearing or sensation are examples of impairment.
- Disability is the consequence of pathology or impairment, and is an inability to undertake an activity to a level or in a manner that is considered normal for a human being; examples of disabilities are difficulties with, or the inability to, walk or control balance.
- Handicap is the social or societal consequence of impairment or disability that limits or prevents the fulfilment of a role that is normal (depending on age, sex, social and cultural factors) for that individual; examples of handicap are difficulties with, or inability to, work, visit friends or go shopping.

DEFINING EVALUATION

The management of physical function varies but McLellan (1997) suggests that successful treatment results from a combination of three approaches: reducing disability; acquiring new strategies and skills, through which the impact of the disability could be minimised; and altering the environment, including the behaviour of non-disabled people, so that impairment and disability no longer confer a handicap. Regardless of which of these approaches or combinations of approaches is used, the ability to quantify physical function is key to successful treatment, as the process involves assessment (identification of the problem), planning goal-directed treatment, provision of intervention, and evaluation of outcome.

THE PRINCIPLES OF EVALUATION

Evaluation includes assessment, which in turn involves observation to produce subjective information as well as measurements providing objective data.

ASSESSMENT

Assessment in physiotherapy refers to the collection of information needed to come to a conclusion about a client's diagnosis or prognosis or a decision on intervention. The aim is to describe the client, and the process involves the interpretation of findings from measurements of the client, in the context of other problems or deficits that the individual may experience. Sadly, assessments may become rituals rather than valuable tools (Wade, 1992) and the purpose of evaluating physical function, which is to record objectively, document and communicate findings about movement disorders and activity levels, can be lost.

Quantitative measures are rarely used by physiotherapists and the meanings of verbal descriptions of subjective observations differ widely according to the experience, expectations and aspirations of assessors and those who read the records. As a consequence, the rules for using phrases such as 'slightly reduced range of movement' or 'has a normal walk' are flexible and interpretations are varied. The purpose of assessment by a physiotherapist in the management of a client with a neurological disorder is: (1) to establish whether there is a movement disorder; (2) to determine what the future status is likely to be; and (3) to detect whether change has occurred over time. Kirschner & Guyatt (1985) suggested that appropriate measures need to be developed for each of these three purposes. Following the identification of a motor problem in a client, it is helpful if future change can be predicted so that realistic treatment goals can be set and evaluated over time.

The prime aim of assessment is to identify what the problem is—a process that involves the interpretation of individual measures of ability or disability, not just in the context of the client but also within the family and society. An ability to analyse movement is an essential prerequisite for the assessment of patients with impairment of movement (Edwards, 1996).

Shumway-Cook & Woollacott (1995) described the process of evaluating a movement disorder as the posing and testing of a series of hypotheses. For example, a client may have a shuffling gait pattern with no heel strike. The hypotheses posed could be that the walking pattern results from a shortened Achilles tendon or a weak tibialis anterior muscle. Findings from the measurement of both of these deficits form the basis to the problem-solving process, the stages of which are below (Edwards, 1996):
1. Identify the problem.
2. Describe the problem.
3. Develop goal-directed therapy.
4. Monitor progress.
5. Follow-up.
6. Measure outcome.

At the initial assessment the client should be encouraged, where appropriate, to list his or her problems and expectations of treatment. Clear statements of the carer's view of the client's situation and the carer's needs and expectations should be gathered also. For the purpose of recording motor activity, standardised tests should be used to measure key deficits of movement, sensation and function. However, there are limitations to classifying function through categories and the unique aspects of each client and situation may be more readily captured by reporting on findings gathered through observation, listening and manual handling skills. These skills are essential to practice but should be viewed as supplementary to measurement when evaluating and communicating movement disorders because of the lack of standardisation and variability of interpretation.

Background information and knowledge about features that may contribute to the movement disorder should be gathered from medical notes and colleagues. A clear, logical process for collecting data should be established to ensure that findings are both complete and transferable to others. A summary at the end of the document can assist interpretation of the client's situation and reinforce key points and problems, allowing for the planning of goal-oriented therapy.

Ward & McIntosh (1993) recommended two stages to the clinical assessment: a survey of abilities and disabilities, followed by careful examination and measurement of features. For the survey they suggested the following check-list: diagnosis and clinical status; signs and symptoms; medical history; home situation; mobility; self-care; communication ability; psychological function; role and occupation in society; physical health; and personal history. The special features they suggested in the neurological assessment for rehabilitation are listed below.

History

This should include:
- Presenting problems: purpose of assessment.
- Medical history and diagnosis.
- Survey of everyday function: home situation; mobility; self-care; communication; psychological function; roles; occupation; and physical function.
- Personal history.

Examination

This should include:
- Functional assessments relevant to presenting problems: e.g. mood; personality; behaviour; cognitive function; functional vision; communication (verbal and non-verbal); functional mobility (e.g. transfers and walking); relevant self-care activities (e.g. dressing); and swallowing.
- Further routine examinations as required to confirm pathological diagnosis and also to establish functional diagnoses.
- Further assessments (if required): nutritional status; special seating requirements or problems related to seating; orthoses and other aids; skin status, especially around the sacral area.

The physiotherapist's concern with movement leads to a particular interest in the assessment of motor function, covering all aspects of motor control, such as: range of movement (ROM); muscle power; pattern of movement of arm, leg and trunk; levels of muscle tone; tests of functional movement; dexterity; and sensation.

In addition, Stillwell & Stillwell (personal communication) have suggested a community outcome scale which features the assessment of:
- Mobility (where can the client go?).
- Occupation (what can the client do?).
- Social integration (with whom can the client spend time?).
- Engagement ('Who are you?', which covers self-esteem and wellbeing).

These may be important issues to explore in the future when objective measures are developed.

In the past, assessment has been largely subjective so there is a dearth of meaningful data and knowledge about movement disorders and normal movement. To be useful, an assessment must be objective, and this requires the use of standardised measurement.

Measurement

Measurement has been defined as the quantification of an observation against a standard (Wade, 1992). The following are examples of a standard: a metal tape measure; stop watch; goniometer; dynamometer; force plate; and a validated functional scale. Measurements can be used for recording: physical and mental or cognitive functions; activities of daily living; global measures of independence and disability; generic and disease-specific health-related quality of life; health status; and vocational behaviour (Wade, 1992).

Physiotherapists who lack the experience of managing or using measures on people with specific long-term neurological problems may find it difficult to gauge what is realistically achievable and which postures and movements may encourage the development of musculoskeletal deformity. Appropriately developed measures to discriminate, predict and evaluate change over time are needed. The future developments of the profession, at an individual client level and through research, rely on the common use and development of objective and valid assessments. Reliable and accurate communications of movement disorders in meaningful and systematic ways, both nationally and internationally, should be adopted.

The first requirement, prior to using measurements, is to establish what needs to be measured. Physiotherapists may wish to measure muscle tone, muscle strength or joint ROM in order to record the impairment of the movement disorder or the resulting secondary biomechanical constraints. They may wish to measure the disability through activities of daily living, gross motor function or levels of mobility, or they may wish to measure handicap by recording quality of life. The evaluation of impairment without reference to functional outcome or the evaluation of functional outcome without reference to quality of life is, however, meaningless.

The next step is to establish the reason for making the measurement: to describe the problem, to predict the outcome, or to evaluate the effect of treatment. The physiotherapist may wish to inform the client and/or carer, or may wish to gain the information for himself or herself and/or other professionals, or may wish to inform the people responsible for paying for the intervention, be they parents, charities, local authorities or government agencies.

With the knowledge of what he or she wants to measure and why, the physiotherapist can look for an appropriately developed and validated measure that satisfies the purpose and population to be measured and is suitable for use in the prevailing clinical situation.

A measure has three key functions:
- To discriminate from normal.
- To predict future status.
- To evaluate change over time.

Discrimination Measures

For a measure to be used in a discriminative way there must be a normal database, adjusted for age and sex, against which the performance of a patient can be compared. Such measures are usually only linked to disability and impairment, as handicap cannot usually be referenced against a norm, though it can be related to the individual's status and may be synonymous with quality of life (Wade, 1992). Commonly used examples of discriminative measures are:
- Peabody Development Motor Scales and Activity Cards (Folio et al., 1983), which measure gross and fine motor skills of children aged from birth to about 6 years.
- Bayley Scales of Infant Development (Bayley, 1969), which measure the developmental status of both mental and motor skills in children aged 2 months to $2^1/_2$ years.
- Denver Development Screening Test (Frankenburg et al., 1970), which measures fine and gross motor, personal –social, language and intellectual skills of children.
- Middlesex Elderly Assessment of Mental State (MEAMS), which measures cognitive function (Shiel & Wilson, 1992).
- Behavioural Inattention Test, which is designed to detect visual neglect (Halligan et al., 1991).
- Balance Performance Monitor, which is a force plate designed to measure static sway and distribution of body weight (Sackley & Lincoln, 1991).
- Box and Block Assessment, which was developed to measure gross manual dexterity; a normal database was developed by Desrosiers et al. (1994).

Predictive Measures

Predictive measures forecast what should happen in the future. If a measure is to be used in that way it must have been validated for that function and the ability to predict confirmed, i.e. client status after the prediction needs to have been validated. There are few scales tested in that way and, as predictive items are usually derived from studies on large populations, unusual phenomena that may influence the outcome of a small minority may not be recognised. Most prognostic items are markers of overall severity and several items may be interrelated, e.g. severe paralysis, sensory and cognitive loss, sitting balance and incontinence have been associated with poor outcome in acute stroke (Wade, 1992). Further studies, which are disease-specific, are required to confirm the predictive value of individual and combined variables.

Three of the following measures are examples of tools developed as predictive scales; the fourth is a scale that has been used to describe patterns of recovery from stroke, the predictive value of which has not been confirmed:
- Bleck Scale (Bleck, 1975), which measures a child's postural and tonic reflex activity on seven specific items at 1 year of age, to predict ambulatory status at 7 years of age.
- Movement Assessment of Infants (Chandler et al., 1980), which measures the motor function of high-risk neonates; however, this has been found not to be as useful a predictor of future status as was originally anticipated (Deitz et al., 1987).
- The Guy's Prognostic Score for functional independence (Allen, 1984) is a scale that has been developed from documented medically recognised signs, but the influence of rehabilitation on outcome has been disregarded.
- Recovery curves were developed from a series of activities tested over time on clients with stroke (Partridge & Edwards, 1988).

Measures of Evaluation

Evaluative measures are based on criterion-referenced data and demonstrate whether the client is different from the last time he or she was measured. Such tools need to be able to show whether change has occurred over time. It is important that the measure has been validated for that task and shown to be sensitive to variations in the performance of individuals. Commonly used examples, for which further references on validity and reliability are given below (see 'Functional measures'), include:
- Gross Motor Function Measure (Russell et al., 1993), which measures gross motor function of children from birth to 16 years.
- Bruininks–Oseretsky Test of Motor Proficiency (Bruininks, 1978), which measures gross and fine motor function of children from $4^1/_2$ to $14^1/_2$ years.
- Klein–Bell ADL Scale (Klein & Bell, 1982), which measures activities of daily living at any age but has been validated for use with children.
- Barthel Index (Mahoney & Barthel, 1965), which measures dependency during activities of daily living in adolescents and adults.
- Functional Independence Measure (FIM; Granger et al., 1986) and the 'Wee-Fim' (Msall et al., 1994), which measure dependency in adults and children, respectively.
- Paediatric Evaluation of Disability Inventory (Haley et al., 1992), which measures adaptive function from the age of 6 months to $7^1/_2$ years in children with physical or a combination of physical and cognitive disabilities.
- Rivermead Stroke Assessment (Lincoln & Leadbitter, 1979), which was developed to record motor ability and disability following stroke.
- The Functional Balance Scale, which was developed by Berg (1993) and consists of 14 activities; it is cited in Shumway-Cook & Woollacott (1995).

In conclusion, the purpose of assessment is to find out whether a client is different from the norm, to predict the natural history of the difference (ailment/problem), and then to evaluate change over time to see whether he or she is progressing as predicted, and whether interventions prescribed are affecting the natural progression.

RECORD KEEPING

As teams of different professionals are increasingly established to consult on the problems of both adult and paediatric patients, there is a move towards multidisciplinary assessment. Such a move towards joint assessment is valuable but does not obliterate the professional obligation of physiotherapists to document their own findings and hold their own records. Where standardised validated measures are used, a score sheet is usually provided and this should be utilised and kept in the physiotherapist's records.

CHARACTERISTICS OF MEASUREMENTS

Various types of measurements exist (e.g. technical, functional) but all must have certain characteristics in order to be valid and reliable tools. A critical review of measures was provided by Wade (1992).

SCALES AND LEVELS OF SCORING

Information produced by different measurement tools can be classified according to levels of refinement of the measures. The different levels are known as nominal, ordinal and interval, and different statistical analyses are applied to the data obtained.

Nominal Measures

The lowest level of classification, nominal measures, refers to naming categories such as male or female, smoker or non-smoker. This type of categorisation does not really measure as there is no value difference but it allows groups to be formed and numbers of subjects to be counted in each group.

Ordinal Measures

Ordinal measures have numbered scores organised in an order of value. The characteristic of this scoring system is that the difference between each of the number scores cannot be assumed to be the same. Most measures used in rehabilitation are ordinal; e.g. unable to achieve = 1, needs the assistance of a person = 2, independent with an aid = 3, independent = 4. The difference between 1 and 2 cannot be assumed to be the same as that between 3 and 4.

Interval Measures

Interval measures refer to numbered scores where the differences between the numbers on the scale are equal and the starting point is zero, e.g. tape measure, goniometer. With this type of measurement the difference between, for example, millimetres 3 and 4 is the same as the difference between millimetres 13 and 14.

Multiple Items

Multiple items are assessed by grouping tasks into scales or indices. The scores of multiple items can be treated in different ways:

- They can be *summed*, to produce a total score, e.g. the Motor Club Assessment (Ashburn *et al.*, 1982).

- Items can be *weighted*, so that when they are added up the more sensitive items have a higher score and make a greater contribution to the total score, e.g. the Nottingham Health Profile (Wade, 1992).
- Items can be arranged in an index in an order of hierarchy of difficulty, thus forming a *Guttman scale*; individual items are scored as 'yes' or 'no' and those that are achieved in order are summed to produce a score, e.g. the Rivermead Stroke Assessment (Lincoln & Leadbitter, 1979).
- A *Likert scale* consists of a number of questions aimed to test opinion or attitude; items and answers are of equal value and scoring can range, for example, from 'strongly agree' to 'strongly disagree', e.g. The Measure of Processes of Care (King *et al.*, 1995).

VALIDITY

A test is considered valid if it measures what it purports to measure. Validation therefore is concerned with understanding what a test measures and what inferences can be drawn from specific scores or findings from the measure (Anastasi, 1986), who the test was developed for, which group of subjects it was evaluated on, and why it was developed. If measures are used for reasons other than those for which they were developed or tested, no assumption can be made about the validity of the findings. Multiple procedures are required to develop and evaluate a test adequately. There are three core types of validity: construct, content, and criterion-related (Wade, 1992; Streiner & Norman, 1993).

Construct Validity

All measurements tools are developed for a purpose and component activities are included for reasons. Each measure, therefore, is built on one or more theories about what the test will measure; this is referred to as the construct. For example, the construct of an ADL measure is that it tests the ability to achieve independence in the basic activities required for everyday living. When an investigator embarks on developing a new measure, it is done with knowledge of the underlying theory of what the test will measure. Construct validity refers to the extent to which results obtained using the outcome measure concur with the results predicted from the underlying theoretical model (Wade, 1992).

Content Validity

Content validity refers to the items included in a measure (Wade, 1992) and validation consists of judgement by experts on whether the items in a scale appear appropriate for the intended use (Streiner & Norman, 1993). Further confirmation of the validity of component items can be sought through cross-referencing with published literature (Wilkin *et al.*, 1993). In addition, the items need to be appropriately and adequately related to the construct or theoretical model of the measure.

Criterion-related Validity

Criterion-related validation is concerned with external validity or comparison of the findings of a new outcome measure with that of an alternative established standardised tool or gold standard. Two further terms are sometimes used under this heading. The first is concurrent validity, which refers to the use of a currently used tool for comparison of findings. The second is predictive validity, which compares the findings of the new outcome measure with a predicted outcome.

RELIABILITY

Reliability is a test of a scale or instrument to measure something in a reproducible manner (Wade, 1992). The degree to which someone can repeat the measurements he or she has obtained is known as intra-tester or intra-rater reliability. The degree to which more than one tester obtains measures from the same subject that agree is inter-tester reliability (Wade, 1992). Test reliability can be improved through training and by ensuring the procedure has been clearly defined and standardised. These processes aim for uniformity of administering and scoring the test (Jones, 1991). Variability of findings from repeated tests may result from differing environmental factors, subjects and procedural differences, or instability of the measure (Jones, 1991). The user of an outcome measure can also introduce elements of variation or error.

Standardisation (use of manuals)

Standardisation is essential for good reliability. Careful documentation, through a manual of how a test should be used, is one recommended way of standardising the test procedure. A standardised measure should have a manual with explicit instructions for both administering and scoring the measure, so that all assessors use the measure in precisely the same fashion. No matter how good a measure is, it is only as good as the way in which it is used.

RESPONSIVENESS

A responsive measure is one that is sensitive to change. It is particularly important that an evaluative measure is sensitive to clinically important changes in a client over time (Kirschner & Guyatt, 1985). Responsiveness can be determined by the test–retest reliability of a measure and by the ability of a measure to detect actual changes which occur in a client over time.

TYPES OF MEASURES

Measures can be technical, functional or relate to quality of life. Many of the tests mentioned below are used more for research than for clinical purposes, but more clinical use could be made of those that require minimal equipment and time. Only those tests that have been shown to be reliable are mentioned. However, some show conflicting reliability in the literature, mainly due to their not being used for the purposes for which they were intended.

Technical Measures

Technical measures are usually of primary interest to the physiotherapist and are often concerned with the level of impairment or resulting secondary biomechanical constraints. Comprehensive reviews can be found in Rothstein (1989) and Greenwood et al. (1993). Commonly used examples include:

- Active and/or passive joint ROM.
- Kinematic, kinetic and EMG gait laboratory measurement.
- Muscle performance measurement, such as those used to test strength using the hand-held dynamometer (Bohannon & Andrews, 1987), or power and endurance using isokinetic devices such as the Cybex or Kin-Com.
- Muscle tone measurement, such as the Modified Ashworth Scale (MAS) which is commonly used in research to assess the severity of muscle spasticity (Bohannon & Smith, 1987; Allison et al., 1996).

Functional Measures

Functional measures are of interest to both the client and the physiotherapist and are usually concerned with the level of disability or dependency. They are more helpful if the client has situational understanding and if the function is relevant to everyday living in the client's normal setting. It is a change in the functional status of a client and in the amount of caring and assistance required by the client that tends to be the aim of most neurological rehabilitation. No gold standard or benchmark exists for measurement and research is needed to establish one. Commonly used examples include:

- Barthel Index (Mahoney & Barthel, 1965), which measures dependency during activities of daily living in people with chronic disability and has been tested for reliability and validity (Loewen & Anderson, 1988); the Barthel Index tends to be used as the standard test in the absence of a more widely applicable test for the wide range of severity of disability; the lower end of the scale is too insensitive to detect change in very severely disabled people and the top end is insensitive to change in mildly affected people.
- The FIM (Granger et al., 1986) and the paediatric version, the Wee-Fim (Msall et al., 1994), which measure dependency over a rather wider range of living activities than the Barthel Index; the FIM has been tested for reliability and validity (Kidd et al., 1995), as has the Wee-Fim (Msall et al., 1994).
- Paediatric Evaluation of Disability Inventory (PEDI), which measures adaptive function in mobility, social interactions, self-care and communication in children with chronic disability (Haley et al., 1992) and has been tested for reliability and validity (Feldman et al., 1990).
- Gross Motor Function Measure (GMFM), which measures gross motor functions in children and adolescents with cerebral palsy (Russell et al., 1993) and has been tested for reliability and validity (McLaughlin et al., 1991; Bower et al., 1996).
- Bruininks–Oseretsky Test of Motor Proficiency (Bruininks, 1978), which measures gross and fine motor function in

children and adolescents, including the non-disabled and those with learning difficulties, and has been tested for reliability and validity (Derstine, 1989).

- The Motor Assessment Scale (MAS), which was developed as a measure of functional motor performance (Carr & Shepherd, 1985) and has been tested for reliability and validity (Loewen & Andersen, 1988).
- Functional Reach, which is a single-item test developed as a quick screen for balance problems (Duncan et al., 1990).
- Rivermead Stroke Assessment (Lincoln & Leadbitter, 1979), which was developed to record motor ability and disability following stroke.
- The Office of Population Censuses and Surveys (OPCS) Disability Scale (Martin et al., 1988), which was devised from the disability classification of the WHO (1980) and validated by McPherson et al. (1993); it can be used across the hospital–community divide.

Quality of Life Measures

Measures of quality of life are of particular interest to the client and are concerned with level of handicap and the client's ability to function in the community and interact with society. In clients with mild involvement, one might measure how often they go out, whereas in clients with more severe involvement one might measure how the carer copes. These measures are used increasingly by sociologists and psychologists but are also of relevance to physiotherapists. Commonly used examples are:

- Vineland Adaptive Behaviour Scale (socialisation domain), which measures personal and social sufficiency in children and adolescents from birth to 18 years in both the disabled and non-disabled population (Sparrow et al., 1984).
- Questionnaire on resources and stress, which measures stress in families caring for an ill or disabled member (Holroyd, 1987).
- The Short Form 36 (SF-36; Stewart et al., 1988; Ware et al., 1992), which is a short questionnaire developed from the Rand Health Batteries (Ware et al., 1980).
- Nottingham Health Profile, which is a widely used measure of quality of life (Hunt et al., 1986).

Measures of quality of life have been reviewed by Spilker (1990), Bowling (1995) and Hughes et al. (1995).

GOALS

Setting goals is appropriate for both adults and children, although the examples given below concern children. Setting treatment goals traditionally provides a framework for treatment, but it can also assist the physiotherapist with evaluation of outcome. Setting goals involves identifying and formulating standards of motor activity that are in advance of the patient's current capacity or that retard deterioration (Bower & McLellan, 1994b). The process consists of assessing the client, setting the goals, undertaking the intervention and, after a set time period, evaluating the goals to ascertain to what extent they have been achieved.

In the case of the disabled child, Bower & McLellan (1992) found that goals could be divided into three broad categories. The first was concerned with relationships between the child and those who handled him or her in daily living situations. This category was called 'achieve a state' and was treated principally by techniques of repeated passive corrective handling and positioning. The second category was concerned with equipment, its use and the generalisation of abilities, and was called 'establish a daily programme'. Goals were encouraged by effective equipment, demonstration and on-going interest on the part of the physiotherapist through the use of such strategies as star charts. Star charts are charts designed by the physiotherapist on to which the child, parent, teacher or carer attaches a star on each occasion on which the prescribed programme has been implemented. They can act as a reward for the child, an aide memoir for the parent, teacher or carer, and a monitoring device for the physiotherapist. The third category was concerned with motor skill acquisition and called 'achieve a motor skill'. These goals were encouraged by repeated active movement (Held & Bauer, 1967) and skill training along functional lines. The specific goals were all compatible with the individual child's disability (Bobath & Bobath, 1975) and within the range of the individual child's developmental motor age (Sheridan, 1975).

Collaborative Goal Setting

Psychologists use goal setting (Herbert, 1987) to solve the problems of individual clients and their families. Educationalists use goal setting to motivate students towards a particular objective and to provide a system of monitoring the progress towards that objective. It is possible that in psychology, education and therapy, the people who are involved in the goal-setting process may also affect the outcome. Three probabilities need to be considered. First, the client concerned needs to understand the purpose of the goal and wish to achieve it, so that it is likely that an understanding of the client's level of cognitive, motivational and social ability is required in addition to the aspects more often considered by physiotherapists. Motor change may be the result of biological, intellectual, emotional or psychological change. Secondly, the carers need to identify the goal as a useful skill not requiring increased assistance from them; and, thirdly, the physiotherapist needs to assess that the goal is realistic.

Setting Goals

In the case of children, setting goals for treatment is at the centre of attempts to reduce disability and resolve handicaps for children and their families. In the past, the reasons for treating children with cerebral palsy have usually been related to symptoms without reference to the associated functional capacity of the child. However, it may be time to reconsider this hierarchical system of treatment and allow the identification of problems to be transferred to the child, the parents and the relevant nursery or school carers. The likely causes of, and possible solutions to, these disabilities can then be discussed between the child and all members of the care team. If appropriate treatments are available and are acceptable to the child, family and carers, these can be instituted and monitored by all concerned, who also participate in judging the success of interventions. Thus, problems that are of immediate concern to the child and his or her carers are addressed and a gradual comprehension of the core neurological problems may be achieved. The acquisition of knowledge covers the treatment options and prognosis, including realistic goals for each aspect of the individual child's disabilities. The process does, however, require a physiotherapist who understands all aspects of the condition and its likely progression, possesses sensitive interpersonal skills, and is sufficiently secure to be willing to learn with the child, the family and other carers (Bower, 1997).

Herbert (1987) suggested that goal setting can help children and parents in four ways:

- By focusing attention and action, providing a vision that offers hope and an outlet for concentrated effort.
- By mobilising energy and helping pull the children and/ or parents out of the inertia of helplessness and depression.
- By enhancing the persistence needed for working at problems.
- By motivating all concerned to search for strategies to accomplish them.

Several points need to be considered by the physiotherapist and discussed with the children and care-givers when setting goals (Bower, 1997). These involve being realistic in terms of what is achievable within the limitations imposed by the neurological impairment, the child's wish to change and the appropriateness of the goal at the time. Children achieve skills in stages, and so goals should be formulated in small, simple steps that are achievable, allowing the child to experience success and not failure. The compensatory strategies used by the child, which may combat secondary biomechanical impairments, can be valuable goals.

Careful thought needs to be given to the reason for physical intervention. The priority should not be the satisfaction of the physician, the physiotherapist or even the family, but should be the possibility of helping the child to become integrated in society. Factors that should be discussed with children, parents and nursery or school carers include (Bower, 1993):

- The realistic aims and rationale of treatment.
- The appraisal of therapy at regular intervals so that it can be stopped if not successful.
- Access to appropriate information, including predictions of outcomes.
- Provision of adequate and sympathetic support.
- An identification of the child's abilities and likely objectives.
- Methods of integrating treatment with the academic and social goals of education.

If this process is completed, the effects of physical therapy on family relationships, children's abilities to integrate socially and their scholastic attainments will have been more carefully considered than is often the case. The steps involved in setting goals for children have been discussed in detail by Bower (1997) and include careful assessment prior to goal setting itself.

The problems identified in assessment can be categorised into: (1) those that may be helped by physiotherapy; (2) those that physiotherapy cannot help; and (3) those that someone else may be able to help. The list may then be ranked in order of priority. The client and care team then agree on useful realistic, short-term goals and a time scale in which they should be achieved. These goals must be specific, measurable and documented.

OUTCOMES

The outcome of rehabilitation refers to the end-point evaluation of treatment effectiveness. Although the end point may seem clear, there is debate over when this measure should take place because rehabilitation for many people can last for several months and sometimes years. In the case of clients with chronic deteriorating conditions, there may not be an end point. Should outcome be recorded when the effect of treatment is expected to be at its greatest (Ward & Mcintosh, 1993), at the point of treatment termination, or through regular surveys to check on situations (McLellan, 1997)? The lack of standardisation of this point means that where outcomes have been measured in research studies there is considerable variability that makes interpretation and comparison of study findings very difficult.

In addition, each individual will start rehabilitation from a different point in the recovery process, and receive different interventions with different treatment objectives. Therefore, to use a general functional scale or an index of dependence in ADL alone as an outcome may not be suitable. The most important feature of an outcome measure is that it measures the objectives of the treatment received. It must also be valid and reliable, as discussed above. In many cases the outcome may best be measured through the achievement of individually set treatment goals, as the poor matching of outcome measures with aim of treatment is a common error.

In conclusion, outcome measurements are tools that are selected to test the effect of treatment and so should match the aim of treatment and must be clear and measurable. If the measures selected are consistently used over periods of time it should be possible to show differences in outcome and to move towards predicting the likely outcome of any particular intervention. However, due to the enormous variation of impairment, disability or handicap presented for treatment this process will require co-operation from a large number of treatment centres and agencies throughout the world with standardised computerised recording to build up a sufficient databank with universal access for clinicians and researchers. Nevertheless, even the consistent use of these measures over regions of the Health Service should help to show whether a particular line of therapy can be shown to be helping a particular client and whether the outcome of one line of therapy appears to be of greater benefit than that of another.

CLINICAL AUDIT

Clinical audit is a process for testing the effectiveness of a clinical service and not simply client satisfaction. The data collected should relate to outcome of treatment and should be collected through objective, systematic procedures. The findings should be fed back to practitioners and managers in order to allow standards to be developed and practice to be improved (McLellan, 1997). McLellan highlighted three elements of audit that are important: effectiveness of specific individual techniques; effectiveness of individual team members; and effectiveness of the team as a whole in meeting its client's needs.

PROCEDURES FOR USING MEASUREMENT TOOLS

Prior to using any tests, the equipment and settings for testing need to be arranged in a standardised fashion, e.g. chair and bed height, quiet room, printed forms for a single or a battery of tests. Before choosing a measure the assessor should consider a number of points but no matter how good the measurement tool is, the findings produced are only as good as the way in which the measurement tool is used.

SELECTING A TOOL

The physiotherapist first needs to establish what it is he or she wants to measure. Is it the impairment or pathophysiological component of the disorder, is it the disability or functional limitation resulting from the disorder, or is it the handicap or societal restriction associated with the disability?

Secondly, the physiotherapist needs to be clear why he or she wants to make the measurement. It may be to inform: the client and/or carer; the physiotherapist himself or herself and/or other professionals; or the people responsible for paying for the intervention. The therapist may wish to discriminate, predict or evaluate. With the knowledge of what he or she wants to measure and why, the physiotherapist can look for an appropriately developed and validated measure that satisfies the purpose and population to be measured and is suitable for use in the prevailing clinical situation.

There is little point in the continued use of a measure if it does not demonstrate standardisation, reliability, validity and responsiveness, as the results obtained will possess no scientific or objective value. Gowland *et al.* (1991) have produced some useful guidelines for reviewing publications describing measurements, which are equally relevant when selecting a measure for clinical use. Six main areas were reviewed:

1. **Purpose and population:**
    *   What is the primary purpose for which the scale was designed?
    *   For which age group and disease or disorder was the scale designed?
2. **Clinical utility:**
    *   Are the instructions clear?
    *   What does the measure cost?
    *   How long does it take to administer?
    *   What is the format?
    *   What qualifications does the examiner require?
3. **Scale construction:**
    *   Are the items well selected?
    *   What is the level of measurement?
4. **Standardisation:**
    *   Is there a manual?
5. **Reliability:**
    *   Have studies been undertaken?
    *   Have appropriate statistics been used?
    *   What is the level of reliability?
6. **Validity:**
    *   Have studies been undertaken?
    *   Is there content validity?
    *   Is there construct validity?
    *   Is there criterion-related validity?
    *   Is the measure responsive?

An example of a review could be as follows.

The Gross Motor Function Measure

1. Purpose and population

The purpose of the Gross Motor Function Measure (Russell *et al.*, 1993) is to evaluate motor changes over time in the following five dimensions: lying and rolling; sitting; crawling and kneeling; standing and walking; running and jumping. There are 88 items in the five dimensions. The measure quantifies whether the child is able to perform the motor function but not how the child performs the motor function. Its weaknesses lie in the measurement of endurance, of hand and arm function, and of some compensatory movements such as sitting on a chair pulling to stand at a bar. The scale was designed to be used for children with cerebral palsy aged from birth to 16 years. Whether this refers to chronological age or developmental age is not clear but the manual does state that all items could be achieved by a normal 5-year-old child. The measure is being developed further for use with developmentally delayed children, in particular children with Down's syndrome and those with head injuries.

2. Clinical utility

The instructions for administration and scoring are clearly set out in a user-friendly manual that must be followed and always kept handy for easy reference. The time taken to complete the test depends on the severity of the symptoms and the type of cerebral palsy. A child with predominantly ataxic or athetoid symptoms usually takes longer than a child with predominantly spastic symptoms. The complete test usually takes between 60 and 90 minutes. Few children can achieve all the items.

The format of the measure is observation. The child is allowed only three tries at each item, which must be achieved with no hands-on help. The child must be seen to perform the function in the test situation and at the test time. A potential problem with scoring only what the child performs in the test situation is that it may sacrifice validity in the non-compliant child. The entire measure does not have to be tested on the same occasion if the child is too tired or non-compliant but previously tested items may not be retested on the second occasion. Items do not have to be tested in a specified order. In order to use the Gross Motor Function Measure, a background of physiotherapy or occupational therapy training is preferable. A training package and videotape are available and courses are held in the USA, Canada and the UK. The equipment required is described in the manual; it is easily standardised, readily available and transportable.

Children are usually tested in shorts and a T-shirt, with shoes off. If aids or orthoses are used, the test is readministered in the relevant dimensions with these on. Scoring is on a four-point Likert scale for each item. The progression of most items is precisely described in the manual. A clear score sheet is supplied and the method of calculating overall dimension and goal scores is well explained.

3. Scale construction
Items are selected and presented in a hierarchical sequence. The level of measurement is ordinal.

4. Standardisation
There is a manual and this must be followed. The scale is criterion-referenced, so that the measurement is designed to establish whether the child has changed since the last time of measurement. There are no normative data. The measure is not designed to establish whether the child is different from the norm.

5. Reliability
Studies have been undertaken to establish reliability. These are described in the manual and more detail about inter-assessor error rates can be found in Bower et al. (1996).

6. Validity
Studies have been undertaken to establish validity and these are again described in the manual. The measure has been compared to the Peabody Developmental Motor Scales (Folio et al., 1983) and found to be more responsive to change over time.

IMPORTANCE OF EVALUATION

As already mentioned, appropriately developed and validated measures are rarely used in the clinical situation. In four recent studies (Bower & McLellen, 1992, 1994a,b; Bower et al., 1996) undertaken in 24 different UK health districts over the period 1989 to 1995, it was found that in the field of community neuropaediatric physiotherapy, virtually no measures were used. Some of the reasons and possible remedies for this may be:
- Physiotherapists are often unaware of the different measures available; the situation could be remedied by reading relevant research journals and undertaking literature searches; most, if not all, well developed measures have been used in research studies and the resulting articles have been published in peer-reviewed journals.
- Physiotherapists often do not know which measure to choose for which purpose; there has been a dearth of appropriately developed measures, and traditionally therapists have often used personally or locally devised checklists; such checklists, although understood in individual local situations, do not provide reproducible or generalisable scientific evidence; the lack of measures is gradually being overcome by the formation of multi-disciplinary professional teams, in both the USA and Canada, who are adequately funded to undertake the development of appropriate measurement tools which are standardised, reliable and validated.

WHY DO PHYSIOTHERAPISTS NEED TO EVALUATE ?
There are five main reasons for taking measurements, as described by Russell & Rosenbaum (personal communication):
- Decision making for the individual client.
- Research into effectiveness of treatments.
- Programme evaluation.
- Quality management.
- Professional and financial accountability.

Decision Making for the Individual Client
Treatments should relate to problems experienced and therefore it is appropriate that individual specific goals should be negotiated with each client and, where relevant, with carers.

Research into Effectiveness of Treatment
The second reason why physiotherapists need measurement is to evaluate the effectiveness of different approaches to treatment in a more generalised way, to establish guidelines to aid in the choice of treatment most likely to suit individual needs. Table 4.1 shows the treatment methods on which individual approaches place particular emphasis and some of these are discussed in Chapter 22. It is very tempting for a physiotherapist to want to know what is the 'right' treatment for a client in a given situation, but what is the basis for this so-called knowledge? Is it a reaction to, or a natural sympathy with, one method or approach, or a synthesis of elements which have been found to be effective from different methods, or is it just self-satisfaction not objectively founded?

Traditional treatments for neurologically affected clients could be classified by their therapeutic rationale and divided into three categories as pointed out by Scrutton (1984). The first category is 'mechanical', which aims to ameliorate musculoskeletal deformity at the periphery. Orthopaedic, orthotic, muscle strengthening procedures and stretching exercises to increase joint ROM are all included in this category. The second category is 'neurophysiological'; it aims to alter patterns of muscular activity that are centrally generated. Bobath and

Table 4.1 Examples of treatment methods on which individual 'schools' place particular emphasis. See Chapter 22 for discussion of some of these approaches.

Examples of treatment methods on which individual 'schools' place particular emphasis

Treatment approach	1	2	3	4	5	6	7	8
Voluntary active movement		✓		✓	✓			
Facilitated automatic movement	✓		✓			✓		✓
Passive movement	✓			✓			✓	
Normalisation of quality of movement	✓							
Functional activities		✓			✓			
Orthopaedic management of secondary biomechanical constraints				✓				
Development sequence of activities O= Ontogenetic (human)						✓		
P= Phylogenetic (creature)						✓		✓

Treatment approach:
Column 1 = Bobath
Column 2 = Conductive education
Column 3 = Kabat
Column 4 = Phelps
Column 5 = Portage
Column 6 = Rood
Column 7 = Temple Fay
Doman Delacato
Column 8 = Vojta

neurodevelopmental therapy are the most commonly used procedures in this category. The third category is 'educational', which is based on learning theory and aims to improve functional performance. Conductive education and Portage are in this category.

All three treatment categories described above are biased towards decisions being made by the physiotherapist giving the treatment as opposed to the client undertaking the treatment. If at all possible, the client undertaking the treatment needs to understand the purpose, the carer needs to find the purpose useful, and the physiotherapist needs to ensure that the purpose is realistic.

Programme Evaluation

The third reason why measurement is needed is to ascertain the best delivery arrangements for the treatment in individual circumstances. Such factors as who should give the treatment or how it should be undertaken, the duration, the frequency, and the locality in which the treatment should ideally take place need to be resolved. Table 4.2 shows the treatment delivery arrangements on which some individual approaches place particular emphasis.

Quality Management

Measurement should ensure the maximum satisfaction of the clients undergoing treatment and their families, within the confines of what can realistically be achieved.

Professional and Financial Accountability

It is necessary to satisfy the people responsible for paying for the treatment that their money is being spent wisely and to satisfy the professionals involved in the treatment that their time is being spent wisely.

It is interesting that the four outstanding biological achievements of humans that separate them from other animals (Sheridan, 1975) are often affected in clients with neurological disorder or disease:
1. Upright posture, which facilitates locomotion whilst leaving hands free.
2. Finely adjusted vision and flexible digits, enabling the construction and use of tools.
3. Spoken language.
4. Structured social behaviour for the benefit of both the individual and the community and for rearing children who remain dependent for a longer period than in other species.

However, it is probably the combination of these four factors, plus their intelligence and reasoning powers, which mark humans' difference from other animals. All of these features need to be measured in an assessment in order to understand the strengths and difficulties experienced by a client with a neurological disorder.

Examples of paediatric treatment delivery arrangements on which individual 'schools' place particular emphasis								
Treatment approach	1	2	3	4	5	6	7	8
Selection of children for treatment		✓						
Group treatment		✓						
Segregation from normal peers through treatment		✓		✓			✓ *	
Involvement of parents in treatment a) at centre = C b) at home = H	✓ C+H	✓ C if child 1½-3½ years			✓ H		✓ H	✓ H
Intensity and duration of treatment by professionals a) more than x3 weekly = 1 b) more than 1 hour per session = 2		✓ 1+2		✓ 1				
Special furniture		✓		✓				

Treatment approach:
Column 1 = Bobath
Column 2 = Conductive education
Column 3 = Kabat
Column 4 = Phelps
Column 5 = Portage
Column 6 = Rood
Column 7 = Temple Fay
              Doman Delacato
Column 8 = Vojta

*by intensity of treatment

Table 4.2 Examples of paediatric treatment delivery arrangements on which individual 'schools' place particular emphasis.

REFERENCES

Allen C. Predicting the outcome of acute stroke: a prognostic score. *J Neurol Neurosurg Psych* 1984, **47**: 475-480.

Allison S, Abraham L, Petersen C. Reliability of the Modified Ashworth Scale in the assessment of plantar flexor muscle spasticity in patients with traumatic brain injury. *Int J Rehab Research* 1996, **19**:67-78.

Anastasi A. Evolving concepts of test validation. *Ann Rev Psychol* 1986, **37**:1-15.

[Anonymous.] *Effective health care: stroke rehabilitation*. Leeds: University of Leeds; 1992.

Ashburn A, Members of Motor Club. A physical assessment for stroke patients. *Physiotherapy* 1982, **68**:109-113.

Bayley N. *Bayley scales of infant development*. New York: The Psychological Corporation; 1969.

Berg K. *Measuring balance in the elderly: valuation of an instrument. [Dissertation.]* Montreal, Canada: McGill University; 1993.

Bleck LE. Locomotor prognosis in cerebral palsy. *Dev Med Child Neurol* 1975, **17**:18-25.

Bobath B, Bobath K. *Motor development in the different types of cerebral palsy*. London: Heinemann Medical Books; 1975.

Bohannon R, Andrews A. Inter-rater reliability of a hand-held dynamometer. *Phys Ther* 1987, **67**:931-933.

Bohannon R, Smith M. Interrater reliability of a Modified Ashworth Scale of muscle spasticity. *Phys Ther* 1987, **67**:206-207.

Bower E. Physiotherapy for cerebral palsy: an historical review. In: Ward C, ed. *Rehabilitation of motor disorders*. London: WB Saunders; 1993:29-55. (Ballière's Clinical Neurology, Vol. 2 (I).)

Bower E. The multiply handicapped child. In: McLellan DL, Wilson B, eds. *The handbook of rehabilitation studies*. Cambridge: Cambridge University Press; 1997:315-355.

Bower E, McLellen DL. Effects of increased exposure to physiotherapy on skill acquistion in children with cerebral palsy. *Dev Med Child Neurol* 1992, **34**:25-39.

Bower E, McLellan DL. Assessing motor skill acquisition in four centres for the treatment of children with cerebral palsy. *Dev Med Child Neurol* 1994a, **36**:902-909.

Bower E, McLellan DL. Measuring motor goals in children with cerebral palsy. *Clin Rehab* 1994b, **8**:198-206.

Bower E, McLellan DL, Arney J, *et al*. A randomised controlled trial of different intensities of physiotherapy and different goal setting procedures in 44 children with cerebral palsy. *Dev Med Child Neurol* 1996, **38**:226-238.

Bowling A. Measuring disease: a review of disease-specific quality of life measurement scales. Buckingham: Open University Press; 1995.

Bruininks RH. *Briuninks-Osertesky Test of Motor Proficiency: examiners manual*. Circle Pines, Minnesota: American Guidance Service; 1978.

Carr J, Shepherd R. Investigation of a new motor assessment scale for stroke patients. *Phys Ther* 1985, **65**:175-180.

Chandler LS, Andrews MS, Swanson NW. *Movement Assessment of Infants: a manual*. Rolling Bay, Washington: Infant Movement Research; 1980.

Deitz JC, Crowe TK, Harris SR. Relationship between infant neurometer assessment and preschool motor measures. *Phys Ther* 1987, **67**:14-17.

Derstine S. Tests of infant and child development. In: Cleary PL, ed. *Paediatric physical therapy*. Philadelphia: Lippincott; 1989:16-39.

Desrosiers J, Bravo G, Herbert R, *et al*. Validation of the box and block test as a measure of dexterity in elderly people: validity and norm studies. *Arch Phys Med Rehab* 1994, **75**:751-755.

Duncan P, Weiner D, Chandler J, *et al*. Functional reach: a new clinical measure of balance. *J Gerontol* 1990, **45**:192-195.

Edwards S. *Neurological physiotherapy: a problem solving approach*. Edinburgh: Churchill Livingstone; 1996.

Feldman AB, Haley SM, Coryell J. Concurrent and construct validity of the paediatric evaluation disability inventory. *Phys Ther* 1990, **70**:602-610.

Frankenburg WK, Dodds JB, Fandel AW. *Denver Developmental Screening Test manual, revised edition*. Denver: University of Colorado Medical Centre; 1970.

Folio R, Fewell R, DuBose RF. Peabody developmental motor scales and activity cards. Hingham, Massachusetts: Teaching Resources Corp; 1983.

Granger CV, Hamilton BB, Keith RA. Advances in functional assessment for medical rehabilitation. *Topic Ger Rehab* 1986, **1**:59-74.

Gowland C, King G, King S, *et al*. Review of selected measures in neurodevelopmental rehabilitation - a rational approach for selecting clinical measures. Research Report 91-2. Hamilton, Ontario: Chedoke McMasters Hospitals Neurodevelopmental Clinical Research Unit; 1991.

Greenwood R, Barnes M, McMillan T, *et al. Neurological rehabilitation*. Edinburgh: Churchill Livingstone; 1993.

Halligan P, Cockburn J, Wilson B. The behavioural assessment of visual neglect. *Neuropsych Rehab* 1991, **1**:5-32.

Haley S, Coster W, Ludlow L. *Pediatric Evaluation of Disability Inventory (PEDI)*. Boston: New England Medical Centre Hospitals Inc; 1992.

Held R, Bauer JA. Visually guided reaching in infant monkeys after restricted rearing. *Science* 1967, **155**: 718-720.

Herbert M. *Behavioural treatment of children with problems: a practice manual, 2nd edition*. London: Academic Press; 1987.

Holroyd J. *Questionnaire on resources and stress for families with chronically ill or handicapped members*. Brandon, Vermont: Clinical Psychology Publishing Co.; 1987.

Hughes C, Hwang B, Kim J, *et al*. Quality of life in applied research: a review and analysis of empirical measures. *Am J Mental Retard* 1995, **99**:623-641.

Hunt S, McEwan J, McKenna S. *Measuring health status*. Beckenham: Croom Helm; 1986.

Jones L. The standardised test. *Clin Rehab* 1991, **5**:177-180.

Kidd D, Stewart G, Baldry J. The functional independence measure: a comparative validity and reliability study. *Disabil Rehab* 1995, **17**:10-14.

King S, Rosenbaum P, King G. *The Measure of Processes of Care. A means to assess family-centred behaviour of health care providers*. Hamilton, Ontario: Chedoke-McMaster Hospitals Neurodevelopmental Clinical Research Unit; 1995.

Kirschner B, Guyatt G. A methodological framework for assessing health indices. *J Chronic Dis* 1985, **38**:27-36.

Klein RM, Bell BB. *The Klein-Bell A.D.L. Scale*. Seattle, Washington: University of Washington Health Sciences Learning Resource Center; 1982.

Lincoln N, Leadbitter D. Assessment of motor function in stroke patients. *Physiotherapy* **65**(2):48-51.

Loewen S, Anderson B. Reliability of the Modified Motor Assessment Scale and the Barthel Index. *Phys Ther* 1988, **68**:1077-1081.

Mahoney F, Barthel D. Functional evaluation: The Barthel Index. *Maryland State Med J* 1965, **14**:61-65.

Martin J, Meltzer M, Elliot D. *The prevalance of disability among adults*. London: HMSO/Office of Population Censuses and Surveys; 1988.

McLauglin J, Bjornson K, Granbert C, *et al*. Ability to detect functional change with the gross motor function measure: a pilot study. *Dev Neurol Child Neurol* 1991, **33**(64):26.

McLellan DL. Introduction to rehabilitation. In: McLellan DL, Wilson B, eds. *The handbook of rehabilitation studies*. Cambridge: Cambridge University Press; 1997:1-21.

McPherson K, Sloan RL, Hunter J, *et al*. Validation studies of the OPCS scale: more useful than the Barthel Index? *Clin Rehab* 1993, **7**:105-112.

Msall ME, DiGandio K, Duffy LC. Wee Fim: normative sample of an instrument for tracking functional independence in children. *Clin Paediat* 1994, **33**:431-438.

Partridge C, Edwards S. Recovery curves as a basis for evaluation. *Physiotherapy* 1988, **74**(3):141-143.

Rothstein J. *Measurement in physical therapy*. New York: Churchill Livingstone; 1989.

Russell D, Rosenbaum P, Gowland C, *et al. Gross Motor Function Measure manual, 2nd edition*. Hamilton, Ontario: Chedoke-McMaster Hospitals Neurodevelopmental Clinical Research Unit; 1993.

Sackley C, Lincoln N. Weight distribution and postural sway in healthy adults. *Clin Rehab* 1991, **5**:81-186.

Scrutton D. *Management of motor disorders of children with cerebral palsy*. London: Spastics International Medical Publications with Blackwell Scientific Publications; 1984. (Clinics in Developmental Medicine, vol. 90: 1-6.)

Sheridan MD. *Child's developmental progress from birth to five years: the STYCAR sequences*. Windsor: NFER-Nelson; 1975.

Shiel A, Wilson B. Performance of stroke patients on the Middlesex Elderly Assessment of Mental State. *Clin Rehab* 1992, **6**:283-289.

Shumway-Cook A, Woollacott M. A conceptual framework for clinical practice. In: Shumway-Cook A, Woollacott M, eds. *Motor control: Theory and practical application*. Baltimore: Williams & Wilkins; 1995:99-116.

Sparrow SS, Balla DA, Cicchetti DV. *Vineland Adaptive Behaviour Scales (survey form)*. Circle Pines, Minnesota: American Guidance Service; 1984.

Spilker B. *Quality of life assessments in clinical trials*. New York: Raven Press; 1990.

Streiner D, Norman G. *Health measurement scales: a practical guide to their development and use*. Oxford: Oxford University Press; 1993.

Stewart A, Hays R, Ware J. The MOS short form general health survey: reliability and validity in a patient population. *Med Care* 1988, **26**:124-135.

Wade D. *Measurement in neurological rehabilitation*. Oxford: Oxford University Press; 1992.

Ward C, McIntosh S. The rehabilitation process: a neurological perspective. In: Greenwood R, Barnes M, McMillan T *et al*., eds. *Neurological rehabilitation*. Edinburgh: Churchill Livingstone; 1993:13-27.

Ware J, Brook R, Davies-Avery A, *et al*. Conceptualisation and measurement of health for adults in health insurance study. *Vol VI. Analysis of relationships using Health Status Measures*. Santa Monica, California: Rand Corporation; 1980.

Ware J, Sherbourne C, Davies A. Developing and testing the MOS 20 item short form health survey: a general population application. In: Stewart A, Ware J, eds. *Measuring functions and well being: the medical outcomes study approach*. Durham, North Carolina: Duke University Press; 1992:3-43.

Wilkin D, Hallam L, Doggett M. *Measures of need and outcome for primary health care*. Oxford: Oxford University Press; 1993.

World Health Organisation. *The international classification of impairments, disabilities and handicaps - a manual of classification relating to the consequences of disease*. Geneva: World Health Organisation; 1980.

ABNORMALITIES OF MUSCLE TONE AND MOVEMENT

CHAPTER OUTLINE

- Muscle tone
- Movement disorders

INTRODUCTION

This chapter presents an overview of the abnormalities of muscle tone and movement seen in patients with neurological disorders. The nature and proposed mechanisms of the abnormalities, the disorders in which they commonly occur and their medical treatment are outlined. Physical management is discussed in Chapter 25. Specialist texts in which further details can be found include Adams & Victor (1989), Weiner & Laing (1989) and Rothwell (1994).

MUSCLE TONE

Muscle tone can be defined clinically as the resistance that is encountered when the joint of a relaxed patient is moved passively. (This is the usual clinical definition of muscle tone, though there is no universally accepted definition. Physiologists, in particular, use 'tone' in a different way—to signify a state of muscle tension or continuous muscle activity.) In practice, the clinician (medical practitioner or physiotherapist) usually assesses muscle tone in one of two ways. He or she may grasp a patient's relaxed limb and try to move it, noting the amount of effort required to overcome the resistance—the muscle tone. Alternatively, the clinician may observe how a limb responds to being shaken or to being released suddenly: the greater the resistance to movement (i.e. the greater the muscle tone), the more rigidly the limb will behave.

The resistance encountered when moving the joint of a relaxed individual is a combination of the passive stiffness of the joint and its surrounding soft tissues plus any active tension set up by stretch reflex contraction. The passive stiffness is dependent upon the inherent viscoelastic properties of the tissues and varies with age and other physiological parameters (e.g. limb temperature, preceding exercise). The contribution of active stretch reflex contractions to overall muscle tone also varies considerably, even in normal individuals, being particularly influenced by the age and emotional state of the person, as well as whether tone is assessed at a proximal or distal joint.

All of the many factors that can affect normal muscle tone need to be taken into account before the clinician decides whether muscle tone is abnormal and this requires considerable skill. The assessment of muscle tone is an important and valuable part of the clinical examination and allows useful deductions to be made about the state of the nervous system.

Clinically, muscle tone may be abnormally increased (hypertonia) or decreased (hypotonia). In principle, hypertonia or hypotonia may arise either as a consequence of changes in the *passive* stiffness of the joint and its surrounding soft tissues or because of changes in the amount contributed by *active* stretch reflex contractions. Most clinical and neurophysiological research has hitherto concentrated on the latter mechanism, but there is increasing awareness of the potential importance of changes in passive joint stiffness.

HYPERTONIA

Two main types of hypertonia are recognised: spasticity and rigidity. These differ in their cause and clinical significance. Two rare types of hypertonia, gegenhalten and alpha-rigidity, are also discussed briefly.

Spasticity

Spasticity may be defined as a velocity-dependent increase in resistance to passive stretch of a muscle, with exaggerated tendon reflexes (Lance, 1990; Parziale et al., 1993).

Clinical Features

Spasticity is recognised clinically by: (1) the characteristic pattern of involvement of certain muscle groups; (2) the increased responsiveness of muscles to stretch; and (3) markedly increased tendon reflexes. Spasticity predominantly affects the antigravity muscles, i.e. the flexors of the arms and the extensors of the legs. As a result, the arms tend to assume a flexed and pronated posture whilst the legs are usually held extended and adducted, but this is not always the case. This posture is commonly seen (on the affected side) in hemiplegic patients following a stroke and should be instantly recognisable to all clinicians (see Chapter 7).

Stretching the muscle of a patient with spasticity results in an abnormally large reflex contraction. This increased responsiveness of muscle to stretch is the result of an increase in the stretch reflex gain (Thilmann et al., 1991) and a reduction in its threshold (Dietz, 1992), and is dependent on the stretch velocity. The more rapidly the examiner moves the limb of a patient with spasticity, the greater the increase in muscle tone. Indeed, the resistance to movement may become so great as to stop all movement, the abrupt cessation of movement being described clinically as a 'catch'. If passive flexion of the arm or extension of the leg continues, the resistance to movement may then disappear rapidly. The 'catch' followed by the sudden melting away of resistance is referred to clinically as the 'clasp-knife phenomenon'.

The pathologically brisk tendon reflexes are further evidence of the increased responsiveness of muscle to stretch. The pathophysiological mechanisms involved in the response to brief phasic stretches almost certainly differ from those involved in the response to slower stretches discussed in the paragraph above. Not only are tendon reflexes pathologically brisk, but there is a tendency for them to spread or 'irradiate' to other muscles or muscle groups (Adams & Victor, 1989). Thus, a tap on the Achilles tendon not only evokes a pathologically brisk ankle jerk but may also produce reflex contractions in the proximal muscles such as the hamstrings, quadriceps and hip adductor muscles.

In certain situations, sustained rhythmic contractions can be generated when a muscle is stretched rapidly and the tension maintained. The rhythmic contractions, which are usually at a frequency of 5–7 Hz, are termed 'clonus'. Clonus is most commonly seen at the ankle when the foot is dorsiflexed (ankle clonus). It can also be seen at the knee (patellar clonus) and occasionally at other sites in the body.

Clinical Significance

Spasticity is one of the cardinal features of an upper motor neurone syndrome. The presence of spasticity should therefore always lead to a search for lesions of the 'upper motor neurone' anywhere from the motor cortex to the spinal motoneurones. Common causes of spasticity include cerebrovascular disease (Chapter 7), brain damage (Chapters 8 & 19), spinal cord compression (Chapters 9 & 20), and inflammatory lesions of the spinal cord such as those found in multiple sclerosis (Chapter 11).

Pathophysiological Mechanisms of Spasticity

The pathological basis of spasticity is the abnormal enhancement of spinal stretch reflexes. What causes the enhancement of spinal stretch reflexes is less certain. In principle, they could be enhanced by increased muscle spindle sensitivity (mediated via increased γ-motoneurone drive) or by increased excitability of central synapses involved in the reflex arc.

Microneurographic studies in humans and neurophysiological studies in experimental animals have found no abnormality in the sensitivity of the muscle spindle in established spasticity (Burke, 1983; Pierrot-Deseilligny & Mazieres, 1985). Muscle spindle sensitivity may be increased in the early stages of an upper motor neurone lesion, but then return to normal. Increased excitability of central synapses involved in the reflex arc therefore appears to be the main factor determining the enhancement of spinal stretch reflexes.

How does an upper motor neurone lesion alter the excitability of central synapses involved in the stretch reflex arc? In the short term, it seems that previously inactive (or silent) spinal synapses can become active following the disruption of descending motor inputs, thereby increasing the efficiency of the reflex arc (Pierrot-Deseilligny & Mazieres, 1985). In the longer term, the synapses of descending motor pathways on spinal motoneurones and interneurones degenerate and are replaced by sprouting of the remaining intraspinal synapses, again increasing the efficiency of the reflex arc (Tsukahara & Murakami, 1983; Noth, 1991).

Reading the preceding paragraphs might lead one to believe that spasticity was simply a release phenomenon, caused by the removal of inhibitory descending influences on the spinal cord. Such an impression, however, would be wrong. The true situation is almost certainly more complicated. Removal of inhibitory descending influences is undoubtedly important but spasticity also occurs in the presence of facilitatory descending influences.

There are many descending pathways that arise in the brainstem and influence spinal cord excitability (see Chapter 1). For simplicity, these descending pathways can be divided into two main groups on the basis of their anatomy and physiology. One group, comprising the pontine and lateral bulbar reticulospinal pathways, along with the vestibulospinal pathways (although the functional contribution of the latter is probably limited in man), descends in the ventral funiculus of the spinal cord and tends to facilitate muscle tone. The other group, comprising mainly the crossed reticulospinal pathways from the ventromedial bulbar reticular formation, descends in the lateral funiculus (just behind the corticospinal tracts) and tends to inhibit muscle tone. Evidence from man and experi-mental animals suggests that normal muscle tone depends on a balance between the facilitatory and inhibitory systems (Brown, 1994). Spasticity may arise if the inhibitory pathways are interrupted or if there is increased activity in the facilitatory pathways. Spasticity following lesions of the frontal cerebral cortex or internal capsule probably results from loss of cortical drive to the bulbar inhibitory centre (thereby reducing activity in the inhibitory crossed reticulospinal pathways and releasing the spinal stretch reflex).

The above discussion has concentrated on the neural and stretch reflex changes that accompany spasticity. Such changes are certainly of prime importance. However, there is increasing awareness that established spasticity is also associated with significant changes in *passive mechanical factors* (Davidoff, 1992; Lin *et al.*, 1994; Given *et al.*, 1995; O'Dwyer *et al.*, 1996). With weakness and disuse, muscles undergo shortening with a reduction in the number of sarcomeres and an increase in collagen content (Williams *et al.*, 1988). They also tend to have a decreasing proportion of type II muscle fibres (Dattola *et al.*, 1993). All of these changes lead to an increase in the passive stiffness of the joint.

The changes in the passive mechanical factors associated with spasticity are of practical importance. All clinicians know of the difficulty of dealing with established contractures in patients with spasticity. It has been proposed that such contractures are the result of a 'vicious circle'. The increased gain of the stretch reflex loop causes the muscle to shorten. The shortened muscle then undergoes remodelling, losing some of its sarcomeres. Unless there is some intervention to stretch or lengthen the muscle, this process will continue, leading to contracture (see Chapter 25). If this model is correct, then the most appropriate treatment would be regular stretching of affected muscles (e.g. stretching exercises). Such treatment might be assisted with the judicious use of muscle relaxants or botulinum toxin injections. In contrast, tendon lengthening operations would not appear to be ideal, since the (released) muscle would continue to lose its sarcomeres and therefore shorten further. However, tendon lenthening operations do allow the joint to assume a more natural position, thereby often increasing limb function and allowing the antagonist muscles to work at less mechanical disadvantage.

The clinical and pathophysiological features of spasticity are summarised and contrasted with those of rigidity in Table 5.1.

Pharmacological Treatment

Details of the drugs mentioned in this section are given in Chapter 28. The mainstay of treatment for spasticity is baclofen. Baclofen is believed to act on inhibitory GABA-B receptors within the spinal cord, reducing the gain of the stretch reflex loop. Like all drugs that are used in the treatment of spasticity, baclofen may uncover or exacerbate muscle weakness. Patients often rely on their spasticity for support and when it is reduced they find that their limbs are floppy and weak. Baclofen also causes drowsiness and tiredness, which can be lessened if the drug is given intrathecally by pump.

Benzodiazepines (e.g. diazepam, clonazepam) are also used in the treatment of spasticity, but are generally less favoured than baclofen because of their potential to produce addiction. They are believed to act on inhibitory GABA-A receptors within the spinal cord.

Dantrolene acts directly on muscle to produce weakness by inhibiting excitation–contraction coupling. It is rarely used on its own but may be used in conjunction with baclofen or benzodiazepines. Hepatotoxicity can be a problem with dantrolene.

Table 5.1 Comparison of spasticity and rigidity.

Comparison of spasticity and rigidity		
	Spasticity	**Rigidity**
Pattern of muscle involvement	Upper limb flexors; lower limb extensors	Flexors and extensors equally
Nature of tone	Velocity-dependent increase in tone; 'clasp-knife'	Constant throughout movement; 'lead pipe'
Tendon reflexes	Increased	Normal
Pathophysiology	Increased spinal stretch reflex gain	Increased long-latency component of stretch reflex
Clinical significance	Upper motor neurone (pyramidal) sign	Extrapyramidal sign

Botulinum toxin injections have been used to weaken muscles selectively. The results in adult patients with spasticity are mixed, but more favourable results have been obtained in children with spastic cerebral palsy (Cosgrove *et al.*, 1994). Experimental work in mice suggests that botulinum toxin injections may reduce the risk of developing contractures (Cosgrove & Graham, 1994).

Intrathecal phenol blocks are occasionally used in patients with severe lower limb spasticity to help control pain or improve posture (Beckerman *et al.*, 1996). The risks of non-specific damage to other neural structures is high, and such treatment is therefore usually restricted to patients who have no useful lower limb function or sphincter control.

Rigidity

Another abnormality associated with increased force is rigidity, which can occur in different forms. It should be noted that the terms decerebrate rigidity and decorticate rigidity describe abnormal posturing associated with coma rather than a specific type of hypertonia. The more correct terms would therefore be decerebrate and decorticate posturing. Decerebrate posturing occurs with a variety of acute and subacute brainstem disorders and consists of opisthotonus, clenched jaws and stiffly extended limbs. The abnormal postures are characteristically triggered by passive movements of the limbs or neck or by any noxious stimulus. Decorticate posturing occurs with high brainstem or midbrain lesions and consists of flexion of the upper limb and extension of the legs similar to that of a spastic tetraplegia.

Clinical Features

Rigidity is recognised clinically as an increased resistance to relatively slowly imposed passive movements. It is present in both extensor and flexor muscle groups. Typically the examiner will flex and extend the wrist slowly and may describe the resistance as being of 'lead pipe' type, reflecting the fact that the resistance is felt throughout the movement (in distinction to spasticity where the resistance initially increases rapidly and then melts away— the so-called clasp-knife phenomenon). It should be emphasised that the imposed movements must be slow: use of more rapid movements, that would be appropriate for examining spasticity, may result in the erroneous conclusion that the tone is normal. Tendon reflexes are normal, in contrast to the hyperreflexia associated with spasticity.

Many patients with rigidity have an additional tremor as part of their extrapyramidal disorder. When this is so, the tremor will be felt superimposed on the rigidity, giving rise to the clinical phenomenon of 'cogwheel rigidity'.

Rigidity may be appreciated in the limbs or axially. One of the best ways of demonstrating axial tone is to rotate the patient's shoulders while he or she stands relaxed. In normal individuals, the examiner will encounter little resistance and the arms will be seen to swing relatively freely. However, in patients with axial rigidity, the examiner has the feeling of trying to move a rigid structure and the arms fail to swing.

Clinical Significance

Rigidity is one of the cardinal features of an extrapyramidal syndrome. The term parkinsonism is synonymous with extrapyramidal syndrome; other synonyms used include parkinsonian syndrome and akinetic–rigid syndrome. Parkinson's disease (see Chapter 12) is a specific disease entity and is but one cause of parkinsonism. The other cardinal feature is hypokinesia/bradykinesia (reduced and slow movements, see below.) Tremor is a frequent finding in parkinsonism, but is not always present. Extrapyramidal syndromes are caused by functional disturbances of the basal ganglia (caudate nucleus, putamen, globus pallidus and subthalamic nucleus).

Common causes of parkinsonism include Parkinson's disease itself, multiple system atrophy, and a number of rarer conditions that are sometimes called 'Parkinson-plus syndromes' (e.g. progressive supranuclear palsy, cortico-basal degeneration). Extrapyramidal syndromes are a not uncommon side effect of drugs, especially the neuroleptic drugs and the so-called vestibular sedatives (e.g. metoclopramide, prochlorperazine, cinnarizine).

Cerebrovascular disease rarely gives rise to true parkinsonism. However, cerebrovascular disease affecting the frontal lobes may give rise to a superficially similar clinical syndrome, with gait dyspraxia (which can be mistaken for the shuffling gait of parkinsonism) and gegenhalten, mentioned below (which may be mistaken for rigidity). The condition can be distinguished from parkinsonism by the relative preservation of upper limb and facial movement, the lack of a significant response to levodopa, and the frequent occurrence of urinary incontinence.

Pathophysiological Mechanisms

The pathophysiological basis of rigidity appears to be enhancement of the long-latency component of the stretch reflex (Rothwell, 1994). The normal stretch reflex can be divided into a short-latency component and a long-latency component (see Chapter 1). In patients with parkinsonian rigidity, the short-latency (spinal) component is normal in size, reflecting the fact that tendon reflexes in the condition are normal. However, the long-latency component, which may take a transcortical route, is enlarged. Furthermore, the size of the long-latency component correlates with the clinical degree of rigidity: the greater the rigidity, the larger the size of the long-latency component.

Pharmacological Treatment

Treatment is usually focused on the underlying extrapyramidal syndrome rather than the rigidity *per se*. It is always important to check whether the patient is taking any neuroleptic medication that could be causing or exacerbating his or her condition.

Parkinson's disease itself is treated with levodopa (Chapter 12). Levodopa is generally given in conjunction with a peripheral dopa-decarboxylase inhibitor to prevent the drug's metabolism in the gut and to increase its availability to the brain. The initial response to levodopa is usually very gratifying. Unfortunately, longer-term treatment may be associated with a less satisfactory clinical response and the development of troublesome side effects, including involuntary movements and psychiatric disturbance. Other drugs used in the treatment of Parkinson's disease include dopamine agonists, anticholinergics and selegiline. The same drugs are also frequently used in the treatment of other (non-Parkinson's disease) extrapyramidal syndromes, but the clinical response is generally less impressive.

Gegenhalten
Some elderly patients find it difficult to 'relax' their limbs during examination. When attempting to examine tone, the patients appear to resist movement voluntarily but they are unable to prevent such movement and it is not therefore voluntary resistance. This phenomenon is usually termed gegenhalten (Adams & Victor, 1989).

Gegenhalten is usually caused by damage to the frontal lobes of the brain, and may be seen in association with cerebrovascular disease or neurodegenerative conditions such as Alzheimer's disease. Cognitive impairment, grasp reflexes and other primitive reflexes are frequent accompaniments.

Alpha-rigidity
In some patients, tone may be increased in a rigid fashion (being present equally in both flexor and extensor muscles), but their tendon reflexes are absent or reduced. It is as though there is increased motor unit excitability in the absence of the spinal reflex arc. Such a condition may be seen in association with spinal cord lesions, particularly those affecting the central grey matter.

HYPOTONIA
In the normal individual, active stretch reflex contractions contribute little to resting muscle tone. Most of the tone arises from the passive viscoelastic properties of the joints and soft tissues. Reduced tone due to central nervous system (CNS) disorders is therefore often difficult to detect clinically (because the viscoelastic properties remain unchanged). Hypotonia due to central lesions may be apparent in certain situations, however. Patients with cerebellar hypotonia characteristically have pendular tendon reflexes because of limb underdamping. Children with hypotonia due to CNS disorders are often described as floppy. Hypotonia is also seen in the acute stage of spinal cord disease or trauma (see Chapter 9). With recovery from this spinal shock, the tone increases and the reflexes return to produce the characteristic upper motor neurone syndrome.

Reduced muscle tone due to peripheral nervous system disorders is usually easier to detect. This is mainly because the associated muscle wasting reduces the passive stiffness of the joint. The absence of stretch reflex contractions in lower motor neurone lesions probably contributes little to the reduction in muscle tone. When hypotonia is unequivocally present, it is usually indicative of a lower motor neurone lesion. Other features of a lower motor neurone lesion include weakness, areflexia and fasciculation.

MOVEMENT DISORDERS

Clinically distinctive patterns of involuntary movements occur in many diseases. Recognising these patterns may help in identifying the underlying disorder. The aim of the remainder of the chapter is to give brief descriptions of the common movement disorders and their clinical significance. First, however, it may be helpful to define some general terms.

GENERAL TERMS FOR MOVEMENT DISORDERS
The terms discussed here describe the amount and speed of movement, as well as some involuntary movements.

Akinesia and Hypokinesia
Akinesia is the absence of movement and hypokinesia describes poverty of movement. Akinesia is often used inaccurately to describe hypokinesia. For example, hypokinesia is one of the cardinal features of extrapyramidal disease, to the extent that some neurologists refer to parkinsonism as an akinetic–rigid syndrome. It should be noted, however, that akinesia or hypokinesia are not used when there is paresis (either upper or lower motor neurone) to account for the lack of movement. Basal ganglia and frontal lobe dysfunction, particularly the supplementary motor area, are thought to underlie akinesia and hypokinesia.

Bradykinesia and Hypometria
Patients with parkinsonism not only show a lack of movement but the movement that they do have is slow. The slowness of movement is termed bradykinesia and is evident in slowness in initiating movement (the patient may take a longer than normal time to respond) and also by slowness in carrying out a task. When such a patient is called from the out-patient waiting room, he or she will often take a long time to rise from the chair and then walk slowly from the waiting room into the clinic room itself. Part of the problem with walking is that people with parkinsonism tend to take shorter steps than is normal. Indeed, the amplitudes of all their movements tend to be smaller than required for optimal performance; this is termed hypometria. In the upper limb, bradykinesia can most easily be demonstrated by asking the patient to open and close his or her fist as quickly as possible.

Dyskinesias and Hyperkinesia
Some neurological diseases are associated with additional (involuntary) movements. Such involuntary movements are best termed dyskinesias and include myoclonus, chorea, ballism, dystonia, tic and tremor (see Table 5.2). Some neurologists describe these conditions as hyperkinesias rather than dyskinesias in order to distinguish them from hypokinetic movement disorders (e.g. parkinsonism). However, confusion may then arise when a patient with (hypokinetic) Parkinson's disease develops (hyperkinetic) tremor or chorea. A further problem with the use of the term hyperkinesia is that it is sometimes assumed that

hyperkinetic movements are faster than normal. This is not the case (and hyperkinesia is not the converse of bradykinesia). Indeed, in most so-called hyperkinetic movement disorders, movement velocities are actually slower than normal. The term dyskinesia is therefore preferred to hyperkinesia.

TREMOR

Tremor is best defined as any unwanted, rhythmic, approximately sinusoidal movement of a limb or body part (Elble & Koller, 1990). The fact that the movement is unwanted distinguishes tremor from voluntary oscillatory movements such as waving or writing. Its rhythmic and approximately sinusoidal character distinguish it from myoclonus and chorea. The term myorhythmia is occasionally used to signify a slow tremor of relatively large amplitude that affects the proximal part of a limb.

Clinically, tremor is usually classified according to the situation in which it occurs (Bain, 1993). Examples of types of tremor and the conditions in which they occur are given in Table 5.2. A tremor that is present when the limb is relaxed and fully supported is called a rest tremor. Action tremors occur when the patient attempts to maintain a posture (postural tremor) or to move (kinetic tremor). Tremor which gets worse at the end of a movement is called an intention or terminal tremor and is associated with cerebellar dysfunction.

There is no satisfactory pathological classification of tremor. A rest tremor almost always suggests parkinsonism. Postural tremors have many causes but are most commonly due to enhanced physiological tremor or essential tremor. All of us have a fine postural tremor (physiological tremor) of which we are usually completely unaware. Physiological tremor may become noticeable however in certain situations (e.g. anxiety, fear, thyrotoxicosis, fatigue, use of adrenergic drugs). This noticeable tremor is called enhanced physiological tremor. Essential tremor is suggested by the finding of a symmetrical postural upper limb tremor that is absent at rest and is not made strikingly worse by movement (and in the absence of factors that might enhance physiological tremor). In a substantial proportion of patients with essential tremor, there is a family history of similarly affected relatives and up to half the patients may find temporary amelioration of their tremor with alcohol. For a discussion of other tremors the reader is referred to Elble & Koller (1990) and Bain (1993).

The pathophysiological mechanisms responsible for tremor are poorly understood. The nervous system, like all mechanical systems, has a natural tendency to oscillate. This tendency is due in part to the mechanical properties of the limbs and in part to neural feedback loops. Neuropathologial studies have demonstrated physical and biochemical changes in brains from patients with different disorders involving tremor but have failed to elucidate the precice changes that can be attributed to the symptom of tremor (Bain, 1993). Recent evidence suggests that cerebellar mechanisms are of central importance to the maintenance and generation of essential tremor (Britton, 1995).

MYOCLONUS

Myoclonus describes brief shock-like jerks of a limb or body part. Myoclonic jerks may be restricted to one part of the body ('focal myoclonus') or may be generalised ('generalised myoclonus'). Jerks can occur spontaneously or with movement, or they may be reflexly triggered by light, sound, touch or tendon taps. Following a myoclonic jerk there is a lapse of posture which is associated with electrical silence in the muscles, lasting for around 200 milliseconds (Shibasaki, 1995). Lapses in posture can sometimes occur without a noticeable preceding jerk. Such postural lapses are called asterixis and typically occur with metabolic encephalopathies (e.g. in respiratory, renal or liver failure).

There are three main types of myoclonus: cortical myoclonus, which arises from the cerebral cortex; reticular reflex myoclonus, which arises from the brainstem; and propriospinal myoclonus, which arises from the spinal cord. Neurophysiological studies are of special help in the assessment of patients with myoclonus (Shibasaki, 1995). Cortical myoclonus is preceded by an electrical 'spike' over the contralateral motor cortex (normal movements, even fast movements, are never preceded by an electrical 'spike'). The jerks are focal and can often be triggered by touching the affected limb (cortical reflex myoclonus). The condition responds to anticonvulsants and piracetam. Occasionally, there may be repetitive bursts of cortical myoclonus. Such repetitive bursts are in essence a focal epileptic discharge.

Neurophysiological studies in reticular reflex myoclonus show that the abnormal electrical activity arises from the brainstem. Such jerks are symmetrical and generalised. They may be triggered by a startle (e.g. unexpected noise or light) and the jerks themselves have a number of similarities to an exaggerated startle response.

Some patients with spinal cord disease have abnormal jerks which begin at one segmental level and then spread to neighbouring segments. Such patients have spinal myoclonus.

Myoclonus is a feature of many neurological diseases. Most patients are found to have a progressive, usually degenerative, encephalopathy. Post-anoxic myoclonus occurs, as its name suggests, after a respiratory arrest, especially in patients with chronic lung conditions. After recovery, such patients develop severe myoclonic jerking, especially in their legs, and they walk with a characteristic bouncy gait. There are often additional cerebellar signs and the condition is presumed to arise because of damage to the large (and hence oxygen-demanding) cerebellar Purkinje cells (see Chapters 1 & 2). The condition is treated with valproate and 5-hydroxytryptamine.

CHOREA

Patients with disease of the basal ganglia may develop frequent jerky movements that constantly flit from one part of the body to another. Such movements are termed chorea. The movements flit randomly around the body, in contrast to myoclonus which tends to affect the same part or parts of the body. The absence of sustained abnormal posturing distinguish the condition from dystonia.

Chorea occurs in a range of basal ganglia diseases including Wilson's disease, Huntington's disease (see Chapter 13), polycythaemia, thyrotoxicosis, systemic lupus erythematosus, cerebrovascular disease and several other rarer neurogenerative conditions. Sydenham's chorea is still occasionally seen following streptococcal infection in the UK. Pregnancy and the oral contraceptive pill are also associated with chorea. Chorea can be a side effect of chronic neuroleptic medication.

Table 5.2 Main causes of some dyskinetic movement disorders. (Abbreviation: MS; multiple sclerosis.)

Main causes of some dyskinetic movement disorders

Tremor

Rest tremor	Parkinson's disease Drug-induced parkinsonism Other extrapyramidal disease
Action tremor	Enhanced physiological tremor (e.g. anxiety, alcohol, hyperthyroidism) Essential tremor Cerebellar disease Wilson's disease
Intention tremor	Brainstem or cerebellar disease (e.g. MS, spinocerebellar degeneration)

Myoclonus

Without encephalopathy	Juvenile myoclonic epilepsy Myoclonic epilepsy
With encephalopathy	
non-progressive	Post-anoxic myoclonus
progressive	Storage disorders (e.g. Lafora body disease) Unverricht–Lundborg disease Metabolic encephalopathies (e.g. respiratory, renal and liver failure) Creutzfeldt–Jakob disease

Chorea

Sydenham's chorea
Pregnancy-associated chorea
Contraceptive pill-associated chorea
Huntington's disease
Thyrotoxicosis
Systemic lupus erythematosus
Drug-induced chorea (e.g. neuroleptics, phenytoin)

Dystonia

Generalised	Idiopathic torsion dystonia Drug-induced Athetoid cerebral palsy Wilson's disease Metabolic storage disorders Dopa-responsive dystonia
Hemidystonia	Basal ganglia lesions (e.g. tumours, vascular, post-thalamotomy)

Where possible, the underlying cause of chorea should be treated. Chorea itself may respond to tetrabenazine, a drug that depletes presynaptic dopamine stores. Neuroleptic medication is also used.

BALLISMUS
Violent, large-amplitude, involuntary movements of the limbs are called ballismus, or, if they affect only one side of the body, hemiballismus. These movements are often so large that they throw the patient off balance. They are continuous and may lead to exhaustion and even death. The usual cause of ballismus is cerebrovascular disease (Berardelli, 1995). It can be treated with tetrabenazine.

DYSTONIA
Dystonia (previously known as athetosis) describes a condition where limbs or body parts are twisted into abnormal postures by sustained muscle activity. Typically, dystonia is brought out by attempted movement. However, despite the contorted posturing, such patients are often able to accomplish remarkably skilled tasks.

Dystonia may be generalised, affecting the whole body, or localised, affecting a single body part or segment. Dystonia affecting just one side of the body is termed hemidystonia and is of clinical significance because its presence should lead to a search for a lesion in the contralateral basal ganglia.

Generalised dystonia is most commonly due to idiopathic torsion dystonia. The condition usually begins in childhood and affects the legs first. It is inherited in a dominanat fashion, and the gene has been linked to chromosome 9 in some families (Warner et al., 1993). Dystonia is also seen following actual or presumed cerebral insults at or around the time of birth; a diagnosis of dystonic (athetoid) cerebral palsy may be made in such circumstances. More rarely, generalised dystonia may be a manifestation of a recognised metabolic disease or storage disorder. There is a rare type of familial dystonia called dopa-responsive dystonia with diurnal fluctuations. This condition responds exquisitely to levodopa. Dopa-responsive dystonia has recently been shown to result from an abnormality in the synthesis of tetrahydrobiopterin (Nygaard, 1995).

Focal dystonias usually begin in adult life and commonly affect the eyes (blepharospasm), neck (torticollis) or upper limb. The legs are rarely affected. Upper limb dystonia may be task-specific and may be the cause of some occupational cramps.

Electrophysiological recordings in dystonia show abnormal patterns of muscle activation with co-contraction of agonist and antagonist muscles (Rothwell, 1994). These abnormalities seem to be due to reduced 'reciprocal inhibition'. When a muscle is activated voluntarily, its antagonist muscles normally relax. The relaxation of antagonist muscles depends in part upon reciprocal inhibition: afferent impulses from the activated muscle inhibits the firing of motoneurones subserving antagonists. In patients with dystonia, reciprocal inhibition is reduced and co-cotraction occurs.

Various treatments have been used in dystonia, including drugs (especially anticholinergics, neuroleptics, tetrabenazine), botulinum toxin injections, and surgery (section of nerves and roots). Botulinum toxin is the treatment of choice for blepharospasm (a focal dystonia of facial muscles causing involuntary eye closure) and is often very beneficial in torticollis.

ATAXIA
Ataxia describes a disturbance in the co-ordination of movement. Movements are clumsy and the gait is unsteady with a wide base and reeling quality. Posture may also be affected, such that there are irregular jerky movements of the trunk when sitting (truncal ataxia or disequilibrium). In addition, there may be a limb tremor which generally gets worse towards the end of a goal-directed movement—so-called intention tremor. The latter can be brought out by asking the patient alternately to touch the examiner's finger and then his or her own nose: the task is one of accuracy and not speed and can be made more difficult by ensuring that the patient touches the examiner's finger as gently as possible.

Although it is relatively easy for an experienced clinician to recognise ataxia, it is much harder to analyse exactly what about the ataxic patient's movements is abnormal. Several features seem to contribute but none is pathognomonic. Patients tend to make hypermetric movements, i.e. their limbs move further than the desired target. They also tend to use too much force. The mechanisms that normally bring a movement to a smooth halt are abnormal and tremor commonly results. The movements of ataxic patients are also slower than normal.

The significance of ataxia is that it is almost invariably associated with disease of the cerebellum or its brainstem connections (Adams & Victor, 1989). Common causes of ataxia include multiple sclerosis (see Chapter 11), Friedreich's ataxia, alcohol, and posterior fossa tumours. Less common causes include paraneoplastic syndromes and a variety of neurodegenerative conditions, some of which are hereditary (e.g. the spinocerebellar ataxias and Friedreich's ataxia).

OTHER DISORDERS OF MOVEMENT
The following are abnormal movements that are associated with different neurological disorders.

Hemifacial Spasm
Hemifacial spasm describes unilateral twitching of facial muscles due to an irritative lesion of the facial nerve. The eye winks and the corner of the mouth on the affected side elevates. There may be mild facial weakness. It responds well to botulinum toxin injections. Some patients have neurosurgery to reposition blood vessels that impinge on the facial nerve.

Orofacial Dyskinesias
Orofacial dyskinesias are commonly seen in the elderly as a complication of neuroleptic treatment. They consist of involuntary lip-smacking and chewing movements,

occasionally associated with tongue protrusion. Neuroleptic medication should be avoided. Tetrabenazine may provide some benefit.

Palatal Myoclonus (Tremor)

Some patients develop involuntary rhythmical elevation of the soft palate, which produces an audible click and interferes with speech. Some cases are associated with hypertrophy of the inferior olivary nucleus in the brainstem.

Tics

Tics are involuntary movements or vocalisations that patients may be able to suppress temporarily at the expense of increasing inner tension. The movements can be simple, e.g. a twitch of the face or arm, or more complex, when they may appear semi-purposeful. Tics are associated with obsessive–compulsive disorders and the Gilles de la Tourette syndrome. Neuroleptic medication may be required.

REFERENCES

Adams RD, Victor M. *Principles of neurology*. New York: McGraw-Hill; 1989.

Bain P. A combined clinical and neurophysiological approach to the study of patients with tremor. *J Neurol Neurosurg Psychiat* 1993, **56**:839-844.

Beckerman H, Lankhorst GJ, Verbeek ALM, *et al*. The effects of phenol nerve and muscle blocks in treating spasticity: review of the literature. *Crit Rev Rehab* 1996, **8**:111-124.

Berardelli A. Symptomatic or secondary basal ganglia diseases and tardive dyskinesias. *Curr Opin Neurol* 1995, **8**:320-322.

Britton TC. Essential tremor and its variants. *Curr Opin Neurol* 1995, 8:314-319.

Brown P. Spasticity. *J Neurol Neurosurg Psychiat* 1994, **57**:773-777.

Burke D. Critical examination of the case for and against fusimotor involvement in disorders of muscle tone. *Adv Neurol* 1983, **39**:133-150.

Cosgrove AP, Corry IS, Graham HK. Botulinum toxin in the management of the lower limb in cerebral palsy. *Dev Med Child Neurol* 1994, **36**:386-396.

Cosgrove AP, Graham HK. Botulinum toxin A prevents the development of contractures in the hereditary spastic mouse. *Dev Med Child Neurol* 1994, **36**:379-385.

Dattola R, Girlanda P, Vita G, *et al*. Muscle rearrangement in patients with hemiparesis after stroke: an electrophysiological and morphological study. *Eur Neurol* 1993, **33**:109-114.

Davidoff RA. Skeletal muscle tone and the misunderstood stretch reflex. *Neurology* 1992, **42**:951-963.

Dietz V. Human neuroneal control of automatic functional movements: interaction between central programs and afferent input. *Physiol Rev* 1992, **72**:33-69.

Elble RJ, Koller WC. *Tremor*. Baltimore: Johns Hopkins University Press; 1990.

Given JD, Dewald JP, Rymer WZ. Joint dependent passive stiffness in paretic and contralateral limbs of spastic patients with hemiparetic stroke. *J Neurol Neurosurg Psychiat* 1995, **59**:271-279.

Lance JW. What is spasticity? *Lancet* 1990, **335**:606.

Lin JP, Brown JK, Brotherstone R. Assessment of spasticity in hemiplegic cerebral palsy. II: Distal lower-limb reflex excitability and function. *Dev Med Child Neurol* 1994, **36**:290-303.

Noth J. Trends in the pathophysiology and pharmacology of spasticity. *J Neurol* 1991, **238**:131-139.

Nygaard TG. Dopa-responsive dystonia. *Curr Opin Neurol* 1995, **8**:310-313.

O'Dwyer NJ, Ada L, Neilson PD. Spasticity and muscle contracture following stroke. *Brain* 1996, **119**:1737-1749.

Parziale JR, Akelman E, Herz DA. Spasticity: pathophysiology and management. *Orthopaedics* 1993, **16**:801-811.

Pierrot-Deseilligny E, Mazieres L. Spinal mechanisms underlying spasticity. In : Delwaide PJ, Young RR, eds. *Clinical neurophysiology in spasticity*. Amsterdam: Elsevier; 1985.

Rothwell JC. *Control of human voluntary movement, 2nd edition*. London: Chapman & Hall; 1994.

Shibasaki H. Myoclonus. *Curr Opin Neurol* 1995, **8**:331-334.

Thilmann AF, Fellows SJ, Garms E. The mechanism of spastic muscle hypertonus. Variation in reflex gain over the time course of spasticity. *Brain* 1991, **114**:233-244.

Tsukahara N, Murakami F. Axonal sprouting and recovery of function after brain damage. *Adv Neurol* 1983, **39**:1073-1084.

Warner TT, Fletcher NA, Davis MB, *et al*. Linkage analysis in British and French families with idiopathic torsion dystonia. *Brain* 1993, **116**:739-744.

Weiner WJ, Lang AE. *Movement disorders: A comprehensive survey*. New York: Futura; 1989.

Williams PE, Catanese T, Lucey EG, Goldspink G. The importance of stretch and contractile activity in the prevention of connective tissue accumulation in muscle. *J Anat* 1988, **158**:109-114.

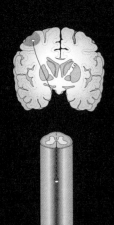

6

M Lowrie

PLASTICITY

CHAPTER OUTLINE

- **Plasticity in development**
- **Plasticity in the adult**

- **Plasticity in injury and disease**

INTRODUCTION

To say that a process is plastic implies that it can adapt readily to changes in external circumstances. In this sense plasticity is the basis of all neural control. Within the normal range of function, the control of movement depends upon the nervous system's responding continuously to the information it receives about the state of the body and the outside world (see Chapter 2). The resulting adjustment to motor patterns combines specificity with speed and requires a degree of flexibility in the functioning of neural and muscle tissue. Sometimes this plasticity is stretched so that neuromuscular function can adapt to external circumstances which fall outside the normal range. These more extreme plastic changes may be physiological or structural but usually require time to form. Two examples are: regular marathon running increases oxidative metabolism in largely anaerobic muscles; and when a peripheral nerve is injured, axons sprout from the cut end and grow towards the muscle.

The concept of plasticity is central to the work of physiotherapists. Many of the problems encountered in practice are the result of too little or too much plasticity. For example, motor axons injured within the spinal cord will not regenerate, causing permanent motor impairment, whilst injured axons in a peripheral nerve will grow easily but indiscriminately, limiting the usefulness of reinnervated muscles. Many of the procedures used in physiotherapy exploit the plasticity inherent in brain and muscles to maximise rehabilitation.

PLASTICITY IN DEVELOPMENT

It is generally believed that developing cells have a higher capacity for adaptability than mature ones. This is necessary to facilitate interaction between different types of cells, and in the neuromuscular system it is particularly important for matching the function of the different components and for promoting specificity of motor control. This has both positive and negative consequences. Greater plasticity may allow children to recover from some disorders which leave adults with permanent disability. Alternatively, some extreme plastic responses may exacerbate a developmental abnormality.

THE MOTOR UNIT

The lower motoneurones and muscle fibres are derived from very different tissues, but the fine control of movement depends upon these two components of the motor unit being precisely matched in size and function. Soon after the motoneurones in the spinal cord and brainstem have contacted the developing muscle cells, they undergo a period of programmed cell death (see Chapter 18) which reduces the number of motoneurones by about 50%. This somewhat aggressive reduction is believed to be necessary to match the number of motoneurones to the muscle, and it is partly regulated by a retrograde signal from the muscle. Motoneurones appear to compete for this signal: increasing the amount of muscle available leads to increased survival of motoneurones, whilst reduction increases motoneurone death (Oppenheim, 1991). Spinal muscular atrophy, a disease involving degeneration of motoneurones during infancy (see Chapter 21), may be partly caused by defective development of the muscle at this critical time, which in turn may extend or reactivate programmed motoneurone death (Braun *et al.*, 1995).

Motor units vary in their size and contractile characteristics but within a motor unit the muscle fibres are highly homogeneous. Their properties are induced largely by the pattern of activity imposed on them by the motoneurone. This was shown initially by cross-innervation between fast and slow muscles in animals: a slow muscle was transformed into a fast one by a 'fast' nerve, and a fast muscle was transformed into a slow muscle by a 'slow' nerve (Buller *et al.*, 1960). Subsequently it was shown that the effects of cross-innervation could be mimicked by electrical stimulation (Salmons & Vrbová, 1969) and that many other aspects of muscle metabolism could be transformed by altering the pattern of electrical activity reaching it (Pette & Vrbová, 1992).

Activity also plays an important part in deciding the final size of the motor unit and its specific innervation. Initially each muscle fibre is innervated by several motoneurones and each motoneurone innervates many muscle fibres; there is, thus, much overlap in force production between units. During later development all but one of the axon terminals withdraw so that individual motor units become separate and the number of muscle fibres in each is reduced. Stimulation of a muscle during this period accelerates the process of synapse elimination while inactivation delays or even stops this process (Vrbová *et al.*, 1995). The decision of which axon terminal remains at an endplate also probably depends upon the differential activity of the competing motoneurones, and the mechanism of withdrawal of the losers involves interaction with the muscle (Vrbová & Lowrie, 1989).

THE CENTRAL NERVOUS SYSTEM (CNS)

Motoneurones receive information from many sources. Sensory information projects from surface, joint and muscle receptors of the body (see Chapter 1). Other inputs consist of various descending pathways from the brain. These inputs synapse either directly with the motoneurone or indirectly through interneurones. There is evidence that initially both sensory and descending inputs innervate their target with a degree of non-specificity but that later inappropriate projections are removed (Stanfield, 1992; Seebach & Ziskind-Conhaim, 1994).

The mechanism that controls the pruning of synapses at the motoneurone may be similar to that which operates at the neuromuscular junction and, by analogy with other neural systems, probably depends upon differential activity. Thus a general principle which operates during the development of the motor system is one of initial overgrowth followed by selective reduction, either by cell death or by terminal withdrawal. This form of plasticity ensures specificity of connection and matches the properties of the individual parts of the motor system. Figure 6.1 indicates some of the sites in the motor system at which plasticity plays a role in normal growth and function.

PLASTICITY IN THE ADULT

In the adult, plasticity occurs in response to muscle use and also plays a role in central nervous system (CNS) function in relation to learning and memory.

ADAPTATION OF MUSCLE TO USE

Activity continues to influence muscle differentiation and size into adulthood and can be exploited in a number of ways. Its use in normal life varies from maintaining muscle tone with moderate exercise, to marked changes in muscle use for sport. Endurance training increases the oxidative metabolism of muscles and tends to convert fast-contracting motor units into slow ones. In body-building, individual muscles are enlarged and strengthened by selective patterns of intensive training. Percutaneous electrical stimulation can assist these programmes. Reduction in usage can lead to muscle wasting and many physiotherapy practices are directed towards counteracting this. Exercise programmes can hasten recovery of muscle function after periods of immobilisation or disuse, and in cases of paralysis or paresis electrical stimulation is useful in supplementing passive exercise (Rose *et al.*, 1989).

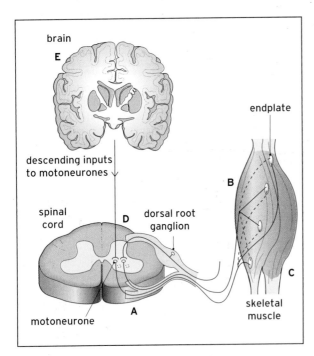

Figure 6.1 Plasticity in normal motor development and function. A: motoneurone survival and maturation during development depends on interaction with the muscle. **B**: motor unit size is determined by retraction of axon terminals. **C**: muscle differentiation is largely determined by motoneurone activity. **D**: inputs to motoneurones are reorganised during development. **E**: synaptic plasticity in motor areas of the brain underlies the learning of motor skills.

LEARNING MOTOR SKILLS

Plasticity of the nervous system is clearly necessary for learning and memory, and much research effort has been directed at finding the sites and processes in the brain which underlie it. The main focus of research has been the hippocampus, a phylogenetically old part of the cerebral cortex which produces a striking amnesia when damaged. This deficit is limited to conscious recollection of factual information and events, however; patients retain the ability to learn new motor and cognitive skills which are remembered unconsciously. Evidence is now accumulating that other parts of the brain, particularly those concerned with motor function, mediate the learning and memory of motor skills. Most of this evidence comes from studying the effects of lesions in man and animals upon the acquisition of motor tasks, and its validity depends upon distinguishing learning from performance deficits. Nevertheless it now seems clear that the cerebellum and basal ganglia play important roles in the timing and sequencing of the component parts of a learned motor programme (Salmon & Butters, 1995). The motor cortex is also implicated as a site of motor learning. Non-invasive techniques have shown localised increases in activity during the learning of motor tasks (Pascual-Leone et al., 1994; Karni et al., 1995).

The cellular process that underlies the learning of motor skills is not known. By analogy with work on conscious memory, it may involve the activity-dependent facilitation of synapses. Long-term potentiation of synaptic transmission is known to occur in the hippocampus and some other brain structures following repeated stimulation (Bliss & Collingridge, 1993). The molecular mechanism subserving long-term potentiation is controversial, but it is known to be mediated by calcium and probably involves changes in both postsynaptic glutamate receptors and presynaptic transmitter release. Recent evidence suggests that structural changes in dendritic spines may also be involved (Hosokawa et al., 1995). In the cerebellum, another form of synaptic plasticity, long-term depression, has been identified and proposed as the substrate for motor learning (Ito, 1993). It has been correlated with learning motor tasks in some studies, but its exact role is controversial (De Schutter, 1995).

In addition to brain structures, the spinal cord may also mediate plastic changes relevant to acquisition of motor skills. The spinal stretch reflex alters in response to reward-driven motor training and is retained independently of supraspinal influences (Wolpaw, 1994). It may be that all structures in the CNS concerned with motor function undergo plastic changes during the learning of motor skills.

PLASTICITY IN INJURY AND DISEASE

From a practical viewpoint, the response of the nervous system to injury can be considered in two ways: there is the response to interruption of axonal tracts, which requires long-distance growth; and there is synaptic plasticity, which operates locally. Often both types of plasticity are necessary for full recovery and the mechanisms responsible for them may be shared. Figure 6.2 indicates the range of plastic responses to injury or disease.

REGENERATION

Most mature neurones that survive injury to their axons respond by attempting to regenerate a new axon. In this sense neurones possess a considerable capability for repair. The vigour with which the outgrowth occurs and the success of reinnervation varies greatly; however, the sharpest distinction being between the peripheral nervous system and the CNS. Neurones that normally project their axons in peripheral nerves are generally successful in regenerating them after injury, if the appropriate non-neuroneal cells, adhesion molecules and growth factors are available (Madison et al., 1991). Axonal sprouts are capable of growing long distances along empty nerve sheaths and will even grow through artificial conduits to reach their synaptic targets. In contrast, axonal injury in the CNS does not lead to regeneration and the consequence of a lesion in a major motor tract, e.g. after a stroke or spinal injury, is permanent motor impairment. The CNS does, however, undergo synaptic plasticity and hence some recovery of motor function is possible (see below).

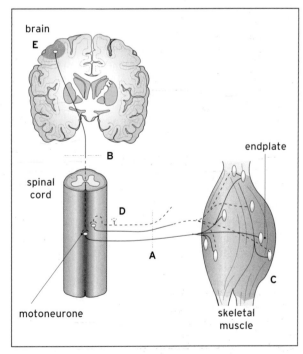

Figure 6.2 Plasticity of the motor system in injury and disease. A: regeneration of injured peripheral nerve. **B**: no regeneration of injured central tract. **C**: sprouting of intact axons in partially denervated muscle. **D**: central synaptic reorganisation after peripheral injury. **E**: synaptic plasticity after a central lesion.

The apparently poor response of central neurones to injury is not due to an inability to grow their axons. This was most dramatically demonstrated by the experiments of Aguayo (Muller & Aguayo, 1992) who used a peripheral nerve graft to bridge across a spinal lesion. Descending axons grew several centimetres through the nerve bridge into the spinal cord beyond the lesion. The current prevailing view as to why CNS neurones do not normally utilise their regenerative capability focuses on the fact that the environment within the CNS is inhibitory as a result of the activities of the neuroglial cells there. Improving CNS regeneration will probably depend upon defining the nature of this inhibitory environment and devising ways to counteract it (Bähr & Bonhoeffer, 1994).

Whether in the CNS or the peripheral nervous system, regeneration of injured axons is only half the battle for recovery. Reinnervation of muscle must be specific if it is to be useful. The general view, derived from clinical studies of peripheral nerve injury and from early animal experiments, is that the mechanisms which guide innervation of appropriate targets during embryonic development do not operate during reinnervation. This means that after section of a large mixed nerve, some sensory axons will innervate muscles and some motor axons will innervate cutaneous receptors. Moreover individual muscles may be reinnervated by motoneurones from other motor pools and will therefore be activated inappropriately. Microsurgical techniques can be applied at the site of nerve injury to optimise specific reinnervation but, even so, recovery of function is often limited (see Chapter 10). In this situation plasticity appears to be a mixed blessing.

More recent studies on reinnervation in animals suggest that although reinnervation may be non-specific initially, the precision of motor reinnervation may improve with time. There is a selective withdrawal of misdirected collateral axonal branches over many weeks. Little is known about the mechanisms involved but presumably it is mediated by differential signals emanating from the appropriate and inappropriate targets (Brushart, 1993; Hennig & Dietrichs, 1994).

SYNAPTIC PLASTICITY

Plasticity in the form of altered synaptic function or growth of novel synapses can be observed at all levels of the neuromuscular system in response to injury or disease. When muscle is partially denervated, either by nerve injury or loss of motoneurones as in motor neurone disease, extensive sprouting occurs from remaining axon terminals to reinnervate the denervated muscle fibres. The motor unit is thought to be able to expand to five times its original size, so considerable deficiencies in innervation can be compensated for. This explains why in motor neurone disease muscle weakness does not become apparent until 50% of motoneurones have already degenerated (see Chapter 14). Sprouting also occurs in the early stages of muscular dystrophy where degenerating muscle fibres are replaced by newly developing ones (see Chapter 16). The trigger for motor neurone sprouting in muscle is not known but probably involves a local signal from inactivated muscle fibres (Brown et al., 1991).

Nerve injury can induce synaptic reorganisation centrally as well as peripherally. In the spinal cord, disruption of dorsal root afferents by peripheral nerve injury can alter dorsal horn connectivity. This may underlie some forms of chronic pain (Woolf et al., 1992). Injury of both sensory and motor axons may cause remodelling of the dendritic tree of motoneurones, leading to their altered activation (O'Hanlon & Lowrie, 1994).

In the brain, plastic changes occur in response to both local and peripheral injuries. It was assumed that such adaptation was possible only when the injury occurred early in development. Transcranial magnetic stimulation of children with cerebral palsy showed evidence that corticospinal axons from undamaged parts of the cortex make connections with inappropriate motoneurones (Brouwer & Ashby, 1991; Farmer et al., 1991). Such connections may be considered counterproductive when they are responsible for coactivation of agonist and antagonist muscles or when they produce mirror movements of the limbs. Substantial plasticity has also been found in corticospinal connections to the muscles proximal to congenital amputations (Hall et al., 1990).

More recent work suggests that substantial reorganisations also occur after injury in the brains of adults (Kaas, 1991; Steward et al., 1992). Most of the evidence is derived from experiments in animals that show that sensory and motor maps in the cerebral cortex change after injury (see Chapter 2). More recently, positron emission tomography of adult patients who have suffered striatocapsular stroke has demonstrated bilateral activation of motor pathways and the recruitment of additional sensorimotor cortical areas associated with recovery of motor function (Weiller et al., 1992).

Several processes probably contribute to cortical plasticity following injury. Some changes occur within hours and are mediated by dynamic changes in synaptic activation (Kaas, 1991), but extensive work on the hippocampus indicates that sprouting of axon terminals can occur in the longer term. Furthermore, in an interesting study of experimentally induced neocortical ischaemia in rats, behavioural recovery was correlated with the sequential enhancement of axonal growth and synapse formation in the adjacent healthy cortex (Stroemer et al., 1995). Whether such processes are triggered by the degeneration invoked by injury or by a change in the activity of the system is not clear. In a recent experiment on intact adult primates, simultaneous tactile stimulation of several fingers of one hand caused cortical neurones, which are normally activated only by touch of a single finger, to respond in a more generalised manner (Wang et al., 1995). After injury it may be possible to direct or reinforce such synaptic plasticity by appropriate manipulation of the system from the periphery in order to aid recovery of motor skills or cognitive function.

SUMMARY

It has long been known that substantial plasticity occurs in development of the nervous system. With improved research methods it is now becoming clear that significant plasticity persists into adulthood. Of particular significance for motor function is the apparent ease with which cortical maps may be altered by peripheral inputs, and the suggestion that some elements of the embryonic guidance mechanism for specific innervation of muscles may still be retained in the adult. Following injury or disease, some plastic responses favour recovery but others are counter-productive. As more is understood about the underlying mechanisms, it should be possible to regulate plasticity more precisely and this would have important implications for physiotherapy.

REFERENCES

Bähr M, Bonhoeffer F. Perspectives on axonal regeneration in the mammalian CNS. *Trends Neurosci* 1994, **17**:473-479.

Bliss TV, Collingridge GL. A synaptic model of memory: long-term potentiation in the hippocampus. *Nature* 1993, **361**:31-39.

Braun S, Croizat B, Lagrange M-C, Warter J-M, Poindron P. Constitutive muscular abnormalities in culture in spinal muscular atrophy. *Lancet* 1995, **345**:694-695.

Brouwer B, Ashby P. Altered corticospinal projections to lower limb motoneurones in subjects with cerebral palsy. *Brain* 1991, **114**:1395-1407.

Brown MC, Hopkins WG, Keynes RJ. *Essentials of neural development.* Cambridge: Cambridge University Press; 1991.

Brushart TME. Motor axons preferentially reinnervate motor pathways. *J Neurosci* 1993, **13**:2730-2738.

Buller AJ, Eccles JC, Eccles RM. Interactions between motoneurones and muscles in respect of the characteristic speeds of their responses. *J Physiol (Lond)* 1960, **150**:417-439.

De Schutter E. Cerebellar long-term depression might normalise excitation of Purkinje cells: a hypothesis. *Trends Neurosci* 1995, **18**:291-295.

Farmer SF, Harrison LM, Ingram DA, *et al.* Plasticity of central motor pathways in children with hemiplegic cerebral palsy. *Neurology* 1991, **41**:1505-1510.

Hall EJ, Flament D, Fraser C, *et al.* Non-invasive brain stimulation reveals reorganised cortical outputs in amputees. *Neurosci Lett* 1990, **116**:379-386.

Hennig R, Dietrichs E. Transient reinnervation of antagonistic muscles by the same motoneurone. *Exp Neurol* 1994, **130**:331-336.

Hosokawa T, Rusakov DA, Bliss TV, *et al.* Repeated confocal imaging of individual dendritic spines in the living hippocampal slice: evidence for changes in length and orientation associated with chemically induced LTP. *J Neurosci* 1995, **15**:5560-5573.

Ito M. Synaptic plasticity in the cerebellar cortex and its role in motor learning. *Can J Neurol Sci* 1993, **20**(3):570-574.

Kaas JH. Plasticity of sensory and motor maps in adult mammals. *Ann Rev Neurosci* 1991, **14**:137-167.

Karni A, Meyer G, Jezzard P, *et al.* Functional MRI evidence for adult motor cortex plasticity during motor skill learning. *Nature* 1995, **377**(6545): 155-158.

Madison RD, Archibald SJ, Krarup C. Peripheral nerve injury. In: Cohen IK, Diegelman F, Lindblad WJ, eds. *Wound healing: Biochemical and clinical aspects.* Philadelphia: WB Saunders; 1991:450-487.

Muller KJ, Aguayo AJ. Views on regeneration in the nervous system. *J Neurobiol* 1992, **23**:467.

O'Hanlon GM, Lowrie MB. Both afferent and efferent connections influence postnatal growth of motoneurone dendrites in the rat. *Dev Neurosci* 1994, **16**:100-107.

Oppenheim RW. Cell death during development of the nervous system. *Ann Rev Neurosci* 1991, **14**:453-501.

Pascual-Leone A, Grafman J, Hallett M. Modulation of cortical output maps during development of implicit and explicit knowledge. *Science* 1994, **263**:1287-1289.

Pette D, Vrbová G. Adaptation of mammalian skeletal muscle fibers to chronic electrical stimulation. *Rev Physiol Biochem Pharmacol* 1992, **120**:115-202.

Rose FC, Jones R, Vrbová G. *Neuromuscular stimulation: Basic concepts and clinical implications.* New York: Demos; 1989.

Salmon DP, Butters N. Neurobiology of skill and habit learning. *Curr Opin Neurobiol* 1995, **5**:184-190.

Salmons S, Vrbová G. The influence of activity on some contractile characteristics of mammalian fast and slow muscles. *J Physiol (Lond)* 1969, **201**:535-549.

Seebach BS, Ziskind-Conhaim L. Formation of transient inappropriate sensorimotor synapses in developing rat spinal cords. *J Neurosci* 1994, **14**:4520-4528.

Stanfield BB. The development of the corticospinal projection. *Prog Neurobiol* 1992, **38**:169-202.

Steward O, Tomasulo R, Torre E, *et al.* Reorganisation of neural connections following CNS injury: Is synaptic reorganisation initiated by the changes in neuroneal activity which occur following injury? *Brain Dysfunct* 1992, **5**:27-49.

Stroemer RP, Thomas AK, Hulsebosch CE. Neocortical neural sprouting, synaptogenesis, and behavioural recovery after neocortical infarction in rats. *Stroke* 1995, **26**:2135-2144.

Vrbová G, Gordon T, Jones R. *Nerve-muscle interaction, 2nd edition.* London: Chapman & Hall; 1995.

Vrbová G, Lowrie MB. The role of activity in developing synapses: search for molecular mechanisms. *News Physiol Sci* 1989, **4**:75-78.

Wang X, Merzenich MM, Sameshima K, *et al.* Remodelling of hand representation in adult cortex determined by timing of tactile stimulation. *Nature* 1995, **378**:71-75.

Weiller C, Chollet F, Friston KJ, *et al.* Functional reorganisation of the brain in recovery from striatocapsular infarction in man. *Ann Neurol* 1992, **31**:463-472.

Wolpaw JR. Acquisition and maintenance of the simplest motor skill: investigation of CNS mechanisms. *Med Sci Sports Exerc* 1994, **26**:1475-1479.

Woolf CJ, Shortland P, Coggeshall RE. Peripheral nerve injury triggers central sprouting of myelinated afferents. *Nature* 1992, **355**:75-78.

SECTION 2

NEUROLOGICAL AND NEUROMUSCULAR CONDITIONS

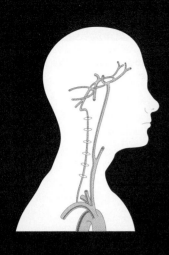

7

B Durward, G Baer & J Wade

STROKE

CHAPTER OUTLINE

- **Definitions**
- **Anatomy and physiology**
- **Types of stroke and their signs and symptoms**
- **The stroke-prone population**
- **Threatened stroke**
- **Medical examination of the stroke patient**
- **Medical management**
- **Recovery following stroke**
- **Physical management**

INTRODUCTION

The stroke patient presents the physiotherapist with a unique complex of physical, psychological and social problems. The onset of stroke is usually sudden, with maximum deficit at the outset, so the shock to patients and their families may be devastating. The prevalence is approximately 2 per 1000, with the outcome being death within the first 3 weeks in approximately 30% of cases, full recovery in 30% and residual disability in 40% (Langton Hewer, 1993).

DEFINITIONS

'Stroke' is synonymous with cerebrovascular accident (CVA), and is a clinical definition. The World Health Organisation definition of stroke is 'a rapidly developed clinical sign of focal disturbance of cerebral function of presumed vascular origin and of more than 24-hours' duration'. This definition does not include 'transient ischaemic attacks'. Hemiplegia is the paralysis of muscles on one side of the body, contralateral to the side of the brain in which the CVA occurred.

ANATOMY AND PHYSIOLOGY

Metabolism in the brain is almost exclusively aerobic, so neurones depend on a continuous blood supply. If the brain is deprived of blood, consciousness is lost within seconds and permanent damage occurs within minutes. Perhaps because of the brain's unique vulnerability, evolution has provided it with a copious and anatomically diverse blood supply (Figure 7.1), a detailed description of which can be found in anatomy texts (e.g. Williams, 1995). A complex physiological mechanism ensures that the blood supply remains stable over a wide range of arterial blood pressure, a phenomenon termed 'autoregulation'.

Blood arrives at the brain via four major vessels. The right carotid artery arises from the innominate artery, and the left carotid artery directly from the aorta; they pass up the front of the neck, and each artery divides into two, the branches (anterior and middle cerebral arteries) supplying the frontal, parietal and temporal lobes. The two anterior cerebral arteries join anteriorly through the anterior communicating artery and this forms the front of the circle of Willis. This safeguard means that severe stenosis, or even occlusion, of one of the internal carotid arteries does not

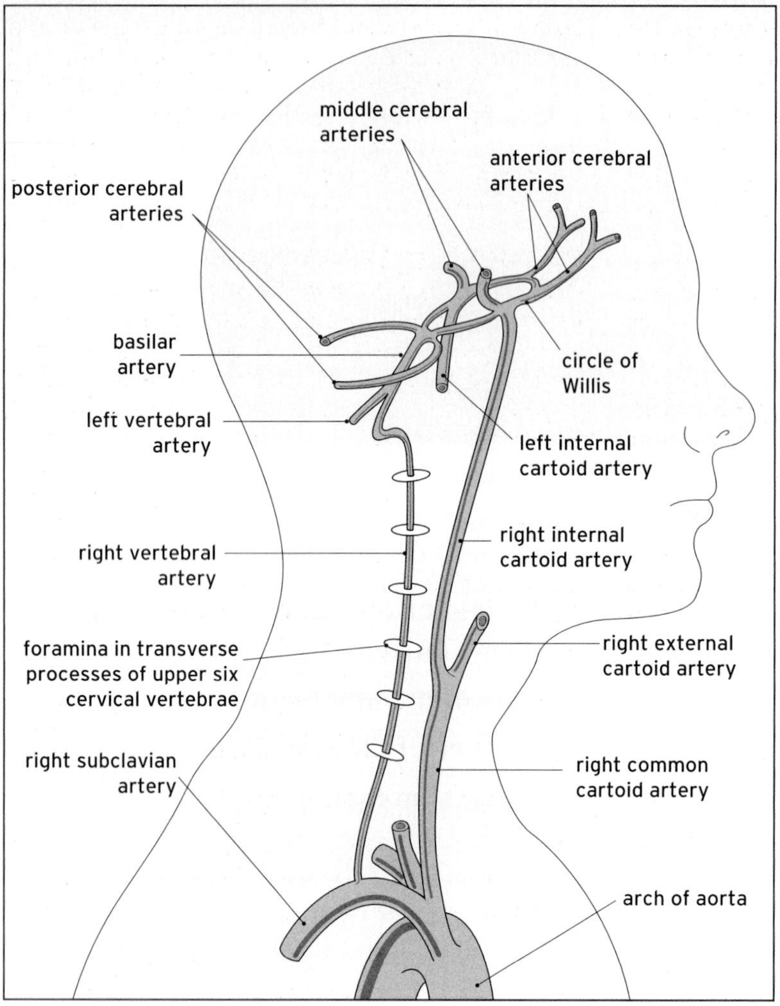

Figure 7.1 Blood supply to the brain, showing the circle of Willis.

usually lead to stroke, since blood can pass from right to left (or vice versa) via the anterior communicating artery.

There are two other arteries, known as the vertebrals, which are smaller than the internal carotids and are branches of the subclavian vessels. These run up the neck through the foramina in the transverse processes of the cervical vertebrae and anastomose in front of the brainstem to form the basilar artery. Branches of that artery supply the medulla, pons, cerebellum and midbrain. At the top of the midbrain, the basilar artery divides into two posterior cerebral arteries that turn backwards to supply the occipital lobes. These two arteries are also joined to the back of the circle of Willis by small posterior communicating arteries and so an anastomosis occurs between the internal carotids and the vertebral circulation. This offers a further safeguard, and it is not uncommon to see patients who are well despite having bilaterally occluded internal carotid arteries.

The branches of the major cerebral vessels (anterior, middle and posterior cerebral arteries) do not, however, anastomose with each other and they are therefore termed end arteries. The parts of the brain they supply are relatively well designated and distinct, although anastomoses do occur at the periphery of each region. If one of these vessels is occluded, then relatively stereotyped brain damage occurs in the area which it supplies (see below) when considering the types of stroke.

TYPES OF STROKE AND THEIR SIGNS AND SYMPTOMS

Knowledge of the functional anatomy of the brain is essential to understanding the effect of stroke on the patient. The functional deficits described below are related to the area of damage, regardless of the cause, e.g. ischaemia or haemorrhage.

ISCHAEMIC STROKE

The most common cause of stroke is obstruction of one of the major cerebral arteries (middle, posterior and anterior, in descending order of frequency) or their smaller perforating branches to deeper parts of the brain. Brainstem strokes, arising from disease in the vertebral and basilar arteries, are less common. Approximately 80% of all strokes are due to occlusion (Bamford *et al.*, 1988), either as a result of atheroma in the artery itself or secondary to emboli (small clots of blood) being washed up from the heart or diseased neck vessels. The patient does not usually lose consciousness but may complain of headache, and symptoms of hemiparesis and/or dysphasia develop rapidly. The hemiplegia is initially flaccid but within a few days this gives way to spasticity of the muscles.

The middle cerebral artery supplies most of the convexity of the cerebral hemisphere and important deeper structures, so there is a dense contralateral hemiplegia affecting the arm, face and leg. The optic radiation is often affected, leading to a contralateral homonymous hemianopia, and there may be a cortical type of sensory loss. Since the main centre for speech is on the left side of the brain, speech prob-lems can be severe in left hemisphere lesions and there may be neglect of the contralateral side. In right hemisphere lesions, parietal damage can lead to visuospatial disturbances and left-sided neglect. If the main part of the middle cerebral artery is not affected, but one of its distal branches is, the symptoms will be less extreme.

The most prominent symptoms following posterior cerebral artery occlusion are visual and usually comprise a contralateral homonymous field defect. More compli-cated disturbances of visual interpretation or complete blindness can follow bilateral infarcts. The posterior cerebral artery also supplies much of the medial aspect of the temporal lobe and the thalamus, so strokes may involve memory and contralateral sensory modalities. The anterior cerebral artery supplies the medial aspect of the frontal lobe and a parasagittal strip of cortex extending back as far as the occipital lobe. Occlusion of this artery may therefore give rise to a contralateral monoplegia affecting the leg, cortical sensory loss and sometimes the behavioural abnor-malities associated with frontal lobe damage.

A more specific subclassification of cerebral infarct has been developed by Bamford et al., (1991). From an analysis of 543 patients with cerebral infarct, classifications were formed based on the areas of anatomical involvement. 17% were found to have large anterior cerebral infarcts with both cortical and subcortical involvement; this group was classified as total anterior circulation infarcts (TACI). The largest group, 34%, presented with more restricted and pre-dominantly cortical infarcts and were classified as partial anterior circulation infarcts (PACI). 24% had infarcts involving the vertebrobasilar artery and were called posterior circulation infarcts (POCI); and 25% had infarcts in the territory of the deep perforating arteries and were called lacunar infarcts (LACI).

Noticeable differences have been identified in the natural history of these sub-types of infarct stroke. The TACI strokes tend to have a poor prognosis for indepent functinal outcome and a high mortality rate. This classifi-cation system has implications for therapeutic intervention. Currently, physiotherapists are investigating the different recovery patterns associated with each subtype of infarct (Smith & Baer, 1997). Work of this type may lead to the development of more specific intervention strategies for individual patients.

Occlusion of the vertebral arteries, or the basilar artery and its branches, is potentially much more damaging, since the brainstem contains centres which control vital functions such as respiration and blood pressure. The nuclei of the cranial nerves are clustered in the brainstem and the pyramidal and sensory tracts course through it (see Chapter 1). Thus, ischaemic brain damage may itself be life-threatening and if the patient survives he or she may be severely incapacitated by cranial nerve palsies, spastic tetraplegia and sensory loss.

HAEMORRHAGIC STROKE

Of all first strokes, 9% are caused by haemorrhage into the deeper parts of the brain (Bamford et al., 1988). The patient is usually hypertensive, a condition which leads to a particular type of degeneration, known as lipohyalinosis, in the small penetrating arteries of the brain. The arterial walls weaken, and as a result small herniations or micro-aneurysms develop. These may rupture and the resultant haematoma may spread by splitting planes of white matter to form a substantial mass lesion. Haematomas usually occur in the deeper parts of the brain, often involving the thalamus, lentiform nucleus and external capsule, less often the cerebellum and the pons. They may rupture into the ventricular system and this is often rapidly fatal.

The onset is usually dramatic, with severe headache, vomiting and, in about 50% of cases, loss of consciousness. The normal vascular autoregulation is lost in the vicinity of the haematoma and since the lesion itself may have considerable mass, intracranial pressure often rises abruptly. If the patient survives the initial ictus, then profound hemiplegic and hemisensory signs may be elicited. A homonymous visual field defect may also be apparent. The initial prognosis is grave but those who do begin to recover often do surprisingly well as the haematoma reabsorbs, presumably because fewer neurones are destroyed than in severe ischaemic strokes. Occasionally, early surgical drainage can be remarkably successful, particularly when the haematoma is in the cerebellum.

Younger, normotensive patients sometimes suffer from spontaneous intracerebral haematoma from an underlying congenital defect of the blood vessels. Such abnormalities are commonly arteriovenous malformations (AVMs); circumscribed areas of dilated and thin-walled vessels which can be demonstrated angiographically. Patients with AVMs are liable to subsequent rebleeding and surgical excision is undertaken when possible.

SUBARACHNOID HAEMORRHAGE

Subarachnoid haemorrhage (SAH) involves bleeding into the subarachnoid space, usually arising from rupture of a berry aneurysm situated at or near the circle of Willis. The most common site is in the region of the anterior communicating artery, with posterior and middle cerebral artery lesions almost as frequent. Congenital factors play some part in the aetiology of berry aneurysms but SAH is not predominantly a disease of the young. Hypertension and vascular disease lead to an increase in aneurysm size and subsequent rupture.

The patient complains of sudden intense headache, often associated with vomiting and neck stiffness.

Consciousness may be lost and about 10% will die in the first hour or two. Of those that remain, 40% will die within the first 2 weeks and the survivors have a substantially increased risk from rebleeding for the next 6 weeks. A hemiplegia may be evident at the outset if the blood erupts into the deep parts of the brain, and other focal neurological signs may evolve over the first 2 weeks because there is a tendency for blood vessels, tracking through the bloody subarachnoid space, to go into spasm leading to secondary ischaemic brain damage.

Early investigation by angiography, followed by a competent neurosurgical procedure to clip the aneurysm and prevent rebleeding, offers the best hope for recovery.

LESS FREQUENT CAUSES OF STROKE

Stroke may occasionally occur in the context of a generalised medical disorder which affects either the arteries or the blood going through them. An arteritis, or inflammation of the arteries, may complicate meningitis, particularly tuberculous, and strokes were relatively common in tertiary syphilis. The collagen vascular diseases, particularly systemic lupus erythematosus and polyarteritis nodosa, may affect medium and small cranial arteries. Temporal arteritis, an inflammatory condition predominantly affecting the extracranial and retinal arteries in the elderly, may also give rise to stroke by intracranial involvement.

Conditions that may cause ischemic stroke include bacterial infection of damaged heart valves (bacterial endocarditis) and atrial fibrillation (particularly if there is coincidental mitral stenosis), and mitral valve prolapse (floppy valve), which is a fairly common congenital abnormality. Echocardiography has demonstrated atrial shunts through which clots in the venous circulation can cross to the arterial supply.

Haematological diseases such as polycythaemia rubra vera, thrombocythaemia and sickle cell disease can provoke stasis in the intracranial arteries, thus leading to ischaemic brain damage. Completed stroke occasionally complicates severe migraine if the vessel spasm which normally produces only temporary symptoms is of such intensity and such duration that ischaemic damage occurs. Finally, there is evidence that women taking the contraceptive pill, particularly if it has a high oestrogen content, suffer a slightly higher incidence of stroke than those not on the pill (Hannaford et al., 1994); the absolute risk is small but is increased by cigarette smoking.

THE STROKE-PRONE POPULATION

A comprehensive epidemiological study found that while the chance of having a stroke increases with age, it should not be considered a natural concomitant of increasing age (Kannel & Wolf, 1983). The most significant risk factor is hypertension, either systolic (>160 mmHg) or diastolic (>95 mmHg), and there is evidence that prophylactic hypotensive therapy reduces this susceptibility but is not solely responsible for the decline in the incidence of stroke in the general population (Whisnant, 1996). In a review,

Whisnant (1996) summarised the results of 17 randomised controlled trials of treatment for hypertension, involving nearly 48,000 patients worldwide, which showed a 38% reduction in all types of stroke and a 40% reduction in fatal stroke, providing evidence which leaves no doubt about the effectiveness of treatment.

Other significant risk factors are ischaemic heart disease, diabetes mellitus, a high-salt diet and smoking, which is a substantial independent risk factor (Whisnant, 1996). The oestrogen-containing contraceptive pill also increases the risk of stroke (Hannaford et al., 1994).

The 'final common pathway' for all these risk factors is the arterial disease atherosclerosis, a disease of the larger and medium-sized arteries, characterised by the deposition of cholesterol and other substances in the arterial wall. The irregular vessel wall provokes clot formation in the lumen of the artery, which may completely occlude the vessel or may dislodge to form emboli. Hypertension and other risk factors therefore predispose to ischaemic strokes, but it will be remembered that the most usual cause for intracerebral haematoma is also hypertension and the associated small vessel disease (lipohyalinosis).

THREATENED STROKE

The conditions mentioned below may predispose to stroke or represent subclinical arterial disease but do not necessarily lead to a stroke.

TRANSIENT ISCHAEMIC ATTACKS

A transient ischaemic attack (TIA) refers to a stroke-like syndrome in which recovery is complete within 24 hours. It is important to recognise TIAs because about 10% of patients will go on to have a completed stroke. The symptoms depend on which part of the brain has been temporarily deprived of blood, e.g. hemisphere or brainstem. Thus, if the left middle cerebral artery has been briefly occluded, symptoms may comprise weakness and clumsiness of the right side and difficulty making oneself understood (dysphasia). The symptoms evolve rapidly, and resolve more gradually, but it is unusual for the whole episode to last more than an hour and there are no permanent sequelae. Sometimes the retinal artery is involved and the patient complains of a unilateral visual field disturbance, or blindness, often descending like a curtain across the vision. Within half an hour or so (often much more rapidly) the veil lifts and vision is restored.

Virtually all patients with TIAs are put on aspirin (150 mg daily) to reduce the chances of subsequent stroke. Risk factors may be amenable to modification (e.g. cessation of smoking, treatment of hypertension) and this can further reduce the risk of stroke (Whisnant, 1996). A few patients will be identified as having severe stenosis (>70%) of the carotid artery and, provided this is considered symptomatic, they may be offered the operation of endarterectomy (Brown & Humphrey, 1992).

LEAKING ANEURYSM
About 40% of patients who have a subarachnoid haemorrhage

have preceding symptoms of minor leaks which usually occur within a month before the major bleed, and often go unrecognised. Symptoms are sudden headache, nausea, photophobia and sometimes neck stiffness which can resolve rapidly and may be incorrectly attributed to migraine.

ASYMPTOMATIC CAROTID BRUIT

A noise (or bruit) may be heard over the carotid artery during routine medical examination. The bruit suggests turbulent blood flow due to underlying atherosclerosis and is an asymptomatic carotid bruit if present in an otherwise healthy individual. Some 5% of patients with a bruit will go on to have a stroke, though not always in the distribution of the diseased artery.

MEDICAL EXAMINATION OF THE STROKE PATIENT

The first objective is to decide which of the three main types of stroke (ischaemic, haemorrhagic or SAH) the patient has had. The history and clinical examination are discussed in Chapter 3. Brain imaging will differentiate between ischaemia and haemorrhage.

When the history suggests SAH, confirmation can be obtained by examining CSF after lumbar puncture. If the CSF is bloodstained, angiography should be undertaken to identify the source of bleeding.

Patients with small ischaemic strokes, who have made a good recovery, are investigated along the same lines as those with TIAs, to try to prevent further strokes. The cause may be immediately apparent, such as severe hypertension, in which case investigations will be limited to those indicated in the evaluation of hypertension. Assuming the patient is normotensive, routine blood tests may be helpful. An ECG and echocardiogram should be performed if there is any chance that the heart is acting as a source of emboli. Patients with carotid-territory TIA or small completed stroke require carotid duplex (or MR) angiography as a non-invasive technique for assessing the presence and degree of carotid stenosis. Those with tight stenosis may have carotid angiography as a prelude to endarterectomy.

MEDICAL MANAGEMENT

Patients with subarachnoid haemorrhage are treated surgically provided they are considered fit enough to withstand surgery. If they are not, then treatment is conservative, with prolonged bed rest (4–6 weeks) and perhaps medication to prevent clot lysis. Some patients with haematomas are also treated surgically, but for the most part the treatment of patients suffering stroke is conservative and is undertaken by GPs. There are no drugs that reduce infarct size convincingly. The neurological deficit is usually maximal at the outset and, if not severe, the patient can be managed at home satisfactorily. In practice, many patients are admitted to hospital for a short period of treatment and investigation. Patients with more severe strokes will require admission to hospital.

In some cases of ischaemic CVA, a secondary deterioration occurs 2 or 3 days after the initial event, usually due to evolving oedema around the infarct; this may respond to drug treatment. Severe hypertension should be treated cautiously and biochemical abnormalities corrected. Most recovery occurs within the first 8 weeks and the time course is discussed below.

Almost all patients with ischaemic stroke are put on aspirin to prevent recurrence or extension. Those with dense hemiplegias should have stockings and warfarin as prophylaxis against deep venous thrombosis (DVT). If the stroke is restricted and recovery good, or if the patient has suffered only from TIA and by definition has no residual deficit, then treatment aimed at preventing recurrence may be more aggressive, depending on the results of the investigations. If the heart is considered a likely source of emboli, then long-term treatment with anticoagulants may be indicated. Atherosclerosis, leading to tight stenosis of the internal carotid artery, can be confirmed angiographically and treated surgically by carotid endarterectomy (Brown & Humphrey, 1992).

RECOVERY FOLLOWING STROKE

The most common physical consequence of stroke is hemiplegia, which is defined as 'complete paralysis of the upper and lower limbs on the same side of the body' (Scottish Office Home and Health Department, 1993). Other sequelae of stroke could include perceptual, cognitive, sensory and communication problems, all of which need to be considered in physiotherapy management.

Whatever the cause of the stroke, a proportion of patients will recover to some degree (Duncan et al., 1994). Recovery is related to the site, extent and nature of the lesion, the integrity of the collateral circulation and the pre-morbid status of the patient. Haemorrhagic and ischaemic strokes present with different patterns of initial recovery (see above). Characteristically, ischaemic infarct lesions present suddenly and the full extent of the initial insult is apparent. In contrast, with haemorrhagic strokes the extent of the impairment initially seems more extensive due to localised inflammation surrounding the site of the bleed. Some of the initial recovery in haemmorhagic stroke can be attributed to the resolution of inflammation (Allen et al., 1988).

Some stroke patients fail to regain conciousness within the first 24 hours following the CVA and it is considered widely that the majority will not regain consciousness. The physiotherapy management of these patients is similar to that after severe brain injury and will include regular chest care, turning and positioning (see Chapter 8).

In patients who regain consciousness within 24 hours, the first 3 months are a critical period when greatest recovery is thought to occur (Wade et al., 1985b), although potential for improvement may exist for many months (Wade et al., 1992). Physiotherapy during this initial period should aim to maximise all aspects of recovery in order to limit residual disability and reduce handicap. Therefore, physiotherapy commences as soon as the patient is admitted to hospital, or is stable, and should continue up to the time when physical recovery ceases.

Hemiplegia as a consequence of stroke is considered to be a recovering neurological condition (Carr & Shepherd, 1989; Bobath, 1990). Although the process of recovery remains unclear, it may be related to one or more of the following (Wade et al., 1985a; Jongbloed, 1986; Anderson, 1994; Duncan et al., 1994):

- The site and extent of the initial lesion.
- The age of the patient.
- The capacity to achieve a motor goal related to functional movement.
- The capacity of the nervous system to reorganise (plasticity; see Chapter 6).
- The premorbid status of the patient.
- The motivation and attitude of the patient towards recovery.

Whilst the specific effects of physiotherapy during rehabilitation remain uncertain, there is increasing evidence that early physiotherapy can maximise physical recovery (Ernst, 1990; Anonymous, 1992; Ashburn et al., 1993).

A recent prospective study attempted to describe the time profile of some physical disabilities in 348 recovering stroke patients with weekly assessment of physical ability following referral for physiotherapy (Partridge et al., 1993). The results indicated that different milestones of recovery occur for different physical tasks (Table 7.1).

Whilst nearly all patients (334/348; 96%) recovered an ability to maintain sitting balance by 6 weeks, the ability to walk inside independently at 6 weeks was achieved by only 195 patients (56%). Whilst the range of motor tasks investigated in this study was incomplete, the results indicated that specific gross movements may require either additional physiotherapy or more time during rehabilitation to ensure the restoration of ability. The time history of recovery is discussed further in relation to rehabilitation below.

PHYSICAL MANAGEMENT OF STROKE

The physical management process aims to maximise functional ability and prevent secondary complications to enable the patient to resume all aspects of life in his or her own environment.

The physiotherapist plays a major role in the physical management of stroke, using skills acquired during education and professional development, to identify and manage the problems of stroke using scientific principles (Durward & Baer, 1995). Operating as a clinical movement scientist, the physiotherapist is able to identify and

Recovery from disability after a stroke						
Milestone items Gross body movements	On referral	Week 1	Week 2	Week 4	Week 6	Not at week 6
1. Lying supine, turn head to both left and right	302 (86.8)	323 (92.8)	331 (95.1)	335 (96.3)	341 (98.0)	7 (2.0)
2. Maintain sitting balance for one minute	234 (67.2)	287 (82.5)	306 (87.9)	326 (93.7)	334 (96.0)	14 (4.0)
3. Lying supine, roll to both left and right side	149 (42.8)	208 (59.8)	240 (69.0)	273 (78.4)	294 (84.5)	54 (15.5)
4. Lying supine, get up to sitting from left to right	99 (28.4)	159 (45.7)	202 (58.0)	241 (69.3)	259 (74.4)	89 (25.6)
5. Stand up to free-standing	102 (29.3)	156 (44.8)	198 (56.9)	230 (66.1)	254 (73.0)	94 (27.0)
6. From sitting, transfer from bed to chair left and right side	84 (24.1)	138 (39.7)	174 (50.0)	217 (62.4)	241 (69.3)	107 (30.7)
7. From standing, take two steps forward	68 (19.5)	120 (34.5)	157 (45.1)	202 (58.0)	228 (65.5)	120 (34.5)
8. From standing, take two steps backwards	52 (14.9)	99 (28.4)	138 (39.7)	186 (53.4)	211 (60.6)	137 (39.4)
9. Independent walking inside	41 (11.8)	86 (24.7)	120 (34.5)	169 (48.6)	195 (56.0)	153 (44.0)

Table 7.1 Recovery from disability after a stroke. A total of 348 patients was studied: the numbers achieving each milestone are shown, with percentages in parantheses. (Data from Partridge et al., 1993, with permission.)

measure the disorders of movement, and to design, implement and evaluate appropriate therapeutic strategies. This process includes dealing with the social and psychological factors which affect the stroke patient.

Within the multidisciplinary team (MDT) of healthcare professionals, the main roles of the physiotherapist include: restoration of function; prevention of secondary complications, such as shortening of soft tissues and the development of painful shoulder; and research. Areas where research is required include development of scientific measurement and assessment techniques, evidence-based intervention strategies, and valid and reliable outcome measures.

TYPICAL TIME HISTORY FOR STROKE REHABILITATION

In the context of stroke rehabilitation, the management of the patient can be considered to take place in four distinct stages (Table 7.2), which are intended to be indicative; not all patients will adhere to these time-related stages and in some instances the stages may overlap.

Typical time history for stroke rehabilitation		
Stage	**Definition**	**Typical management**
Acute	The immediate period following the cerebrovascular accident	Initial assessment of basic systems, e.g. • swallowing, coughing and respiration • recognition of consciousness level • skin and pressure areas • muscle tone and soft tissue shortening • determination of medical stability Physiotherapy intervention for respiratory problems Initial dialogue with patient and carers regarding the nature of stroke Assessment of the patients' environment and social milieu
Intermediate	The period which commences once the patient is medically stable, conscious and actively engaged in the rehabilitation process	Regular identification and assessment of agreed rehabilitation objectives Active engagement in a physiotherapy intervention programme Formulation and adherence to self-treatment strategies
Discharge and transfer	The period immediately prior to, and following, discharge from formal rehabilitation	Assessment of residual disability Physiotherapy intervention for agreed discharge objectives Modifications to the patients' environment Management of transfer of skills between environments Review and monitoring of self-treatment strategies Determine the pattern of rehabilitation once the patient has returned home or when community physiotherapy stops
Long term	The period following the cessation of formal regular rehabilitation	May include: • Regular review of patient status • Task specific treatment sessions • Review and modification of self-treatment strategies

Table 7.2 Typical time history for stroke rehabilitation.

Acute Stage

In the acute stage the physiotherapist concentrates on basic problems such as respiratory function and the ability to cough and swallow. The patient may be unconscious and therefore require assistance to maintain normal respiratory function and removal of secretions from the upper airway (Carter & Edwards, 1996).

Communication with members of the MDT will be necessary to ascertain any complicating medical factors that may influence physiotherapy management. Routine skin, soft tissue and joint care may be required, in conjunction with advice regarding positioning (Ada & Canning, 1990; Lynch & Grisogono, 1991). The physiotherapist should endeavour to communicate with the patient and carers regarding the nature of stroke, and provide an explanation of the aims and nature of rehabilitation.

Intermediate Stage

The intermediate stage may commence as early as 24 hours following CVA, when it is important to complete a physiotherapeutic assessment that represents an extensive database comprising a range of details pertaining to the patient (see 'Assessment'). The initial assessment serves as a baseline against which recovery or effectiveness of physiotherapeutic intervention can be gauged (see Chapter 4).

Where possible, the patient and carers should participate actively in the identification and agreement of realistic and achievable physiotherapy objectives, in collaboration with all members of the MDT (see 'Treatment planning').

Tasks related to functional movements that the patient can practise independently should be identified to involve the patient as an active participant in his or her own rehabilitation (Ada & Canning 1990), as discussed below (see 'Self-practice'). The home or ward may need to be adapted to enable the patient to participate safely in independent practice.

Discharge and Transfer Stage

This is a critical period in the rehabilitation of the stroke patient and requires specific physiotherapy management. In the case of the patient in hospital or a Stroke Rehabilitation Unit, the decision is made to return him or her home or into residential care. For the patient in the community, this is the time when formal contact with physiotherapy ceases.

An important feature of this stage is the careful management of skill transference. Home visits should be carried out and discharge goals set to enable motor skills to be maintained when the patient is at home (see 'Transfer of learning'). After leaving hospital, regular contact with the physiotherapist may continue on either an out-patient or community basis.

The self-treatment strategies devised during the intermediate stage should be reviewed. The physiotherapist should deliberately withdraw directed treatment and place emphasis on assisting the patient to adhere to an independent practice regimen. The patient and carers should also be guided in developing a record of self-practice strategies.

Long Term

Management issues in the long term will need to reflect the residual disability and handicap status of the patient. If resources allow, it may be desirable to plan regular but low-frequency reviews of the patient's status to confirm his or her continued independence or highlight the need for limited task-specific treatment sessions for certain functional disabilities. It will also allow the physiotherapist to review and modify self-treatment strategies if required.

PHYSIOTHERAPY DELIVERY FOR STROKE PATIENTS

The location, mode and pattern of intervention need to be considered when planning the delivery of physiotherapy for stroke.

Location of Treatment

Treatment may be given in a number of locations: home; Stroke Rehabilitation Unit; hospital ward; day hospital; or nursing home.

The optimal environment for the physical management of stroke provides the patient with continuous stimulation and challenges directed towards maximising recovery. This environment should be organised to allow regular periods of activity under the direction of the physiotherapist and other healthcare professionals, regular periods for organised self-practice, periods of rest and relaxation, and opportunity for social interaction. Observational studies of recovering stroke patients in hospital rehabilitation settings in the UK, however, have shown that the patient may be inactive for much of the day, with only 11–17% of the working day spent in therapy and around 40% spent in recreation (Tinson, 1989; Ellul, et al., 1993; Lincoln et al., 1996).

The environment of the patient will affect the provision of physiotherapy. Evidence from a number of studies suggests that stroke patients treated in a specialist Stroke Rehabilitation Unit may live longer than those cared for in a hospital ward and that recovery may be greater in terms of mobility and return to independent living (Kalra 1994).

The advocates for Stroke Units have proposed a number of specific benefits that may positively affect outcome (Kalra, 1994; Wood & Wade, 1995). A Stroke Unit provides highly trained staff with expertise and interest in stroke and a capacity to manipulate the environment to provide an appropriate challenge for each patient. Also, the physical organisation, daily timetables and the involvement of carers are more easily managed within a Stroke Unit.

The management of the patient in his or her own home offers some unique opportunities but also presents specific difficulties. Familiarity with the surroundings assists orientation and ensures that physiotherapy and self-practice tasks are specific to the functional demands of the home environment. Problems include co-ordination of the different rehabilitation professionals, the potential for less frequent physiotherapy, lack of access to specialised equipment, and a less challenging environment.

Modes of Intervention

Intervention may be given in a number of ways and by a variety of persons: physiotherapist alone; physiotherapist and carer; carer alone; organised self-practice; physiotherapist with other professionals.

Assessment will enable selection of: treatment techniques to be administered directly by the physiotherapist; strategies to enable the carer to participate in rehabilitation; and activities conducive to organised self-practice. The nature of each mode of intervention will vary at different stages of rehabilitation. During the long-term stage, the emphasis should be on carer involvement and self-practice. Combined intervention from more than one professional may be appropriate. For example, the physiotherapist and occupational therapist may work together in re-educating the patient to be able to dress. While the occupational therapist teaches components of dressing tasks, the physiotherapist could re-educate the patient's balance and prevent abnormal adaptive or compensatory activity.

Pattern of Intervention Delivery

The frequency of intervention refers to the number of interactions between a patient and physiotherapist over a prescribed time interval, such as a day or week. The duration of intervention indicates the length of time allocated to each interaction. Factors such as exercise tolerance and concentration, in terms of attention and memory, are likely to influence the pattern of intervention.

Factors Leading to Modification of Intervention

Factors that might lead to the need to modify physiotherapy intervention need to be identified. These may be linked to the patient's age, other pathologies that can cause reduced exercise tolerance (cardiovascular fitness), and altered mental or cognitive states. When identifying these, it is important to separate true or chronological age from 'pathological age'. Pre-morbid status and the presence of other pathologies are more likely than age to affect the final outcome and recovery from stroke. Modification of intervention is discussed below.

STROKE MANAGEMENT: A PROBLEM-SOLVING PROCESS

Problem solving is a process that provides the physiotherapist with a structured and efficient system of interlinked decision-making levels for the management of patients. Figure 7.2 represents a problem-solving model appropriate for the management of stroke (Salter & Ferguson, 1991). The objectives of this model are: to establish physiotherapy objectives; to facilitate selection of therapeutic intervention strategies; and to provide a decision-making algorithm that will lead the physiotherapist to determine whether intervention has been effective.

Assessment

The assessment process should be both formal and structured. It should include the collection of patient data, the formation of a documented record of the information, and an analysis that will lead to the identification of physiotherapy objectives and the selection of appropriate therapeutic techniques. Initially, the assessment should be completed prior to any form of intervention and then repeated at regular and predetermined intervals thereafter. The provision of treatment before the initial assessment process could result in ineffective or possibly even harmful intervention.

An initial database should comprise personal details such as the age and address of the patient and the medical history, together with physical (functional and motor ability), psychological, family and social issues. The organisation and analysis of patient data, and the identification of problems need to be documented in a systematic manner. Record systems such as Problem-Oriented Medical Records (POMR) offer an appropriate method for structuring, retrieving and reviewing patient data (Kettenbach, 1990).

There are many assessment tools available for stroke and some examples are discussed in Chapter 4. Despite an extensive range there is limited research evidence supporting the validity and reliability of these assessment tools. Most stroke assessment tools use ordinal scales to establish the status of the patient but measurement at this level may have inherent 'ceiling' effects; at a certain point in recovery, the scale becomes insensitive to changes in the patient's status (Ashburn, 1986). The opposite may also be true, in that a 'floor' effect may exist where the scale cannot reflect initial recovery.

Examples of commonly used stroke assessment tools that have been tested to establish levels of validity and reliability include the Rivermead Stroke Assessment (Lincoln & Leadbitter, 1979) and the Motor Assessment Scale (MAS; Carr et al., 1985). Whilst both provide ordinal data derived using rating scales that can reflect the physical status of the patient, the MAS is directly linked to a specific physiotherapeutic approach for stroke (Carr & Shepherd, 1987). This close association between an assessment tool and a specific treatment approach may lead to bias in the data collected. This bias may be negative; i.e. the assessment tool may be insensitive to changes in the patient that are anticipated as part of the expectations of the treatment approach. Alternatively, bias may be positive; in this case the assessment tool may reflect the expectations of the treatment approach but be insensitive to other unexpected aspects of recovery or deterioration.

Treatment Planning

Following assessment, short- and long-term physiotherapeutic objectives and the mode and pattern of intervention should be determined, and appropriate therapeutic techniques selected. An example of where assessment data inform planning might be using the findings of measurement of impairments such as muscle strength and balance to plan re-education of gait. A systematic review of 24 studies found that certain impairments were highly correlated

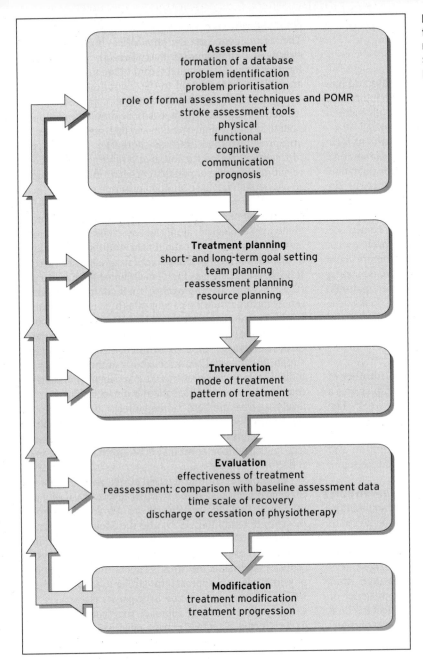

Figure 7.2 Problem-solving model for the physiotherapeutic management of patients after stroke. (Abbreviation: POMR, problem-oriented medical records.)

with gait performance and thus serve as appropriate targets for treatment and evaluation (Bohannon *et al.*, 1995).

Communication between members of the MDT is central to the process of treatment planning and, whenever possible, the patient (and carers when appropriate) should also participate in this process (Draper *et al.*, 1991; Ehrlich *et al.*, 1992). During planning, the MDT may function in both a retrospective and prospective manner. On a regular basis, the MDT will review the patient's progress in terms of achieving established short- and long-term objectives. The MDT should aim to establish common rehabilitation goals with short- and long-term treatment objectives. An example of a short-term objective might be 'achievement of

independent sitting balance for a period of 30 seconds', which the patient might achieve within the next 7 days. This prospectively agreed objective will serve to unify the MDT and co-ordinate their separate interactions with the patient.

The planning process should also include strategic plans to prevent secondary complications such as painful shoulder or oedematous hand. Early identification of potential for secondary trauma, and the deliberate inclusion of plans to prevent its occurrence, can ensure that there is minimal disruption to the rehabilitation process.

A pattern for regular reassessment should be established during treatment planning to monitor the overall status at different stages during rehabilitation, concentrating on aspects of functional recovery that relate to current short-term objectives.

Resources that need to be considered include: the availability of staff; potential for involvement of carers; and resources for direct patient treatment and self-practice in the institutional setting, home and community. Availability and involvement of external agencies such as social workers, stroke support workers, carer support and stroke clubs may also need to be considered.

Intervention

Initial assessment data may indicate that some patients are more suitable for intensive rehabilitation whilst others, possibly the patient with complicating pathologies, may require less intensive intervention. The aims of intervention are to maximise functional ability and prevent secondary complications such as contractures and painful shoulder.

The modes of intervention may alter during rehabilitation in order to make the best use of available resources. For example, in striving to meet the short-term objective of holding a glass in order to drink, the patient may need to interact with the physiotherapist alone, the carer, or a combination of occupational therapist and physiotherapist. In addition, the patient will also have a task-specific programme of organised self-practice related to this short-term goal.

Different treatment approaches are discussed in Chapter 22 and actual physiotherapeutic intervention techniques are discussed in Chapter 24; the management of abnormal muscle tone is discussed in Chapter 25.

Evaluation

A central feature of the problem-solving model is the need to ensure that physiotherapeutic intervention is effective, as both an immediate and long-term component of patient management.

A single physiotherapy treatment, irrespective of location, mode or pattern, should produce a positive therapeutic effect. Effectiveness is determined either by testing the patient with reference to time or performance criteria, or by observing their immediate response to the treatment. This immediate evaluation may indicate that a specific therapeutic technique may need to be either modified or replaced.

While day-to-day physiotherapy may appear to have an immediate effect, review of patient progress with regard to the specified short- and long-term physiotherapy objectives is necessary. This estimate of 'true' progress, or otherwise, can be established by comparing current assessment data with the initial baseline status of the patient. It follows that this process of evaluation may indicate the rate of progress during rehabilitation. An important aspect of evaluation is to determine whether the patient is capable of returning home and whether formal contact with a physiotherapist is no longer required.

Modification

Evaluation may reveal uncertainty regarding the effectiveness of intervention and should lead to the physiotherapist revisiting one or more levels of the problem-solving model. The section above on 'Factors leading to modification of intervention' is relevant to this process. Modification of treatment may include changing the mode or pattern of intervention, or the treatment techniques.

GENERAL MANAGEMENT ISSUES

This section will deal with a range of issues which need to be addressed in the overall management of stroke, and which may arise at any stage of recovery.

Respiratory Care

Respiratory care includes both prophylactic and terminal care. Respiratory problems are most likely to occur in the acute and intermediate stages following stroke. Initial assessment should include the examination of rate, depth and pattern of respiration, in conjunction with chest auscultation, to prevent secondary complications such as atelectasis and pneumonia (Hough, 1991; Smith & Ball, 1998). The patient may be predisposed to these problems due to relative immobility, prolonged supine positioning and altered tone in the respiratory muscles. Also, the cough reflex may be suppressed or weak, resulting in difficulties with removal of secretions from the airways.

Altered breathing patterns may be characteristic of a stroke patient whose condition is considered to be terminal. A serious complication following a severe stroke with brainstem involvement may be the presence of Cheyne–Stokes breathing, in which periods of apnoea alternate with a series of respirations which increase and decrease in amplitude. In the general management of stroke, the physiotherapist will aim to maintain a clear airway, stimulate the cough reflex, assist effective removal of secretions and encourage a normal respiratory pattern (Hough, 1991; Smith & Ball, 1998).

Positioning

Positioning of the patient needs to be considered with respect to the environment as well as a suitable bed and chair.

The controlled orientation and position of the patient in the immediate environment can provide useful stimulation when problems of visual and perceptual dysfunction exist (see 'Perceptual Problems'). In these instances, effort should be made to ensure that the environment provides a challenging stimulus and the immediate surroundings should be organised so as to encourage the patient to look over his or her affected side (Davies, 1985; Riddoch et al., 1995).

The management of stimulation may be clarified if a distinction between visual and perceptual problems is established. During the acute stage, for a patient with visual and perceptual dysfunction, it may be reasonable to advise carers, relatives and members of the MDT to address the patient and provide stimulation from the midline (i.e. by standing directly in front of the patient). As the visual and perceptual problems start to resolve, stimulation may be provided from the affected side.

Strategies exist for positioning the hemiplegic patient when seated in a chair and lying on a bed (Lynch & Grisogono, 1991). These strategies are designed to optimise sensory stimulation and encourage the adoption of effective weight bearing. In addition, these positions attempt to prevent secondary complications such as soft tissue shortening and the development of a painful shoulder, and inhibit the development of abnormal muscle tone (Ada & Canning, 1990; Bobath, 1990). For further discussion of positioning strategies see Carr & Kenney (1992), as well as Chapter 25.

Continence
Physiotherapy intervention has a role to play in the management of urinary and faecal continence. Early encouragement and assistance to enable the patient to adopt weight-bearing standing and sitting positions may help overcome these problems. Special attention should be given to the patient with communication difficulties who may be unable to ask for either a bedpan or bottle. Regular offers to assist the patient to the toilet or to use a bedpan or bottle may help to preserve continence and maintain the patient's self-esteem.

Communication
Issues of communication include: the types of problems encountered; strategies for combatting them; and the roles of the patient, the MDT and carers.

The communication problems commonly associated with stroke include: dysarthria (problems of articulation); dysphasia (either a receptive or expressive problem which affects the understanding and use of correct words); aphasia (inability to express oneself in speech or writing or to understand written or spoken language); orofacial dysfunction; and loss of facial expression and gesture. Dysphasia may result in the patient's being unable to understand what has happened or to ask questions regarding the stroke. The physiotherapist and the MDT should allow additional response times during verbal communication and use clear and simple speech. A designated member of the MDT should allocate time to give the patient information about the nature of the stroke, the recovery process and rehabilitation. The MDT, with guidance from a speech and language therapist, should determine clear and consistent approaches for communication with individual stroke patients.

Carer Support
Carer support may involve education, counselling and access to support agencies.

The involvement of carers as active members of the MDT can facilitate the overall management of the stroke patient. Immediately following stroke, it is important to inform carers of the nature of stroke, the rehabilitation process and their involvement in it, and the prospects of recovery. The carer may also require professional counselling.

The problems facing carers of the patient who remains at home may require quite different management strategies. Following discussion with the patient and carers, a designated member of the MDT, who is often the physiotherapist, should initiate access to appropriate support agencies. In the UK, many stroke services routinely involve agencies such as Meals on Wheels, Stroke Clubs, Crossroads (a carer respite agency), Chest, Heart and Stroke Association (Scotland) or The Stroke Association (England and Wales), and a designated Stroke Support Worker (see 'Associations and Support Groups').

Re-education of Movement
The physiotherapist should advise the MDT regarding the potential for recovery of functional movement, strategies for movement re-education, the extent to which each patient is susceptible to secondary trauma, and intervention strategies to prevent their occurrence.

Learning strategies for the re-education of movement are selected for the individual patient and the variables that can be manipulated include aspects of practice, feedback, the self-practice programme and the environment.

Organised Practice
Part or whole practice–A decision should be made as to whether the patient should attempt to practice some components of a task as a pretraining for performance of the whole task (Winstein, 1991).

When the amount of practice time is greater than the rest period, this is termed massed practice. Conversely, when the rest period is greater than or equal to the time taken for the task, this is distributed practice (Shumway-Cook & Woollacott, 1995). Whilst massed practice may lead to greater fatigue there is evidence that it may have a greater effect on learning. Blocked practice refers to consistent practice of a single task. Random practice is varying practice amongst distinctly different tasks (Van Sant, 1991).

Self-practice–The patient should be considered to be an active learner during rehabilitation (Ada et al., 1990). It is the responsibility of the physiotherapist to devise and teach self-practice schedules that reflect the ability of the patient, the environment and the aims and objectives of rehabilitation. The physiotherapist should monitor performance to ensure that compensatory or adaptive strategies do not develop. Carers may play a crucial part in assisting with self-practice sessions.

Feedback
Information about the success of movement is a critical ingredient of motor learning, where the learner cannot establish this information independently (Schmidt, 1991). Feedback may be provided in many forms.

Knowledge of results (KR) normally entails providing verbal information, after the attempt to move, to augment other forms of feedback indicating whether the goal has been achieved. Knowledge of performance (KP) is feedback related to the patterns of actions that led to the achievement, or not, of the goal. The bandwidth of feedback is the acceptable margin of error (bandwidth) that may occur before feedback is provided. Decisions regarding bandwidth can relate to the strategic withdrawal of feedback during rehabilitation (Schmidt, 1991).

The frequency of feedback needs to be considered, as patients may become dependent upon continual verbal feedback (Schmidt, 1991). The physiotherapist should consider reducing the frequency of feedback to enhance learning.

Transfer of Learning

When the patient is considered to be capable of living at home, motor skill acquisition must be maintained in that environment (Shumway-Cook & Woollacott, 1995). Strategies to assist in the transfer of learning include home visits involving the patient and carers, early involvement and education of carers themselves and ensuring self-practice strategies are well established prior to returning home.

In addition to assessing the patient's living environment, home visits provide an opportunity for performance and practice of established functional skills, such as moving from a lying position to sitting up over the edge of the bed, standing up from a chair, and walking. During a home visit the patient should be directed to attempt all self-practice programmes and, wherever possible, with the involvement of carers. Strategies for assisting the transfer of learning between environments should be planned well in advance of the patient's return home. This includes identifying the need for any modifications to the home.

A similar management strategy should be implemented when the decision has been reached that physiotherapy should stop for the patient in his or her own home. Treatment by the physiotherapist should be reduced, while the emphasis is placed on self-practice programmes.

Sexual Dysfunction

Because of the sensitive nature of sexual dysfunction and the age of most stroke patients, these problems are seldom discussed or considered by the MDT. Sexual problems may be linked to physical disability and emotional factors in the patient, or fear and anxiety in the sexual partner. Counselling or referral to agencies such as SPOD (Sexual and Personal Difficulties of the Disabled) may be appropriate.

Sociological Issues

The patient's race and cultural background may affect how treatment can be given. The role of gender also needs consideration.

Direct physical contact from the physiotherapist or the need to undress the patient may be unacceptable to members of certain religious or ethnic groups. Effort should be made to identify these concerns at an early stage and to make appropriate modifications to physiotherapeuic intervention. These modifications may include physiotherapy outside the normal treatment area, inviting relatives to act as chaperones, and alteration of the techniques used. Many hospitals employ representatives from ethnic groups to assist in communication between the patient and carers and healthcare professionals.

Within a pleuralistic society, religious, ethnic and gender issues that may influence the participation in rehabilitation must be considered. In some cultures, gender roles and responsibilities are quite distinct. It may be that the woman's role is to be a carer and the man to be the provider. These traditional roles may have a powerful influence on the individual following stroke with respect to motivation to become independent or to adopt a passive acceptance of the 'sick role'.

Lifestyle

In forming a rehabilitation programme, full consideration should be given to important lifestyle factors such as the patient's hobbies, pastimes and leisure interests. It may be possible to relate specific components of directed treatment or self-practice to these activities, and therefore increase motivation. Modifications to the home, for example the construction of raised flower beds, may enable the patient to continue the pursuit of specific hobbies.

To determine if a patient can return to work a number of factors need to be considered, such as the nature of the occupation, the extent of physical handicap, the attitude of the employer, the capacity to travel to and from work, and the potential to make adaptations to the work environment. It may be possible to alter the nature of the employment, with minimal retraining, to allow a return to work. In a longitudinal study of 183 patients, all of whom were under the age of 65 at the time they had a stroke, it was found that the most significant predictors of a return to work were normal muscle strength and the absence of dyspraxia (Saeki, et al., 1995).

PROBLEMS INFLUENCING PHYSICAL MANAGEMENT

Various physical and psychological problems may affect physical management and the physiotherapist must be aware of these in order to modify the management programme. Psychological problems are discussed further in Chapter 27.

Soft Tissue Complications

Soft tissue problems may involve the skin, contractures, or a painful shoulder.

Pressure sores or skin breakdown and contractures are avoidable secondary complications of stroke. Strategies for preventing skin breakdown include appropriate positioning of the patient in a bed or chair, regular assistance to enable the patient to alter position, the provision of appropriate equipment such as special seat cushions (see Chapter 8) and mattresses, and careful management of urinary and bowel incontinence.

The development of soft tissue shortening and contractures due to disuse, immobility or spasticity will inevitably affect motor function. The effects of muscle length on sarcomere loss are well documented (see Chapter 25); the physiotherapist should ensure that the patient is positioned to avoid prolonged shortening of soft issues and initiate a regimen of stretching for vulnerable tissues (see Chapter 25). Shoulder pain is common in patients with stroke and has been reported to affect rehabilitation (Van

Langenberghe *et al.*, 1988; Wanklyn *et al.*, 1996). There is no clear picture of the scale or nature of the problem but shoulder pain has been reported as being present at least once during rehabilitation or follow-up in 72% of stroke patients (Van Ouwenaller *et al.*, 1986). A number of causes of shoulder pain in hemiplegia have been suggested and include trauma, altered muscle tone, glenohumeral subluxation, contracture of capsular structures and shoulder–hand syndrome (Van Langenberghe *et al.*, 1988). Prevention of a painful shoulder should be of prime concern to the physiotherapist. This may be achieved by careful assessment of the biomechanical integrity of the glenohumeral joint and shoulder girdle, and by ensuring careful positioning and handling of the patient by members of the MDT.

Feeding Problems

Dysphagia

Dysphagia is a problem with swallowing and may occur in approximately one third of patients after stroke (Barer, 1989). For most, dysphagia may resolve in the first few days after stroke. Initial attention should determine if the patient can eat and drink independently without fear of aspiration. Assessment by the MDT should include the integrity of the swallowing and cough reflexes and the ability to co-ordinate breathing with swallowing.

Effective management of dysphagia should involve the combined intervention of the speech and language therapist, nurse and physiotherapist. The physiotherapist should assist in the control of upright posture and head position, and facilitate lip, tongue and jaw movements that may enable the patient to eat and drink.

Tube and Parenteral Feeding

Feeding by means of a nasogastric tube may be required when a patient is unable to swallow, process food within the mouth or protect the airway with an effective cough reflex. If these patients are not fed via a tube, they may become dehydrated and/or malnourished. In the long term, if problems of dysphagia continue, feeding may be delivered via a gastrostomy tube (see Chapter 8).

Orofacial Dysfunction

Orofacial dysfunction should be considered a major focus for physiotherapy following stroke. Muscle paralysis may lead to an inability to close the lips, move food in the mouth and swallow effectively, and the patient may also experience considerable embarrassment. Specific techniques to assist feeding may include: stimulation of lip closure; activation of buccinator contractions and tongue movements; and facilitation of the swallowing reflex. Attempts should be made to stimulate activity in the facial muscles, in particular those surrounding the eyes and mouth. The patient may be encouraged to practise these facial activities with a mirror. Problems such as hypersensitivity of the mouth or abnormal reflex activity, e.g. a positive bite reflex, may require desensitising techniques.

Psychological Problems

Psychological problems may include: depression; unrealistic state; labile state; and personality changes.

There is considerable evidence that a number of psychological problems may be associated with stroke. Mood disorders may affect intellectual capacity (Robinson *et al.*, 1986) and adversely affect rehabilitation (Sinyor *et al.*, 1986). The physiotherapist should be aware of any existing psychological problems and take them into account throughout the rehabilitation process. The direct management of psychological problems is the responsibility of the medical doctor and referral to a clinical psychologist may be required.

The incidence of depression may be greater in stroke patients admitted to hospital than in those who remain at home (House *et al.*, 1991). This difference may be a function of severity of stroke and reflect the greater likelihood of being admitted to hospital with a severe stroke. Some patients may have had episodes of depression prior to the stroke (Gordon, 1997).

A patient may have unrealistic rehabilitation goals that are inappropriate for the stage of recovery. The physiotherapist should discuss realistic goals with the patient and encourage him or her to recognise successful achievements.

Emotional lability is a common problem following stroke (House *et al.*, 1991) and there appears to be either a reduced threshold for, or inappropriate control of, emotions such as crying or laughing. The physiotherapist should discuss the problem sensitively with the patient.

Relatives or carers may notice personality changes—either aggressive or passive behaviour—in a person following a stroke. Carers and relatives may require counselling to help cope with feelings of fear, embarrassment, inadequacy and guilt.

Cognitive Problems

Many forms of cognitive problems can arise following stroke and the initial physiotherapy assessment may identify difficulties that require further assessment by the clinical psychologist or occupational therapist. Reduced attention span may be a problem at any stage of rehabilitation and should be considered in the design of rehabilitation programmes.

The stroke patient may have difficulties with short-term memory recall (Wade, 1985a) that will affect the ability to relearn functional movement tasks. Repetitive simple instructions, visual and verbal cues, involvement of carers, part practice of tasks and the use of practice books or task performance diaries may be helpful (Ada *et al.*, 1990).

Perceptual Problems

Problems of perception are considered to be one of the main factors limiting functional motor recovery following stroke (Turnbull, 1986). Patients who have had a right-sided CVA, and therefore have left hemiplegia, have the most severe perceptual problems.

Visuospatial Neglect

In visuospatial neglect the patient fails to respond appropriately to stimuli presented on the hemiplegic side. It is more common and often severe following right parietal lesions but may be present with damage to the left hemisphere. Management strategies include addressing the patient from the affected side, deliberate placement of items such as tissues or drinks on that side, and advice to carers regarding the position they should adopt whilst talking to the patient (Robertson & North, 1992; Riddoch et al., 1995).

Agnosia

Agnosia has been defined as loss of knowledge or inability to perceive objects through otherwise normally functioning sensory pathways (Kandel et al., 1995). This group of perceptual disorders, related to the inability to recognise previously familiar objects, may affect the patient in a number of ways. Patients may deny or disown the existence of their own affected arm or leg, and in severe instances they may exhibit an inability to recognise familiar faces (prosopagnosia). During any form of intervention, the patient should be assisted to observe his or her own limbs in an attempt to promote recognition.

Dyspraxia

Difficulty in executing volitional purposeful movements is termed dyspraxia. This phenomenon may be exposed in the patient who appears to have good comprehension, normal sensation and some recovery of ability to move.

Dyspraxia may influence the completion of any functional task. For example, a patient who is able to flex and extend the joints in a hand may be unable to grasp a cup when attempting to drink. Dressing dyspraxia is a recognised example of this perceptual impairment: the patient understands the purpose of dressing but is unable to complete the task appropriately. Typically, he or she may attempt to place the head in the sleeve of a shirt, or put a jacket on back-to-front. The literature provides little direction as to the management of these problems. The physiotherapist should reassure the patient and devise simple movement sequences that might facilitate the completion of functional tasks.

SUMMARY OF PHYSICAL MANAGEMENT

The main components of physiotherapeutic management for stroke have been reviewed and linked to current understanding of recovery. In the light of this knowledge, stages of physiotherapeutic management have been proposed, reflecting important episodes and processes inherent within physiotherapy management. Delivery of physiotherapy has been elaborated, with the intention of making appropriate use of finite resources. A problem-solving model, designed to facilitate decision making and establish effectiveness of practice, has been detailed. Finally, key aspects of general management have been introduced and placed in the overall context of stroke rehabilitation.

REFERENCES

Ada L, Canning C, eds. Key issues in neurological physiotherapy. Oxford: Butterworth Heinemann; 1990.

Ada L, Canning C, Westwood P. The patient as an active learner. In: Ada L, Canning C, eds. Key issues in neurological physiotherapy. Oxford: Butterworth Heinemann; 1990:99-124.

Allen CMC, Harrison MJG, Wade DT. The management of acute stroke. Tunbridge Wells: Castle House Publications; 1988.

Anderson C. Baseline measures and outcome predictors. Neuroepidemiology 1994, 13:283-289.

[Anonymous] Stroke rehabilitation. Leeds: Leeds Evaluation Unit; 1992. (Effective Health Care Series).

Ashburn A, Partridge CJ, DeSouza L. Physiotherapy in the rehabilitation of stroke: a review. Clin Rehab 1993, 7:337-345.

Ashburn A. Methods of assessing the physical disabilities of stroke patients. Physiother Pract 1986, 2:59-62.

Bamford J, Sandercock P, Dennis M, et al. A prospective study of acute cerebrovascular disease in the community: the Oxfordshire Community Stroke Project 1981-86. 1. Methodology, demography and incident cases of first-ever stroke. J Neurol Neurosurg Psychiat 1988, 51:1373-1380.

Bamford J, Sandercock P, Dennis M, et al. Classification and natural history of clinically identifiable subtypes of cerebral infarction. Lancet 1991, 337:1521-1526.

Barer DH. The natural history and functional consequences of dysphagia after hemispheric stroke. J Neurol Neurosurg Psychiat 1989, 52:236-241.

Bobath B. Adult hemiplegia: Evaluation and treatment, 3rd edition. London: Heinemann; 1990.

Bohannon RW, Williams Andrews A. Relationship between impairments and gait performance after stroke: a summary of relevant research. Gait Posture 1995, 3:236-240.

Brown MM, Humphrey PRD. Carotid endarterectomy: recommendations for the management of transient ischaemic attacks and ischaemic stroke. Br Med J 1992, 305:1071-1074.

Carr EK, Kenney F. Positioning the stroke patient: a review of the literature. Int J Nurs Stud 1992, 29:355-369.

Carr JH, Shepherd RB. A motor relearning programme for stroke, 2nd edition. Oxford: Butterworth Heinemann; 1987.

Carr JH, Shepherd RB. A motor learning model for stroke rehabilitation. Physiotherapy 1989, 75:372-380.

Carr JH, Shepherd RB, Nordholm L, et al. Investigation of a new Motor Assessment Scale for stroke patients. Phys Ther 1985, 65:175-180.

Carter P, Edwards MS. General principles of treamtent. In: Edwards MS, ed. Neurological physiotherapy: A problem solving approach. Edinburgh: Churchill Livingstone; 1996:87-112.

Davies P. Steps to follow. Berlin: Springer Verlag; 1985.

Draper BM, Poulos CJ, Cole AM, et al. Who cares for the carer of the old and ill? Med J Aust 1991, 154:293.

Duncan PW, Goldstein LB, Horner RD, et al. Similar motor recovery of upper and lower extremities after stroke. Stroke 1994, 25:1181-1188.

Durward BR, Baer GD. Physiotherapy and neurology: towards research-based practice. Physiotherapy 1995, 81:436-439.

Ehrlich F, Bowring G, Draper BM, et al. Caring for carers - a rational problem. Med J Aust 1992, 156:590-592.

Ellul J, Watkins C, Ferguson N, *et al.* Increasing patient engagement in rehabilitation activities. *Clin Rehab* 1993, **7**:297-302.

Ernst E. A review of stroke rehabilitation and physiotherapy. *Stroke* 1990, **21**:1081-1085.

Gordon WA, Hibbard MR. Post-Stroke Depression: an examination of the literature. *Arch Phys Med Rehabil* 1997, **78**:658-663.

Hannaford PC, Croft PR, Kay CR. Oral contraception and stroke. *Stroke* 1994, **25**:935-942.

Hough A. *Physiotherapy in respiratory care: a problem solving approach.* London: Chapman & Hall; 1991.

House A, Dennis M, Morgridge L, *et al.* Mood disorders in the year after first stroke. *Br J Psych* 1991, **158**:83-92.

Jongbloed L. Prediction of function after stroke: a critical review. *Stroke* 1986, **17**:765-776.

Kalra L. The influence of stroke unit rehabilitation on functional recovery from stroke. *Stroke* 1994, **25**:821-825.

Kandel ER, Schwartz JH, Jessell TM. *Essentials of neural science and behavior.* USA: Appleton & Lange; 1995:701.

Kannel WB, Wolf PA. Epidemiology of cerebrovascular disease. In: Ross Rusell RW, ed. *Vascular disease of the central nervous system.* Edinburgh: Churchill Livingstone; 1983:1-24.

Kettenbach G. *Writing SOAP notes.* Philadelphia: FA Davis; 1990.

Langton Hewer R. The epidemiology of disabling neurological disorders. In: Greenwood R, Barnes MP, McMillan TM, *et al.*, eds. *Neurological rehabilitation.* London: Churchill Livingstone; 1993:3-12.

Lincoln NB, Leadbitter D. Assessment of motor function in stroke patients. *Physiotherapy* 1979, **65**:48-51.

Lincoln NB, Willis D *et al.* Comparison of rehabilitation practice on hospital wards for stroke patients. *Stroke*, 1996; **27**:18-23.

Lynch M, Grisogono V. *Strokes and head injuries: A guide for patients, families, friends and carers.* London: John Murray; 1991.

Partridge CJ, Morris LW, Edwards MS. Recovery from physical disability after stroke: profiles for different levels of starting severity. *Clin Rehab* 1993, **7**:210-217.

Riddoch MJ, Humphreys GW, Bateman A. Cognitive deficits following stroke. *Physiotherapy* 1995, **81**:465-473.

Robertson IH, North N. Spatio-motor cueing in unilateral left neglect: the role of hemispace, hand and motor activation. *Neuropsychology* 1992, **30**:553-563.

Robinson R, Bolla Wilson K, Kaplan E, *et al.* Depression influences intellectual impairment in stroke patients. *Br J Psych* 1986, **148**:541-547.

Saeki S, Ogata H, Okubo T, *et al.* Return to work after stroke: a follow-up study. *Stroke* 1995, **26**:399-401.

Salter PM, Ferguson RM. A process of physiotherapy: an analysis of the activities of the physiotherapist. *Proceedings of the World Confederation for Physical Therapy.* London: 11th International Congress; 1991:1704-1706.

Schmidt RA. Motor learning principles for physical therapy. In: Lister MJ, ed. Contemporary management of motor control problems. *Proceedings of the II STEP Conference.* USA: Foundation for Physical Therapy; 1991:49-63.

Scottish Office Home & Health Department. *The Management of Patients with Stroke.* Edinburgh: HMSO; 1993.

Shumway-Cook A & Woollacott M. *Motor Control, Theory and Practical Applications.* Baltimore City: Williams and Wilkins; 1995.

Sinyor D, Amato P, Kaloupek DG *et al.* Post stroke depression: relationships to functional impairment, coping strategies and rehabilitation outcomes. *Stroke*, 1986 **17**:1102-1107.

Smith M, Ball V. *Cardiovascular/Respiratory Physiotherapy.* London: Mosby; 1998. In progress.

Smith MT, Baer GD. Measuring the outcome of specific stroke subtypes using simple mobility milestones. *Physiotherapy*, 1997; **83**:354.

Tinson DJ. How stroke patients spend their days. *Int Disabil Stud* 1989, **11**:45-49.

Turnbull GI. The application of motor learning theory. In: Banks M, ed. *Stroke.* Edinburgh: Churchill Livingstone; 1986.

Van Langenberghe HVK, Partridge CJ, Edwards MS *et al.* Shoulder pain in hemiplegia - a literature review. *Physiother Prac* 1988, **4**:155-162.

Van Ouwenaller C, LaPlace PM, Chantraine A. Painful shoulder in hemiplegia. *Arch Phys Med Rehabil* 1986, **67**: 23-26.

VanSant AF. Motor control, motor learning and motor development. In: Montgomery PC, Connolly BH, eds. *Motor Control and Physical Therapy: Theoretical Framework and Practical Applications.* Tennessee: Chattanooga Group Inc; 1991:13-28.

Wade DT, Collen FM, Robb GF *et al.* Physiotherapy intervention late after stroke. *Brit Med J* 1992, **405**:609-613.

Wade DT, Langton Hewer L, Skilbech CE *et al. Stroke: a critical approach to diagnosis, treatment and management.* London: Chapman Hall; 1985a.

Wade DT, Wood VA & Langton Hewer R. Recovery after stroke - the first 3 months. *J Neurol Neurosurg Psychiat* 1985b, **48**:7-13.

Wanklyn P, Forster A, Young J. Hemiplegic Shoulder Pain (HSP); natural history and investigation of associated features. *Disability and Rehab,* 1996;**18**:497-501.

Whisnant JP. Effectiveness versus efficacy of treatment of hypertension for stroke prevention. *Neurol* 1996, **46**: 301-307.

Williams P. *Gray's Anatomy.* London: Churchill Livingstone; 1995.

Winstein CJ. Designing practice for motor learning: clinical implications. In: Lister, MJ, ed. Contemporary Management of Motor Control Problems. *Proceedings of the II STEP Conference* USA: Foundation for Physical Therapy; 1991:65-76.

Wood J & Wade J. Setting up stroke services in district general hospitals. *Brit J Ther Rehabil* 1995, **2**:199-203.

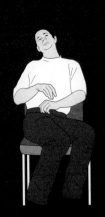

8

C Collin & G Daly

BRAIN INJURY

CHAPTER OUTLINE

- Brain injury assessment scales
- Epidemiology
- Risk factors and prevention
- Pathophysiology
- Early general management of brain injury

- Later general management of brain injury
- Post concussional syndrome after mild head injury
- Physical management
- Case history

INTRODUCTION

Head injuries are a major health problem: they can cause death or disability, change permanently the abilities and prospects of the injured, and disturb the lives of their family members. Where there is no family able to care for the patient, society pays the price for the damaged survivor.

Head trauma may cause extracranial injuries of the scalp and face, maxillofacial and skull fractures, and cranial nerve and brain injury. Skull fractures may be simple or compound, undisplaced or depressed. Brain injury may be primary (immediate), occurring in the moment of the injury, or secondary, occurring as a result of other injuries or at a later point in time; secondary brain injury may be avoidable. Head injury can be caused by an incident as apparently trivial as two people knocking their heads together when stooping to pick up some fallen fruit in a supermarket, or by a serious event such as a high-speed crash on a motorway. Serious head injury may lead to coma and severe physical and cognitive deficits that require months of in-patient rehabilitation.

BRAIN INJURY ASSESSMENT SCALES

Brain injury may be classified according to the worst level of coma observed, by the length of post-traumatic amnesia, or by an outcome scale such as the Glasgow Outcome Scale. Coma is usually measured by the Glasgow Coma Scale (GCS), first described by Teasdale & Jennett in 1974 (Table 8.1). This scores behavioural responses to verbal command or painful stimuli in three areas of activity: eye opening, best motor response and best verbal response. Each scale is hierarchical and has been shown to have a high level of interobserver agreement. The verbal response score can be modified for children under the age of 5 years (Table 8.2).

Brain injury can also be classified retrospectively into severity using Ritchie Russell's categorisation based on post-traumatic amnesia (PTA)—the length of time between injury and the restoration of continuous day-to-day memory (Russell & Smith, 1961). There are three categories: mild, <1 hour; moderate, 1–24 hours; and severe or very severe, >24 hours. Length of PTA can only be judged retrospectively by interviewing the patient; a judgement on continuous memory might be made by presenting a picture recognition test at 24-hour intervals (Artiola *et al.*, 1980) or an orientation questionnaire like the Galveston Orientation and Amnesia Test (GOAT; Levin *et al.*, 1979).

The Glasgow Coma Scale	
Eye opening	
Spontaneous	4
To sound	3
To pain	2
No response	1
Best motor response	
Obeys	6
Localises	5
Withdraws	4
Flexion - abnormal (decorticate rigidity)	3
Extends (decerebrate rigidity)	2
No response	1
Best verbal response	
Oriented and converses	5
Disoriented and converses	4
Inappropriate words	3
Incomprehensible sounds	2
No response	1
Total score	3-15

Table 8.1 The Glasgow Coma Scale. (Devised by Teasdale & Jennett, 1974.)

Modified GCS for vocal responses from children under 5 years			
2-5 years		**<2 years**	
Words of any sort	5	Coos, smiles, cries	5
Monosyllables	4	Cries only	4
Cries or screams	3	Unstimulated screaming	3
Grunts	2	Grunts	2
None	1	None	1

Table 8.2 Modified Glasgow Coma Scale (GCS) for vocal responses from children under 5 years.

Another retrospective scale of severity of brain injury is the aforementioned Glasgow Outcome Scale (GOS) which was developed by Jennett & Bond (1975). It is a simple 5-point scale describing the following levels of recovery:
1. Death.
2. Persistent vegetative state.
3. Severe disability—conscious but disabled and dependent for daily support.
4. Moderate disability—disabled but independent (these patients can travel by public transport, work in a sheltered environment).
5. Good recovery (this implies resumption of normal life although there may be minor neurological and psychological deficits).

The vegetative state (VS), referred to in Stage 2 of the GOS scale, has been defined as: 'clinical condition of unawareness of self and environment in which the patient breathes spontaneously, has a stable circulation and shows cycles of eye closure and eye opening which may stimulate sleep and waking' (Black *et al.*, 1996). The state may be considered persistent or permanent (PVS) if it continues for more than 12 months after head injury.

In 1981 Jennett *et al.* subdivided each of the grades 3, 4 and 5 into a higher and a lower level, converting the GOS into an 8-point scale, with greater sensitivity, but lower reliability.

Severity of head injury, including injury to the brain, might alternatively be classified according to the nature of the skull fracture or the findings on CT scan, based on intracranial measurements of amount of midline shift, compression of the cisterns, or size of intracerebral lesions. Some knowledge of the inclusion criteria is required before the results of outcome studies can be interpreted fairly. The most widely accepted criteria of severity appear to be the GCS score and the length of PTA, plotted from the moment of injury and including the period in coma. These are both measures of cerebral function, rather than anatomical disruption. Scores on the GCS scale need to be interpreted more carefully if there is any metabolic disturbance present at the time of injury. The most common substance found at this stage is alcohol, and is implicated in 30–80% of all head injuries.

EPIDEMIOLOGY

The incidence and prevalence of all head injury is unknown because much goes unreported, but the number of head injuries that attract medical attention has been counted. The numbers vary around the world, but figures demonstrate that young men are the most likely victims in all societies. The overall reported incidence of head injury resulting in hospital admission, at all ages, in England and Wales is 270/100,000 per annum (Jennett & MacMillan, 1981) with a ratio of admission to death of 30:1. This is five times lower than the numbers with head injury attending hospital (1800/100,000 per annum), suggesting that in the

UK approximately 1 million people visit Accident and Emergency Units with a head injury each year. Small babies and children attend most frequently but men aged 15–24 have the most serious injuries (Field, 1976).

RISK FACTORS AND PREVENTION

Head injury accounts for 15% of all deaths in childhood. The commonest causes in children are falls, followed by road traffic accidents, sporting accidents, and assaults. In adolescents and adults, alcohol is reported as a contributory cause in 30–80% of all head injuries, and road traffic accidents are a more prominent cause of injury than in childhood. Men aged 15–24 have the highest personal risk and >30% of deaths in this group are due to head injury; this falls to <5% after the age of 40 in both sexes (Field, 1976).

Reduction of injury in childhood can be achieved by separating play areas from roads with physical barriers (Sharples *et al.*, 1990) and by recognising and reducing the risk factors for non-accidental injury. Improved control of alcohol use might be expected to reduce the incidence of head injury in adolescents and adults. The introduction of compulsory helmet use by motorcyclists was associated with a fall in death rate and non-fatal head injuries. The results of helmet use in cyclists have been difficult to monitor because where their use has been made compulsory, there has been an overall reduction in cycling use. McDermott (1995) in Australia reported a 48% reduction in serious head injury in the first year after legislation was introduced for compulsory helmet use and a reduction of 70% in the second year. Similar findings have been reported by Thompson *et al.* (1989) in the USA. The introduction of front-seat airbags into cars may further reduce injuries in line with the reduction caused by seat-belt use. A reduction of driving speed to 20 miles/h in urban areas might help reduce the number and severity of head injuries. Segregated car-free cycle lanes have been introduced but not widely enough.

Some sports, e.g. rugby and football, are associated with a risk of head injury and it may never be possible to legislate the risk away even though strenuous efforts may be made. In the case of boxing, in which the purpose of the sport is to render one player unconscious, severe head injuries or cumulative severe head injury will continue to occur.

PATHOPHYSIOLOGY

Injury to the brain may be primary, due to direct insult, or secondary, caused by indirect effects from injuries to other structures or by complications after head injury.

PRIMARY BRAIN INJURY
The brain is enclosed in a rigid container, the cranium. In injury the brain may be subject to a direct crushing blow, as in an assault. In a motorway crash, the brain may be brought to a sudden standstill in a few seconds. This produces a combination of a twisting deceleration injury and a direct impact, and exerts a mixture of linear and rotational forces on the gel-like substance of the brain. This contains millions of nerve fibres and a complex vascular system, which are deformed as the brain is shaken within or torn against the sharp edges of the sphenoid wings, the petrous temporal bones or the falx. These forces may be strong enough to tear or disrupt cranial nerves from brain tissue. The cortex of the brain may be damaged either by a direct blow or by shearing forces against the internal surface of the skull, producing localised contusions with haemorrhage. These characteristically affect the undersurface of the frontal lobes or the front of the temporal lobes.

Acute deceleration injuries are usually associated with diffuse axonal injury. This was first reported by Strich (1956), after post-mortem examination of brain tissue revealed shearing injuries of white matter, and has been confirmed by others. It is now best demonstrated with immunocyto-chemical staining techniques (Grady *et al.*, 1993). Small retraction balls or axonal swellings were seen amongst normal axons. Where axoplasm had continued to flow along a disrupted axon, a ball had formed at the point of disruption. Later (after days) a cellular reaction took place that produced an appearance of microglial stars. Weeks later, marked atrophy was observed, with relative expansion of the ventricles. Diffuse axonal injury has been shown to occur in mild head injury (Povlishock *et al.*, 1983).

Coup/contrecoup lesions are seen as a result of falls or, occasionally, direct blows. These are focal cortical contusions at the site of impact and also on the opposite side of the brain, or there may even be no contusion at the site of impact. The classic example is the individual who falls over backwards and strikes the occiput, doing little or no posterior damage but sustaining haemorrhagic contusions of one or both frontal lobes. The explanation is probably that the frontal lobes are more prone to damage on the orbital ridges; in a fall, the injury is still a deceleration injury, with a linear or rotational vector that causes deformation of the brain against the internal surfaces of the skull.

Vascular damage is one of the main components of both primary and secondary brain damage. In primary damage there is often evidence of subarachnoid bleeding on computerised tomography (CT) scanning, and angiography studies have shown that vasospasm may be a major feature. Small areas of petechial haemorrhage in subcortical white matter are observed on CT scanning, in association with diffuse axonal injury, and are thought to represent shearing injuries. The size of these traumatic haemorrhages is usually an indicator of severity. Intracerebral and subdural haematomas may form acutely at the time of primary injury and are usually associated with primary brain damage.

SECONDARY BRAIN INJURY
Secondary brain injury is to some extent avoidable or treatable. It may be due to extracranial or intracranial factors. Avoidable deaths are thought to be those in which the patient is conscious or talks after the injury but then lapses back into coma, usually with an extradural haematoma

and little underlying brain damage. Secondary brain damage can be classified into extracranial and intracranial.

Extracranial

Extracranial causes of secondary brain damage include chest and other multiple injuries that may lead to cardiac arrest or hypotension or hypoxia. These require urgent treatment to prevent a secondary hypoxic insult to the brain.

Hypoxia and Hypotension

Hypoxia produces an increase in cerebral blood flow but this regulatory mechanism eventually fails, and will fail more quickly if there is accompanying hypotension, which causes a reduced cerebral perfusion pressure (CPP). CPP is affected by mean arterial blood pressure (BP) or by an increased intracranial pressure (ICP) and can be calculated using the equation CPP = BP – ICP (Ada *et al.*, 1990). In major trauma with head injury, there is nearly always a period of time when blood pressure falls and intracranial pressure rises; if CPP falls below a critical level, the cerebral blood flow regulatory mechanisms are lost and ischaemic damage takes place (Mendelow *et al.*, 1983).

Intracranial

Intracranial causes of secondary brain damage include acute traumatic haematomas, infection and raised intracranial pressure.

Acute Traumatic Haematomas

These haematomas may be classified according to site: extradural, subdural and intracerebral. Extradural haematomas are usually associated with a skull fracture caused by an injury due to a fall or an assault. The typical case is of a young man admitted late at night after a fight, with a scalp wound and an underlying skull fracture, initially talking or shouting, but with repeated GCS scores documenting a falling level of consciousness. A CT scan will typically demonstrate an extradural haematoma that requires urgent neurosurgical evacuation or immediate burr-hole surgery. There may have been few initial physical signs followed by a rapidly increasing hemiparesis. Underlying serious brain injury is often minimal and if it is detected early enough these patients can make a full recovery.

Subdural and intracerebral haematomas are usually associated with high-velocity injuries and serious underlying brain damage, with cortical contusions and lacerations. They can collectively be called intradural haematomas because a more specific diagnosis is not helpful (Galbraith & Teasdale, 1982). They are usually associated with a raised ICP and secondary hypoxia. Bleeding into the ventricles or subarachnoid spaces is often associated with acute hydrocephalus, requiring external cerebrospinal fluid (CSF) drainage.

Infection

Infection is a serious event after traumatic brain injury, often associated with compound fracture and leakage of CSF. Meningitis or cerebral abscess may occur, and may in turn cause further brain injury due to local swelling and hypoxia. Infection may also predispose to the development of hydrocephalus.

Raised ICP

Raised ICP occurs after severe head injury, and the increasing use of monitoring devices shows that it remains raised for much longer periods of time than was previously expected (Bullock & Teasdale, 1990). It is caused by oedema of the brain and an increase in its blood volume. It is influenced adversely by routine nursing procedures, adjustment of posture, catheter care, and physiotherapy. Its relationship with cerebral blood volume can be likened to the 'chicken and egg' situation: experimentally, a raised ICP can be shown to increase cerebral blood volume by compression of veins, and increased cerebral blood volume may be the cause of raised ICP. Oedema of the brain includes cytotoxic oedema, a swelling of damaged brain cells, and interstitial oedema, a collection of fluid between the cells. Vasogenic oedema has also been described (Crockard, 1985). Early after brain injury a CT scan may reveal only what is described as a 'tight looking' brain, with loss of contrast due to brain swelling, and compression of the ventricles and basal cisterns. Magnetic resonance (MR) imaging may reveal greater detail and show haemorrhagic lesions in subcortical white matter and the brainstem.

Children under the age of 2 years who present with altered level of consciousness due to a fall in the home may be the victims of non-accidental injury. Occurrence of a lucid interval followed by neurological deterioration may be associated with intracranial haematoma formation as in adults, and in children a greater proportion of these are extradural and treatable. Deterioration after quite mild injury may be due to cerebral oedema or increased cerebral blood volume, both of which will be demonstrated by raised ICP. There may also be cerebral arterial vasospasm and ictal activity (i.e. focal seizures).

Monitoring of ICP in children and adults has demonstrated that it can remain raised for many days and is also subject to wide fluctuations on movement of the patient for nursing or physiotherapy procedures (Unterberg *et al.*, 1993).

EARLY GENERAL MANAGEMENT OF BRAIN INJURY

Management in the immediate post-injury stage involves emergency procedures, assessment, possibly neurosurgery, and nutritional and fluid balance care.

GENERAL MEASURES

Early assessment must proceed alongside treatment for any life-threatening situation. Standard procedures for general resuscitation, including maintenance of an adequate airway and ventilation, correction of hypotension and control of major haemorrhage, and other life-support measures, should be followed (Jennett & Teasdale, 1981; Morgan,

1994). Level of consciousness should be measured using the GCS. If the patient is not paralysed or ventilated then the GCS should be reassessed frequently. The history of the injury should be recorded from observers or ambulance crew, including the level of consciousness from the moment of injury onwards. If there was a lucid interval preceding coma, then the patient may require urgent neurosurgical evacuation of haematoma. Focal neurological signs may be present to suggest the localisation of brain injury, but other injuries, e.g. brachial plexus lesions, may confuse the overall picture. Changes in pupillary reactions in the absence of local eye trauma may be helpful in detecting a deterioration due to midline shift or pressure on the brainstem.

ASSESSMENT OF SEVERITY

In addition to the subjective assessment scales mentioned above, objective investigations can also be carried out.

Skull X-ray

Guidelines have been developed to reduce the amount of radiography performed because it is often not helpful in diagnosis of brain injury. A normal skull X-ray can be compatible with severe brain injury leading to death, but detection of a closed fracture identifies those patients with an increased tendency to later complications due to haematoma formation. Loss of consciousness, clinical signs suggesting fracture, focal neurology, confused behaviour or a significant history of a deceleration injury are all indicators for skull X-ray, and, in many cases, spinal X-rays to detect neck injuries commonly associated with head injuries.

CT and MR Imaging

Where readily available, CT scanning has replaced skull radiography as the investigation of first choice. A CT scan can adequately demonstrate a skull fracture, particularly where there is displacement of bone fragments. Its great importance lies in its ability to define fluid collections and midline shift. Parenchymal haemorrhages appear as areas of increased density on CT scan; MR imaging provides higher definition of these lesions and will detect haemorrhages unsuspected on CT scan. Unfortunately, CT scans are not freely available and patients may have to be moved to the facility where the investigation is available and then moved again to a neurosurgical centre for treatment. Those patients at high risk of intradural and extradural haemorrhage must be selected for early CT scan to ensure that there is an opportunity to treat before fatal brain compression occurs. The two main risk factors are: skull fracture; and loss or change in level of consciousness after a lucid interval. The risk of significant haemorrhage is of the order of 1:4 when both these factors are present and as low as 1:8000 when neither is present (Mendelow et al., 1983; Teasdale et al., 1990).

Electroencephalography (EEG)

This has little part to play in the assessment of acute head injury but may be useful in the longer term in patients who

have remained in coma (see Chapter 3).

Somatosensory evoked potentials have been the subject of investigation as prognostic indicators but have not become a clinically useful tool and are not widely available (see Chapter 3). Inability to demonstrate a cortical response to peripheral stimuli suggests a uniformly bad prognosis.

ICP Monitoring

Originally, ICP monitoring was performed to derive a reading which was normal or raised, but monitoring is now continuous. The intraventricular route is considered best for ICP monitoring and provides a means of draining CSF, but this is performed only in neurosurgical centres. Many serious head injuries are managed in the District General Hospital (DGH) because of inadequate availability of neurosurgical beds. CT scans taken in the DGH can often be faxed to the local neurosurgical centre and if there is no possibility of useful neurosurgical intervention these patients will remain in the DGH. It is now possible to monitor the ICP of these patients in the Intensive Care Unit in a DGH with the development of subarachnoid bolts which do not require neurosurgical expertise for accurate placement (Addy et al., 1996). Raised ICP can be lowered by a variety of techniques including sedation, hyperventilation and osmotic diuretic drugs. The indications for ICP monitoring in patients not requiring neurosurgery include a GCS score of 8 or less, a midline shift on CT scan of more than 0.5 mm and compression of the basal cisterns.

Use of ICP monitoring can predict when it is safe to reduce sedation and wean the patient off ventilation. The use of ICP monitors appears to lengthen the period of elective ventilation significantly but it is too early to say whether it is associated with a significant reduction in mortality or morbidity.

Positron Emission Tomography (PET) and Single Photon Emission Computed Tomography SPECT)

PET is used for producing functional rather than anatomical or structural brain images (Herscovitch, 1996). It provides information about regional blood flow and oxygen or glucose metabolism, depending on the isotope used, e.g. ^{15}O, ^{18}F or ^{11}C.

SPECT uses more readily available, longer lasting isotopes and conventional rotating gamma cameras to produce images that are related to blood flow, and can show hyper- and hypoperfusion. SPECT requires a much smaller investment in equipment but produces data of lower resolution than does PET.

Neither of these sophisticated techniques, which remain expensive research tools, is yet of practical value in the management of brain injury. A global reduction of cortical blood flow is usually associated with a very poor outcome and has been demonstrated using both procedures. They have been used as the gold standard for the development of functional MR imaging.

NEUROSURGICAL INTERVENTION

Neurosurgery is not described in any detail in this book and the reader is referred to Black & Rossitch (1995). Neurosurgical opinion should be sought in all head injuries associated with skull fracture, seizures, neurological signs, deteriorating level of consciousness, depressed or compound skull fractures, basal skull fractures and persisting (>8 hours) coma or confusion. Intervention may include ICP monitoring, evacuation of a clot through a craniotomy or burr hole, surgical debridement of dirty wounds, and elevation of bone fragments. Antibiotics are no longer used routinely in all compound skull fractures but are selectively used when the risk of infection is high, e.g. in basal skull fractures where there is communication between the brain and sinuses around the nose or middle ear. Meningitis or brain abscess may occur. Superficial wound infections are not uncommon but bone infections are rare.

NUTRITION

Patients with head injuries still arrive in rehabilitation facilities with varying degrees of cachexia, suggesting that their nutritional requirements are often underestimated. After severe head injury, many patients have hyperpyrexia and sweating due to autonomic dysregulation, hypercatabolism and hypermetabolism (Clifton *et al.*, 1984). There is evidence of increased loss of nitrogen, calcium and protein. Major weight loss may increase morbidity and mortality, impair tissue healing and contribute to the development of pressure sores and other complications. Early after the head injury there may be paralytic ileus, and feeding via a nasogastric tube may need to begin slowly. Gastric erosions are common and H2 receptor drugs may be necessary. If gastric stasis is prolonged, then a motility stimulant such as metoclopramide might be useful. If nasogastric feeding is prolonged, conversion to percutaneous endoscopic gastrostomy (PEG) is recommended as it is aesthetically more acceptable and less likely to be pulled out. If a PEG tube is pulled out, a small Foley catheter should immediately be inserted and the bulb inflated to keep the PEG site patent until a new gastrostomy tube can be sited. At least 3000 kcal should be given daily; weekly weighing will indicate whether more is required.

FLUID BALANCE

In the acute stage, accurate fluid balance records must be kept, the patient being catheterised so that urine volume can be measured. Insensible loss due to sweating may be high. There may also be excessive loss due to the use of mannitol to lower ICP. Parenteral fluid replacement is required initially and daily plasma electrolytes are required.

Overhydration or the use of too much dextrose may lead to hyponatraemia, which can itself cause brain swelling. Inappropriate antidiuretic hormone (ADH) secretion is probably overdiagnosed, low plasma sodium more often being due to overhydration, or failure to replace sodium losses. Hyperglycaemia should also be avoided because of its potential to increase the severity of ischaemic neuroneal cell death.

LATER GENERAL MANAGEMENT OF BRAIN INJURY

The commonest medical complications requiring treatment will now be discussed. The patient should have been moved from the acute sector and be commencing a period of intensive rehabilitation with supervision by a multidisciplinary neurorehabilitation team experienced in head injury management. Goal-oriented interdisciplinary practice, with regular evaluation of impairment and disability using recognised measures, is recommended. There should be regular team meetings, including the patient and family at intervals. The family or friends should gain confidence in the multidisciplinary team (MDT) and see that change is taking place in the head-injured person. A small number of patients may remain in prolonged coma and their placement will depend on local facilities and resources, but they should have an active rehabilitation programme to prevent complications and enhance recovery if it occurs.

The head injury rehabilitation team will usually include a medical specialist, a neuropsychologist, an occupational therapist, a speech and language therapist, a dietician, a seating specialist, a rehabilitation nurse, a social worker, and a physiotherapist. One of these may be the patient's keyworker or care manager but this may be a separate appointment.

Impairment and disability depend on which areas of the brain are damaged but often follow typical patterns according to right or left hemisphere or brainstem involvement. Infarction of an arterial territory may be superimposed on severe diffuse axonal injury in the brainstem. Temporal lobe damage may be associated with epilepsy or mood dysequilibrium. Occipital lobe damage may be associated with visual field loss or cortical blindness.

Physical disability is rarely the cause of the greatest handicap. Cognitive impairment, poor memory, lack of initiative, motivation or drive, and personality change seem to provide the greatest personal morbidity and lead to family breakdown, isolation and grief. Executive function, decision making and concentration may be seriously impaired after quite mild head injury and this may be relatively resistant to treatment. Specialised input is required to help individuals cope with these aspects of head injury (McMillan & Greenwood, 1993).

CRANIAL NERVE DAMAGE

This may be temporary or permanent, depending on the site and severity of brain trauma, and may initially produce confusing physical signs. Bilateral facial and oculomotor paresis produces an expressionless face with little opportunity for meaningful eye contact but full recovery may occur over months. From the patient's point of view, bilateral oculomotor and facial palsies mean that everything is seen in duplicate and blurred images; he or she cannot blink or open the eyes fully, and the face feels stiff and no longer moves. There may also be troublesome tinnitus, vertigo or deafness if the eighth nerve is affected.

The olfactory nerve is very prone to damage where it passes through the cribriform plate; such damage produces partial or complete loss of smell and an associated reduction in taste. Visual acuity may be reduced or vision lost altogether due to direct damage to the optic nerve, either from fracture of the orbit or from the effect of raised ICP on the blood supply of the nerve. More posteriorly, the optic tract or its radiations through to the occipital cortex may be damaged, producing characteristic hemianopic or quadrantanopic field losses. Recovery of these rarely occurs. The nerves controlling eye movement are often affected early in head injury, producing diplopia which gradually resolves. The oculomotor and abducens nerves are most commonly affected by raised pressure, or by fracture of the middle cranial fossa.

The trochlear nerve is rarely reported as damaged but it is possible that it may have recovered by the time its function is fully tested when looking down whilst walking downstairs. Initially, diplopia should be prevented when doing close work by the use of an eye patch, used alternately on each eye. Focusing and pupillary reactions may also remain sluggish. If diplopia is persistent it may be reduced or abolished by the introduction of prismatic lenses. The orthoptist should undertake regular review of patients with traumatic diplopia. Rarely, opthalmological intervention may be necessary to reduce diplopia when looking straight ahead.

The auditory system may be affected due to direct trauma to the middle ear and disruption of the ossicles, which may be surgically remediable, or to cochlear damage producing deafness and tinnitus. Labyrinthine or vestibular nerve damage is likely to cause vertigo or dizziness. Benign paroxysmal positional vertigo is common after quite mild head injury and is thought to be due to calcium debris breaking off and floating freely in the semicircular canals. Specific head manoeuvres may be taught to minimise the symptoms but specialist assessment is recommended; symptoms often resolve over months. The trigeminal nerve and lower cranial nerves (ninth to twelfth) rarely attract clinical attention although they are undoubtedly damaged in some cases.

EPILEPSY

Post-traumatic epilepsy is relatively uncommon, occurring in <5% of all head injuries. It is reasonable to wait until the individual has had two fits before recommending treatment, although in some patients with a known high risk treatment may be introduced after one fit. Until recently most patients sustaining head injury requiring neurosurgical input were started on prophylactic anticonvulsants. There is no good evidence that this policy reduced the incidence of post-traumatic epilepsy. The risk factors for epilepsy after head injury were established by Jennett (1975) and include: early fits occurring in the first week after injury; depressed skull fracture; and intracranial

haematoma. Post-traumatic amnesia for >24 hours also increases the risk. Risk tables drawn from Jennett's work are used by the Driver and Vehicle Licensing Authority who decide whether to withdraw a driving licence when the holder has had a head injury.

Phenytoin has been superseded by newer less-sedative antiepileptics. Carbamazepine is useful in monotherapy and may also act as a mood stabilizer. Lamotrigine is a new antiepileptic licensed for monotherapy and appears to be much freer of sedative side effects. It requires a gradual introduction and may also be used in reduced dosage in combination with sodium valproate for epilepsy that is difficult to control. Other new agents are not yet licensed for monotherapy.

SPASTICITY

Head injury is often associated with very severe spasticity (see Chapter 5). This usually develops after a few days or in the first few weeks. The aims of treatment are improvement of function, prevention of complications such as contractures, and prevention of pain.

Physiotherapy techniques, positioning, splinting and stretching have a large part to play (see below and Chapter 25). The avoidance of certain stimuli, e.g. constipation, bladder infection, skin irritation, and poor seating, will all help to reduce muscle tone. Oral medication for spasticity is currently not recommended because of inadequate evidence of effectiveness, but it is sometimes used when physical or local measures appear to be failing (Barnes et al., 1993).

Drugs currently used in spasticity include those that act at the level of peripheral muscle, suppressing the release of calcium ions, e.g. dantrolene, and those that act centrally at spinal cord level, e.g. baclofen (see Chapter 28). Both are limited by side effects and are not specific for cerebrally mediated spasticity. The mechanism of production of spasticity is not clearly understood but, if drugs are necessary, it seems more logical to try the peripherally acting drug first. Diazepam is not recommended because use may be long term. Drugs should be introduced gradually and carefully titrated to high dosage with the doctor, physiotherapist and patient working in partnership, then gradually discontinued if effec-tiveness is in question.

Botulinum toxin injection is an alternative way of relieving local spasticity and can be beneficial, allowing exposure of returning muscle control and enhancing treatment opportunities. The advantage of botulinum toxin is that its effect wears off after 2–3 months, sometimes sooner. It is an easy technique as long as one can easily feel the spastic muscle that one is trying to weaken. It is beneficial in improving head posture, and reducing upper and lower limb spasticity early in brain injury recovery.

Nerve blocks with alcohol or phenol injected through a needle electrode may be useful for long-term spasticity when there is no hope of useful recovery, but are not usually considered in the early phase of recovery. If spasticity has already resulted in severe contractures which cannot be recovered by physiotherapy or splinting techniques, then surgical release may be required.

HETEROTOPIC OSSIFICATION

This is also known as periarticular new bone formation and is seen commonly in brain injury associated with prolonged coma. The large joints are most often affected and clinical signs vary from pain, swelling, warmth and reduced range of movement to the presence of a large hard mass around an ankylosed joint. It is not usually observed radiologically until a month after the injury and may progress for a year or more before becoming quiescent. Treatment is difficult. Some physiotherapy must be continued to try and prevent contractures, but may cause more local trauma and exacerbate the condition. Treatments used are intended to reduce new bone formation and have included radiotherapy, disodium etidronate and, most recently, indomethacin. Surgical correction is not usually contemplated until 2 years after the injury.

DIABETES INSIPIDUS

Diabetes insipidus is a rare complication of head injury due to damage to the posterior pituitary. It is eminently treatable with synthetic vasopressin, which can be taken intranasally. Symptoms include polyuria, nocturia and compensatory polydipsia. Investigations demonstrate a high or high-to-normal plasma osmolality with a low urine osmolality.

MOOD DISORDERS, PSYCHOSES AND SLEEP DISORDERS

These problems are all observed in the head-injured population and many will respond to pharmacological intervention. There are a few rules worth following in this group of patients. When selecting medication it is worth remembering the old adage 'Start low and go slow'. Some patients with brain injury react adversely to antidepressant or antipsychotic medication; others seem nearly resistant to its effects. Drugs should be selected that have a low (or no) potential for triggering epilepsy. Cognitive techniques should be used where appropriate (see Chapter 27). Expressing anger and grief is appropriate quite late after severe head injury and may indicate that the patient is moving successfully, though slowly, through an adjustment phase. If difficulty is experienced, counselling may be appropriate.

Psychostimulants have been used on the basis that their use may improve attentional skills. There are no outstanding trials confirming their effectiveness and policing the use of these drugs would be difficult in this population, who as a group have an increased incidence of substance abuse. The use of psychostimulants is therefore not recommended.

POSTCONCUSSIONAL SYNDROME AFTER MILD HEAD INJURY

Most mildly injured patients eventually make a full recovery although many will have decreased attentional skills, impaired memory, mood disturbance and a plethora of other symptoms lasting several weeks (Levin *et al.*, 1989).

These symptoms are more likely if the PTA is longer than 1 hour; if resources are scarce, it is worthwhile concentrating on this group. Help can be provided by accurate assessment and advice on managing the symptoms successfully (Powell *et al.*, 1996).

This usually means encouraging the individual to slow down his or her lifestyle for a period of time, using memory strategies, delaying important meetings or seeking dispensation from examination boards for increased response times. Most patients will be back to their normal efficiency in 3–6 months, though a few may have permanent changes. Schoolchildren seem particularly vulnerable to mild head injury and should be advised to avoid contact sports for at least 3 months or until they are completely recovered (Levin *et al.*, 1989).

PHYSICAL MANAGEMENT

The need for specialist rehabilitation services for brain-injured patients has increased, particularly over the past decade. Many major reports on rehabilitation needs have been produced (e.g. Royal College of Physicians, 1986; Medical Disability Society, 1988).

The majority of head injuries (95%) are described as minor, with coma of <6 hours and PTA of <24 hours (Medical Disability Society, 1988). The remaining 5% of brain injuries may be described as severe, and as such will exhibit some specific problem areas. These include :

- Physical disability.
- Dependency in activities of daily living.
- Cognitive impairment.
- Behavioural disorder.
- Emotional problems.
- Psychiatric problems.

These problems may vary in their levels of severity, and may inevitably overlap.

It is important to emphasise that within the group of injuries described as severe, there will be a wide range of outcome. Some patients will achieve good functional levels of recovery, and perhaps return to some form of independent living and employment, whilst others will remain severely disabled and dependent upon others for care and management.

As we are looking at the physical management of the brain-injured patient, we will be mainly addressing the first two problems; those of physical disability (which may be long term) and dependency. The initial process of recovery after trauma will have been managed, but the physical disability may extend over months and years. This text will concentrate on the long-term physical management after giving a brief overview of early management from intensive care to the subacute stage.

Specific physiotherapy techniques used to treat patients after head injury are mentioned in Chapter 24 and the management of spasticity and other abnormalities of muscle tone in Chapter 25. Many similarities exist between the management of head injuries and stroke (see Chapter 7).

EARLY PHYSICAL MANAGEMENT

As mentioned above, the patient will be managed on a trauma unit in the acute phase after head injury, and the priority is to achieve a stable medical condition. Early post-injury physiotherapy will emphasise the promotion of good respiratory function and the prevention of contractures, and will manage the consequences of spasticity and abnormalities of movement and muscle tone (McMillan & Greenwood, 1993).

Sensory stimulation assessment and treatment (coma arousal therapy) may be carried out to aid diagnosis and maximise the potential for recovery (Rader & Ellis, 1994; Burke, 1995; Gill-Thwaites, 1997) and are usually carried out by the occupational therapist.

Respiratory physiotherapy while the patient is in intensive care will not be discussed here as it is covered in the respiratory book in this series (Smith & Ball, 1998) as well as by Ada et al. (1990) and Hough (1991). Hough (1991) suggested that respiratory physiotherapy in patients with head injury should involve maximum involvement but minimum intervention. This is important, as intervention can induce complications such as decreased clearance of secretions and increased risk of infection (Ellis, 1990). Frequent assessment and monitoring of the patient's medical status are necessary in order to decide whether or how to intervene. Respiratory physiotherapy aims to prevent build-up of secretions, possible infection and respiratory failure, and to enhance oxygenation of the brain.

During this early phase the patient must be handled appropriately, avoiding overstimulation, and appropriate positioning in bed must be ensured. The patient in coma or a post-coma state should be assumed to be able to hear and understand, so explanations and continued verbal communication are essential. Range-of-motion exercises for all limbs should be carried out daily (see Chapters 24 & 25) and plaster casts may be applied serially (Conine et al., 1990), perhaps combined with peripheral nerve blocks (Keenan et al., 1990) or intramuscular injections of botulinum toxin (see Chapter 28). These would be regarded as proactive techniques.

The benefits of early intervention (post-acute) in the rehabilitation of head-injured patients has been discussed by Cope & Hall (1982), Brooks (1991) and Mackay et al. (1992). The assumption is made that prevention of respiratory and musculoskeletal complications, and sensory deprivation while the patient is unconscious, will improve the chances of rehabilitation being more effective when the patient becomes conscious.

LONG-TERM PHYSICAL MANAGEMENT AFTER SEVERE HEAD INJURY

For patients who will experience long-term physical disability, management of the whole physical condition in all environments is necessary (Pope, 1992). This entails devising an integrated programme of 24-hour care, which is incorporated into the patient's lifestyle (Burke, 1995; Cope, 1995). The objectives of such a programme are to limit secondary complications, whilst maximising any remaining ability.

The complications frequently found in the patient with severe motor dysfunction include :

- Contractures producing fixed postural deformity.
- Pressure sores.
- Masked ability, i.e. ability which cannot be used due to the dominance of positive neurological signs such as spasticity.
- Tiredness/discomfort.
- Potential for the bedfast state.

If we acknowledge that instability from loss of postural control is at the core of the physical problems experienced by patients with severe head injuries, the above-mentioned complications may occur. Pope et al. (1991) suggested that such complications increase the time and effort of care required. It is therefore necessary to implement an effective, but realistic, programme of care that can be sustained in the long term by an MDT of therapists, carers and relatives.

Assessment

A full physical assessment of the patient is undertaken to enable an individual physical management plan to be devised. Assessment is essential for identifying problems, establishing goals and implementing appropriate care (see Chapter 4). Assessment forms are designed and developed in different institutions by the clinicians to meet the needs of a particular patient group. Clearly, there is a need for multicentre trials to establish gold-standard assessments which will be understood by all physiotherapists so that appropriate and understandable information is transferred with the patient.

A form for use with severely brain-injured patients, based on the work of Hare (1990), is suggested below, and is divided into three parts :

A. **General information.**
- Vision.
- Hearing.
- Comprehension.
- Speech/communication.
- Behavioural state.
- Orthopaedic complications.
- Sensation.
- Drug profile.
- Family support.

B. **Negative factors—Static assessment.**
- Preferred posture.
- Pattern of deformity.
- Joint contracture.
- Neurological release phenomena (Martin, 1967).
- Neurological reactions.
- Respiratory status.
- Pressure sores.
- Positioning in wheelchair.
- Positioning in bed.

C. **Positive factors—Dynamic assessment.**
- Postural ability—Assessed in lying, sitting and standing.
- Motor ability—Also assessed in lying, sitting and standing.
- Mode of transfer, e.g. lift/hoist, stand transfer.

From the negative and positive factors it is possible to identify problems requiring specific intervention, indicators for deterioration, existing abilities and potential for enhanced motor function.

This information can then be used to set short-term and long-term objectives for the patient, to state the physical management needs, and to implement a plan of care.

Plan of Care

The purpose of the plan of care is to maintain an optimal physical condition, thus providing a basis from which learning and relearning may be enhanced (see 'Physiotherapeutic approaches') and nursing care facilitated. The components of a plan of care are:
• Control of posture—in lying, sitting and standing.
• Maintenance of range of motion (ROM) in joints.
• Respiratory care.
• Encouragement of remaining ability.

Control of Posture

Management of posture forms a major part of the physiotherapist's role in caring for the brain-injured patient. A comprehensive review of the subject by Pope (1996) is widely illustrated, giving practical details which it is not possible to go into in the present chapter.

Posture while Lying

Many patients with complex physical disability present with asymmetrical, decerebrate postures and are unable to accept the support of the surface of the bed. This results in unequal loading of tissues which makes the patient vulnerable to joint contractures, pressure sores and respiratory complications.

The presenting posture may be modified by providing additional support (pillows, foam rolls, wedges) and thus stability to the body segments. For example, a T-roll provides improved alignment in a patient with adductor spasticity (see Figure 25.2). Additional support also results in greater body symmetry and improved ability to conform to the supporting surface.

Posture while Sitting

When a patient with complex disability is placed in the sitting position, he or she becomes very unstable. This is the result of a small base of support and altered postural tone. Consequently, patients have often failed to be adequately and safely seated in a wheelchair. The base of support should be increased, and appropriate support given to the trunk to maintain it in alignment over the base. This can be achieved by the provision of suitable seating systems (see below).

It should be noted that an inappropriate wheelchair can serve to exaggerate a patient's physical problems. It is important to remember that all activity is posture-dependent, and that the organisation of posture is under central control. The central postural control mechanism is disturbed in the patient with head injury, who cannot remain erect against the force of gravity and presents with postural disorder and disarray.

There are three typical postural patterns in sitting:
1. C-shaped posture. This is a slumped, kyphotic pattern (Figure 8.1A).
2. Arched posture. The body is arched backwards from the coccyx, with an exaggerated lumbar lordosis. Legs tend to flex, and arms to extend. Inevitably the buttocks will tend to lift and slide forwards (Figure 8.1B).
3. Asymmetrical posture. In this position the legs may be windswept, the pelvis tilted and rotated, and the trunk and the side of the head flexed and rotated (Figure 8.1C).

The patient may display a combination of these postures and most will adopt a preferred position in sitting. If a patient is unable to provide his or her own postural support, it must be provided externally to provide a stable, balanced, symmetrical and functional position, whilst relieving pressure and shearing forces.

Posture while Standing

Standing makes an effective contribution to the general physical management of the patient in the following ways:
• When included in a programme with the correct use of prone lying, standing counteracts the flexed posture displayed in sitting and lying.
• When the body is correctly aligned, and weight bearing is even over the feet, plantigrade position is achieved.
• The effect of gravity on the body in the standing position is helpful in the promotion of improved renal function and urinary drainage. It may also improve bowel function.
• There may also be a psychological benefit.

Standing is achieved by the mechanical support of a tilt-table or standing frame, when the joint range of the lower extremities allow this to be a safe and achievable procedure.

Special Seating Systems

A suitable seating system can be a very positive tool for providing the much needed support in sitting. This subject is discussed in detail by Pope (1996). In order to identify the appropriate wheelchair for the patient, a full physical and environmental assessment must be made, ideally by the physiotherapist and occupational therapist.

Providing a brain-injured patient with a suitable seating system should be achieved as soon as possible in the course of rehabilitation as it allows the patient to interact safely, to explore the environment and to re-establish some level of orientation. It also enhances the use of communication aids such as communication boards and computers.

Patients with severe head injury will often present with postural problems that cannot be successfully managed by seating available through commercial companies and it may be necessary to provide customised seating such as the Matrix system (Cousins et al., 1983; Sharman & Ponton, 1990) to provide adequate support and control. Conversely, a standard wheelchair may be appropriate, but only in combination with a profile of removable adaptations.

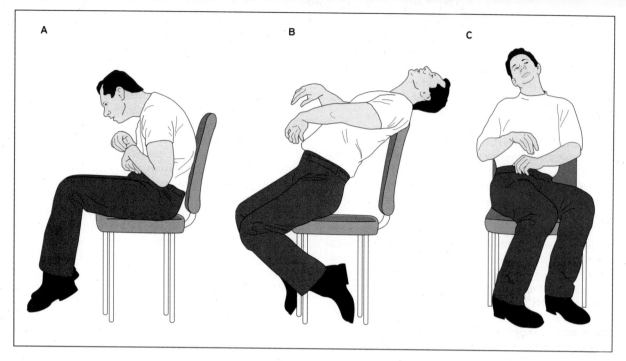

Figure 8.1 Typical postural patterns in sitting. (A) The 'C'-shaped posture. (B) 'Arched' posture. (C) The asymmetrical posture.

Maintenance of Joint ROM

Reduced ROM can lead to contractures and contribute to asymmetrical postures and an unstable position. It can also impede general nursing care and influence the physical management programme. When joint ROM is limited but does not impede care or positioning, it should be maintained or improved by a regimen of stretching exercises (see Chapter 25). If decreased ROM limits the patient's potential for progress (e.g. decreased ability to be positioned in lying, sitting or standing) physiotherapeutic measures may be initiated to stretch contracted tissues, e.g. splinting and serial casting (see Chapter 25). If this fails to be effective, surgical intervention, i.e. tenotomy, may be considered for contractures of the lower extremities. Prior to such intervention, assurance of appropriate assessment and postsurgical physiotherapeutic management should be obtained.

Respiratory Care

The patient will have limited lung excursion due to loss of function of respiratory muscles and poor postural control, and this will predispose to chest infection. Postural drainage may be used prophylactically or to treat chest infections should they occur. Improving posture and position allows improved air entry to the lungs and effective coughing should be taught where possible. If the chest is productive and a tracheostomy site is still open, suction may be necessary. Care must be taken at all times when treating patients, that a clear airway is ensured and that there is freedom for head movement.

If the patient has the physical and cognitive ability to learn to improve his or her own respiratory function, a regimen of breathing exercises can be taught and the patient placed in a position of forward lean that allows improved lung expansion. Increased levels of physical activity and assuming good sitting and standing positions will also aid respiratory function. Respiratory physiotherapy for the head-injured patient is discussed by Ellis (1990), Hough (1991) and Smith & Ball (1998). The importance of understanding the relationships between brain and lung function for effective therapy is stressed by Ellis (1990).

Encourage Remaining Ability

When a patient is well managed physically the potential for motor recovery may be enhanced, but this will also be dependent on the degree of recovery of brain function. Discrete movement of a body segment, e.g. the head, requires stability of base and adjacent segments (Butler & Major, 1992). If the patient cannot achieve stability of posture it must be provided.

Stimulating interest in a task, providing an element of competition and frequent repetition, may enhance performance of even the most simple task. Leisure activities such as swimming should be encouraged and wheelchair activities such as archery and table tennis. Social activities are also important, e.g. visits to sporting events or the theatre. Of course, these activities will depend on the patient's ability to enjoy and/or take part in them.

If a patient is to return home with some level of independence, time spent in a transitional living unit may be invaluable. This will not only provide the opportunity to gain skills in certain daily living activities such as self-care, shopping and cooking, but also increases the patient's confidence. Where a patient has the capacity to return to employment, opportunities for return to previous work or for retraining should be given. Multidisciplinary support will be necessary for this to be achieved (Wehman *et al.*, 1990).

If a physically disabled patient displays some, or all, of the secondary complications mentioned earlier, the physical management programme may be considered to have 'failed', but if many of the complications have been prevented it may be regarded as a 'static success'. If further ability can be superimposed on that, the outcome may be seen to be a 'dynamic success' (Pope, 1992).

The overall objective of a management programme for the brain-injured patient with severe long-term physical disability is to ensure that the patient enjoys the best possible quality of life, in terms of general wellbeing and control of adverse secondary complications, whilst exploiting to the full any independence available.

Physiotherapeutic Approaches

Several options exist for the management of motor dysfunction and these are discussed in Chapter 22. As in many areas of physiotherapy, management of the head-injured patient draws on the different approaches to provide a treatment programme which is appropriate to the individual patient. Aspects of the Bobath approach, motor relearning (or Carr & Shepperd) approach, the Hare approach (see Chapter 19; and Hare, 1990) and others may be employed.

Specific physiotherapy techniques used to manage the head-injured patient, such as ice and heat, are described in Chapter 24, and those related to the management of spasticity and movement abnormalities are discussed in Chapter 25. Physiotherapy is undertaken within the MDT to achieve structured and appropriate management of the patient (McGrath *et al.*, 1995).

Outcome Measures

The effectiveness of rehabilitation programmes needs to be measured for the individual patient and for research purposes. This usually involves the measurement of disability, which is a very difficult task; several measurement scales exist (see Chapter 4). There is a lack of validated scales and those which exist do not meet the needs of all patient groups, particularly those who are very severely disabled in whom only subtle changes may occur. Disability scales therefore need to be sensitive enough to detect small changes. The effect of rehabilitation on outcome in head injury has been examined (e.g. Spivack *et al.*, 1992; Cope, 1995) as have the merits of outcome measures themselves (e.g. Hall *et al.*, 1985; Whiteneck *et al.*, 1992). However, reliable and valid outcome measures, ideally producing an international benchmark, need to be established (see Chapter 4). Rehabilitation of the patient with head injury could then be based on evaluated treatments.

CASE HISTORY

Patient A was 22 years old when he was involved in a road traffic accident as a pedestrian. He sustained a severe traumatic brain injury, with a left temporal subdural haematoma which was evacuated surgically. He was intubated and ventilated and managed on an Intensive Care Unit for several days, and a tracheostomy was performed. He had remained in a coma for approximately 8 weeks and at the time of his arrival at the Brain Injury Unit he was emerging from the comatose state. He presented with very low muscle tone, no active movement and no response to command. He was being fed via a nasogastric tube and was considered underweight. During the time at the acute hospital he had been managed in bed, and had received passive ROM exercises for all limbs.

A full assessment was made at the Brain Injury Unit, problems identified, objectives set, and a treatment plan implemented by the MDT. The two most immediate needs were to improve Patient A's nutrition (a PEG tube was promptly put in place) and to get him up out of bed for periods of the day. Within the first week of admission, a wheelchair assessment was completed, recommendations made and applications sent to his local wheelchair service for provision of appropriate seating. In the interim, he was seated in a 'loan wheelchair' and began to build up his sitting tolerance. Initially his lean build made him vulnerable to developing pressure areas in sitting. This was monitored closely but there were no problems and with improved nutrition he reached his 'target weight'.

When he was able to sit up and be in a position to be in touch with his environment, he began to keep his eyes open, to 'track' objects and people, and to respond to verbal commands. He was standing regularly on a tilt-table and work was aimed at increasing his low muscle tone and isolating any active movement.

About a month after admission to the Brain Injury Unit, following intensive stimulation therapy from the occupational therapists, his level of awareness improved dramatically. He began to respond consistently to commands and to be able to hold his head up against gravity. He developed active movement in his left arm and it was soon discovered that he was able, with great effort, to write with his left hand.

Patient A's physical progress was slow but ongoing. His right arm remained essentially non-functional but the ability of the left arm increased and some months later he was able to use this arm to manipulate a powered wheelchair. He was also able to walk short distances with maximal support.

Written communication continued to improve and he also developed the skill to use a computerised communication aid. During this time he also began to verbalise, although it was difficult to comprehend, and writing remained his preference for communication. At this point, consideration needed to be given to his future. After assessment for suitability, he was discharged to a residential educational programme which specialised in the needs of neurologically damaged patients, and his progress continued.

Patient A was still on the programme 1 year after discharge from the Brain Injury Unit. He was able to walk with assistance but for practical reasons used his powered wheelchair. His speech had improved, although was still impaired. He was doing well with his educational programme and had regained his great sense of humour and outgoing personality.

REFERENCES

Ada L, Canning C, Paratz J. Care of the unconscious head-injured patient. In: Ada L, Canning C, eds. *Key issues in neurological physiotherapy.* London: Butterworth Heinemann, 1990:249-287.

Addy EV, Waldmann CS, Collin C. Review of the use of intracranial pressure monitoring in a district general hospital intensive care unit. *Clin Intens Care* 1996, **7**:87-91.

Artiola L, Portuny I, Briggs M. Measuring the duration of post traumatic amnesia. *J Neurol Neurosurg Psychiat* 1980, **43**:377-379.

Barnes M, McLellan L, Sutton R. Spasticity. In: Greenwood R, Barnes MP, McMillan TM *et al.*, eds. *Neurological rehabilitation.* London: Churchill Livingstone; 1993:161-172.

Black D, London D, Bates D, *et al.* Working Group convened by the Royal College of Physicians: The permanent vegetative state. *J Roy Coll Phys Lond* 1996, **30**:119-121.

Black P, Rossitch E. *Neurosurgery: an introductory text.* Oxford: University Press; 1995.

Brooks N. The effectiveness of post-acute rehabilitation. *Brain Inj* 1991, **5**:103-109.

Bullock R, Teasdale G. Head injuries, I. *Br Med J* 1990, **300**:1515-1518.

Burke CD. Models of brain injury rehabilitation. *Brain Inj* 1995, **9**:735-743.

Butler RP, Major RE. The learning of motor control. Biomedical conditions. *Physiotherapy* 1992, **78**:6-11.

Clifton GL, Robertson CS, Grossmand RG, *et al.* The metabolic response to severe head injury. *J Neurosurg* 1984, **60**:687-696.

Conine TA, Sullivan T, Mackie T, Goodman M. Effects of serial casting for the prevention of equinovarus in patients with acute head injury. *Arch Phys Med Rehab* 1990, **71**:310-312.

Cope DN. The effectiveness on traumatic brain injury rehabilitation. *Brain Inj* 1995, **9**:649-670.

Cope DN, Hall K. Head injury rehabilitation: benefit of early intervention. *Arch Phys Med Rehab* 1982, **63**:433-437.

Cousins SJ, Jones KN, Ackerley KE. Aids in prevention and treatment of pressure sores: cushion fabrication using the shapeable Matrix. In: Barbenel JC, Forbes CD, Lowe GDO, eds. *Pressure sores.* London: Macmillan Press; 1983:151-156.

Crockard A. Brain swelling, brain oedema and blood brain barrier. In: Crockard A, Hayward R, Haff J-T, eds. *Neurosurgery: the scientific basis of clinical practice.* Oxford: Blackwell; 1985:333-349.

Ellis E. Respiratory function following head injury. In: Ada L, Canning C, eds. *Key issues in neurological physiotherapy.* London: Butterworth Heinemann; 1990:237-248.

Field JH. *A study of the epidemiology of head injury in England and Wales with particular application to rehabilitation.* London: HMSO; 1976.

Galbraith S, Teasdale GM. Head injuries. In: Russell RCG, ed. *Recent advances in surgery.* Edinburgh: Churchill Livingstone; 1982:71-84.

Gill-Thwaites H. The sensory modality assessment rehabilitation technique – A tool for assessment and treatment of patients with severe brain injury in a vegetative state. *Brain Inj* 1997, **11**:723-734.

Grady MS, McLaughlin MR, Christman CW, *et al.* The use of antibodies targeted against the neurofilament subunits for the detection of diffuse axonal injury in humans. *J Neuropath Exp Neurol* 1993, **52**:143-152.

Hall K, Cope DN, Rappaport M. Glasgow Outcome Scale and Disability Rating Scale: comparative usefulness in following recovery on traumatic head injury. *Arch Phys Med Rehab* 1985, **66**:35-37.

Hare N. The analysis and measurement of physical disability. In: Hare N, ed. *What the hare tortoise.* London: Hare Association for Physical Ability; 1990, I:2-27.

Herscovitch P. Functional brain imaging - basic principles and application to head trauma. In: Rizzo and Tranel, eds. *Head Injury and post concussive syndrome.* London: Churchill Livingstone; 1996:89-119.

Hough A. *Physiotherapy in respiratory care: a problem solving approach.* London: Chapman & Hall; 1991:183-186.

Jennett B. *Epilepsy after non-missile head injuries.* London: Heinemann; 1975.

Jennett B, Snoek J, Bond MR, *et al.* Disability after severe head injury: observations on the use of the Glasgow Outcome Scale. *J Neurol Neurosurg Psychiat* 1981, **44**:285-293.

Jennett B, Bond M. Assessment of outcome after severe brain damage: a practical scale. *Lancet* 1975, **i**:1031-1034.

Jennett B, MacMillan R. Epidemiology of head injury. *Br Med J* 1981, **282**:101-104.

Jennett B, Teasdale G. *Management of head injuries.* Philadelphia: FA Davis; 1981.

Keenan MA, Thomas ES, Stone C, Gersten LM. Percutaneous phenol block of the musculocutaneous nerve to control elbow flexion spasticity. *J Hand Surg* 1990, **15**:340-346.

Levin HS, Ewing-Cobbs, Fletcher JM. Neurobehavioural outcome of mild head injury in children. In: Levin HS, Eisenberg HM, Benton AL, eds. *Mild head injury.* Oxford: Oxford University Press; 1989:189-213.

Levin HS, O'Donnell VM, Grossman RG, *et al.* The Galveston Orientation and Amnesia Test. *J Nerv Ment Dis* 1979, **167**:675-684.

Mackay LE, Bernstein BA, Chapman PE, *et al.* Early intervention in severe head injury: long term benefits of a formalised program. *Arch Phys Med Rehab* 1992, **73**:635-641.

Martin JP. *The basal ganglia and posture.* London: Pittman Medical; 1967.

McDermott FT. Bicyclist head injury prevention by helmets and mandatory wearing legislation in Victoria, Australia. *Ann Roy Coll Surg Engl* 1995, **77**:38-44.

McGrath JR, Marks JA, Davis AM. Interdisciplinary rehabilitation: further developments at Rivermead Rehabilitation Centre. *Clin Rehab* 1995, **9**:320-326.

McMillan T, Greenwood R. Head injury. In: Greenwood R, Barnes MP, McMillan TM *et al.*, eds. *Neurological rehabilitation.* London: Churchill Livingstone; 1993: 437-450.

Medical Disability Society. *Report of a working party on the management of traumatic brain injury.* London: The Development Trust for the Young Disabled; 1988.

Mendelow AD, Teasdale GM, Teasdale E, *et al.* Cerebral blood flow and intracranial pressure in head injured patients. In: Ishii S, Nagai H, Brock M, eds. *Intracranial pressure.* Berlin: Springer Verlag; 1983:495-500.

Morgan AS. The trauma centre as a continuum of care for persons with severe brain injury. *J Head Trauma Rehab* 1994, **9:**1-10.

Pope PM. Management of the physical condition in patients with chronic and severe neurological pathologies. *Physiotherapy* 1992, **78:**896-903.

Pope PM. Postural management and special seating. In: Edwards S, ed. *Neurological physiotherapy: a problem solving approach.* London: Churchill Livingstone; 1996:135-160.

Pope PM, Bowes CE, Tudor M, *et al.* Surgery combined with continued post-operative stretching and management of knee flexion contractures. *Clin Rehab* 1991, **5:**15-23.

Povlishock JT, Becker DP, Cheng CLY, *et al.* Axonal change in minor head injury. *J Neuropathol Exp Neurol* 1983, **42:**225-242.

Powell TJ, Collin C, Sutton K. A follow-up study of patients hospitalised after minor head injury. *Disabil Rehab* 1996, **18:**231-237.

Rader MA, Ellis DW. The sensory stimulation assessment measure (SSAM): a tool for early evaluation of severely brain-injured patients. *Brain Inj* 1994, **8:**309-321.

Royal College of Physicians. Physical disabilities in 1986 and beyond. *J Roy Coll Phys Lond* 1986, **20:**30-37.

Russell WR, Smith A. Post traumatic amnesia in closed head injury. *Arch Neurol* 1961, **5:**16-29.

Sharman A, Ponton T. The social, functional and physiological benefits of intimately-contoured customised seating; the Matrix body support system. *Physiotherapy* 1990, **76:**187-192.

Sharples PM, Aynsley-Green A, Eyre JA. Causes of fatal childhood accidents involving head injury in the Northern Region 1979-1986. *Br Med J* 1990, **301:**1193-1197.

Smith M, Ball V. *Cardiovascular/Respiratory Physiotherapy.* London: Mosby; 1998. In progress.

Spivack G, Spettle CM, Ellis DW, *et al.* Effects of intensity of treatment and lengths of stay on rehabilitation outcomes. *Brain Inj* 1992, **6:**419-434.

Strich SJ. Diffuse degeneration of the cerebral white matter in severe dementia following head injury. *J Neurol Neurosurg Psychiat* 1956, **19:**163-185.

Teasdale G, Jennett B. Assessment of coma and impaired consciousness: a practical scale. *Lancet* 1974, **ii:**81-84.

Teasdale G, Murray G, Anderson EM, *et al.* Risks of acute traumatic intracranial haematoma in children and adults: implications for managing head injury. *Br Med J* 1990, **300:**363-367.

Thompson RS, Rivara FP, Thompson DC. A case control study of the effectiveness of bicycle safety helmets. *N Engl J Med* 1989, **320:**1361-1367.

Unterberg A, Kiening K, Schmiedex P, *et al.* Long term observations of intracranial pressure after severe head injury. The phenomenon of secondary rise of intracranial pressure. *Neurosurgery* 1993, **32:**17-24.

Wehman PH, Kreutzer JS, West MD, *et al.* Return to work for persons with traumatic brain injury: a supported employment approach. *Med Rehab* 1990, **71:**1047-1052.

Whiteneck GG, Charlifue SW, Gerhart KA, *et al.* Quantifying handicap: a new measure of long-term rehabilitation outcomes. *Arch Phys Med Rehab* 1992, **73:**519-526.

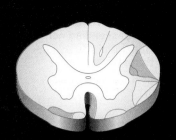

9

S Rowley, H Forde, S Glickman & FRI Middleton

SPINAL CORD INJURY

CHAPTER OUTLINE

- Terminology
- Types of spinal cord injury
- Incidence and aetiology
- Pathogenesis
- Spinal cord shock

- Spinal cord plasticity
- Effect of cord injury on the respiratory system
- General management
- Physical management

INTRODUCTION

Traumatic spinal cord injury is a life-transforming condition of sudden onset that can have devastating consequences. Clinical management involves trauma management in the acute phase and rehabilitation which is lifelong. The objectives of management are to produce a healthy person who can choose his or her own destiny.

TERMINOLOGY

Terms used to describe these patients indicate the general level of the spinal injury and loss of function.

PARAPLEGIA

Paraplegia refers to the impairment or loss of motor and/or sensory function in thoracic, lumbar or sacral segments of the spinal cord. Upper limb function is spared but the trunk, legs and pelvic organs may be involved.

TETRAPLEGIA

The term tetraplegia is preferred to quadriplegia. Tetraplegic patients have impairment or loss of motor and/or sensory function in cervical segments of the spinal cord. The upper limbs are affected as well as the trunk, legs and pelvic organs. The term does not include the brachial plexus or injury to

peripheral nerves (see Chapter 10). Quadraparesis and paraparesis are terms that were used to describe incomplete lesions but their use is now discouraged.

TYPES OF SPINAL CORD INJURY

Spinal cord injury damages a complex neural network involved in transmitting, modifying and co-ordinating motor, sensory and autonomic control of organ systems. In effect, post-traumatic dysfunction of the spinal cord causes loss of homoeostatic and adaptive mechanisms which keep people naturally healthy. The American Spinal Injury Association motor and sensory assessments are used for establishing injury level (ASIA, 1992; Dittuno *et al.*, 1994). The relative incidence of levels of injury are: 58% cervical, 35% thoracic, and 7% lumbar and sacral. Lesion patterns vary widely and classically recognisable patterns are presented below.

COMPLETE INJURY

This describes the case where all neural communication across the lesion is interrupted, as in complete spinal cord transsection.

INCOMPLETE LESIONS

There are recognised patterns of incomplete cord injury which tend to present clinically as combinations of

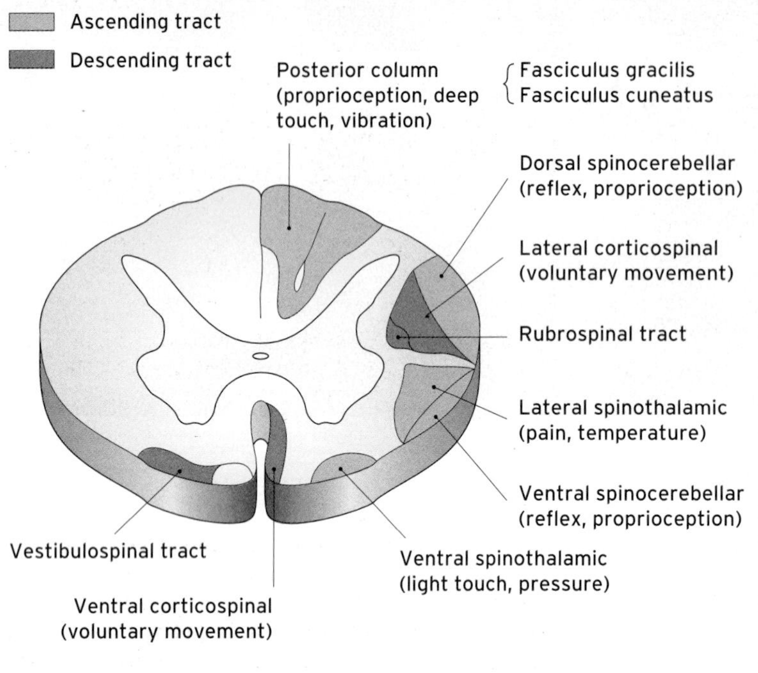
Ascending tract
Descending tract
Posterior column
(proprioception, deep
touch, vibration)
Fasciculus gracilis
Fasciculus cuneatus
Dorsal spinocerebellar
(reflex, proprioception)
Lateral corticospinal
(voluntary movement)
Rubrospinal tract
Lateral spinothalamic
(pain, temperature)
Ventral spinocerebellar
(reflex, proprioception)
Vestibulospinal tract
Ventral spinothalamic
(light touch, pressure)
Ventral corticospinal
(voluntary movement)

Figure 9.1 Cross-section of the spinal cord illustrating the main ascending and descending nerve tracts. The functions affected by damage to these tracts are indicated.

syndromes rather than in isolation. The signs and symptoms are related to the anatomical areas of the cord affected (Figure 9.1). Clinically, incomplete lesions are referred to as either a syndrome or injury.

Anterior Cord Injury

Anterior cord injury describes the effects of ventral cord damage; there is complete motor loss caudal to the lesion, and loss of pain and temperature sensation as these sensory tracts are located anterolaterally in the spinal cord. Preservation of the posterior columns means that perception of vibration and proprioception on the ipsilateral side are intact. This syndrome can arise from anterior spinal artery embolisation.

Brown-Séquard Syndrome

Originally described by Galen, this syndrome describes saggital hemicord damage with ipsilateral paralysis and dorsal column interruption with contralateral pain and loss of temperature sensation. The relatively normal pain and temperature sensation on the ipsilateral side is due to the spinothalamic tract crossing over to the opposite side of the cord. This hemisection injury of the cord is classically caused by stabbing.

Central Cord Injury

The upper limbs are more profoundly affected than the lower limbs and the condition is typically seen in older patients with cervical spondylosis. A hyperextension injury compresses the cord between the vertebral body and intervertebral disc. The central cervical tracts are predominatly affected. There is flaccid weakness of the arms, due to lower motor neurone lesions, and spastic patterning in the legs due to upper motor neurone injury. Bowel and bladder dysfunctions are common but only partial.

Conus Medullaris

Conus medullaris describes damage to the most caudal portion of the spinal cord; bladder and bowel dysfunctions occur with variable symmetrical lower limb deficits.

Cauda Equina Lesion

This produces flaccid paralysis as there is peripheral nerve damage at this level of the spine, usually affecting several levels with variable sacral root interruption.

Posterior Cord Injury

This rare condition produces damage to the dorsal columns (sensation of light touch, proprioception and vibration) with preservation of motor function and pain and temperature pathways. However, the patient presents with profound ataxia due to loss of proprioception.

INCOMPLETE VERSUS COMPLETE INJURY

The American Spinal Injuries Association (ASIA, 1992) reviewed standards for assessing and classifying functional levels of spinal cord injury, including the definitions of complete and incomplete lesions. The strict criteria for these classifications will not be entered into here but reference should be made to the ASIA classification, which includes the zone of partial preservation, and the Frankel classification of degree of incompleteness. For general guidance, the term 'incomplete' indicates there is some neurological sparing below the level of the lesion.

The statistical trends show an increase in incomplete lesions and a significant reduction in mortality, mainly due to medical advances (Grundy & Swain, 1993; Whalley Hamilton, 1995). The distribution varies between centres and the current pattern at the authors' unit at Stanmore Hospital is: 29% complete, 63% incomplete, 8% no neurological deficit.

INCIDENCE AND AETIOLOGY

The Spinal Injuries Association (SIA, 1995) estimated that approximately 13 people per million of the population in the UK suffer a spinal cord injury per annum (see Mendoza *et al.*, 1993, for a review).

The ratio of male to female cases is approximately 5:1, and varies with age. The greatest incidence is in the age range of 20–39 years (45%), then 40–59 years (24%), and 0–19 years (20%), with those over 60 years showing the lowest incidence of 11% (Gardner *et al.*, 1988). The incidence and aetiology vary greatly from country to country (Soopramanien, 1994), North America being the only region to produce any clear analysis (Whalley Hamilton, 1995).

Spinal cord damage can result from trauma (84% of cases) or non-traumatic causes (16%). The main causes of traumatic injury are shown in Figure 9.2; gunshots and stabbings also make small but increasing contributions (Mendoza *et al.*, 1993; Whalley Hamilton, 1995). Occasionally, patients with antecedent pathology, such as depression or schizophrenia, will sustain injury from jumping from a height.

Non-traumatic causes include: developmental anomalies (e.g. spina bifida); congenital anomalies (e.g. angiomatous malformations); inflammation (e.g. multiple sclerosis); ischaemia (e.g. cord stroke); infection arising extrinsically to the spinal cord (e.g. osteomyelitis of the vertebral column), or intrinsic to the cord (transverse myelitis); and space-occupying lesions both benign and malignant, extrinsic or intrinsic to the spinal cord. Each condition and each individual has its own distinct management needs and features. Their management will benefit from the knowledge and skills derived from an understanding of traumatic spinal cord injury, which is the focus of this chapter.

PATHOGENESIS

A brief outline of the pathological changes which occur with spinal cord injury is now given; further details can be found in other texts such as Hughes (1988).

IMMEDIATE/PRIMARY DAMAGE

The commonest clinical presentations are fractures and dislocations of the vertebral spine, with associated soft tissue damage. This trauma impacts on the spinal cord, producing primary direct cellular and/or vascular damage.

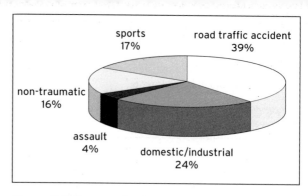

Figure 9.2 Causes of spinal cord injury from traumatic and non-traumatic aetiologies. The percentages illustrated were obtained from the references cited in the text.

SECONDARY DAMAGE

Secondary damage arises from cellular swelling and the exudation of chemicals that destroy adjacent cells and neural tracts. These changes are associated with acute inflammation. The blood vessels feeding the spinal cord can react by vasospasm to produce ischaemic tertiary damage. The relative contribution of each type of damage is unknown.

LATER PROBLEMS

After some weeks, there is evidence of astroglial scarring with cyst formation producing distorted neural architecture. In some cases, months or years later, a syrinx, arising from cystic degeneration of the cord, will extend rostrally to produce further spinal cord damage. This post-traumatic syringomyelia may require drainage by shunt to prevent further extension. In view of the possibility of syringomyelia, the neurological status should be reassessed periodically (Illis, 1988).

SPINAL CORD SHOCK

This is the phenomenon of cessation of all nervous system function below the level of damage to the cord and may be due to the loss of descending neural influences. After several seconds to months, the flaccid paralysis and areflexia of spinal shock are replaced by hyperexcitability, seen clinically as hyper-reflexia, spasticity and spasms. Lesions from lower thoracic levels persist distally, with flaccid paralysis. The return of muscle tone and involuntary activity can mislead patients into believing there is functional neural recovery. Therapists need to anticipate such reactions in order to avoid subsequent confusion and disappointment.

SPINAL CORD PLASTICITY

When a peripheral nerve is cut, if the nerve sheath is placed in apposition, regeneration of the axons will occur leading to significant return of function. It is hypothesised that there is no spontaneous regeneration in the CNS. Research into a nerve growth factor or genetic marker which might act as a guide to successful linkage is proceeding, but as yet without significant success. Plasticity is discussed in detail in Chapter 6.

EFFECT OF CORD INJURY ON THE RESPIRATORY SYSTEM

Respiration is a complex motor activity using muscles at various levels (see 'Physical management'). Patients with lesions of T1 and above will lose some 40–50% of their respiratory function but most patients with cervical injuries have an initial vital lung capacity of only 1 litre or less, which is approximately 20% of that expected. Thus, all patients with cervical injuries should be fully evaluated for respiratory efficiency with frequent vital capacity, peak flow and partial pressure of oxygen (pO_2) measurement in the initial weeks after injury. For an overview of respiratory physiology with an explanation of the tests mentioned here and normal values, the reader is referred to relevant text-books (e.g. Hough, 1991; Smith & Ball, 1998).

Given the aetiology of spinal cord injury in the UK, many patients sustain associated deceleration injuries affecting the lungs. They present at 24–48 hours post-injury with deteriorating respiratory function, with a falling pO_2 and rising pCO_2. This is a serious development and mechanical ventilation may be required, occasionally for a number of weeks. It is one of the situations where early steroid administration is thought to be helpful.

In other patients, deterioration of respiratory function in the first days after injury may be associated with an ascending cord lesion due to oedema or extending hypoxia in the cord. This again may lead to the need for mechanical ventilation for a period and then subsequent weaning from the ventilator as cord function returns. Occasionally the higher ascended level may become the permanent level.

If significant hypoxia persists, particularly with associated low blood pressure, further damage to the cord may occur. Once respiratory stability has been achieved, a maintenance programme will be required to compensate for the lack of full excursion of the lungs in patients without the use of intercostal or abdominal muscles (see 'Physical management').

Atelectasis is common in patients with spinal cord injuries. Subsequent infection and pneumonia still account for considerable morbidity and some mortality in tetraplegics. Contusion to the lungs or pneumo- or haemo-pneumothorax is common in patients with thoracic lesions, often associated with steering wheel impact in road vehicle accidents. The recognition of such a situation in Accident and Emergency Units is crucial and insertion of a chest drain may be required.

Another complication that may occur over the few days after injury and remain a risk for some months is the development of pulmonary emboli associated with deep venous thrombosis (DVT). Prophylactic measures, including frequent passive movement, the wearing of pressure stockings and early mobilisation, are important. The use of anticoagulants remains contentious with, as yet, no strong research evidence of their prophylactic effectiveness. Extreme vigilance with regard to leg size and other signs of DVT by all team members is important, as there is a 1–2% incidence of mortality from massive pulmonary embolus each year.

GENERAL MANAGEMENT

Although the primary damage is to the spinal cord, every organ system can be affected. Antecedent and post-traumatic psychological and social conditions also must be given full consideration as they play their inevitable parts in the success or failure of rehabilitation. In other words, management of people with traumatic spinal cord injury demands an holistic approach in which all rehabilitation team members work towards common goals, agreed amongst the team and with the patient.

TRAUMA MANAGEMENT

Spinal cord injury presentation must remain a key issue for all of us and we, as professionals, should be vigilant about the risks of activities in which we may be involved, such as on rugby fields or at swimming pools.

Immediate Management

When an accident occurs a spinal injury should be suspected, and in a spinal accident other injuries should be suspected. The incident history should be recorded. Pain, bruising and/or palpable spinal deformity are likely features.

Proper handling will avoid unnecessary further damage, and the following simple advice can be immensely valuable. The patient should be advised not to move. The airway and breathing should be checked. If he or she needs removal to another site, the transfer should be gentle, avoiding any twisting. Lifting should be performed by at least four people, with one acting as leader to co-ordinate the team.

The patient should be placed in a supine position with the head and body kept strictly in alignment. If unconscious, the patient should be strapped to, and supported on, a board to allow tilt and avoid aspiration. Normal spinal curvature should be supported by a rolled-up cloth. The skin should be protected from pressure and ulceration by removing objects from pockets or by removing clothes. Point pressure from heels on hard surfaces, or 'knocking knees', should be avoided. Various spinal immobilisation boards, e.g. the scoop stretcher, and collars are available in ambulances for moving patients. If possible, a motor and sensory charting should be performed for a baseline neuro-assessment with diagrammatic recording.

Admission to Hospital

Currently in the UK, after sustaining a spinal cord injury the person is admitted to the local Accident and Emergency or Trauma Unit. A full physical and neurological assessment is carried out and a decision is made about referral to a specialist unit. The decision to manage the patient conservatively or surgically will be influenced by the results of imaging, via X-ray, MRI and/or CT, and the policy of the hospital.

Spinal Stabilisation versus Conservative Management

Spinal fractures may be classified as stable, unstable or quasi-stable (i.e. currently stable but likely to become unstable in the course of everyday activity). Disagreement continues between protagonists and antagonists of surgical stabilisation of the spine but surgery is increasingly used (Collins, 1995). Definition of instability or stability of a spinal lesion has now achieved substantial agreement based on the three column principles (Dennis, 1983). There is general agreement that restoration of the anatomy of the canal is sensible in terms of giving the cord the best opportunity of recovery. There is no evidence that the neurological recovery or degree of spinal stability in the long term differs with surgical or conservative management. From a psychological point of view, strong argument is made in favour of early mobilisation, which can take place 7–10 days after surgery, and shorter in-patient stay.

Acute Hospital Management

Acute trauma management guidelines are well established (Moore et al., 1991). The 'ABCs', which are ensuring a patent Airway, Breathing and maintenance of Circulation, are enshrined in all emergency practice, as is the importance of taking a history and performing an examination. Acute management of the patient with a spinal cord injury has special features resulting from spinal cord shock.

Breathing

Paralysis of intercostal muscles can occur, depending on the level of the lesion. Patients with acute cervical cord injuries can be fatigued in their breathing as a result. Pulse oximetry is a crude indicator of respiratory distress because it measures only haemoglobin saturation and not pO_2 (Hough, 1991). Any evidence of desaturation or of falling saturation should be reported to medical staff. Monitoring patients' breathing rate and pattern and their colour, and noting agitation or distress behaviour, is vital. Arterial blood gas analysis can be useful for confirming or refuting clinical judgement and may be the critical factor in deciding whether to provide ventilatory support.

Circulation

The sympathetic nerve supply to the heart is via cervical, cervical thoracic and upper thoracic branches of the sympathetic trunk. Cervical and upper thoracic injuries may produce denervation, with impaired ability to produce a needed tachycardia. Therefore, pulse rate may mislead in the presence of circulatory shock. There is skin vasodilation within the dermatomes caudal to the injury. This causes a lowering of blood pressure. Injudicious fluid replacement to augment the blood pressure can cause pulmonary oedema. Pharyngeal suction, urethral catheterisation, or simply repositioning of the patient can produce vagal overstimulation and lead to bradycardia; intravenous atropine may be required to restore normal heart rate.

Skin Care

Denervated skin is at risk from pressure damage within 20–30 minutes of injury. If this occurs, it can cause distress and delay in the rehabilitation process if there is ulceration. Clinical staff attending immediately after admission should be vigilant to protect the skin and should report red marks.

Gastrointestinal Tract

Spinal cord injury can produce ileus and gastric distension that can restrict movement of the diaphragm, further compromising breathing. A nasogastric tube should be placed for decompression if bowel sounds are absent. Gastric stress ulcers can occur and prophylactic treatment with mucosal protectors is recommended.

Bladder

Spinal shock causes retention of urine; the bladder should therefore be catheterised routinely in order to monitor fluid output and to protect it from overdistension damage.

Management of Acute Lesions at T4 and Above

Surgical stabilisation may be achieved by anterior or posterior fixation, or a combination of the two (e.g. Collins, 1995). Patients managed conservatively are immobilised with bedrest; depending on the degree of instability, they may have to be maintained in spinal alignment by skull traction. Traction is applied usually by Halo Traction, Crutchfield Calipers, Gardner–Wells or Cone Calipers (Grundy & Swain, 1993), depending on the preference of the surgeon and the individual's requirements.

Early mobilisation may be indicated and can be achieved using a Halo-brace. Care in handling and positioning during physiotherapy are discussed below under 'Physical management—passive movements'.

Length of immobilisation will vary depending on the extent of bony injury and ligamentous instability, and whether surgery has been performed. There may be several spinal segments affected and this will also influence the length of bedrest. Multiple level fractures in the cervical spine are usually treated conservatively by halo traction and a period of immobilisation in a hard collar. Bedrest is usually for 3 months. On starting mobilisation, patients with all levels of injury will usually wear a collar of some type, depending on their stability.

Management of Acute Lesions at T4 and Below

Spinal fractures in the thoracolumbar region are most common at the L1 level, this being the level of greatest mobility. Patients with unstable lesions at T9 and below must not have their hips flexed greater than 30 degrees in order to avoid lumbar flexion.

Stable wedge fractures are usually treated conservatively with a brace or plaster of Paris (or similar) jacket. Unstable burst fractures, with cord compression, will justify surgical decompression and fixation. Generally, an anterior and posterior fixation technique will require the wearing of a brace for 3 months postoperatively. If the spine is stable anteriorly, it may be sufficient to stabilise posteriorly. In this situation, a brace will be recommended for 6 months.

Bracing techniques vary greatly between institutions. A moulded hard plastic (subortholen) jacket can be made from an individual casting of plaster. Many braces are commercially available 'off the shelf' or other materials are used to form a brace, e.g. leather jackets or Neofract.

Spasticity: A Reminder!

Since the spinal cord is shorter than the vertebral column, lower vertebral injuries will not involve damage to the cord, but there will be nerve root damage which will determine the presence of spasticity. The spinal cord usually extends to the first or second lumbar vertebra (Williams, 1995). Below this level, the nerve roots descend as the cauda equina and emerge from their respective vertebral levels. Injuries at these lower levels, therefore, are peripheral nerve (or lower motor neurone) injuries.

A patient with an upper motor neurone injury, i.e. at the level of T12 or above, may present with a varied amount of spasticity. Weakness occurs but there may be sparing of muscle bulk to some extent due to the increased tone. A patient with a lower motor neurone injury, i.e. below the level of T12, will present with flaccid paralysis or weakness only. Obviously, this cut off level of T12 is a general rule as an individual's anatomy may vary from the usual.

REHABILITATION MEDICINE

After the acute phase, when rehabilitation takes place, special attention is paid to care of the skin, bladder and bowel and to sexual function. For further details than space allows for the overview given below, the reader is referred to specialist texts (e.g. Buchanan & Nawoezenski, 1987; Zedlik, 1992; Grundy & Swain, 1993).

Skin Care

Common sites of pressure sores are ischial (from prolonged sitting), sacral (from sheer loading), trochanteric, malleolar, calcaneal and plantar surfaces from prolonged loading or direct trauma. Spasticity producing contractures and postural deformity are potential risk factors. Although poor nutrition, incontinence and co-morbid factors increase the risk of decubitus ulceration, without ischaemia the ulcers do not arise. Therefore, patients are taught about risk management and provided with pressure re-distributing mattresses and cushions.

The Bladder

Urological complications of traumatic spinal cord injury are major mortal and morbid risks and the reader is referred to Fowler & Fowler (1993) for a review. Spinal cord damage disrupts the neural controls for storing and voiding urine. The objectives of definitive bladder management are to provide a system which ensures safety as well as minimal infection, handicap and cost.

In the acute stage the bladder is catheterised to allow free drainage, to accommodate any fluid input and output fluctuations, and to avoid bladder distension. After spinal shock passes, urodynamic studies are used to identify the emergent bladder behaviour. An appropriate form of catherisation is selected for long-term use.

Functional electrical stimulation, where anterior sacral root stimulators are implanted, may be used and is primarily for controlling urinary voiding but also facilitates defecation and penile erection separately. Reflex micturition (by tapping the abdominal wall or stroking the medial thigh) is not favoured because the bladder is unprotected from hyper-reflexic complications.

The Bowel

Although morbid complications rarely arise in the bowel, handicap is common and often perceived by patients as more devastating than limb paralysis. With laxatives, most people can achieve a bowel frequency within the normal range. For intractable constipation, occasional enemas can be useful. Increasing use of anterior sacral root stimulators and colostomies may reduce handicap. The mainstay of bowel care is to produce a predictable pattern which will minimise incontinence, impaction and interference with activities of daily living.

Fertility

Fertility is usually maintained in women, with the ovulatory cycle being normal within 9 months after injury. Fertility in men is, however, a problem (Brindley, 1984). Improvements in fertility rates for men after spinal cord injury have been made due to several important technical advances. These include improved methods in the retrieval and preparation of sperm, such as electro-ejaculation, and improved means of achieving fertilisation with limited quality and sperm numbers through *in-vitro* techniques.

SPECIAL PROBLEMS IN SPINAL CORD INJURY

Problems which are specifically prominent in patients with spinal cord injury are discussed briefly below.

Autonomic Dysreflexia

Autonomic dysreflexia can be described as a sympathetic nervous system discharge producing hypertension, bradycardia, sweating, pallor below the lesion level, skin vaso-constriction, headache, pilo-erection and capillary dilation. Some or all of these can result from such stimuli as bladder or rectal distension, or any afferent stimulus. If it occurs, the patient should be sat up, given appropriate medication, and the underlying cause treated. Patients and therapists should be aware that the hypertension can rise sufficiently to induce cerebral haemorrhage, so this should be treated as an emergency. In some cases, mild autonomic dysreflexic symptoms act as signals to patients for toileting. Induction of autonomic dysreflexia has been used foolishly, in the authors' view, to enhance sporting performance.

Increased Muscle Tone

This is an important issue in the management of patients with spinal cord injury (Young & Shahani, 1986; Priebe *et al.*, 1996); it is a very large subject and requires more consideration than this chapter allows (see also Chapters 5 & 25). Spasticity is essentially an abnormal increase in muscle tone, associated with increased stretch reflexes. In complete spinal cord lesions, it most commonly becomes apparent about 3 months after the injury and some weeks after the end of spinal shock. It tends to reach a maximum between 6 and 12 months after injury and then to diminish and become manageable. However, in a minority it remains at a high level and presents a major problem of management, affecting function, posture and joint movement.

In incomplete cord lesions, depending on the pattern, spasticity tends to occur earlier and may be present almost from the outset. It may be severe and render any underlying voluntary movement useless. Unfortunately, reduction in the spasticity does not always improve voluntary movement.

A moderate amount of spasticity will assist with standing transfers, maintain muscle bulk, protect the skin to some extent and may contribute to prevention of osteoporosis. It is when the spasticity is excessive that problems occur.

Spasticity Management

The best management is prevention and this takes place in the first few months after spinal cord injury. The basis of prevention comprises good posture and positioning, regular stretching of muscles, maintaining ROM at joints, and early weight bearing (see Chapter 25). It is also important to avoid triggering factors such as urinary tract infection or skin breakdown. When spasticity is established as a problem, physiotherapy remains the major component for treating it (see below).

The main medical approach is through pharmacology, although none of the drugs commonly used (baclofen, dantrolene and diazepam) is universally effective or indeed predictable in its effect. Nerve blocks of accessible nerves, such as the femoral nerve, have been used for many years, usually using either phenol or alcohol. All the above drugs have significant and numerous side effects (see Chapter 28). As the use of intramuscular botulinum toxin increases, the use of other nerve blocks will probably diminish.

Surgery has some place in treatment, in the form of tendon release and nerve divisions, such as obturator neurectomy. These techniques can be successful, particularly where the procedure has been carried out for hygiene and posture reasons.

Osteoporosis

Osteoporosis is a loss in bone mass without any alteration of the ratio between mineral and the organic matrix. A text by Riggs & Melton (1995) provides a comprehensive overview of osteoporosis. It is thought that immobilisation for long periods and a sedentary life lead to an increase in bone resorption, thus causing osteoporosis.

It is not known how quickly osteoporosis develops after spinal cord injury, but at 2 years after injury most patients will demonstrate a significant reduction in bone density in the lower limbs, though the spine tends to be spared. The osteoporosis may be sufficient to cause fractures of long bones during relatively simple manoeuvres, such as transfer or passive movements.

The issue of whether the patient should bear his or her weight when osteoporosis is present is a difficult one. It is not known how much effect weight bearing has on reducing established osteoporosis. The question is frequently asked whether a patient who has not stood for several years should recommence standing. Currently the advice of the unit at Stanmore is to start the weight-bearing programme with tilt-tabling for 2 or 3 months before standing in a frame. Such advice is empirical and it may be that better information from controlled studies will become available in the future.

Heterotopic Ossification

Calcification in denervated or upper motor neurone-disordered muscle remains an ill understood process and commonly occurs in patients with spinal cord injuries (David *et al.*, 1993). It may be confused in the early stages with DVT when it presents as swelling, alteration in skin colour and increased heat, usually in relation to a joint. It is a process which occurs over many months and the end result is the presence of mature bone within the tissue, demonstrable on radiography. During the active process, analysis of plasma biochemistry shows a raised alkaline phosphatase.

Effect on joint movements may be dramatic and lead to difficulty in posture, particularly in sitting. If ossification occurs around the hips it may lead to further skin pressure problems. Treatment of this condition, in which the aetiology and pathogenic process are uncertain, remains empirical. Management includes maintaining ROM with gentle stretching, and monitoring of the skin and posture to prevent as much deformity as possible. It must be emphasised that stretching should be gentle, as over-stretching may be a predisposing factor for this condition (David *et al.*, 1993). Pharmacological treatment has not yet been fully evaluated.

Psychological Aspects

Management of psychological and social issues must take place in parallel with early medical and rehabilitation aspects. In the early weeks and months after injury, the patient may present with rapid and dramatic changes in mood state and may express denial of his or her situation, anger at what has happened and depression, which may include stating the desire to die. A persisting underlying anxiety state may also occur and may become acute at times, with dramatic symptoms of 'out of body' experiences and dramatic autonomic physical effects.

Although all the members of the MDT will play a role in supporting a patient, advice and guidance from a qualified psychologist is essential and at times one-to-one direct patient therapy by the psychologist is necessary. The process of adaptation to spinal paralysis, reflected as integration back into the community, is a gradual one. Maintaining a positive approach with realistic expectations is essential for the patient's wellbeing (see Chapter 27).

PHYSICAL MANAGEMENT

As with medical and general management, care can be divided into the acute and rehabilitation stages; it must be integrated with those other aspects (CSP, 1997).

ACUTE CARE

In the early post-injury phase, physical management will mainly involve prevention of respiratory and circulatory complications, and care of pressure areas.

Principles of Assessment

Assessment must be carried out as soon after admission as possible to obtain an objective baseline measurement of function, to see whether specific problems are likely to develop and to set up a prophylactic treatment programme. Current history of the injury is taken from the patient's notes, including the results of relevant tests, e.g. lung function. Medical history is also noted. It is important to be aware of associated injuries, as these may influence management. The principles of assessment are discussed in Chapter 4.

The therapist needs to assess:

- Respiratory state.
- Passive range of movement of all joints above and below the level of injury.
- Muscle function—i.e. strength using a muscle chart and the Oxford Grading System, Medical Research Council (MRC) scale or ASIA (1992) assessment; and tone using the Ashworth Scale or another assessment tool (Bohannon & Smith, 1987).
- Extent of sensation and proprioceptive loss.

Respiratory Function

Extreme ventilatory compromise in spinal injury is caused by one or more of the following:

- Inspiratory and expiratory muscle paralysis leading to decreased lung volume.
- Loss of effective cough.
- Diminished chest wall mobility.
- Reduced lung compliance.
- Increased energy cost of breathing and paradoxical chest wall movement.

Chest and head injuries are commonly associated with spinal injury and provide their own respiratory problems which must also be assessed and treated appropriately.

Muscles Affecting Respiratory Function

The abdominal muscles (innervated by T6–T12 spinal nerves) are essential for forced expiration and effective coughing. They also stabilise the lower ribs and assist the function of the diaphragm. The intercostal muscles (innervated by T1–T11 spinal nerves) have a predominantly inspiratory function as prime movers but also as fixators for the diaphragm. These muscle groups comprise about 40% of respiratory motor effort.

The diaphragm (innervated by C3–C5, phrenic nerves) is the main inspiratory muscle but relies on other muscles to maximise efficiency. The accessory muscles (innervated by C1–C8 nerves and cranial nerve XI) include the trapezius, sternomastoid, levator scapulae and scalenii muscles; they can act as sole muscles of inspiration for short periods, but if the diaphragm is paralysed they cannot maintain adequate ventilation unassisted.

Chest Movement

The use of accessory muscles and diaphragm function can be assessed by palpation at the lower costal border. Muscle paralysis results in altered mechanics of respiration. In lesions involving paralysis of the abdominal and intercostal muscles, the lower ribs will be drawn in on inspiration in a paradoxical movement (Webber & Pryor, 1993). These abnormalities reduce the efficiency of the diaphragm in producing negative intrathoracic pressure, hence causing reductions in lung volume and efficiency of ventilation. Any asymmetry of movement, as well as respiratory rate, is noted.

Routine Auscultation

This is as for any other patient. However, one must remember that problems such as added breath sounds, pneumothorax or haemopneumothorax severely affect the injured person's ability to maintain adequate ventilation and perfusion.

Forced Vital Capacity (FVC)

This is a readily available objective measurement of respiratory muscle function, as is peak inspiratory flow rate. It is essential that FVC is recorded on a regular basis, especially in the first 24–48 hours. This is because cord swelling in the initial stage may cause symptoms higher up the spinal cord by two or three spinal levels. A progressive fall in FVC may be indicative of an impairment in diaphragmatic function.

If the FVC is <1 litre, the therapist may choose to instigate either intermittent positive pressure breathing (IPPB), e.g. the Bird respirator, or bilevel intermittent positive airway pressure (BIPAP) as discussed by Hough (1991). This assisted ventilation can be used prophylactically to maintain and increase inspiratory volume and aid clearance of secretions. It is a useful adjunct to active manual techniques for patients with sputum retention and lung collapse, and can be used to administer bronchodilators (Webber & Pryor, 1993).

In cases of severe pain from rib fractures and associated soft tissue injuries, a mixture of nitrous oxide and oxygen (Entonox) may be used and, if applicable, entrained into the IPPB circuit. Breathing exercises and respiratory muscle training may also include the use of

IPPB. However, as explained by Webber & Pryor (1993), continuous training would be necessary to maintain improvement. Elective ventilation is normally undertaken if the FVC falls below 500 ml.

Cough
A patient with a lesion above T6 will not have an effective cough as he or she will have lost the action of the abdominal muscles. The physiotherapist can compensate for this loss by the use of assisted coughing in order that the patient can clear secretions (Bromley, 1998).

Pain
This can cause splinting and further reduction in function of the diaphragm. Transcutaneous nerve stimulation is useful for pain relief (see Chapter 24). In the case of rib fractures, stimulation appears to be most effective if electrodes are positioned directly along the intercostal nerves but this suggestion is based on clinical observation only.

Treatment Objectives in the Acute Phase
The main objectives are:
- To institute a prophylactic respiratory regimen and treat any complications.
- To achieve independent respiratory status where possible.
- To maintain full ROM of all joints within the limitations determined by the fracture (i.e. type, stability, severity and level).
- To monitor neurological status and manage appropriately.
- To involve/educate the patient, carers, family and staff.
- To maintain/strengthen all innervated muscle groups.

Respiratory Care and Management of Complications
If no other respiratory complications are present, the physiotherapist will teach prophylactic breathing exercises to encourage chest expansion and improve ventilation. This will assist in strengthening any recovering respiratory muscles as spinal shock subsides. Incentive spirometry is useful for patients with midthoracic lesions and above, to give the patient and family positive feedback of breathing function. Care is necessary to maintain stability of the spine. It is advised that shoulders are held for patients with unstable lesions of T4 and above when performing an assisted cough. In these circumstances, bilateral techniques should always be used in order to maintain spinal alignment. Adapted postural drainage for an unstable lesion is performed using specialised turning beds that allow spinal alignment to be maintained.

Ventilation–Assisted ventilation may be necessary, and such intervention before the patient becomes exhausted will make subsequent management easier. Elective intubation is potentially less damaging to the spinal cord than intubation following cardiac arrest. Respiratory therapy for the spinal-injured ventilated patient is similar to that for other ventilated patients (Ada *et al.*, 1990; Hough, 1991; Smith & Ball, 1998), apart from added vigilance to protect the fracture site.

Weaning from the ventilator should start as soon as the patient's condition stabilises. It is important to avoid fatigue whilst weaning, so careful monitoring ensures that FVC does not fall by more than 20%, or respiratory rate rise above 25–30 breaths per minute. For those patients who fail to wean, usually those with a greater degree of diaphragm paralysis, long-term ventilation is required (see 'The long-term ventilated patient').

Suctioning–Secretions should be removed by suction; this should always be undertaken with care in patients with spinal cord injury. Suctioning is not recommended in the cervical non-intubated patient as the neck cannot be extended to open the airway. It is important to assist the cough when stimulating the cough reflex, as merely stimulating the reflex will not produce an effective cough.

In patients with lesions above T6, the thoracolumbar sympathetic outflow is interrupted. During suction the vagus nerve is unopposed and the patient may become hypotensive and bradycardiac, possibly resulting in cardiac arrest. Endotracheal intubation may produce a similar response. Suction causes vagal stimulation via the carotid bodies, which pass impulses to the brain via the glossopharyngeal nerves and are sensitive to lack of oxygen (Williams, 1995). It is therefore wise to preoxygenate the patient and monitor heart rate.

Passive Movements
As discussed in Chapter 24, the aims of passive movements are to:
- Assist circulation.
- Maintain muscle length, therefore preventing soft tissue shortening of all paralysed structures.
- Maintain full ROM of all joints.

Passive movements are commenced from the first day of injury and features which are specifically important in patients with spinal cord injuries are now discussed. Shoulder movements are usually performed at least twice a day and leg movements once a day, in order to monitor any return of movement. For lumbar and low thoracic fractures, hip flexion should be kept to below 30 degrees, to avoid lumbar flexion, until stability is established. Knee flexion must, therefore, be performed in Taylor's position, i.e. 'frogging' (see Figure 9.3). If there is sparing of muscle function, these movements should be performed as active assisted exercises.

Special emphasis should be put on the following:
- Stretch finger flexors with wrist in neutral to preserve tenodesis grip (Bromley, 1998).
- Ensure a full fist can be attained with wrist extension.
- Pronation and supination in both elbow flexion and extension.
- Full elevation and lateral rotation of the shoulder from day one.
- Stretch long head of triceps—arm in elevation with elbow flexion.

- Stretch rhomboids bilaterally—avoid twisting cervical spine.
- Stretch upper fibres of trapezius muscle.

Where there is no active flexion of the fingers and thumb, it is appropriate to allow shortening of the long flexors. However, the ROM of individual joints at the wrist, fingers and thumb must be maintained. When the wrist is actively extended, the fingers and thumb are pulled into flexion to produce a functional 'key-type' grip, the 'Tenodesis grip'. If this contracture does not occur naturally, it can be encouraged by splinting whilst in the acute phase.

During the period of spinal shock, care must be taken not to overstretch structures. Once reflex activity returns, limbs must be handled with care so as not to elicit spasm and re-enforce the spastic pattern. Extreme ROM must be avoided, especially at the hip and knee, as micro-trauma may be a predisposing factor in the formation of

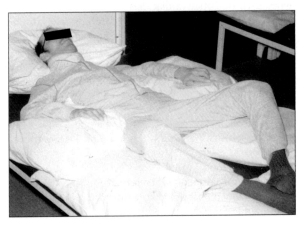

Figure 9.3 A patient in the 'frogging' or Taylor's position. This position is used to prevent movement of the lumbar spine during passive movements of the knees. It is used here to reduce mass extensor tone.

periarticular ossification (see above). Passive movements of paralysed limbs are continued until the patient is mobile and thus capable of ensuring full mobility through their own activities, unless there are complications such as excessive spasm or stiffness.

Pain can be a problem during passive movements in patients with spinal cord injury, notably due to adverse neural tension (see Chapter 23). The presence of DVT is also a problem, so passive movements should be performed only if the patient is fully heparinised.

During the recovery phase, the physiotherapist should use the principles of facilitation of normal movement in handling and moving the patient. Normal movement patterns are used during exercises rather than isolated muscle activities, to encourage functional movement.

Turning and Positioning

Whilst patients are managed with bedrest they will require frequent turning. A pictorial turning chart can be used to assist staff with the turning regimen over each 24-hour period. This is to avoid pressure marking of anaesthetic skin and gives an opportunity to check skin tolerance. This turning regimen is used in conjunction with postural drainage positions. Turning beds can be used for repositioning a patient, and the choice of bed depends on the individual unit's policy.

Upper limb positioning in the tetraplegic patient is very important during bedrest. Where increased flexor tone is a problem, the patient is placed in the crucifix position, with elbows extended and shoulders alternated between lateral and medial rotation (Figure 9.4).

Incomplete cervical lesions are particularly prone to shortening of soft tissues due to muscle imbalance, resulting in partial subluxation and pain. Length of the medial rotators of the shoulder should be maintained to reduce this problem.

Positioning is used to minimise spasticity as in patients with other conditions. When the patient is exhibiting mass muscle tone in flexion or extension, the limbs may be placed into a reflex-inhibited position, or whole trunk and

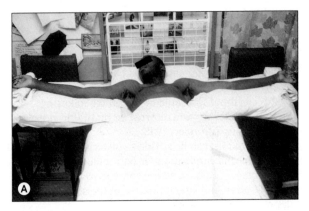
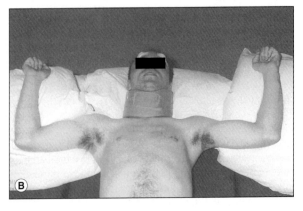

Figure 9.4 Upper limb positioning in the tetraplegic patient. (A) The crucifix position. (B) A modified crucifix position with the shoulders in lateral rotation.

limb positions may be used. Positioning is also discussed in Chapters 7 & 8 and in further detail by Pope (1996).

Preparation for Mobilisation
Patient education begins during the acute phase and explanation of treatment interventions is vital to encourage the patient to take control of rehabilitation.

Initiation of mobilisation—Once check radiographs have been performed, mobilisation is initiated by sitting the patient up gradually. Postural hypotension will be the main problem and patients with lesions at T6 and above will require an elasticated abdominal binder. This helps to maintain intrathoracic pressure to reduce pooling of the blood from lack of abdominal action. Once the patient starts to sit up, he or she will be supported in a hard or soft collar, or a brace. Anti-embolism stockings may be worn as prophylaxis against DVT. Special adaptations to wheelchairs can be used to help reduce hypotensive fainting, e.g. reclining back and raised leg supports.

Pressure lifting—This is a technique in which patients lift themselves in their wheelchairs to relieve pressure. It is recommended that they lift every half hour, for approximately 30 seconds. Where a patient cannot lift, a modified position in forward leaning is used.

REHABILITATION
The following section outlines physiotherapy management from the start of the rehabilitation phase through to discharge. Much of this information has been gained from the experience of the authors' unit at Stanmore; procedures can vary between centres but the principles are similar (Bromley, 1998; Whalley Hamilton, 1995).

Aims of Rehabilitation
- To establish an interdisciplinary process which is patient-focused, comprehensive and co-ordinated.
- Early intervention and prophylaxis to prevent further complications.
- To achieve functional independence, whether physical or verbal, appropriate to the level of injury.
- To achieve and maintain successful reintegration into the community.

Goal Planning
Rehabilitation can be evaluated by reviewing the achievement of goals, which should be patient-focused, appropriate and objective. Subjective goals are difficult to evaluate. The goals can be set in many ways but it is recommended that they are created in a team environment, led by the patient, with interdisciplinary co-operation to ensure that they are achievable. Regular review and resetting of goals are required.

Objectives of Rehabilitation
The progression of objectives as the patient gains more ability is outlined below. These objectives need to be set in relation to the level of spinal injury and the appropriate functional goals (Table 9.1).

Bed Mobility
Rolling from side to side is taught first, then lying to sitting, and sitting to lying. Function is achieved dependent upon the level of the lesion, e.g. C5, rolling side to side, C6, rolling, lying to sitting and sitting to lying, C7, independent in all aspects of bed mobility.

Sitting Balance
Starting with sitting balance in the wheelchair, this is progressed to sitting on a plinth supported, unsupported, static and then dynamic. Balance is practised in short and long sitting, hamstring length determining the ability to long sit independently.

Lifting
Lifting starts with pressure lifts in the wheelchair, and progresses to lifts on blocks on a plinth and then unaided without blocks.

Wheelchair Mobility
Wheelchair mobility and safety are taught. Adaptations such as extended brakes and a modular supportive backrest are required for higher lesions.

Transfers
Depending on the level of the lesion and functional ability, a sliding board may be used for legs-up and legs-down transfers on to the bed. This can then be progressed without a board where possible. Transfers are then progressed to lifting from various levels: high to low; low to high; between two plinths; floor to plinth; floor to chair; chair to car; chair to easy chair.

Standing Programme
Unless contraindicated, standing is commenced as soon as possible using a tilt-table. This has many benefits: respiratory and psychological, maintenance of bone density, and improved systemic body functions. An abdominal binder is recommended for patients with lesions of T6 and above. Once the patient can stand with no ill effect, progression is made to standing in a frame such as the Oswestry Standing Frame, working up to standing for 1 hour, 3 times a week. Patients with lesions of C5 and below should be capable of standing in the Oswestry Frame. Whilst standing, trunk balance work can start by, for example, removing hand support, throwing and catching a ball. There are many standing devices available commercially, some with electric hoist adaptations to assist standing from sitting. Once good balance is achieved, the patient can prepare for caliper walking by standing in backslabs, where appropriate.

Upper Limb Strengthening
This is started whilst still in bed in the acute phase using a variety of techniques, e.g. resisted exercises,

Functional goals of rehabilitation in relation to the level of the spinal cord lesion

Level	Key muscle control	Movement	Functional goals
C1-3	Sternocleidomastoid Upper trapezius Levator	Neck control	Ventilator-dependent Electric wheelchair Verbally independent
C4	C3 plus diaphragm	Shoulder shrug	Electric wheelchair Verbally independent
C5	Biceps Deltoid Rotator cuff	Elbow flexion, supination Shoulder flexion, abduction	Manual wheelchair with capstans Electric wheelchair for long distance Independent brushing teeth/hair and feeding with feeding strap
C6	Wrist extensors Supinator	Wrist extension, pronation Tenodesis grip	Manual wheelchair (+/-capstans) Independent feeding, grooming, dressing top half, simple cooking May transfer same height, bed to chair, bed to toilet
C7	Triceps Latissimus dorsi Flexor digitorum Flexor carpi radialis	Elbow extension Finger flexion/extension	Manual wheelchair Independent ADL, simple transfers, i.e. bed, car, toilet, may drive with hand controls
C8	All upper limbs except lumbricals, interossei	Limited fine finger movements	Manual wheelchair Independent ADL, simple transfers, i.e. bed, chair to toilet, chair to car and chair to bath
T1-T5	Varying intercostals and back muscles	Trunk support No lower limb movements	Full wheelchair independence Orthotic ambulation
T6-T12	Abdominals	Trunk control	Orthotic/caliper ambulation
L1-L2	Psoas major Iliopsoas	Hip flexion	Caliper ambulation
L3-L4	Quadriceps Tibialis anterior	Knee extension Foot dorsiflexion	Ambulation with orthoses and crutches/sticks
L5	Peronei	Eversion	Ambulation with relevant orthoses
S1-S5	Glutei Bladder, bowel, sexual function	Hip extension	Normal gait

Table 9.1 Functional goals of rehabilitation in relation to the level of the spinal cord lesion.

biofeedback, electrical stimulation and PNF (see Chapter 24). Once the patient begins mobilisation in the wheelchair there are many options for strengthening, e.g. weight circuits and sporting activities. This is an enjoyable adjunct to rehabilitation and encourages reintegration.

Hydrotherapy is used for strengthening and as preparation for swimming. Patients are taught how to roll in the water and to swim. If the patient is wearing a brace, this will limit activities in the water. Anyone with an FVC of <1 litre will need careful consideration before swimming is introduced.

Pain Management
Pain management is continued through from acute care. The physiotherapist will use any relevant modalities, such as ultrasound, interferential, ice and positioning, electrical stimulation, stretches and acupuncture, unless otherwise contraindicated (see Chapter 24).

Cardiovascular Fitness
The arm-powered ergonomic bike may be used, and progressed. Wheelchair slalom, with increasing speed of

circuit, and more active sporting activities are encouraged. Hydrotherapy and swimming can also be used to improve cardiovascular fitness. Activities can eventually progress to more competitive sports and clubs. Cardiovascular fitness after spinal cord injury has been reviewed by Davis & Glaser (1990).

Education/Advice to Carers/Family
Carers are advised on how to handle and lift the patient whilst paying attention to skin care, their own safety and back care. They are also taught how to assist if necessary with putting on and taking off calipers, and lifting to stand and sit in calipers. These activities should be carried out in accordance with the unit's lifting and handling policy.

Wheelchairs
The variety of wheelchairs available increases each year, including those which enable the patient to rise into standing. Initially, patients are mobilised in a 'standard' wheelchair, which offers greatest support and stability. Following a comprehensive assessment, the wheelchair is correctly fitted and adjusted. Adaptions are made to provide a well supported, evenly balanced seating position (Pope, 1996).

The key to good sitting stability is achieved by support and alignment at the pelvis. The cushion is equally important and should be assessed in a similar way, also taking into account the need for protection of pressure areas. Various methods can be used to assess pressure areas and skin viability when sitting and these can aid cushion prescription (Barbenel *et al.*, 1983). At a later stage in rehabilitation, it will be useful to try out a variety of wheelchairs which can offer greater mobility and independence according to an individual's needs.

Functional Electrical Stimulation
Functional elecrtrical stimulation (FES) aims to assist paraplegic patients to walk and is still at an experimental stage. Despite promising advances in technology, the physiological limitations of the neuromuscular system prohibit the clinical use of FES to achieve a realistic and successful functional outcome. Further research is required to overcome these problems. Principles of the technique are discussed in Chapter 24.

Discharge Plan
A home visit is made by the occupational therapist and community team and may include school or workplace. The physiotherapist may be involved in this visit to assess accessibility for wheelchair and calipers.

Coping in the event of a fall from the wheelchair or out of bed is reviewed, as well as safety of all handling techniques by the carers. A home programme is devised to ensure maintained fitness, stressing that standing should be continued. Throughout rehabilitation, the team provides psychological support in overcoming functional difficulties. Goal planning will ensure that this is continued after discharge.

On discharge, all patients will require further close follow-up and reassessment, which may involve the community physiotherapist. Ideally this will be a multidisciplinary review to maintain continued support and to monitor physical well-being and thus facilitate reintegration into society.

Rehabilitation of Incomplete Lesions
Emphasis is placed on managing muscle imbalance, spasticity and tone, and proprioception and sensory loss. As incomplete lesions cover a wide range of disability, treatment will depend on the level of disability and specific physical problems. The treatment techniques mentioned below are discussed in Chapter 24, except where indicated.

Treatment may include: facilitation of normal movement; muscle strengthening; reduction of muscle imbalance (see Chapter 23); and inhibition of spasticity (see Chapter 25). Balance re-education may include: use of the gymnastic ball; mat and plinth work; and use of a wobble board. Gait re-education, wheelchair skills and functional activities are performed as appropriate to the patient's level of ability.

ASSISTED GAIT, CALIPERS AND ORTHOSES
During the middle phase of rehabilitation, the patient is assessed for suitability for walking with calipers. Depending on the type of fixation, gait training will normally commence about a year after surgery, or earlier if no fixation surgery was indicated.

It should be recognised that, even if a patient has the ability to walk with calipers, he or she may not choose to or may be advised not to try. Techniques used for gait training have been discussed in detail by Bromley (1998) and an outline of the progression of training is given below.

The gait training process is physically demanding and requires commitment. There are several criteria which should be considered :
- Sufficient upper limb strength to lift body weight.
- Full range of movement of hips and knees, and no hip flexion contracture.
- Cardiovascular fitness sufficient to sustain walking activity.
- Assessment of spinal deformity, e.g. scoliosis, that may hinder standing balance.
- Motivation of the patient to complete the training.
- Assessment of spasticity that may make walking unsafe.

Experience has shown us that many patients complete their training with calipers, only to discard them a few months or years later as walking has become too much effort. Wheelchair use may be preferable, as the hands are free for functional activities whereas they are not when walking with calipers.

Orthoses
The ability to walk with calipers and the degree of support required depend on the functional level of injury. The following are examples of orthoses used for different levels of injury:
- C7–L1: Douglas brace, HGO (hip guidance orthosis), ARGO (advanced reciprocal gait orthosis), RGO, Walkabout.

- T6–T12: Caliper walk/Walkabout with parawalker/rollator; progress to crutches depends on patient's function.
- T9–L3: Caliper walk with comfortable handle crutches.
- L3 and below: Appropriate orthoses or walking aid.

Initial Gait Work

To commence caliper training, backslabs of plaster of Paris, Dynacast or similar casting material are made for the individual. The backslabs are bandaged on and toe springs applied. Standing balance is achieved in the parallel bars, in front of a mirror, by standing in extension and resting back on the tension of the iliofemoral ligaments. The lifting technique is taught in the standing position, lifting the whole body weight with full control. Lift from sitting to standing and back to sitting is also taught.

Once the patient has achieved standing balance and the appropriate degree of support required, dynamic balance work is started. This includes swinging the legs forwards and backwards, turning safely, swing-to and swing-through gait patterns, and the four-point gait technique for stepping practice.

Transfers

Transferring in backslabs is then practised, from plinth to chair, chair to plinth, and from chair to standing.

Middle Stage of Gait Work

Progression to a rollator or crutches is begun at this stage. Balance is achieved using one parallel bar and one crutch, or with a rollator and one person assisting the patient. Gait patterns and transfers (described above) are then practised. Depending on the functional level, four-point gait with crutches is taught, then kerbs, slopes and stairs. Video assessment for problem solving and improvement of gait techniques may be useful at this stage.

Late Stage of Gait Work

On completion of backslab training, the patient is measured for calipers. For patients using reciprocal gait orthoses, gait re-education is practised in the parallel bars and progressed to a rollator and possibly crutches, as outlined above.

A home standing programme for all patients is devised to improve confidence. This entails using backslabs daily to maintain strength and cardiovascular fitness and to improve mobility. Goals are decided mutually as to how calipers and walking aids will be used at home and at work, to achieve optimum function.

THE LONG-TERM VENTILATED PATIENT

Survival of patients with high lesions is now more common. Resettlement into the community requires domiciliary ventilation and a complex care package. Specialised wheelchairs are available which can be controlled by the mouth or head. Prophylactic chest care is vital, with regular bagging and suction, to reduce atelectasis and prevent infection. These patients are managed with a tracheostomy, which allows easy chest care.

Some patients may be appropriate candidates for diaphragmatic pacing by electrical stimulation of the phrenic nerve. Suitability for this technique is determined by careful assessment involving nerve conduction studies and may include fluoroscopic examination to visualise diaphragmatic excursion (Zedlik, 1992).

Initially, physiotherapy will aim to maximise strength in all innervated muscles to assist in head control and strengthen accessory respiratory muscles. The tilt-table is used for regular standing to prevent contractures and to promote physical wellbeing. Passive movements to prevent contractures and maintain joint range for skin and personal care are continued.

Management of spasticity is also an important consideration and may involve antispasticity medication (see Chapter 28). The aim for these patients is to achieve verbal independence and control of their environment. Various control devices can be operated by the head or mouth, or by voice activation.

POST-DISCHARGE MANAGEMENT AND REINTEGRATION

The discharge of a person with a spinal cord injury will require a full team handover to local community services to ensure that all areas of the person's needs are met. If home adaptations or rehousing are not completed but the patient is ready for discharge, transfer to an interim placement may be required.

The Spinal Injuries Unit will always be available as a resource back-up should any complications or problems arise. During rehabilitation, patients are introduced to special organisations to assist in the reintegration process. These groups can offer social and leisure activities, whilst others have a support and advisory role (see 'Associations and Support Groups').

CONCLUSION

The management of the person with a spinal cord injury is complex and lifelong. This chapter has outlined the care of adults and space did not allow discussion of paediatric care. The principles are essentially similar but children require special consideration in certain aspects (Osenback & Menezes, 1992; Short et al., 1992; also see other childhood conditions in Section 3 of the present book). A multidisciplinary, functional goal-oriented rehabilitation programme should enable the patient with spinal cord injury to live as full and independent a life as possible.

REFERENCES

Ada L, Canning C, Paratz J. Care of the unconscious head-injured patient. In: Ada L, Canning C, eds. *Key issues in neurological physiotherapy*. London: Butterworth Heinemann; 1990:249-287.

American Spinal Injuries Association (ASIA). *International standards for neurological and functional classification of spinal cord injury*. Chicago: ASIA; 1992.

Barbenel JC, Forbes CD, Lowe GDO. *Pressure sores*. London: Macmillan Press; 1983.

Bohannon RW, Smith MB. Interrater reliability of a modified Ashworth scale of muscle spasticity. *Phys Ther* 1987, **67**:206-207.

Brindley GS. The fertility of men with spinal injury. *Paraplegia* 1984, **22**:337-348.

Bromley I. *Tetraplegia and paraplegia, 5th edition*. London: Churchill Livingstone; 1998. In preparation.

Buchanan LE, Nawoezenski DA. *Spinal cord injury concepts and management approaches*. London: Williams & Wilkins; 1987.

Chartered Society of Physiotherapy (CSP). *Standards of physiotherapy practice for people with spinal cord lesions*. London: CSP; 1997.

Collins W. Surgery in the acute treatment of spinal cord injury: a review of the past forty years. *J Spinal Cord Med* 1995, **18**:3-8.

David O, Sett P, Burr RG, *et al*. The relationship of hetertopic ossification to passive movements in paraplegic patients. *Disabil Rehabil* 1993, **15**:114-118.

Davis G, Glaser R. Cardiorespiratory fitness following spinal cord injury: In: Ada L, Canning C, eds. *Key issues in neurological physiotherapy*. London: Butterworth Heinemann; 1990:155-196.

Dennis F. Three column spine and its significance in the classification of acute thoracolumbar spinal injuries. *Spine* 1983, **8**:817-831.

Dittuno JF, Young W, Donovan WH. The International Standards Booklet for neurological and functional classification of spinal cord injury. *Paraplegia* 1994, **32**:70-80.

Fowler CJ, Fowler CG. Neurogenic bladder dysfunction and its management. In: Greenwood R, Barnes MP, McMillian TM *et al*., eds. *Neurological rehabilitation*. London: Churchill Livingstone; 1993:269-277.

Gardner BP, Theocleous F, Krishnan KR. Outcome following acute spinal cord injury: a review of 198 patients. *Paraplegia* 1988, **26**:94-98.

Grundy D, Swain A. *ABC of spinal cord injury, 2nd edition*. London: British Medical Association; 1993.

Hough A. *Physiotherapy in respiratory care: a problem solving approach*. London: Chapman & Hall; 1991.

Hughes JT. Pathological changes after spinal cord injury. In: Illis LS, ed. *Spinal cord dysfunction assessment*. Oxford: Oxford University Press; 1988:34-40.

Illis LS. *Spinal cord dysfunction assessment*. Oxford: Oxford University Press; 1988.

Mendoza N, Bradford R, Middleton F. Spinal injury. In: Greenwood R, Barnes MP, McMillan TM *et al*., eds. *Neurological rehabilitation*. London: Churchill Livingstone; 1993:545-560.

Moore EE, Mattox KL, Feliciano DV. *Trauma, 2nd edition*. Connecticut: Appleton & Lange; 1991.

Osenback RK, Menezes AM. Paediatric spinal cord and vertebral column injury. *Neurosurg* 1992, **30**:385-390.

Pope P. Postural management and special seating. In: Edwards S, ed. *Neurological physiotherapy: a problem-solving approach*. Edinburgh: Churchill Livingstone; 1996:135-160.

Priebe MM, Sherwood AM, Thornby JI, *et al*. Clinical assessment of spasticity in spinal cord injury: a multidimensional problem. *Arch Phys Med Rehab* 1996, **77**:713-716.

Riggs BL, Melton LJ III. *Osteoporosis: etiology, diagnosis and management*. Philadelphia: Lippincott-Raven; 1995.

Short DJ, Frankel HL, Bergström EMK. *Injuries of the spinal cord in children*. London: Elsevier Science; 1992. (Handbook of Clinical Neurology, vol. 17(61): Spinal cord trauma).

Smith M, Ball V. *Cardiovascular/Respiratory Physiotherapy*. London: Mosby; 1998. In progress.

Soopramanien A. Epidemiology of spinal injuries in Romania. *Paraplegia* 1994, **32**:715-722.

Spinal Injuries Association (SIA). *Statistics supplied for year 1994/1995*. London: SIA; 1995.

Webber BA, Pryor JA. *Physiotherapy for respiratory and cardiac problems*. Edinburgh: Churchill Livingstone; 1993.

Whalley Hamilton K. *Spinal cord injury rehabilitation*. Canada: Chapman & Hall; 1995.

Williams P. *Gray's anatomy, 38th edition*. Edinburgh: Churchill Livingstone; 1995.

Young RR, Shahani BT. Spasticity in spinal cord injured patients. In: Block RF, Basbaum M, eds. *Management of spinal cord injuries*. Baltimore: Williams & Wilkins; 1986:241-283.

Zedlik CP. *Management of spinal cord injury, 2nd edition*. Boston: Jones & Bartlett Publishers; 1992.

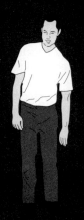

10 R Birch, J Armistead, D Horne, M Nurse & E Hunter

PERIPHERAL NERVE INJURIES

CHAPTER OUTLINE

- **Anatomical and functional features**
- **Causes and incidence of nerve injuries**
- **Clinical presentation and general management**
- **Principles of physical management**

INTRODUCTION

The consequences of an injury to a peripheral nerve can include: loss of sensation, with risk of damage to skin and joint; paralysis, causing atrophy and fixed deformity; and pain. This chapter outlines the work of the multidisciplinary team(MDT), in particular in the treatment of brachial plexus injuries in adults and in children. Specialist centres for the management of these injuries are rare and experience has evolved from them. There is a lack of literature on this subject and much of the content of this chapter is produced from the experience of the authors' Rehabilitation Unit which was set up over 35 years ago to treat patients with severe injuries to peripheral nerves. Wynn Parry's 1981 book is suggested as a comprehensive reference on this subject.

SOME ANATOMICAL AND FUNCTIONAL FEATURES

PERIPHERAL NERVES

The peripheral nerves consist of bundles or fascicles of nerve fibres embedded in connective tissue and a rich longitudinally oriented network of blood vessels. The axons are cytoplasmic extensions of cells lying within the dorsal root ganglia, the autonomic ganglia or the spinal cord itself. Axons are enveloped by satellite Schwann cells. This composite structure of the axon and a sheath of Schwann cells is the nerve fibre. The axons range in diameter from <1 to 20 micrometers. The smallest axons, surrounded by columns of Schwann cell processes, are the non-myelinated nerve fibres and are the most common. Larger axons are surrounded by a sheath of myelin, a lamellar condensation of the Schwann cell cytoplasm and are hence termed myelinated nerve fibres. The characteristics of nerve fibres and the transmission of neural impulses are described in Chapter 1.

THE CONNECTIVE TISSUES

Numbers of nerve fibres are surrounded by the endoneurium, a tightly packed tissue containing collagen, fibroblasts and capillary blood vessels. Surrounding these clusters of nerve fibres is an envelope termed the perineurium, a sheath of flattened cells. This is the most discrete of the connective tissue envelopes of a peripheral nerve. The peri-neurium together with its contents is called a fascicle or bundle. Numbers of fascicles are grouped together by the epineurium, a condensation of areolar connective tissue. There is a rich network of blood vessels within this tissue, which forms the greater part of the cross-sectional area of a peripheral nerve. One of the functions of the epineurium is to protect nerve fibres from pressure and its smooth glistening structure permits gliding of the nerve across joints. Scarring or entrapment inhibits nerve gliding by tethering of the epineurium and this is a common source of pain and disturbance of function. Physiotherapists commonly encounter examples of this, such as entrapment of spinal nerves by an osteophyte encroaching within the intervertebral foramen.

CAUSES AND INCIDENCE OF NERVE INJURIES

The causes of peripheral nerve injuries are summarised in Table 10.1. Most open wounds, in civilian practice, are caused by such sharp objects as knives or glass, and in the majority of these early repair of the nerve is preferred. Injury to a nerve from a missile or from an open fracture is much more severe. Closed traction injury is usually the result of a high-energy injury and the patient may have suffered multiple and even life-threatening injuries. The main cause is road traffic accidents, typically in young motor cyclists who sustain a brachial plexus injury (Rosson, 1987). Another type of brachial plexus damage is irradiation neuritis (IN), a condition caused by radiotherapy for cancer of the neck and axilla (Birch, 1993). Birth injuries occur, leading to a condition termed obstetric brachial plexus palsy (OBPP). The incidence of brachial plexus injuries in the UK is reported to be 1000 cases per year (Birch, 1993); over 500 cases are closed traction injuries, and there are about 200 cases of IN and at least 100 cases of OBPP.

CLINICAL PRESENTATION AND GENERAL MANAGEMENT

The cause and severity of damage will determine the type of injury, which can be classified as described below. Various nerves which are commonly injured are also outlined below. The principles of management apply to all nerves, although the brachial plexus is generally used as an example in the following sections.

CLASSIFICATION OF NERVE INJURIES

The most clinically useful classification of nerve injuries is that described by Seddon (1975) and is based on the behaviour of the axon after different types of injury (Table 10.2). In neurapraxia, a conduction block, there is no interruption of the axon and the architecture of the nerve is more or less undisturbed. It is relatively uncommon in clinical practice and most cases rapidly recover if the cause has been removed. In axonotmesis and neurotmesis, the axon is cut across. The distal part undergoes a process called Wallerian degeneration in which the axoplasm fragments and disappears and myelin gradually disintegrates (Lundborg, 1993). In axonotmesis, the connective tissues of the nerve are more or less intact and there is a high chance of spontaneous recovery. For details on the process of neural regeneration see Mitchell & Osterman (1991). In neurotmesis the whole nerve trunk is cut and there is separation of the stumps. Spontaneous recovery does not occur in humans, and surgical repair is necessary.

Neurapraxia is characterised by absence of pain, preservation of sweating and normal vasomotor tone in the extremities, preservation of some modalities of sensation such as deep pressure sense, and by rapid recovery. In the degenerative lesions, axonotmesis and neurotmesis, there is complete loss of all nerve function distal to the level of the injury. The distinction between these two lesions can be made only by waiting for recovery, which may not occur, or by surgical exploration of the injured nerves (Seddon, 1975).

COMMON SITES OF PERIPHERAL NERVE INJURY

Injury to the brachial plexus is the most severe of upper limb nerve injuries since it affects the innervation to the whole limb. The reader should refer to an anatomy text for a reminder of the structure of the brachial plexus (e.g. Williams, 1995). Briefly, the plexus is formed by the anterior branches of the fifth to eighth cervical nerves and the first thoracic nerve. It extends from the lower lateral aspect of the neck to the axilla and then divides into numerous branches to form the nerves of the upper limb.

The axillary nerve may be injured in association with fractures of the neck of the humerus and shoulder dislocation. Injuries to the ulnar and median nerves commonly occur at the wrist, as a result of putting a hand through a

Table 10.1 Causes of peripheral nerve injuries.

Causes of peripheral nerve injuries		
Lesion	**Characteristic**	**Agent**
Open	Tidy	Knife, glass or scalpel
	Untidy	Missile, burn, open fracture-dislocation
Closed	Compression–ischaemia	Pressure neuropathy in the anaesthetised patient
		Compartment syndrome
	Traction–ischaemia	Fracture dislocation
	Thermal	Acrylic cement, electrical burn
	Irradiation	Irradiation neuritis
	Injection	Regional anaesthetic block, intravenous or intra-arterial catheterisation

Classification of nerve injuries				
Seddon (1975)	**Sunderland**	**Functional loss**	**Anatomical lesion**	**Neurophysiological**
Neurapraxia (non-degenerative)	Grade I	Muscle power, gnosis	Axon and nerve fibre sheath intact	Distal conduction maintained – no fibrillation
Axonotmesis (degenerative)	Grade II, III	All modalities	Interruption of axon and distal Wallerian degeneration	Conduction lost; fibrillation
Neurotmesis (degenerative)	Grade IV, V	All modalities	Interruption of the nerve trunk; Wallerian degeneration	Conduction lost; fibrillation

Table 10.2 Classification of nerve injuries.

window, or from elbow injuries. The ulnar nerve can also be damaged in fractures of the medial epicondyle of the humerus. The median nerve can become damaged in carpal tunnel syndrome.

The radial nerve is most often damaged in fractures of the humerus, at the point where it wraps around the humerus. It is also damaged in the axilla by pressure from axillary crutches or by the arm being left hanging over the edge of a chair for a long period (i.e. 'Saturday night palsy' when a person falls asleep after drinking alcohol).

In the lower limb, common nerve injuries include: the sciatic nerve, from pelvic and thigh wounds or dislocation of the hip; the common peroneal nerve, from fractures of the neck of the fibula or pressure from a plaster cast; and the posterior tibial nerve, from supracondylar fractures of the femur. Many of these occur in sporting injuries (Lorei & Hershman, 1993).

DIAGNOSIS, SIGNS AND SYMPTOMS
A reasonable knowledge of anatomy contributes to accurate diagnosis in most clinical situations and the Medical Research Council Atlas (MRC, 1982) is an invaluable aid. The motor and sensory loss which occurs with specific nerve injuries will not be discussed in detail here.

Muscle Function and Sensation
The extent of paralysis is described using the MRC system for measuring muscle strength (see Chapter 4). One deficiency of the MRC system is that it does not record endurance and stamina, which is a significant defect when one is choosing muscles for transfer or when assessing a patients' ability to do certain types of work. Recording loss of sensation is best achieved by the examiner working with the patient; the complete area of anaesthesia is marked out by a skin marker pen and then, using a different colour, the surrounding area of impaired sensation is similarly marked. The sensory loss can be recorded by a standard chart, photographed or both.

Differential Diagnosis
There are three features which enable the examiner to distinguish between neurapraxia and the degenerative lesions of axonotmesis and neurotmesis. The first of these is sympathetic paralysis. The sympathetic fibres controlling sweating and the tone of the smooth muscles within the skin blood vessels pass with the trunk nerves of the limbs. The median, ulnar and tibial nerves are richly endowed with such nerve fibres and they pass into the nerves of cutaneous sensation in the hand and foot. Loss of sweating and vasomotor tone after wounding of a nerve is indicative of a degenerative lesion. A diagnosis of neurapraxia cannot be made in the face of this evidence.

Pain
Severe pain indicates that the nerve has been badly damaged. The characteristics of neuropathic pain are so clear that an accurate diagnosis of the extent of nerve injury can often be made. A classic example of this is causalgia, burning pain, which follows partial injuries (usually from missiles) of the brachial plexus and the proximal median and ulnar nerves, or of the sciatic and tibial nerves. Causalgia is severe pain which usually occurs with an incomplete lesion of major trunk nerves with a large number of sympathetic fibres and is a term associated with the syndrome of reflex sympathetic dystrophy (see below). Pain is overwhelming; the patient will not permit examination or handling of the part; there is usually excessive sweating of the afflicted skin with instability of vasomotor control. Some nerves of cutaneous sensation are notoriously prone to cause severe pain, notably the superficial radial nerve, the medial cutaneous nerve of the forearm and the sural nerve. These patients show remarkable hypersensitivity of the skin, to the extent that they cannot tolerate light touch. They have allodynia, in which normal sensations are perceived as painful ones. Furthermore, there is often spread of this hypersensitivity to adjacent skin innervated by other nerves. Hyperpathia is a severe example of

abnormal pain following injury to nerves. It is the deep burning pain provoked by gentle examination, a pain which is disproportionate to the stimulus supplied to the skin, which spreads throughout the hand or foot and persists after examination.

Pain after traction lesion of the brachial plexus is common and severe, particularly with preganglonic injuries. These patients describe two sorts of pain. There is a constant crushing or burning pain felt throughout the hand. This may be described as feeling as if the hand is being held in a hot vice, or as if needles are being driven into the hand, or as if the joints are bursting. This constant pain is caused by rupture of the rootlets of the spinal nerves between the dorsal root ganglion and the spinal cord and is deafferentation pain. Superimposed on this is another type of pain, which is convulsive and typically described as like being struck by bolts of lightning. This 'electrical' pain is excruciating and passes down the whole of the limb, each bolt of pain lasting for a few seconds, coming in surges of up to 30 or 40 episodes in every hour. This is avulsion pain; it occurs when the spinal nerves have been torn directly from the spinal cord.

These types of pain were reviewed by Birch (1993). Some patients have such severe pain as to cause addiction to opiates or even suicide.

Special Investigations
Neurophysiological investigations, measuring nerve action potentials and detecting the response of muscle to the insertion of concentric needles, distinguish between conduction block (neurapraxia) and the degenerative lesions axonotmesis and neurotmesis (Misulis, 1993). Recording of nerve action potentials from electrodes attached to the skin of the scalp or neck after stimulation of the nerve trunk in the neck or arm establishes whether there is continuity of the rootlets within the spinal canal. These investigations are particularly important in the accurate diagnosis of injuries of the brachial plexus in adults and in babies. However, such neurophysiological work can be applied only after allowing time for degeneration, i.e. after about 3 weeks from the injury (Friedman, 1991).

Radiological investigations are particularly useful in demonstrating the state of the spinal nerves within the spinal canal. Myelography is certainly useful and accuracy is increased when it is combined with CT scanning (Marshall & de Silva, 1986). Magnetic Resonance (MR) imaging gives valuable information about the state of the spinal cord but as yet it does not provide precise information about the situation of the spinal nerves themselves. These investigations are often necessary in the analysis of cases of injury to the brachial and lumbosacral plexuses.

MEDICAL AND SURGICAL MANAGEMENT
Early repair of damaged nerves and prompt and adequate treatment of the associated injuries to blood vessels, skeleton, muscle and skin are essential. Injuries of the brachial plexus are the most serious of all peripheral nerve

lesions. In many cases the damage lies within the spinal canal, and spinal nerves are either ruptured or torn directly from the spinal cord. A Brown-Séquard syndrome is found in 2–5% of complete lesions (see Chapter 9) and rupture of the subclavian or axillary arteries is found in about 20% of cases (Birch, 1993). Life-threatening associated injuries to the head, chest and viscera are common, and associated fractures of long bones are almost the rule.

The treatment of life-threatening injuries must take priority but urgent surgical exploration to confirm diagnosis and to repair damaged nerves is advocated. Results of repair of the fifth, sixth and seventh cervical nerves are a great deal better than they were 20 years ago but restoration of function of the hand in a complete lesion remains exceptional in rare cases of urgent repair in the younger patient or the stab wound.

Surgical procedures were reviewed by Birch (1993); early surgery includes treatment of open wounds, repair of vascular damage (i.e. ruptured vessels) and repair of torn nerves which may involve grafting. Later surgical procedures include sympathectomy or deafferentation for severe pain, reconstructive surgery such as tendon transfers to restore function, and amputation in cases where other means of treatment have failed and the limb is a hazard to the patient during daily activities. Surgery is only one step in the rehabilitation of the patient.

PROGNOSIS AFTER REPAIR
Various factors influence the prognosis and important ones include: age, the wound, nerve repair, level of the lesion, and delay between injury and repair.

Age
Children generally do much better than adults after repair of a nerve but shortening of the limb and severe fixed deformity from muscular imbalance are striking features of lesions of major trunk nerves in the growing child.

Nature of the Wound
The more destructive the wound, the worse the prognosis. An unrepaired injury to a major artery usually causes ischaemic fibrosis of muscle and may threaten the survival of the limb so that amputation is necessary. The destruction of tissue caused by a close-range shotgun is devastating, with loss of skin, muscle and bone and extensive damage to the nerves. Results of nerve repairs in such cases are generally poor.

Nerve Repair
A good result can generally be expected after repair of nerves such as the musculocutaneous or posterior interosseous, whose major function is the control of muscles. Useful recovery can occur in nerves which have a more mixed motor and sensory function such as the median, ulnar or sciatic nerves but recovery is always imperfect. Results after repair of nerves of cutaneous sensation in the adult, such as the superficial radial, are often poor and complicated by severe pain.

Lesion Level

The importance of the level of the lesion is shown by recovery of function after repair of median and ulnar nerves. Recovery is better when the nerves are injured at the wrist than when they are injured in the axilla. It is unusual to see useful recovery of function of the intrinsic muscles of the hand after repair of the high lesion of either nerve.

Delay

The opinion that delay between injury and repair is harmful is now overwhelming (Birch, 1995). This is because the effects on the target organs, and particularly on muscle and skin, of longstanding denervation may become irreversible. There are also changes within the parent cell bodies of the axons. In severe traction lesions of the brachial plexus, many of the parent ventral motor neurones within the spinal cord die; this has been shown to occur after amputation of limbs for malignant tumours (Birch, 1995).

THE MULTIDISCIPLINARY TEAM (MDT)

A team approach to management is desirable. In the Rehabilitation Unit within the Royal National Orthopaedic Hospital (RNOH), the work of the physiotherapy and occupational therapy departments is integrated, the orthotist provides function splints, the surgeon may be required at any stage, the clinical psychologist becomes involved with patients with cognitive defects following head injury, and the disablement resettlement officer is an essential member of the team in guiding patients back to their original occupation or in helping them to retrain for another occupation. The roles of the physiotherapist and occupational therapist vary in different institutions and overlap greatly.

The majority of patients with peripheral nerve injuries, other than those sustaining multiple injuries, do not require complex nursing care, although they may need physical and emotional support. The physical problems will be dealt with by appropriately trained therapists but there may be difficulties in coming to terms with the consequences and implications of the injury. Nursing staff with suitable experience can give appropriate support and counselling. The senior nursing staff are in a particularly good position to detect significant psychological problems or they become alert to the financial implications of injury and so point the way to retraining or to further education. Only the role of the physiotherapist is elaborated in this chapter.

PSYCHOLOGICAL SUPPORT

Patients with lesions of the brachial plexus will present not only with upper limb sensory and motor deficits but also with special needs relating to the associated effects of the injury on independence, employment and lifestyle. Patients may become self-conscious about physical appearance and will require reassurance to assist in coping. They may suffer cognitive defects from an associated head injury and may require help from a clinical psychologist.

PRINCIPLES OF PHYSICAL MANAGEMENT

As mentioned above, brachial plexus injuries are the most serious of peripheral nerve injuries and this section will concentrate on their management in adults and children. The principles of treatment can be applied to other nerve injuries and treatment of fixed deformities is a major priority.

MANAGEMENT OF THE ADULT BRACHIAL PLEXUS LESION

The patient with a brachial plexus lesion (BPL) presents with a wide variety of problems and challenges for the therapist. The consequences of the injury will usually last for the rest of the individual's life, and the patient may present to a physiotherapist at any time following injury (Frampton, 1984).

Early Management

Since BPLs are usually caused by high-energy injuries, the damage to the brachial plexus is commonly accompanied by damage to the head, chest and viscera. Initial assessment and management are therefore as varied as the patient's medical condition and brachial plexus damage cannot be considered in isolation.

Assessment

The initial physiotherapeutic assessment is ideally carried out together with the occupational therapist. Specific aspects of this assessment are discussed in Chapter 4. Areas which require particular attention when assessing patients with nerve injuries are: pain (including night pain); sensation; oedema; range of active and passive movement (ROM); and muscle power. Horner's (or Bernard–Horner's) sign is a common feature of BPL and indicates a preganglionic injury of T1. The signs are constriction of the pupil and ptosis (drooping of the eyelid) on the affected side, and these inform the therapist that the lesion is severe and that pain may be a major problem.

Evaluation of sensation to light touch should include all of the upper quadrant. Areas of hypersensitivity are recorded; cutaneous sensitivity without pain may be a sign of reinnervation. It is difficult to distinguish this from the hypersensitivity of partial denervated skin where there is an abnormal pain response to light touch (Frampton, 1982) which can be disabling. Pain distribution can be recorded on a body chart. Subjective assessment can be made with a visual analogue scale (0–10). Questions are asked about the pattern of pain, and about aggravating and mitigating factors. Night pain is a useful indication of both the type and the severity of pain experience.

Treatment Aims

The aims of early treatment cover several areas:
- Pain control.
- Maintain/increase the ROM of the affected limb.

- Maintain/increase muscle power.
- Control oedema.
- Teach postural awareness.
- Teach care of the limb.
- Prevent and manage deformity.

Pain control–Adequate control of pain with drugs is vital in the early stages and analgesia should be timed to be effective during physiotherapy sessions. If adequate analgesia cannot be achieved, transcutaneous nerve stimulation (TENS) or acupuncture can be used (see Chapter 4). Whilst healing is taking place, pain caused by stretching to soft tissues to regain ROM slowly eases over time.

Maintain/increase ROM of the affected limb–The patient should be shown self-assisted movements for all joints of the affected limb. Active exercises should be encouraged. The patient should attempt to stretch and to do exercises hourly. Self-assisted abduction and lateral rotation of the shoulder are awkward to carry out effectively, and it is therefore important to involve the family members and friends in the treatment programme and to teach them the passive stretches if this is indicated. A continuous passive mobiliser (CPM), if this is available, and if other medical conditions allow, is an ideal adjunct to the treatment to maintain and improve ROM.

Maintain/increase muscle power–The early exercise programme should include active exercises for all intact muscle groups, including the shoulder girdle. Adapting the exercises to match the grade of muscle power may be required, e.g. using weights.

Oedema–Oedema of the limb can be a problem in the initial stages following injury. If accompanying bone and soft tissue injuries permit, elevation in a roller towel with active or passive exercises of the wrist, hand and fingers can be carried out. Compression garments must be used with caution because of the already altered circulation and sensation of the limb. The CPM is also useful in the control of oedema.

Postural awareness–Correction of the abnormal posture commonly seen in these patients (Figure 10.1) should begin as soon as possible, by raising awareness in the patient and his or her family, and by the start of active correction as part of the early exercise programme.

Care of the limb–Early advice and education in care of a limb with no, or reduced, sensation is important. The patient and the family must be involved.

Prevent and manage deformity–Early application of wrist and hand splints is useful if deformity is present or likely to occur. When the wrist and hand are paralysed, splinting, combined with passive stretches, should be started as soon as possible. The patient should be taught about skin care with splints to prevent pressure areas developing.

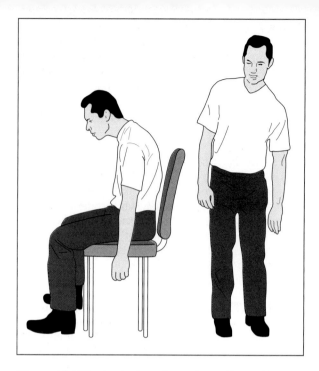

Figure 10.1 The typical posture of a patient with a lesion of the brachial plexus.

Treatment after repair of the brachial plexus
After repair of the brachial plexus by nerve grafting, the patient's arm is immobilised in a Hunter sling for up to 6 weeks. Movements of the shoulder are restricted during this time but movements of all other joints are encouraged to diminish stiffness. These movements should be performed at least daily to maintain ROM or more frequently if improving ROM or controlling oedema is necessary. These movements are done actively in cases where the eighth cervical and first thoracic nerves are spared; otherwise they must be carried out as passive movements, using the other hand or calling on the aid of a relative or friend.

Slings
Slings are usually provided by the occupational therapist. Following operation to the brachial plexus, a fitted Hunter sling is usually used to hold the affected upper limb securely against the trunk, maintaining the shoulder in adduction and medial rotation, with the elbow flexed. At 6 weeks after operation the Hunter sling may be replaced with a Ministry of Pensions sling. This assists in the reduction of oedema and, by supporting the weight of the affected limb, prevents further glenohumeral joint subluxation. When there is some shoulder control and no subluxation, the patient is encouraged not to wear the sling, so allowing the elbow to regain further extension. For patients wishing to return to active sports, a poly sling is recommended. This sling holds the arm firmly against the body with the aid of a waist strap, preventing any uncontrolled movement of the shoulder which would impede function or aggravate pain.

Later Rehabilitation

The principles of treatment are the same for each individual but, since patients may present at any time following injury, the therapist should be familiar with regeneration times of nerves repaired. This will provide an indication of the expected outcome so that the patient can be approached with reasonably accurate expectations of final recovery.

Assessment

In addition to the assessment principles discussed in Chapter 4, specific aspects relating to nerve injuries are outlined here. It is important to know details of the injury, any repair performed and how long after the repair the patient is presenting. Examination should include posture, deformity, appearance of the limb (including oedema, colour and skin condition), presence of Horner's sign, pain, sensation, ROM and muscle power.

Posture

Many of these patients adopt a typically flexed posture, as shown in Figure 10.1. This is particularly obvious in those recently injured. Patients with longstanding injuries are often found to have shortening and reduced flexibility in the side flexors of the trunk of the affected side. The posture should be observed in sitting and standing, and from anterior, posterior and lateral aspects. The degree of active and passive correction should be noted to establish whether the problem is largely that of changes in trunk tone or whether there are established associated soft tissue changes.

The posture of the limb should be examined while standing. Muscle wasting occurs rapidly after injury and the extent of loss of muscle bulk in upper limb and shoulder girdle is noted. Depending on the extent and level of injury, subluxation of the shoulder may be observed. The arm commonly hangs in medial rotation and forearm pronation.

Deformity

The most common fixed deformities are medial rotation of the shoulder and extension of the metacarpophalangeal joints with flexion of the proximal interphalangeal joints.

Deformity is also seen at the elbow, as a flexion deformity, as well as in the wrist. Damage to the eighth cervical and first thoracic nerves can produce deformities similar to those seen in other peripheral nerve injuries, such as the claw hand of the ulnar nerve lesion. Prevention of deformity is mentioned below when discussing complications.

Treatment of the Late Case

Later treatment concentrates on regaining ROM, muscle power and good posture, as well as controlling pain which may still be a significant problem. The treatment techniques mentioned below are discussed in Chapter 24.

ROM–Stretches should be performed as soon as possible if there is limitation in ROM in the upper limb. It is important to stress to the patient that, even if there is no recovery in the hand for example, maintaining range in the joints is important for cosmetic and hygienic reasons.

Stretches are taught for all joints of the shoulder girdle and upper limb, in all directions of movement.

After removal of the Hunter sling at 6 weeks after exploration and repair, stretches every 2 hours are suggested to regain range as quickly as possible. Once ROM is achieved, a daily stretching session will maintain passive range. Family or friends should be involved with the programme and they should be taught the necessary exercises; ideally they should do abduction and lateral rotation of the shoulder with the patient, since these are the most awkward to perform independently. Lateral rotation is the movement that is most frequently lost and it is the most difficult to regain.

Muscle power–An exercise programme should be devised to strengthen the functioning muscles. As each presentation is different, the programme has to be individually designed. Each muscle group will have to be strengthened within the limitations of its grade, i.e. gravity-assisted, neutral or resisted. Electromyographic (EMG) biofeedback can be very useful when starting to strengthen muscles and it can provide an objective method for monitoring progress. Facilitation techniques, such as proprioceptive neuromuscular facilitation (PNF), are particularly useful for upper limb and single joint strengthening. The patient should be encouraged to use the limb as functionally as possible. Introduction to the flail arm splint can augment the strengthening programme. General strengthening and fitness is important. This can involve specific exercises (shoulder girdle exercises, trunk strengthening) as well as a general fitness programme. Swimming is an ideal sport for these patients; it is quite possible for the patient who was a competent swimmer prior to injury to return to a good level of swimming, even with a complete BPL. For the first session after injury, patients ought to be accompanied and encouraged to start swimming on their back while they get used to the altered weight in the water.

Oedema–This is a problem in the early stages and is best managed by elevation of the limb at night, use of a sling during the day, active exercises, massage, and careful use of a compression bandage. The pressure garment can be worn for long-term use in persistent oedema. If compression is to be used, then regular checks on skin condition and monitoring of sudden onset of new pain or even oedema must be performed.

Pain–Pain in the post-acute stage is caused by the nerve injury (see above) and may persist as an extremely disabling problem (Wynn Parry et al., 1987). Many patients respond to TENS, and specific placement of electrodes has been described by Frampton (1982). The high-frequency low-intensity modes are used for 20 minutes prior to the start of the physiotherapy session. Low-frequency high-intensity modes (Eriksson et al., 1979) during stretches can result in a marked decrease in discomfort and corresponding improvement in passive range. Needle acupuncture and electrical acupuncture have been useful in these patients.

Treatment of points on the sensate area of the painful limb can be used as well as the opposite limb and auricular points. When hypersensitivity is a serious problem, the Niagara massaging hand unit is useful.

Sometimes compression of the limb eases pain and a pressure garment can be tried. Persistent shoulder pain can result from subluxation at the joint and this can be improved by subluxation cuffs or support. It is important to be fully aware of the nature and behaviour of the patient's pain. Patients often notice that the pain is worse when they have little else to think about but that it improves when they are busy or distracted. Activities, such as taking up a new hobby, sports such as swimming, or resuming or taking up new employment are important. As well as being central to the overall restoration of a normal lifestyle, these activities act as an effective means of pain control.

Postural awareness–The rehabilitation programme should include some form of balance and proprioceptive work in the form of wobble-board and gym ball stretches and exercises. The extreme example of the typical BPL-related posture has already been shown (Figure 10.1). Postural education should be supplemented with visual feedback. Poor ability to extend laterally and poor control of trunk or pelvis should be addressed using general trunk re-education exercises.

Care of the limb–As with any area of the body with reduced or no sensation, the principles of skin care must be taught. The patient should check his or her skin regularly and become 'limb-aware'. They must get into the habit of knowing where the arm is, because the normal withdrawal response to pain or extremes of heat or cold is lost. The patient should be taught about the consequences of not taking care of the limb, such as prolonged healing time, and the increased risk of sores from reduced circulation.

Deformity–Splints are useful, particularly in the early stages. Night splints are required for the hand and wrist and serial splinting is a valuable component of an active programme to treat deformities which have already occurred.

Activities of daily living–Patients are encouraged to utilise any available function in their affected limb in their daily activities. As well as promoting independence, this provides exercise to the weak muscles and stimulation for sensorily impaired areas. Patients with no functional use in the affected arm are trained in one-handed techniques and, when appropriate, assistive appliances are used. Leisure pursuits need to be addressed, including the feasibility of returning to previous sports. Use of splints or assistive equipment may be an option and often specific appliances for participating in the sport will need to be constructed if they are not commercially available. Occupational aspirations are dis-cussed and the patient must be reassured that the loss of arm function does not lead to loss of employment and financial security. Referral to an employment advisor provides the patient with the necessary support.

Monitoring–The nature of this injury means that it is inappropriate and unnecessary to have longstanding and constant physiotherapy. Indeed this may be counter-productive. The ultimate aim of rehabilitation for these patients is a return to maximum function within the limitations of the injury. Physiotherapy should always include realistic treatment goals and should not be continued once these goals have been achieved. Monitoring of progress at intervals and reviewing management if the situation changes is the most appropriate method of long-term care for these patients.

Muscle and Tendon Transfers

Restoration of function often requires surgical transfer of musculotendinous units to provide or augment poor active movement (see Birch, 1993, for review). Some common transfers include pectoralis major-to-biceps and flexor-to-extensor transfer in the forearm. The transferred muscle should be at least Grade 4 on the MRC Scale (since it will lose a grade in transfer) and have flexibility. The affected limb should be mobile, without contractures of relevant joints. Pre-operatively, physiotherapy may be necessary to ensure the limb is as strong and as mobile as possible. Maintaining ROM in the free joints during the period of immobilisation postoperatively is vital to the overall success of the transfer. Postoperatively, following the period of immobilisation, rehabilitation can begin.

The aims of treatment after transfer include increasing ROM, re-educating muscle to perform new functions, and management of adherent scars using massage.

Increase ROM–Active work may commence 3 weeks after the operation, but passive stretching at the transfer site must be avoided for a further 3 weeks. Patients continue to wear a sling for at least 6 weeks after transfer.

Facilitation of the muscle action–The transferred muscle must now learn to work in a different way; the patient must understand the original action of the muscle transferred and the new desired action. PNF techniques using minimal resistance at first and within the range of the muscle can provide an effective way of initiating this. Active work, initially in the gravity-eliminated positions, and with the arm supported, using EMG biofeedback, and introducing funct-ional use of the limb is a useful method of treatment and can be adapted as the active power and ROM improve. It is always important to remember the patient's social and occupational background and, if this is relevant, focus rehabilitation with this in mind.

With lower limb transfers, such as transfer of tibialis posterior to tibialis anterior, rehabilitation must include gait and balance re-education with a graduated weight-bearing regimen, as well as re-education similar to that in the upper limb.

Splintage

Splints are prescribed, usually by the occupational therapist, after thorough upper limb assessment. The purposes of splinting are: (1) to position the limb correctly and thus prevent secondary complications; and (2) to increase functional use of the affected limb. The design of the splint must take into consideration the individual patient's needs, and available function should be utilised to avoid dependency on a splint. Splintage cannot be used in isolation and it must be supplemented by an exercise programme. When sensation is impaired, checking for any potential pressure areas is crucial following the fitting of the splint.

For those patients with no active wrist extension, a neoprene wrist brace or thermoplastic wrist cock-up splint may be fitted. This should be worn whilst the upper limb is in the sling, so as to discourage the wrist from being held in flexion and ulnar deviation. A night-resting splint, which maintains the hand in the functional position, may be appropriate for the patient with no active movement distal to the forearm, to prevent contractures of the wrist and fingers. A thumb spica may be prescribed for patients with reduced thumb control to allow opposition to fingers, and thumb stability for grasp.

Dynamic splints may be required for exercise purposes as well as for functional use. For example, a patient whose function is impaired by weak wrist extensors may be fitted with a dynamic wrist extension splint, to enhance hand power without restricting movements. At the RNOH, patients with complete lesions of C5–T1 are fitted with the Stanmore flail arm splint (Birch, 1993). The splint is basically a skeleton of an upper limb prosthesis fitting around the paralysed arm. It consists of: a shoulder support allowing rotation, flexion and abduction; an elbow-locking device; forearm shelf or gutter with wrist support; removable terminal appliances; and a cable which allows operation of the hand appliance by protraction and retraction of the unaffected shoulder (Figure 10.2). The splint is fitted by the orthotist and training in its use is given by the occupational therapist.

MANAGEMENT OF COMPLICATIONS

The most common complication of peripheral nerve injuries is fixed deformity. Reflex sympathetic dystrophy can also occur after fractures and is difficult to manage.

Fixed Deformity

The prevention of fixed deformity is one of the first priorities in treatment. Many cases of fixed deformity are a reflection of neglect of elementary principles in the treatment of paralysed limbs. Pain is an important cause of fixed deformity; in the upper limb it leads to severe flexion deformity of the wrist with extension of the metacarpophalangeal joints. Fixed deformity can occur with post-ischaemic fibrosis of muscle and this is seen particularly involving flexor muscles of the forearm, the small muscles of the hand and the deep flexor compartment of the leg. In children, the unopposed action of muscles during growth is an important cause; the effect

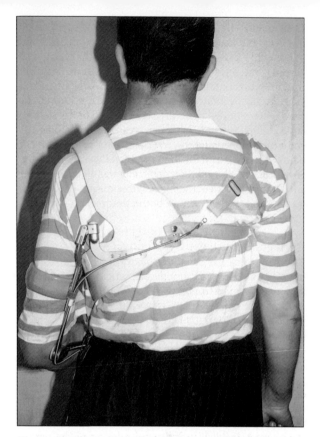

Figure 10.2 The Stanmore flail arm splint. View from the back, on a patient with a complete lesion of the brachial plexus. This view shows the shoulder support, the elbow lock and the cable passing to the undamaged shoulder, which transmits movement to the appliances attached to the wrist support.

on the posture of the foot after irreparable tibial or common peroneal lesion in the growing child is severe. Serial splinting is very useful in treatment of many of these deformities.

Serial Splinting or Fixed Deformity

This technique can be used to correct flexion deformity of the elbow, wrist, fingers, knee and ankle, and is discussed in Chapters 24 & 25. The skin should be healthy and radiographs taken to ensure that the skeleton is sound. Splinting is applied in collaboration with the physiotherapist who will achieve a few more degrees of correction before the new splint is applied each time, and the technique is continued in this way until the required extension is gained. It is important to avoid trying to gain too much correction at one time. Splints are worn at night and in some cases for an hour or two during the day. The technique depends entirely on the co-operation of the patient, who should maintain flexion and gentle stretching of the joint during the day when the splint is not worn.

Case Report

A 44-year-old man was referred with 90° flexion deformity at the elbow and 70° flexion deformity at the wrist, with severe contracture of the thumb web space. Multiple fractures throughout the upper limb had been treated successfully by internal fixation but prolonged immobilisation, complicated by severe pain, had led to this serious contracture. The pain had been treated. The deformities were treated by using three serial plaster splints, for the elbow, the wrist and for the thumb and web space. After 3 months the elbow flexion deformity was 10 degrees with a full range of active flexion; active extension of the wrist was 40° and the contracture of the thumb web space was fully corrected.

Reflex Sympathetic Dystrophy

This syndrome has been ascribed various terms, including Sudeck's atrophy, causalgia, shoulder-hand syndrome, and algoneurodystrophy (van Laere & Claessens, 1992; Veldman *et al.*, 1993). Its cause and pathogenesis are poorly understood but it is often associated with fractures or crush injuries of the wrist and hand. Characteristic symptoms are inflammation (which increases after exercise), pain, limited range of movement, vasomotor instability, trophic skin changes and patchy bone demineralisation. The foundation of treatment in these difficult cases is encouragement towards functional activity. In some cases, guanethidine blocks and/or other drugs are helpful. Forceful manipulation of the part is damaging.

BIRTH INJURY OF THE BRACHIAL PLEXUS

Obstetric brachial plexus palsy (OBPP) is a serious complication of childbirth which appears to be increasing in incidence. Although accurate figures are not available in the UK, the centre at the RNOH now sees over 150 new cases a year (the majority of cases seen in the UK). There are two significant risk factors. Injuries in children born by breech delivery are serious and may be bilateral. Disproportion in the birth canal is a much more common cause; we have found that shoulder dystocia was a complication in 70% of our cases. The weight of the child is the single most significant risk factor and heavy babies are at risk.

A relatively simple classification of OBPP has evolved amongst surgeons in the field and consists of four groups (Narakas, 1987):

Group 1 The fifth and sixth cervical nerves are damaged, and the shoulder and elbow flexor muscles are paralysed. About 90% of these babies make a full spontaneous recovery; this usually begins within 3 months of birth and is complete by 6 months.

Group 2 The fifth, sixth and seventh cervical nerves are damaged. There is paralysis of the shoulder, elbow flexors, and extensor muscles of the wrist and digits. About two thirds of these children make a full spontaneous recovery, though serious defects of the shoulder persist in the remainder. Recovery is slower than in Group 1, with activity in the deltoid and biceps muscles becoming clinically apparent at 3–6 months.

Group 3 Paralysis is virtually complete; there is some flexion of the fingers at or shortly after birth. Full spontaneous recovery occurs in <50% of these children. Most are left with substantial impairment of function at the shoulder and elbow, with deficient rotation of the forearm, and wrist and finger extension does not recover in about 25% of cases.

Group 4 The whole plexus is damaged; paralysis is complete. The limb is atonic and Bernard–Horner syndrome is present. No child makes a full recovery, the spinal nerves have either been ruptured or avulsed from the spinal cord, and there is permanent and serious defect within the limb.

Operations to repair the plexus are indicated in severe cases where there is no clinical evidence of recovery, or operation is necessary to overcome secondary fixed deformities. The most serious of all these secondary deformities is medial rotation contracture of the shoulder which, if untreated, progresses to posterior dislocation of the shoulder.

Of 78 patients assessed in the unit at the RNOH in a 12-month period in 1995/1996, there were 6 patients with Group 1 injuries (8%), 36 with Group 2 (46%), 23 with Group 3 (29%), and 13 with Group 4 (17%).

Physical Management of OBPP

The information in this section is original and has evolved from the experience gained at the authors' centre. Since there is a lack of literature to draw from, more detail is given in this section than is generally given in this book.

The therapist may become involved at any stage in the life of a child with OBPP. The therapeutic needs of the child will change with growth but the approach must be holistic and acknowledge the key role played by the family.

Assessment

In the baby–The assessment is most relevant at 2–3 weeks after birth, since mild cases can improve within a matter of days. The following should be assessed: asymmetry of posture; normal active spontaneous movements of the limb as appropriate to the developmental level of the baby (see Chapter 18); range of movement of the upper limb; and muscle power, though this cannot be performed very accurately in the newborn.

In the older child–The birth history and operative procedure should be noted to obtain an idea of predicted recovery. The therapist should evaluate how the child is performing functionally in relation to the stage of development; this includes activities ranging from clapping, eating and dressing to participation in sports. Any deformity of the limb should be observed.

Formal assessment of sensation is difficult in toddlers, but a child who chews, burns or traps his or her fingers without noticing and cannot handle objects without looking is likely to have a considerable deficit. Occasionally hypersensitive areas occur; they usually resolve with time. Pain is not usually a problem in OBPP.

The scapulohumeral angles are important to record because of the rapid development of contractures within this complex. Three of these are significant: medial rotation contracture; posterior glenohumeral contracture, which is shown by winging of the scapula when the child protracts the arm; and inferior glenohumeral contracture so that the scapula moves away from the chest when the arm is elevated. Most of these deformities are caused by contractures of soft tissue rather than bony deformity. Posterior dislocation is, on the whole, developmental and is preventable in the majority of cases.

Observation of function is a more useful assessment tool than trying to grade the strength of specific muscles. Activities such as crawling, reaching out, throwing and catching provide a good guide to muscle power.

Treatment

The principles of treatment are the same as those for adults. Regardless of the age of the child, the aims of therapy are:
- To educate and involve the child and family in the management of the lesion.
- To prevent deformity.
- To maintain and increase the range of movement.
- To encourage function along with the normal development of the child.

It is essential to ensure full involvement of the family to achieve the child's full potential. Formal physiotherapy is given for only short periods, to educate the parents who carry out most of the treatment.

In all cases, stretching to prevent deformity is the most important aspect of treatment. In the newborn baby, stretches should be encouraged at every nappy change; in older children they are usually performed 3–5 times a day. The parents should be guided about the sensation of the end feeling of the movement but they can be reassured that their baby will also be able to tell them!

Exercise to improve ROM and strength can be incorporated into play activities. The child should be encouraged to use the limb as normally as possible and when of school age to take part in swimming, gym and games activities. The child's teacher may need to be involved with the rehabilitation at this stage. Independence in normal functional tasks (washing, eating) should be promoted. Splinting may be appropriate at night for the child with the more severe lesion with limited recovery or if contracture develops

Maximising Function

Parents often need to be reminded that children are very adaptable and will use their unaffected hand quite spontaneously, even if it is their non-dominant hand. It is not until the child needs to perform bilateral activities, at the age of 4 or 5 years, that he or she will fully utilise what function there is. The more the affected arm and hand can be used,

the better, but parents need to find the right balance between encouragement and frustration. Dressing presented the greatest functional problem for the 78 children reviewed. Dressing can be practised, away from the early morning rush, using large dressing-up clothes. Feeding activities can also be simulated through play. A problem-solving approach to overcome functional difficulties should be encouraged. Use of the imagination can be very helpful, so parents and children should be encouraged to think of alternative approaches and be assured that if it works for them, it is all right.

Continuing Care

For those patients diagnosed with lesions of Groups 1 and 2, follow-up should continue until they have regained full function. For the child with the more severe injury, in Groups 3 and 4, review should be regular in the initial stages but may become less frequent as recovery plateaus. Intermittent checks that the parents are performing the appropriate stretches effectively should be made and, if required, short bursts of treatment carried out should a contracture develop.

Parents can be put in touch with a self-help group for parents of children with OBPP so that they do not feel so isolated. (These groups exist locally and a national contact address cannot be given.) Parents can also be reassured that their child's function will improve over time, or in a more severely affected child that surgery is available and may increase function. They also need reassuring that by allowing a child to struggle, they are encouraging independence even though they may find this difficult.

Encourage a Positive Self-Image

If parents are encouraged to refer to the affected arm as 'special' as opposed to 'bad', the child should grow up with a more positive self-image. These children may require support in dealing appropriately with other children's curiosity or remarks about their arm once they start school, and again in adolescence when the appearance of the arm will be increasingly important. Encouragement from therapists and parents is essential to help these children maintain a positive view of themselves and maximise their potential so that they are able to lead full and active lives.

CONCLUSION

Rehabilitation of the patient with a peripheral nerve injury requires a multidisciplinary approach. The focus is on function, assessing and managing the patient's problems with the long-term goal of facilitating a return to the home, work and social environment.

REFERENCES

Birch R. Management of brachial plexus injuries. In: Greenwood R, Barnes MP, McMillan TM *et al.*, eds. *Neurological rehabilitation*. London: Churchill Livingstone; 1993:587-606.

Birch R. Surgical disorders of peripheral nerves. In: Harris NH, Birch R, eds. *Post graduate textbook of clinical orthopaedics*. Oxford: Blackwell Scientific; 1995:935-980.

Eriksson M, Sjolund B, Nielzen S. Long term results of peripheral conditioning stimulation as an analgesic measure in chronic pain. *Pain* 1979, **6**:335-347.

Frampton V. Pain control with the aid of transcutaneous nerve stimulation. *Physiotherapy* 1982, **68**:77-81.

Frampton V. Management of brachial plexus lesions. *Physiotherapy* 1984, **70**:388.

Friedman WA. The electrophysiology of peripheral nerve injuries. *Neurosurg Clin N Am* 1991, **2**:43-56.

Lorei MP, Hershman EB. Peripheral nerve injuries in athletes: treatment and prevention. *Sports Med* 1993, **16**:130-147.

Lundborg G. Peripheral nerve injuries: pathophysiology and strategies for treatment. *J Hand Ther* 1993, **6**:179-188.

Marshall RW, de Silva RD. Computerised tomography in traction lesions of the brachial plexus. *J Bone Joint Surg* 1986, **68B**:734-738.

Misulis KE. *Essentials of clinical neurophysiology*. London: Butterworth Heinemann; 1993.

Mitchell JR, Osterman AL. Physiology of nerve repair: a research update. *Hand Clin* 1991, **7**:481-490.

Medical Research Council. *MRC atlas: aids to the examination of the peripheral nervous system*. London: HMSO; 1982.

Narakas A. Obstetrical brachial plexus injuries. In: Lamb DW, ed. *The paralysed hand*. Edinburgh: Churchill Livingstone; 1987:116-135.

Rosson JW. Disability following closed traction lesions of the brachial plexus - an epidemic among young motor cyclists. *Injury* 1987, **19**:4-6.

Seddon HJ. *Surgical disorders of peripheral nerves, 2nd edition*. Edinburgh: Churchill Livingstone; 1975.

van Laere M, Claessens M. The treatment of reflex sympathetic dystrophy syndrome: current concepts. *Acta Orthop Belg* 1992, **58**(1):259-261.

Veldman PH, Reynen HM, Arntz IE, *et al*. Signs and symptoms of reflex sympathetic dystrophy: prospective study of 829 patients. *Lancet* 1993, **342**:1012-1016.

Williams P. *Gray's anatomy, 38th edition*. Edinburgh: Churchill Livingstone; 1995.

Wynn Parry CB. *Rehabilitation of the hand, 4th edition*. London: Butterworth; 1981.

Wynn Parry C, Frampton V, Monteith A. Rehabilitation following traction injuries of the brachial plexus. In: Terzis JK, ed. *Microreconstruction of nerve injuries*. Philadelpha: WB Saunders; 1987:483-498.

11

L DeSouza, D Bates & G Moran

MULTIPLE SCLEROSIS

CHAPTER OUTLINE

- Pathology
- Aetiology and epidemiology
- Clinical manifestations
- Diagnosis

- Medical treatment
- General management
- Physical management

INTRODUCTION

Very few people have not heard of multiple sclerosis or its more commonly used acronym MS. It is the major cause of neurological disability in young and middle-aged adults, and therefore a disease of unrivalled importance. However, there is probably no other condition with such an unpredictable outcome or with such protean manifestations; the course of the disease may range from a single transient neurological deficit to, in its most severe form, death within weeks or months of its onset.

PATHOLOGY

MS is the principal member of a group of disorders known as demyelinating diseases. There are many conditions which have demyelination as part of their disease process, but currently the term demyelinating disease is reserved for those conditions which have an immune-mediated destruction of myelin, with relative sparing of other elements of nervous tissue, as an essential pathological finding. The other conditions that fulfil this classification are rare but have many features in common with MS. These include: 'diffuse cerebral sclerosis of Schilder' and 'concentric sclerosis of Balo', possibly both variants of MS; the acute disseminated encephalomyelitides, which may occur either after infection or after vaccination; and acute necrotizing haemorrhagic encephalitis, which is also a post-infective

phenomenon, probably herpetic. Demyelinating diseases with a known underlying infection or metabolic cause are classified according to their underlying aetiology.

Within the central nervous system (CNS), myelin is produced by oligodendrocytes. Each oligodendrocyte gives off a number of processes to surrounding axons. These processes envelop the axons in specialised membranous organelles—the myelin segments. A myelinated fibre has many such segments, all of similar size, arranged along its length (see Chapter 1). Between the myelinated segments there lies a small area of exposed axon plasma membrane known as the node of Ranvier. The myelin segment is alternatively known as the internode (Figure 11.1). With the conduction of an action potential along the axon, ionic transfer predominantly occurs across the neural membrane at the node of Ranvier. The lipid-rich myelin of the internode inhibits ionic transfer at this site. It is this arrangement of segmental myelination that is integral to the phenomenon of saltatory conduction, whereby rapid and efficient axonal conduction is achieved. With loss of myelin, an action potential fails to be conducted normally and function of the nerve effectively ceases.

Gross examination of the brain and spinal cord reveals the characteristic plaques of MS. These are found predominantly, though not exclusively, in the white matter, since it is within the fibre tracts that most myelin is deposited. Lesions are scattered randomly throughout the

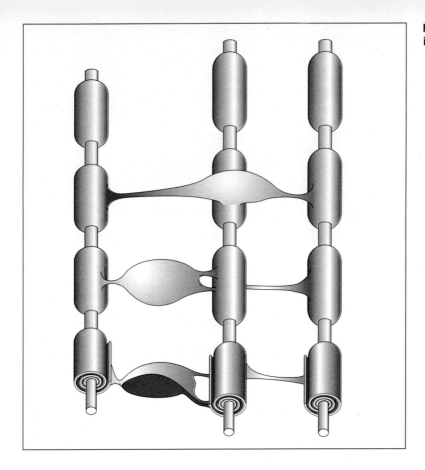

Figure 11.1 Myelinated nerve fibres in the central nervous system.

cerebral hemispheres, brainstem, cerebellum and spinal cord, though there is a preponderance of lesions in the periventricular white matter, particularly of the anterior and posterior horns of the lateral ventricles, and within the optic nerves and chiasm.

The microscopic appearance of a plaque depends on its age. A recent lesion shows a marked inflammatory reaction, with a perivascular infiltration of mononuclear cells and lymphocytes. There is destruction of myelin and a mild degeneration of oligodendrocytes, with relative sparing of nerve cell bodies and axons. With time, the lesions become infiltrated with phagocytes (macrophages), there is proliferation of astrocytes and the subsequent laying down of fibrous tissue. This results in the production of an acellular scar which has no potential for remyelination. Partial remyelination has been observed at autopsy but is of limited extent and is predominantly confined to the edges of the plaques (Prineas & Connell, 1978). For further reading on the pathology of MS see Matthews *et al.* (1991).

AETIOLOGY AND EPIDEMIOLOGY

Although the cause of MS remains obscure, there are a number of well established epidemiological and genetic facts which must be incorporated into any unifying aetiological hypothesis of the disease. A most curious but reproducible finding is the variability of the prevalence of MS with latitude. In equatorial regions, the disease has a prevalence of <1 per 100,000, whereas in the temperate climates of Northern Europe and North America this figure increases to >100 per 100,000 (see Langton Hewer, 1993, for a review). There is also a similar but less clearly defined relationship of increasing prevalence with latitude in the Southern Hemisphere. The increasing prevalence with distance from the Equator is not uniform, however. Regions with the same latitude may have widely differing prevalences of MS. Japan has a relatively low level of MS, as do most oriental countries, whereas Israel has an unexpectedly high level of the disease (Kurtzke & Kurland, 1983). It has been suggested that such a correlation may be accounted for by factors such as the degree of economic development. To address this question, studies have been performed on mainland USA with its wide range in latitude but uniform standards of health care and industrial sophistication. The relationship of prevalence and latitude has been confirmed (Kurtzke *et al.*, 1979).

When migration occurs between areas of differing prevalence of MS, then subsequent generations take on the risk of the adoptive region. In the migrating generation itself, if migration occurs in childhood then the person assumes the risk of the country of destination. When migration occurs in adulthood, then the individual retains the relative risk of the country of origin. The critical age appears to be around 15 years (Dean & Kurtzke, 1971).

'Epidemics' of MS have occurred in several island groups in the North Atlantic. Islands affected in this way include the Faroes (1943–1960; Kurtzke & Hyllested, 1986), the Orkney and Shetland Isles (1940–1969) and Iceland (1945–1954; Kurtzke et al., 1982). It is well known that small isolated populations are subject to a pattern of disappearance, reintroduction and epidemic spread for certain viral illnesses. Each of the 'epidemics' occurred in the 15–25 years following the beginning of World War II. During the War, each of the islands was occupied by allied troops. It has been hypothesised that allied troops reintroduced a viral agent which, with an assumed incubation period of 2–20 years, accounts for the postwar epidemic. It should be emphasised that despite extensive search, no such infective agent has ever been isolated.

A familial tendency towards MS is now well established but no clear pattern of Mendelian inheritance has been found. About 15% of MS patients have an affected relative, which is much higher than expected from the population prevalence (Ebers, 1983). The highest concordance rate is for identical twins—about 30%; non-identical twins and siblings are affected in 5% of cases (Ebers et al., 1986). A genetic factor is further supported by the excess of certain histocompatibility antigens found in MS. HLA-DR[2], -DR[3], -B[7] and -A[3] are all over-represented and are thought to be markers for an MS 'susceptibility gene' (Compston, 1991).

Current thinking hypothesises that MS is the product of both environmental and genetic factors. Exposure to some external agent, possibly viral, during childhood in those genetically susceptible, results in an autoimmune response mounted against native myelin. Like many autoimmune diseases, MS is 2 to 3 times more common in women. However, other diseases with a known autoimmune origin are no more prevalent in MS patients than in the general population.

CLINICAL MANIFESTATIONS

The fundamental clinical characteristic of MS is that episodes of acute neurological deficit affecting non-contiguous parts of the CNS are separated by periods of remission. Initially, resolution following a relapse is usually complete but with time, as the burden of disease increases, recovery from further attacks become partial and patients are left with permanent neurological disability. As the disease progresses the disability increases, either due to the cumulative effects of multiple relapses or as the disease enters a phase of secondary progression, whereby deterioration occurs without definite exacerbation. More rarely the disease is steadily progressive from the outset. This is termed 'primary progressive' MS and is more common when onset occurs in later life (Table 11.1).

Alternatively, MS may be classified according to the certainty of diagnosis (Table 11.2). This is of particular advantage in the construction of drug trials or for epidemiological purposes.

ONSET OF SYMPTOMS

It is a common misconception that the first attack of MS strikes as 'a bolt out of the blue' in a young adult enjoying robust good health. In fact, many patients will complain, on direct questioning, of vague feelings of ill health over the preceding months or years. These 'feelings' usually take the form of odd sensory disturbances, aches and pains, or lethargy. Commonly there is a history which clearly suggests a previous episode of demyelination, such as double vision, blindness, vertigo or limb weakness. These episodes may have been dismissed as trivial by the patient and, as such, may be poorly remembered but eliciting this history may be very helpful in supporting the diagnosis at presentation.

Demyelination may occur anywhere throughout the white matter of the CNS. Consequently, the initial presentation of MS may be highly variable and atypical. The diagnosis is usually suggested when a young or middle-aged adult presents with a clearly defined episode of neurological deficit, e.g. weakness and/or numbness affecting one or more limbs. The onset of the symptoms may develop acutely over minutes or chronically over months. More typically, symptoms evolve over hours or days. Such a presentation, with or without sphincter involvement, usually reflects an area of spinal demyelination. Lhermitte's phenomenon is the experience of a sudden shooting, electric shock-like sensation felt down the back and into the legs when the neck is suddenly flexed. This is a symptom of cervical myelopathy and is commonly seen when there is an area of demyelination within the cervical cord.

In about 25% of cases, the presentation is of acute or subacute visual loss in one or, more rarely, both eyes. Eye movements are painful. This is due to a lesion of the optic nerve known as optic neuritis or retrobulbar neuritis. Improvement usually begins spontaneously within weeks.

Classification of multiple sclerosis (MS)	
Relapsing remitting MS	Characterised by a course of recurrent discrete relapses, interspersed by periods of remission when recovery is either complete or partial
Secondary progressive MS	Following a period of relapse and remission, the disease enters a phase where there is progresive deterioration with or without identifiable superadded relapses
Primary progressive MS	Typified by progressive and cumulative neurological deficit from the onset

Table 11.1 Classification of multiple sclerosis.

Classification of multiple sclerosis according to certainty of diagnosis	
Clinically definite MS	Two attacks and clinical evidence of two separate lesions Two attacks; clinical evidence of one lesion and paraclinical evidence of another separate lesion
Laboratory-supported definite MS	Two attacks; either clinical or paraclinical evidence of one lesion; and CSF oligoclonal bands One attack; clinical evidence of two separate lesions; and CSF oligoclonal bands One attack; clinical evidence of one lesion and paraclinical evidence of another, separate lesion; and CSF oligoclonal bands
Clinically probable MS	Two attacks and clinical evidence of one lesion One attack and clinical evidence of two separate lesions One attack; clinical evidence of one lesion and paraclinical evidence of another, separate lesion
Laboratory-supported probable MS	Two attacks and CSF oligoclonal bands

Table 11.2 Classification of MS according to certainty of diagnosis. Paraclinical evidence is derived from MR imaging, CT scanning or evoked potentials measurement. (CSF: cerebrospinal fluid)

In a third of cases recovery will be complete, with the remainder having some reduction of visual acuity. Following an episode of optic neuritis, the optic disc becomes pale and atrophic (optic atrophy). More than one half of those presenting with optic neuritis will go on to develop other signs of MS. It is undecided whether the others have suffered a single attack of MS or if they have some other disease entity.

Not infrequently, the disease begins with the signs and symptoms of cerebellar dysfunction, with nystagmus, ataxia and cerebellar dysarthria. The combination of nystagmus, slurring speech and intention tremor is known as Charcot's triad and is one of the classic features of MS.

Brainstem demyelination can cause a wide variety of brainstem syndromes with cranial nerve palsies and long tract signs. Diplopia (double vision) is a particularly common presenting complaint. This may be due to palsies of the third, fourth and sixth cranial nerves or their internuclear connections. A very characteristic abnormality is an internuclear ophthalmoplegia due to a lesion of the medial longitudinal fasciculus. With this deficit there is failure of adduction on lateral gaze, with nystagmus of the abducting eye. Bilateral internuclear ophthalmoplegia in a young adult is virtually diagnostic of MS. Trigeminal neuralgia is rare in young adults but when it occurs it suggests underlying brainstem pathology such as demyelination.

SIGNS AND SYMPTOMS OF ESTABLISHED MS

During the established phase of the disease, most patients have a number of symptoms and signs in common. Typical signs include optic atrophy with associated decreased visual acuity, central scotoma and pupillary abnormalities. Bilateral internuclear ophthalmoplegia, with facial sensory disturbances or weakness, and brisk jaw jerk are common. There is almost always evidence of cerebellar disease, with nystagmus, ataxia, dysarthria and tremor. In its most severe form, the tremor can be extremely incapacitating with any attempt to move precipitating violent, uncontrollable movements of head, trunk and limbs. In the limbs there is a spastic tetraparesis with increased tone and weakness in a pyramidal distribution. There is loss of dexterity in the hands and patients commonly complain of difficulty with delicate tasks such as handling coins, buttons and zip fasteners. Walking becomes increasingly difficult owing to progressive weakness, fatigue, spasticity and ataxia. Patients usually come to rely increasingly on walking aids and eventually many become wheelchair-bound.

In the presence of disease of the spinal cord, symptoms of sphincter disturbance are common. These may range from mild urgency and frequency to acute retention of urine, constipation or double incontinence. Sexual dysfunction is common, with erectile and ejaculatory difficulties in men and general weakness and fatigue affecting the expression of sexuality in both sexes.

Psychiatric and psychological disturbances are common (see Chapter 27). Many patients show evidence of emotional instability or affective disorder. Euphoria or an inappropriate cheerfulness in the face of obvious neurological disability is said to be a classic feature of the disease. This is, in fact, quite rare and is probably the result of lesions affecting the subcortical white matter of the frontal lobes. Much more common is depression, which may compound the underlying physical disability, exaggerating symptoms of lethargy and reduced mobility. With diffuse disease, some patients exhibit features of a frank dementia whilst others become psychotic. Seizures occur in 2–3% of cases and may be focal as a result of cortical irritation by a subjacent plaque.

Propagation of an action potential along a neurone is greatly affected by temperature. Nerve condition in an area of partial demyelination is in a critical state of decompensation, whereby a further small increase in temperature may result in conduction block. This is manifest clinically as Uhtoff's phenomenon. Patients frequently complain that their symptoms are much worse in warm weather or, more dramatically, that they are able to get into a hot bath but find they are unable to get out again. Patients should be warned to avoid extremes of temperature and overexertion. It is possible that an attack may be precipitated in this way.

DIAGNOSIS

To make a clinically definite diagnosis of MS there must be a history of at least two attacks and clinical evidence of at least two separate lesions (Paty *et al.*, 1993). At presentation, these criteria are often not fulfilled and corroborative paraclinical, laboratory and radiological evidence is sought.

MAGNETIC RESONANCE (MR) IMAGING

MR scanning of the head and spinal cord is very useful in demonstrating the lesions of MS. Typical high-signal lesions on T2-weighted sequences are seen, distributed throughout the white matter (see Figure 3.2). Gadolinium enhancement emphasises the areas of active inflammation, which are associated with an acute relapse. In particular circumstances, e.g. acute optic neuritis or cervical myelopathy, the demonstration on MR imaging of disseminated asymptomatic lesions is particularly helpful in securing the diagnosis (Paty *et al.*, 1988).

LUMBAR PUNCTURE

Analysis of the cerebrospinal fluid (CSF) in a suspected case of MS is very valuable diagnostically as there is a local production of immunoglobulin (mainly IgG) within the CNS. These antibodies may be detected on biochemical analysis of the CSF. Electrophoresis of CSF shows that the immunoglobulin fraction separates out into a few discrete bands, so-called 'oligoclonal bands'. The blood–brain barrier prevents protein from passing between the blood and the CSF. Electrophoresis of a

paired blood sample reveals that these bands are unmatched in serum, i.e. that immunoglobulin is being synthesised locally within the CNS (Tourtellotte & Booe, 1978). The antigens provoking this antibody response have never been identified, nor is it known whether this response is integral to the underlying pathogenetic process or a secondary phenomenon. Normally, or during a quiescent phase of the disease, CSF contains very few cells. However, during an acute exacerbation there is usually a moderate CSF lymphocytosis that is, in some part, a measure of disease activity. The finding of a raised lymphocyte count may, on occasions, influence the decision to treat an exacerbation.

EVOKED POTENTIALS

In a typical history, signs of more than one lesion of the CNS, together with disseminated white matter lesions on MR imaging and the presence of unmatched oligoclonal bands, put the diagnosis beyond reasonable doubt. When one or more of these findings are inconclusive, further support for the diagnosis may be obtained by performing evoked potentials (EP) tests which include visual, auditory and somatosensory evoked potentials (Misulis, 1993). These EP tests may lend support to evidence of a subclinical lesion which has so far remained undetected (Halliday & McDonald, 1977). Results of a visual EP test are shown in Figure 11.2. The demonstration of more than one lesion is essential in making a secure diagnosis of MS.

MEDICAL TREATMENT OF MS

The drug treatment of MS may be divided into two broad categories:
1. Specific disease-modifying agents that are aimed at reducing the underlying pathological process.
2. Supportive therapy using treatments that are aimed at alleviating the symptoms of MS.

Details of the important drugs mentioned below are given in Chapter 28.

DRUG TREATMENTS TO MODIFY UNDERLYING PATHOLOGY

Just as the cause of MS has remained elusive, so the search for an effective cure has been equally unsuccessful. Much energy has been directed at seeking such a cure and numerous therapies, many of which may seem bizarre to us today, have been investigated without success. In recent years, however, some progress has been made. We now have some therapies which, whilst not curative, indicate that they may have a beneficial effect on disease progression – though further controlled trials are needed. One of the problems of assessing the efficacy of treatments in MS is the relapsing–remitting nature of the disease that creates a particularly strong placebo effect.

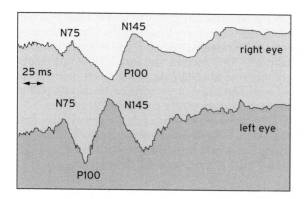

Figure 11.2 Evoked potentials. A visual EP study showing the typical prolonged latency and poor waveform in a lesion of the right optic nerve, such as optic neuritis, in a patient with MS.

Corticosteroids

The treatment of acute exacerbation of MS with corticosteroids hastens the recovery that usually takes place following an attack. There are a number of preparations used, including intravenous methylprednisolone, intramuscular ACTH and oral prednisolone.

Steroids have many significant and potentially serious side effects, including aseptic necrosis of the femoral head, immunosuppression, diabetes mellitus, osteoporosis, muscle weakness and atrophic skin changes, all of which may be particularly disastrous in the patient with MS. The use of long-term steroids has no effect on the natural history of the disease and the risks outweigh any perceived benefit. In the treatment of exacerbations, a total yearly dose of 6 g of methylprednisolone should not be exceeded.

β-Interferon

The interferons are naturally occurring polypeptides that are produced by the body in response to viral infection and other insults. There are three types: α, β and γ, previously known as leucocyte, fibroblast and immune interferon, respectively. They all have antiviral, antiproliferative and immunomodulatory properties. Since a preliminary viral infection has been postulated in the pathogenesis of MS, each of the interferons has been studied as a potential disease-modifying agent. α-Interferon has little effect, whilst γ-Interferon has been shown to have a deleterious effect. β-Interferon has, however, been shown to be beneficial.

In 1993, the results of a large randomised double-blind placebo-controlled multicentre trial of ambulatory relapsing–remitting MS patients showed that high doses of β-Interferon given subcutaneously on alternate days reduced clinical relapses of MS by one third over 2 years compared to a placebo (IFBN Multiple Sclerosis Study Group, 1993). Serial MR scans of these patients also showed that there was a significant reduction in disease activity in the treatment group (Paty et al., 1993). Despite the MR findings, the study did not show any significant reduction in the severity of the attacks, nor was there any effect on the progression of disability. Further studies are currently under way to determine whether β-Interferon has any effect on disease progression either in the relapsing–remitting or secondary progressive subgroups. β-Interferon is currently licensed for use in relapsing–remitting MS in the USA and Europe. The most common side effects are injection-site reactions and flu-like symptoms on the day of injection. These may be troublesome but subside with continued use. Fifty percent of subjects develop antibodies to the drug and this may have an adverse effect on relapse rate.

Immunosuppresion

Despite our incomplete understanding of the pathogenesis of MS, there is strong circumstantial evidence of an autoimmune process and this has prompted considerable interest in treating MS with immunosuppressive agents. A number of agents have been evaluated, including azathioprine (Yudkin et al., 1991), methotrexate (Goodkin et al., 1995), cyclophosphamide (Weiner et al., 1993) and total lymphoid irradiation. With each of these agents, claims of initial success have been encouraging but unfortunately these have not stood up to more rigorous trials. In our anxiety to treat what is often a progressive, crippling disease it is well to remember that the first principle of therapeutics is to do no harm. Each of these agents is associated with severe and potentially life-threatening side effects. These agents must therefore be used with extreme caution and only with the informed consent of the patient.

SUPPORTIVE THERAPY TO RELIEVE SYMPTOMS

MS remains an incurable disease. The therapies listed above for the specific treatment of the underlying process are, at best, only partially effective. Therefore the importance of symptomatic treatment in making life more tolerable cannot be overstated.

Spasticity

Spasticity is one of the most common symptoms of MS, often in association with painful cramps and spasms. There are a number of agents available that may be very effective. Baclofen, a GABA receptor agonist, acts centrally by inhibiting transmission at spinal level. Dantrolene reduces contraction of skeletal muscle with its direct action on excitation–contraction coupling by decreasing the amount of calcium (Ca^{2+}) released from the sarcoplasmic reticulum. Its action is more pronounced on fast fibres than slow fibres, which results in a relative diminution of reflex activity and hence spasticity compared to voluntary contraction. Its major side effect, a generalised muscular weakness, limits it usefulness.

Benzodiazapines such as diazepam and clonazepam may have a role to play in the management of spasticity, though they are more likely than other agents to result in drowsiness because of their non-selective depressive action upon the CNS. Sedation may be an advantage if spasms are a particular problem at night.

In severe painful spasticity, where the aim is to alleviate the distressing symptoms or to aid nursing care rather than to restore function, there are a number of more invasive procedures which may be useful. Local injection of botolinum toxin causes flaccid paralysis in the muscles injected, with minimal systemic side effects. The effect usually lasts for 3 months and may be repeated indefinitely (Snow et al, 1990). As a last resort, irreversible intrathecal or peripheral nerve chemical blocks with phenol or alcohol or surgery may be considered.

It is important to remember that spasticity may often be aggravated by underlying infection, especially urinary tract infection or bed sores. These causes should be sought whenever there is an unexplained deterioration.

Pain

There are a number of reasons why the patient with MS may complain of pain. Very common is the unpleasant 'dysaesthesia' secondary to interruption of the ascending sensory pathways. This can be notoriously difficult to treat but usually responds, at least partially, to centrally acting analgesics such as the antiepileptics carbamazepine, phenytoin and sodium valproate, or to other medications such as tricyclic antidepressants or baclofen. Alternatively, electrostimulation either by transcutaneous nerve stimulation (see Chapter 24) or by dorsal column stimulation may be effective (Tallis et al., 1983). Chronic lower back pain of uncertain aetiology frequently accompanies MS and is best treated with physiotherapy and simple analgesics. Some acute relapses of MS, especially optic neuritis, may be painful and are treated with steroids in the usual way (see above). In a young person, the typical lancinating pain of trigeminal neuralgia may be symptomatic of MS and carbamazepine is very effective in controlling this symptom. Cannabis is thought to be helpful for MS patients but is not used widely. Principles of pain management are discussed in Chapter 26.

Urinary and Bowel Symptoms
These are very common in patients with spinal disease (see Barnes, 1993, for a review). Therapy is best guided by formal urodynamic assessment. In those patients with detrusor instability causing frequency and urgency, the anticholinergic agents oxybutynin and propantheline are helpful. Incomplete bladder emptying is very effectively treated with intermittent self-catheterisation. Patients are often very reluctant to start this practice. However, once trained, they usually agree that it transforms their lives, enabling them to enjoy a more outgoing life without the constant need to be in the vicinity of a lavatory. The use of nasal desmopressin (an analogue of antidiuretic hormone) at night reduces nocturnal frequency and enuresis, and ensures a less disturbed night. Urinary infection should be treated with appropriate antibiotics and, if necessary, with long-term prophylaxis. Bowel problems are less frequent than urinary dysfunction. Constipation is best treated by properly spaced enemas or, in less severe cases, by ensuring adequate fibre intake and the judicious use of aperients.

Fatigue
Virtually all patients with MS will at some time complain of fatigue, and in the majority of cases it is regarded as one of the most disabling symptoms. Pharmacological treatment of this complaint is disappointing. Amantadine and premoline are amongst the more commonly used agents which may have some marginal effect. Reassurance and regular graded exercise programmes are at least as effective (see 'Physical management').

Tremor
Tremor can be a very disabling symptom (see Chapter 5) and its treatment in MS is difficult. Minor action tremors may be helped by beta blockade with propranolol or a low dose of barbiturate, usually primidone. The severely disabling 'dentatorubrothalamic' tremor, present at rest but made worse by the slightest movement, is particularly refractory to treatment. There are reports of the benefit of several agents, including clonazepam, carbamazepine, choline chloride and, curiously, the antituberculous drug isoniazid. None of these treatments is universally effective and the benefit achieved is usually no better than marginal. Unilateral tremor may be treated by stereotactic ventrolateral thalamic ablation, again with often disappointing results.

Sexual Dysfunction
Erectile difficulty is the most common complaint in men. Under expert guidance, therapies are available including oral yohimbine, intracorporeal injection of papaverine and surgically implanted prostheses. In women there are many factors which may deleteriously affect the expression of sexuality. Neurological symptoms from sacral segments, such as diminished genital sensitivity, reduced orgasmic capacity and decreased lubrication are common (Hulter & Lundberg, 1995). Both sexes are affected by leg spasticity, ataxia, vertigo and fatigue, all of which may impair the enjoyment of sexual intercourse. A caring and sensitive clinician may, with practical advice and reassurance, do much to resolve sexual problems and restore the patient and partner to a satisfying and fulfilling lovelife. Counselling may be appropriate in some cases and referral to a specialist counselling service such as SPOD may be useful (see 'Associations and Support Groups').

Psychological Problems
Classically the MS patient is said to become euphoric secondary to lesions of the white matter of the frontal lobes. This certainly does occur but is infrequent. Depression is far more common and is treated in the usual way with tricyclic antidepressants or with the selective 5-hydroxytryptamine reuptake inhibitors. Frank psychotic reactions are treated in the usual way. Psychological issues and behavioural management are discussed in Chapter 27.

Epilepsy
Epilepsy is rare in MS but still more common than in a normal population. It is treated with anticonvulsants. An electroencephalogram (EEG) is ideally obtained first as a guide to the most suitable agent.

GENERAL MANAGEMENT

In general terms, patients should be advised and enabled to enjoy as full and active a life as possible. There is no proven benefit from dietary restriction of any kind. Alcohol is often not tolerated as well as prior to the onset of the disease because of cerebellar involvement. However, there is no harm in a moderate intake of alcohol if desired.

Patients need to be fully informed about their disease, the prognosis, the treatments and support available, and the impact the disease will have on them and their families. Although there is a genetic predisposition, it should be emphasised that the risk of members of the family being affected is low, and if the patient and partner wish to start a family this should not be discouraged. It is recognised that

MS has no effect on fertility, the course of pregnancy or fetal outcome (Birk & Rudick, 1986). Furthermore, during pregnancy, the patient may experience a decrease in relapse rate; however, this is offset by a relative increase in disease activity in the puerperium (Korn-Lubetzki *et al.*, 1984). Many patients find the use of support groups such as the MS Society to be helpful in allowing a forum for meeting other people with MS to share experiences and information (see 'Associations and Support Groups'). Others prefer not to be involved with such societies but patients should be aware that they exist so that they can make their own choice.

As with many chronic and debilitating diseases, a multidisciplinary approach, utilising the skills and expertise of a whole range of health professionals in an integrated MS Clinic, is likely to improve the quality and continuity of care of the MS patient. It is essential that members of the care team develop a good rapport with both the patient and his or her carers in what is likely to be a prolonged, or indeed lifelong, relationship.

PHYSICAL MANAGEMENT

People with MS will usually be referred for physiotherapy, or request it for themselves, when they experience loss of movement skill or the ability to perform functional activities. By this stage, the disease has caused irreversible damage to the CNS and created a level of impairment which results in noticeable and persistent disability.

The loss of movement ability not only has a physical effect on the patient but also often a psychological effect. Whereas, in the early stages of the disease, the MS attacks would resolve and leave the person relatively fit and functional, the first signs of residual disability will underline the physical and psychological vulnerability of having MS. This often unwelcome realisation may bring with it experiences of changed self-image; from that of a healthy fit young person to that of a sick disabled person who needs to have physiotherapy.

The attitude of the physiotherapist towards the person with MS during their initial encounters is crucial, as it will set the scene for the therapist–patient relationship and any ensuing programme of physiotherapy. From the patient's point of view, the hope is that the physiotherapist will help him or her to overcome physical disabilities, and the fear is that the therapist may expose further physical weaknesses and insufficiencies. Physiotherapists need to be aware that the same professional skills that can help the patient can also undermine self-confidence and create feelings of resentment and anger.

The success of treatment should not be determined by whether or not the patient with MS improves, but rather by whether he or she achieves the best level of activity, relevant to lifestyle, at each stage of the disease (De Souza, 1990). In order to achieve this, the treatment of those with MS is best approached with a philosophy of care (Ashburn & De Souza, 1988).

APPROACHES TO PHYSIOTHERAPY

Physiotherapy for those with MS acts mainly at the level of disability and is unlikely to modify the lesions or change the progression of the disease. For the majority of people with MS, it is likely that physiotherapy will be one of several treatments and should, therefore, address the issues of disability within the context of the aims of other treatments and the needs of the individual.

An approach to physiotherapy that views the individual in his or her social, family, work and cultural roles, informs the physiotherapist about the impact of disablement on the individual's lifestyle. This is important in the case of MS as it affects mostly young adults who, when diagnosed, will face an average of 35–42 years living with this progressively disabling disease (Poser *et al.*, 1989). A shift in focus away from 'problems' and towards a more positive attitude which considers disablement as just one of a variety of ways in which a normal life may be pursued has been called for (Oliver, 1983). An understanding of the priorities of individuals with disability, the value they attach to different activities, and their choices for conducting their lives in certain ways should have a profound influence on the physiotherapy which is provided (Williams, 1987).

The approach to physiotherapy should therefore be patient-centred, with the patient taking an active participatory role in treatment. This will include consultation for joint decision making and goal setting, the opportunity to exercise choice, and the provision of information so that the patient has feedback on progress and knowledge of his or her level of ability.

PRINCIPLES OF PHYSIOTHERAPY

As MS is a long-term disease, treatment plans should be flexible and responsive to the needs of the patient as they change over time. Therapy should encompass not only the changes due to the progression of the MS, but also life changes such as employment, pregnancy and childbirth, parenthood, and ageing. The principles of physiotherapy have been described by Ashburn & De Souza (1988) and further by De Souza (1990). These include:
- Encourage development of strategies of movement.
- Encourage learning of motor skills.
- Improve the quality of patterns of movement.
- Minimise abnormalities of muscle tone.
- Emphasise the functional application of physiotherapy.
- Provide support to maintain motivation and co-operation, and reinforce therapy.
- Implement preventive therapy.
- Educate the person towards a greater understanding of the symptoms of MS and how they affect daily living.

Four primary aims of physiotherapy were also identified:
1. Maintain and increase range of movement (ROM).
2. Encourage postural stability.
3. Prevent contractures.
4. Maintain and encourage weight bearing.

The underlying principle for all the above is one of building on, and extending, the patient's abilities. Emphasis during assessment and treatment should be on what the individual can and does achieve, rather than on what he or she fails to achieve.

ASSESSMENT

Assessment is discussed in Chapter 4 but aspects of specific importance to MS will be addressed here.

Fatigue

As mentioned above, fatigue is a well documented symptom of MS; it is reported to occur in 78% of patients (Freal *et al.*, 1984). It is neither related to the amount of disability nor to mood state (Krupp *et al*, 1988). The assessment of fatigue should include:
- The daily pattern of fatigue.
- Times of the day when energy is high, reasonable, and low.
- Activities or occurrences (e.g. hot weather) which worsen or alleviate fatigue.
- The functional impact of fatigue on everyday activities.
- Whether fatigue is localised to specific muscle groups (e.g. ankle dorsiflexors), a body part (e.g. hand or leg), or functional system (e.g. vision or speech).
- Whether central fatigue is causing overall excessive tiredness.

The results of any physical assessments carried out on people with MS can easily be influenced by their fatigue. It is not unusual for MS patients to have a worse outcome when undergoing a battery of tests, and a better one when tests are distributed over time or rest periods are given.

Activities of Daily Living (ADL)

It is important to know exactly what information is required from an assessment of ADL. If the information needed concerns what the MS person can do overall, then the assessment requirement is one of the physical capacity of the individual to complete the tasks in the ADL instrument. However, if the information needed is about what the person does on a daily basis, it will require an exploration of the person's social, family and cultural roles. Once again, the effects of fatigue may have profound influence on how choices are made. For example, a person may choose to have help to wash and dress in the morning in order to save energy for the journey to work, or may elect to have shopping done so as to have sufficient time and energy to collect the children from school.

It should be noted that many of the domestic (e.g. changing and bathing the baby, or playing with children) and social (e.g. talking on the telephone, or 'surfing' the Internet) activities carried out by young adults are not reflected in the available standardised ADL assessments.

Patient Self-Assessment

Participation of the patient in assessment should be encouraged by the physiotherapist so that self-evaluation is instrumental to the process. This evaluation should address the following issues:

- The individual's perception of his or her abilities and limitations.
- Ability to cope.
- Willingness to change.
- Personal priorities and expectations of physiotherapy.

The self-assessment should be formally documented, dated, and form part of the assessment record in the physiotherapy and/or medical notes.

PLANNING TREATMENT

The assessment forms the basis for developing a plan of treatment, deciding the goals and priorities, and formulating a process which will put the plan into action. All these issues must be negotiated with the patient, who provides the context within which physiotherapy must operate from his or her experience of living with the disease and preferred lifestyle. A scheme for negotiating a goal-directed plan of physiotherapy has been suggested by De Souza (1997). It highlights the active roles played by both the physiotherapist and the patient and advocates shared responsibility for the actions to be taken in order for the plan to be operational.

In order to have a good chance of succeeding, a plan of physiotherapy should have the following features:
- Meets the patient's needs.
- Provides a focus on agreed goals.
- Is a feasible and negotiated plan of action.
- Is progressive in nature.
- Harmonises with other concurrent treatments.
- Is acceptable to the individual and carers, as appropriate.
- Is flexible to changing circumstances.

The need for good communication and interpersonal skills employed throughout the process of therapy cannot be overemphasised.

PHYSIOTHERAPY INTERVENTIONS

Physiotherapy is a widely used treatment for MS patients, who often demand it and have high expectations of its value. As Matthews (1985) stated: 'Every account of the rehabilitation of patients with multiple sclerosis includes physiotherapy and every physician uses it.' However, research evidence of the specific benefits of physiotherapy is scarce despite widespread recommendations for its use. This is not surprising as the majority of physiotherapy treatments for a wide range of conditions, including MS, have developed *ad hoc* from an empirical base rather than from a scientific research base. Nonetheless, all have the underlying aim of reducing disability and increasing ability. Two issues are pertinent in planning physiotherapy: (1) timing—when should therapy be given? and (2) content—what therapy should be given?

Timing of Intervention

The issues here concern when therapy should be given in the course of the disease, how long it should continue, and how often it should be given. Early intervention was seen by some authors as desirable, though not always possible

(Todd, 1986; Ashburn & De Souza, 1988). However, there were few suggestions advocating therapy on the basis of disease duration; rather, patients are referred for physiotherapy, or seek it for themselves, when MS has resulted in a noticeable disability rather than at the time of diagnosis (De Souza, 1990).

It is not known whether rest or exercise is more appropriate during a relapse and the lack of research in this area may be due to the random nature of attacks and the wide fluctuations in symptoms seen in relapsing patients. Despite this, some authors have recommended therapy during recovery from relapse and considered it effective (Alexander & Costello, 1987), but evidence of effectiveness was not provided. Another argument could be that maintenance of ability during relapse might enable the patient to maximise the benefit of remission.

Several authors have favoured long-term intervention (Greenspun et al., 1987; Ashburn & De Souza, 1988; Sibley, 1988) but optimum frequency of treatment was not examined. One study reported significant benefits of long-term intervention in a prospective group study of non-relapsing MS subjects (De Souza & Worthington, 1987). Those gaining benefit received on average 8 hours of physiotherapy a month for 18 consecutive months. Patients receiving less physiotherapy did not show significant improvements in function. On the basis of the scant information available, the issue remains open regarding frequency and timing of treatment.

Type of Intervention

Very little research is available to indicate what type of physiotherapy should constitute the content of a treatment programme, although many opinions have been expressed.

Stretching

A clear consensus, and some experimental evidence, exists in favour of muscle stretching (see Chapter 25). Research on a small number of patients has shown that muscle hypertonus can be reduced, and voluntary range of lower limb movement increased, by muscle stretching (Odeen, 1981). In addition, muscle stretching was considered valuable by many authors (e.g. Alexander & Costello, 1987; Sibley, 1988; De Souza, 1990; Arndt et al., 1991) and no reports have so far come to light which counsel against its use.

Active Exercise

Active exercises have been advocated in the treatment of MS but for varying reasons. They have been suggested for retraining function (De Souza, 1984), muscle strengthening (Alexander & Costello, 1987), retraining of balance and co-ordination (De Souza, 1990; Arndt et al., 1991), and maintaining ROM (Ashburn & De Souza, 1988).

Despite the support for active exercises for MS, only a few studies have investigated their use. One reason for such general agreement may be the predilection of physiotherapists for exercise regimens for a wide variety of conditions. However, it has been shown that chronic disuse of muscles in MS causes not only weakness but also extreme fatiguability (Lenman et al., 1989) as it does in normal muscle. This could imply that active exercises are beneficial for maintaining and increasing strength and endurance, but this needs to be examined in MS patients.

A physiotherapy programme utilising both muscle stretching and free active exercise was evaluated in a prospective long-term study of MS patients (De Souza & Worthington, 1987) which showed that whilst the motor impairments worsened, subjects who had an intensive physiotherapy programme deteriorated significantly less than those who had had less treatment. In addition, functional, balance and daily living activities were also significantly improved in the group receiving more treatment. This study is one of the few which has provided research-based evidence for the efficacy of a physiotherapy programme for MS.

Therapeutic exercises causing fatigue were widely thought to be damaging and the consensus is that moderate exercise is appropriate but that too much, which precipitates fatigue, is inappropriate. However, few studies have been carried out to determine the appropriate quantities of active exercises, and fatigue thresholds may differ between individuals.

Resisted Exercises

Weight-resisted exercises were advocated by Alexander & Costello (1987) for MS, despite an earlier finding that a large proportion of patients deteriorated (Russell & Palfrey, 1969). This type of treatment would seem to be inappropriate for inclusion in a physiotherapy programme.

Use of Walking Aids

Physiotherapy to maintain ambulation has been considered beneficial by many authors (e.g. Burnfield & Frank, 1988) but no agreement on the use of lower limb bracing could be determined (Alexander & Costello, 1987; Arndt et al., 1991). Walking aids were also widely recommended by the above authors but care must be taken to avoid postural instability and deformity with long-term use (Todd, 1982). It would seem, therefore, that opinion is generally in favour of patients using aids if required, but warns against overreliance. Walking aids are discussed further below.

Hydrotherapy, Heat and Cold

Many anecdotal reports exist as to the usefulness or otherwise of hydrotherapy and heat or cold therapy. Burnfield (1985), as both a doctor and an MS patient, recommended avoiding hydrotherapy as 'it may make things worse and bring on fatigue'. Conversely, Alexander & Costello (1987) stated that exercises in a pool could be beneficial. However, these reports lack specificity as they do not refer to any particular symptoms or signs being affected by the treatment.

With respect to heat and cold, Forsythe (1988), another doctor with MS, reported that warm baths aided muscle stretching exercises. Burnfield (1985), however, found that cool baths were beneficial, but also described one case where this treatment had a 'disastrous' result. Descriptions were not given as to what constituted either the benefit or the disaster, but these anecdotal reports serve to highlight the individual nature of responses to intervention experienced by some MS patients.

Clear warnings against heat therapy in MS were given by Block & Kester (1970) who thought that it caused severe exacerbation of clinical and subclinical deficits, while De Souza (1990) warned against the use of ice, or ice-cold water, in patients with compromised circulation, as this can cause vasoconstriction and further reduce the circulation.

Electrical Stimulation
Low-frequency neuromuscular electrical stimulation can be beneficial for some MS patients (Worthington & De Souza, 1990) but the need for careful selection of patients for this form of treatment is emphasised as it does not benefit all MS patients. In addition, neuromuscular stimulation is recommended as an adjunct to other physiotherapy, mainly active exercise and muscle stretching (see Chapter 24).

Conclusions—In the absence of any sound evidence, and no consensus of clinical opinion regarding hydrotherapy, heat, or cold therapy, and the small amount of evidence available on muscle stimulation, these treatments may not be appropriate for general application in MS, but may prove helpful to some individuals. On the basis of evidence available, the two components of physiotherapy likely to be the most useful in MS are muscle stretching and active exercises. It is further suggested that the exercises should incorporate training to improve ambulation, and also be paced so as to account for fatigue. These treatment components may be appropriate for a physiotherapy intervention programme for the majority of people with MS, and are further described by De Souza (1984, 1990), and Ashburn & De Souza (1988), and are summarised below.

A PHYSIOTHERAPY TREATMENT PROGRAMME
The programme proposed by Ashburn & De Souza (1988) consisted of active and active-assisted free exercises based upon 12 core exercises, and a simple muscle stretching regimen. The emphasis of the active exercise programme was on functional activities, and the use of the exercises to achieve a functional goal was taught. For example, a sequence which incorporated knee rolling, side sitting (stretch exercise), low kneeling, high kneeling, half kneeling and standing, would achieve the functional activity of rising up from the floor. Other gross body motor skills, such as transferring, may be retrained in a similar way.

The active exercise programme could also be adjusted so that the emphasis moved towards balance activities. This incorporated 'hold' techniques into the basic exercise programme to encourage postural stabilisation and stimulate balance reactions. Patients were required to hold certain positions and postures for a few seconds to begin with and subsequently gradually to increase the period. For example, the position of high kneeling was required to be held for a 10-second period without the patient using any upper limb support, while an upright standing posture utilising a narrow base of support and no upper limb aid was required to be held for 30 seconds. Patients could self-monitor their progress and were encouraged to note their levels of achievement.

The programme may be adjusted to individual levels of ability, e.g. by diversifying exercises in a variety of sitting or kneeling positions if the individual is unable to stand. The emphasis of the different exercises may also be adjusted according to the needs of individuals. Those whose major problems are spasticity, and muscle and joint stiffness, require an emphasis on stretching and increasing active and passive ROM. Those with problems of ataxia and instability need more emphasis on the smooth co-ordination of movements, and on balance and postural stability. The majority of MS patients will have a combination of different motor symptoms, and a balanced programme will need to be constructed.

Management of the MS Person with Mainly Spastic Symptoms
Physiotherapy for an MS patient with predominantly spastic symptoms is generally similar to that for other neurological patients with the same problem (see Chapter 25). However, some specific issues need to be attended to in MS, and the progressive nature of the disease borne in mind. Most importantly, any decision to reduce the level of muscle tone must have a clear objective, and an identifiable and achievable functional benefit. A high level of tone is useful for some MS patients, e.g. those who use their spasticity for standing, transferring, or for utilising a 'swing to' or 'swing through' gait pattern for crutch walking (De Souza, 1990). For these people, spasticity should not be reduced at the expense of their mobility.

For other MS patients, spasticity will hinder their ability, causing movement to be masked and adding to the effort required for voluntary actions, so reduction of muscle tone may be appropriate for these patients. However, careful monitoring of any movement is required during the reduction of tone, as in MS the spasticity often overlies other symptoms, such as weakness or ataxia, which are more difficult for the patient to cope with than the spasticity (De Souza, 1990).

Some MS patients exhibit an extremely changeable distribution of tone in different positions, e.g. lower limb extensor hypertonus in standing and flexor hypertonus in lying. These features are probably due to lesions disrupting CNS pathways which control limb and trunk postural responses to muscular information. Irrespective of the variability of spasticity in MS patients, there are certain muscle groups which tend to exhibit the symptom more than others. It should be recalled that where there is a hypertonic muscle group, there is also generally another muscle group, often the antagonists, which exhibits low tone. These imbalances, if allowed to become permanent, will result in contractures and deformity. The muscle groups most often developing contracture in people with MS are:

- Trunk rotators.
- Trunk lateral flexors.
- Hip flexors.
- Hip adductors.
- Knee flexors.
- Ankle plantar flexors.
- Inverters of the foot.

Spasticity in the upper limbs is less common than in the lower limbs; the muscle groups most often affected are the wrist and finger flexors, and the shoulder adductors and internal rotators. Occasionally, the forearm pronators and elbow flexors are affected, but the full flexion pattern of spasticity, as seen in the hemiplegic arm, is rare, though not unknown, in MS.

Physiotherapy for spasticity is described in Chapter 25. It should be remembered, however, that MS symptoms are bilateral, and the absence of any reference for 'normal' tone in an individual may make the management of spasticity more difficult. With MS, simple strategies to alleviate spasticity, which patients can carry out for themselves, are preferable. The techniques of choice are muscle stretching and the use of positions which retain prolonged muscle stretch (Ashburn & De Souza, 1988; De Souza, 1990).

Management of the MS Person with Ataxia

Ataxia is one of the major motor symptoms affecting people with MS. It rarely occurs in isolation, and is most commonly seen with other motor symptoms, notably spasticity. It is a disturbance that, independently of motor weakness, alters the direction and extent of a voluntary movement and impairs the sustained voluntary and reflex muscle contraction necessary for maintaining posture and equilibrium.

The main problem that ataxic MS patients show is an inability to make movements which require groups of muscles to act together in varying degrees of co-contraction. The difficulty is easily observed during gait as the single-stance phase requires the co-contraction of leg muscles in order to support body weight, whilst at the same time a co-ordinated change in the relative activity of the muscles is needed to move the body weight forward (e.g. from a flexed hip position at 'heel strike', to an extended hip position at 'toe off'). The ataxic patient has greatest difficulty with this phase of gait and either uses the stance leg as a rigid strut, or staggers as co-ordination is lost. Compensation is often afforded by walking aids which reduce the need for weight support through stance, whilst providing at least two (one upper and one lower limb) points of support in all phases of gait. The reduction of upper-limb weight bearing has been considered an essential component for retaining functional gait in ataxic patients (Brandt *et al.*, 1981). Using walking aids, the ataxic patient can ambulate with the hips remaining in flexion, thus eliminating the need to effect a co-ordinated change from hip flexion to extension while bearing weight through the stance leg.

The aim of physiotherapy is to counteract the postural and movement adjustments made by the ataxic patient in order to encourage postural stability and dynamic weight shifting, and to increase the smooth co-ordination of movement. It is also to prevent the preferred postures of ataxic patients, adopted to eliminate their instability, from becoming functional or fixed contractures (De Souza, 1990). The features of postural abnormality are:

- An exaggerated lumbar lordosis.
- An anteriorley tilted pelvis.
- Flexion at the hips.
- Hyperextension of the knees.
- Weight towards the heel parts of the feet.
- Clawed toes (as they grip the ground).

The different types of ataxia have been reviewed by Morgan (1980) and are summarised in Table 11.3 with the main features of motor dysfunction. In MS there may be a mixture of cerebellar, vestibular and sensory components depending on the sites of the lesions.

Ataxia is a very complex movement disorder and there is little research evidence to inform the content of physiotherapy programmes to treat this symptom. However, there are some indications that physiotherapy can help (Brandt *et al.*, 1986) and indeed may be essential for preventing unnecessary inactivity and dependency, and for reducing the risk of falls. The key issue in the treatment of ataxia is to identify the predominant problem to guide the primary aims of treatment. This should be achieved by

Types of ataxia and associated motor disorders	
Sensory ataxia	A 'high stepping' gait pattern More reliance on visual or auditory information about leg or foot position
Vestibular ataxia	Disturbed equilibrium in standing and walking Loss of equilibrium reactions A wide-based, staggering gait pattern
Cerebellar ataxia	Disturbance in the rate, regularity and force of movement Loss of movement co-ordination Overshooting of target (dysmetria) Decomposition of movement (dyssynergia) Loss of speed and rhythm of alternating movements (dysdiadochokinesia) Inco-ordination of agonist-antagonist muscles and loss of the continuity of muscle contraction (tremor, e.g. intention tremor)

Table 11.3 Types of ataxia and associated motor disorders.

careful observational assessment of the ataxic patient carrying out a range of activities. Generally, patients should progress from simple movements to more complex ones as they master the ability to co-ordinate muscle groups.

Assessment and treatment strategies for the ataxic MS patient are summarised in Table 11.4. As there is little research evidence to indicate the most useful way forwards for treatment, however, physiotherapy for ataxia must by necessity take a pragmatic approach.

Therapy techniques that could be used to good effect include: weight shifting in different positions (e.g. kneel walking, step stride and side stride standing); lowering and raising the centre of gravity (e.g. by knee bending and straightening in standing; or moving from high kneeling to side sitting and back to high kneeling); proprioceptive neuromuscular facilitation techniques (see Chapter 24); and the use of slow reversals, rhythmic movements and stabilisations. Whichever techniques are employed, due attention must be given to fatigue. Within a therapy session, frequent periods of rest are generally required and the work performed in a session may be wasted if the patient has been exhausted by the treatment.

Aids for Mobility

Mobility is perhaps the major functional disability in MS. Scheinberg (1987) stated that when patients are asked about their main problem with MS, 90% will cite a walking difficulty. Therefore maintaining walking ability for as long as possible is a priority and should form a primary aim of physiotherapy.

Walking aids have both advantages and disadvantages (Table 11.5) and therapists need to be aware of both in order to discuss the issues with their patients (De Souza, 1990). The main detrimental effects of using a walking aid and the ways by which physiotherapy can reduce the disadvantages have been identified by Todd (1982). Once a mobility aid has been provided, regular review is essential, as the fluctuating and progressive nature of MS may indicate a need to change the type of aid used or the type of gait pattern employed. Follow-up is also essential if a mobility aid has been provided for a patient during a relapse, as any recovery of movement must be maximised and not compromised by the patient's retaining an inappropriate aid or gait pattern for his or her level of recovery (De Souza, 1990).

Assessment and treatment approaches for patients with ataxia		
Predominant problem	**Dysfunction expressed in**	**Primary aims of treatment**
Maintaining equilibrium	Weight bearing and weight transference	Increase postural stability Enhance control of the centre of gravity in weight shifting Encourage maintenance of the control of the centre of gravity in movement from one position to another Progress from a wide to a narrow base of support
Co-ordination of dynamic movement	Patterns of movement	Enhance smoothness of control of movement patterns Progress from simple to complex patterns Progress from fast to slow movements
Located in body axis and trunk	Gross body movements (e.g. transfers)	Independent and free head movement Increase control of movement to, from and around the midline (body axis) Encourage movement of limb girdles in relation to body axis (especially rotation)
Located in limbs	Voluntary body movements	Enhance proximal limb stabilisation Encourage co-ordinated activity of agonist and antagonist muscle groups Progress from large-range to small-range movements Reduce the requirement for visual guidance of movement

Table 11.4 Assessment and treatment approaches for patients with ataxia.

Although the therapy issues surrounding the provision and use of mobility aids focus mainly on lower limb movement and gait, the upper limbs should not be neglected. Regular use of mobility aids may have a detrimental effect on the upper limbs and the physiotherapist should include an examination of them in the review process. The major issues to be addressed are:

- Loss of upper limb function.
- Injury to soft tissue, particularly of the shoulders.
- Joint and muscle pain, including neck pain.
- Loss of joint ROM.
- Compromised skin integrity, especially of the palmar surfaces of the hands.

This section has focused primarily on the physical aspects of walking and the need for aids. However, 'walking' is not only a physical function but also has social, emotional and cultural meanings. For some, the personal disadvantages outweigh the physical advantages, and they decide not to use recommended mobility aids. This could be interpreted, mistakenly, as non-compliance with professional advice, or non-acceptance of the disability if the physiotherapist has not explored and understood the social, cultural and emotional needs of the patient.

Management of the Immobile Person with MS

People with MS may become immobile, either due to progression of the disease causing severe disablement or

Advantages and disadvantages of aids to mobility	
Advantages	**Disadvantages**
Increased safety and stability	Less lower limb weight bearing
Reduced risk of falls	Loss of lower limb muscle strength
Increased walking distance	Reduced head and trunk movements
Increased walking speed	Reduction of balance reactions
Increased gait efficiency	Alteration of muscle tone
Improved quality of gait pattern	Postural abnormality (e.g. hip flexion, trunk lateral flexion)
Reduced fatigue	Upper limb function may be compromised

Table 11.5 Advantages and disadvantages of aids to mobility.

during a relapse. It is essential that when immobile in relapse, the patient is managed in a way that will not disadvantage functional ability after relapse, or prolong unnecessarily the duration of immobility and dependency. Physiotherapy should provide preventive treatment, maintenance regimens and appropriate, staged active exercises when recovery first becomes apparent. Table 11.6 illustrates a typical preventive and maintenance physiotherapy programme.

Attention should also be directed to the general good health and wellbeing of the patient. For example, if immobility lasts over several days or weeks, help may be needed to retain a sound level of nutrition, a social support network or for continence management.

HELPING CARERS

People with MS generally have a number of family members and friends who will also have to learn to live with MS. As Soderburg (1992) stated, '...the diagnosis of MS will affect every aspect of family life. Its impact will extend to work roles, economic status, relationships within the family, and relationships between the family and the larger community.' Professional carers, such as physiotherapists, have an important role in helping the informal carers. Teaching safe and efficient moving, lifting and handling techniques is a major area where direct physiotherapeutic intervention can bring substantial benefits.

Over the long and progressive course of MS, family members may well constitute the most consistent resource for the person with MS. As such, carers should be valued participants of the healthcare team, and be part of the decision-making process (McQueen Davis & Niskala, 1992). Tasks that may be required of carers should not compromise their long-term support in order to achieve a short-term goal. Just as the person with MS is identified and treated as an individual with specific needs, so should the uniqueness of the carer's needs be acknowledged. Recognition must also be given to the social and family role of the carer, and the environmental and emotional settings within which caring takes place. It should be remembered that care giving takes place throughout the day and night (Spackman et al., 1989).

The co-operation of carers cannot be assumed, but must be negotiated. When a carer consents to carry out a task, it is inappropriate to assume that a blanket consent has been obtained for all tasks. The carer should have the opportunity to exercise choice, discretion and judgement about what is best for him or her. Even in situations where carers consent, their willingness to help must be consonant with their apparent physical, psychological and emotional abilities to do so. This issue deserves particular attention where the main carer is an elderly parent, and even more so when the carer is a child (Blackford, 1992; Segal & Simpkins, 1993). Physiotherapists must be aware of the current local and national recommendations, and demonstrate that they have executed their duty of care to both patient and carer.

Table 11.6 Preventive and maintenance physiotherapy for immobile patients with multiple sclerosis

Prevent	Treatment
Respiratory inadequacy Partial lung collapse Chest infections Accumulation of sputum Cyanosis	Establish correct breathing pattern Teach deep breathing exercises in recumbent and sitting positions Promote effective cough Ensure air entry to all areas of lung
Circulatory stasis Deep vein thrombosis	Active rhythmic contraction and relaxation of lower limb muscles Massage, passive movement or use of mechanical aids if no activation of muscles possible
Contractures	Ensure full passive range of movement at all joints Correction and support of posture in lying and sitting Prolonged stretch of hypertonic muscles
Pressure sores	Distribute loading over weight-bearing body surfaces Avoid pressure points Change position frequently and regularly Support correct posture Implement moving and handling techniques that protect skin integrity
Muscle atrophy	Encourage active contraction in all able muscle groups Use passive and assisted movements as appropriate Implement assisted or aided standing when safe and within patient tolerance

CONCLUSIONS

MS is probably one of the most complex conditions encountered by physiotherapists. There is no 'typical' MS patient, nor a 'typical' presentation of the disease, and its variability often astounds even the most experienced practitioners. Although physiotherapists will be concerned primarily with sensorimotor dysfunction, the wider context within which disability is expressed and experienced must also be taken into account.

An interdisciplinary team approach to the management of MS appears to be the best way forward, with the patient and carer being integral to the team. As a team member, the physiotherapist will be required to have high levels of assessment, treatment, and interpersonal skills. Successful management should provide the opportunity for the patient to achieve the best level of activity relevant to his or her lifestyle at every stage of the disease. Best practice does not consist of a series of interventions, but embodies a cohesive care plan which allows the patient to develop skills for living.

A philosophy of care encompasses an understanding that functions, such as walking and transferring, reach far beyond the physical issues. The significance of dysfunction reaches into the realms of social, cultural, psychological and emotional meanings of loss and limitation. The physiotherapist, therefore, cannot just offer treatment, but must also offer care and support to all those who need to learn to live with MS.

REFERENCES

Alexander J, Costello E. Physical and surgical therapy. In: Scheinberg LC, Holland NJ, eds. *Multiple sclerosis: a guide for patients and their families, 2nd edition.* New York: Raven Press; 1987:79-107.

Arndt J, Bhasin C, Brar SP, *et al.* Physical therapy. In: Schapiro RT, ed. *Multiple sclerosis: a rehabilitation approach to management.* New York: Demos; 1991:17-66.

Ashburn A, De Souza LH. An approach to the management of multiple sclerosis. *Physiother Pract* 1988, **4**:139-145.

Barnes M. Multiple sclerosis. In: Greenwood R, Barnes MP, McMillan TM, *et al.*, eds. *Neurological rehabilitation.* London: Churchill Livingstone; 1993:485-504.

Birk K, Rudick R. Pregnancy and multiple sclerosis. *Arch Neurol* 1986, **43**:719-726.

Blackford KA. Strategies for intervention and research with children or adolescents who have a parent with multiple sclerosis. *Axon* 1992, **Dec**:50-55.

Brandt T, Buchele W, Krafczyk S. Training effects on experimental postural instability: a model for clinical ataxia therapy. In: Bles W, Brandt T, eds. *Disorders of posture and gait*. Amsterdam: Elsevier, 1986:353-365.

Brandt T, Krafczyk S, Malsbenden J. Postural imbalance with head extension: improvement by training as a model for ataxia therapy. *Ann NY Acad Sci* 1981, **374**:636-649.

Burnfield A. *Multiple sclerosis: a personal exploration*. London: Souvenir Press; 1985.

Burnfield A, Frank A. Multiple sclerosis. In: Frank A, Maguire P, eds. *Disabling diseases - physical, environmental and psychosocial management*. London: Heinemann Medical; 1988.

Compston DAS. Genetic susceptibility to multiple sclerosis. In: Matthews WB, *et al.*, eds. *McAlpine's multiple sclerosis, 2nd edition*. New York: Churchill Livingstone; 1991:301-319.

De Souza LH. A different approach to physiotherapy for multiple sclerosis patients. *Physiother* 1984, **70**:429-432.

De Souza LH. *Multiple sclerosis: approaches to management*. London: Chapman & Hall; 1990.

De Souza LH. Physiotherapy. In: Goodwill J, Chamberlain MA, Evans C, eds. *Rehabilitation of the physically disabled adult, 2nd edition*. London: Chapman & Hall; 1997:560-575.

De Souza LH, Worthington JA. The effect of long-term physiotherapy on disability in multiple sclerosis patients. In: Clifford Rose F, Jones R, eds. *Multiple sclerosis: immunological, diagnostic and therapeutic aspects*. London & Paris: John Libbey; 1987:155-164.

Dean G, Kurtzke JF. On the risk of multiple sclerosis according to the age at immigration to South Africa. *Br Med J* 1971, **3**:725-729.

Ebers GC. Genetic factors in multiple sclerosis. *Neurol Clin* 1983, **1**:645-654.

Ebers GC, Bulman DE, Sadovnick AD. A population-based study of multiple sclerosis in twins. *N Engl J Med* 1986, **315**:1638-1642.

Forsythe E. *Multiple sclerosis: exploring sickness and health*. London & Boston: Faber & Faber; 1988.

Freal JE, Kraft GH, Coryell JK. Symptomatic fatigue in multiple sclerosis. *Arch Phys Med Rehabil* 1984, **65**:135-138.

Goodkin DE, Rudick PS, Vanderbrug Medendorp S, *et al.* Low dose (7.5 mg) oral methotrexate reduces the rate of progression of chronic progressive multiple sclerosis. *Ann Neurol* 1995, **37**:30-40.

Greenspun B, Stineman M, Agri R. Multiple sclerosis and rehabilitation outcome. *Arch Phys Med Rehabil* 1987, **68**:434-437.

Halliday AM, McDonald WI. Pathophysiology of demyelinating disease. *Br Med Bull* 1977, **33**:21-27.

Hulter BM, Lundberg OL. Sexual function in women with advanced multiple sclerosis. *J Neurol Neurosurg Psychiat* 1995, **59**:83-86.

IFBN Multiple Sclerosis Study Group. Interferon beta-1b is effective in relapsing-remitting multiple sclerosis. I. Clinical results of multicentre, randomised, double-blind, placebo-controlled trial. *Neurology* 1993, **43**:655-661.

Korn-Lubetzki I, Kahana E, Cooper G, *et al.* Activity of multiple sclerosis during pregnancy and puerperium. *Ann Neurol* 1984, **16**:229-231.

Krupp LB, Alvarez LA, LaRocca NG, *et al.* Fatigue in multiple sclerosis. *Arch Neurol* 1988, **45**:435-437.

Kurtzke JF, Beebe GW, Norman JE Jr. Epidemiology of multiple sclerosis in US veterans: I. Race, sex and geographic distribution. *Neurology* 1979, **29**:1228-1235.

Kurtzke JF, Gudmundsson KR, Bergmann S. Multiple sclerosis in Iceland: I. Evidence of a post-war epidemic. *Neurology* 1982, **32**:143-145.

Kurtzke JF, Hyllested K. Multiple sclerosis in the Faroe Islands: II. Clinical update, transmission and the nature of MS. *Neurology* 1986, **36**:307-312.

Kurtzke JF, Kurland LT. The epidemiology of neurologic disease. In: Baker AB, ed. *Clinical neurology*. Philadelphia: Harper & Row; 1983:1-143.

Langton Hewer R. The epidemiology of disabling neurological disorders. In: Greenwood R, Barnes MP, McMillan TM, *et al.*, eds. *Neurological rehabilitation*. London: Churchill Livingstone; 1993:3-12.

Lenman JAR, Tulley FM, Vrbová G, *et al.* Muscle fatigue in some neurological conditions. *Muscle Nerve* 1989, **12**:938-942.

Matthews WB, Acheson ED, Batchelor JR, *et al. McAlpine's multiple sclerosis, 2nd edition*. Edinburgh & London: Churchill Livingstone; 1991.

McQueen Davis ME, Niskala H. Nurturing a valuable resource: family caregivers in multiple sclerosis. *Axon* 1992, **March**:87-91.

Misulis KE. *Essentials of clinical neurophysiology*. London: Butterworth Heinemann; 1993.

Morgan MH. Ataxia–its causes, measurement and management. *Internat Rehab Med* 1980, **2**:126-132.

Odeen I. Reduction of muscular hypertonus by long-term muscle stretch. *Scand J Rehab Med* 1981, **13**:93-99.

Oliver MJ. Social work with disabled people. London: Macmillan Press; 1983.

Paty DW, Li DKB, UBC MS/MRI Study Group, IFNB Multiple Sclerosis Study Group. Interferon beta-1b is effective in relapsing-remitting multiple sclerosis. II. Clinical results in a multicentre, randomised, double-blind, placebo-controlled trial. *Neurology* 1993, **43**:662-667.

Paty DW, Oger JJF, Kastrukoff LF, *et al.* MRI in the diagnosis of MS: a prospective study with comparison of clinical evaluation, evoked potentials, oligoclonal banding and CT. *Neurology* 1988, **38**:180-185.

Poser S, Kurtzke JF, Schaff G. Survival in multiple sclerosis. *J Clin Epidemiol* 1989, **42**:159-168.

Poser CM, Paty DW, Scheinberg L, *et al.* New diagnostic criteria for multiple sclerosis: guidelines for research protocols. *Ann Neurol* 1983, **13**:227-231.

Prineas JW, Connell F. The fine structure of chronically active multiple sclerosis plaques. *Neurology* 1978, **28**:68-75.

Russell WR, Palfrey G. Disseminated sclerosis: rest-exercise therapy - a progress report. *Physiother* 1969, **55**:306-310.

Scheinberg LC. Introduction. In: Scheinberg LC, Holland NJ, eds. *Multiple sclerosis: a guide for patients and their families, 2nd edition*. New York: Raven Press; 1987:1-2.

Segal J, Simpkins J. '*My Mum needs me*': Helping children with ill or disabled parents. London: Penguin Books; 1993.

Sibley W. *Therapeutic claims in multiple sclerosis*. New York: Demos; 1988:104.

Snow BJ, Tsui JKC, Bhatt MH, *et al.* Treatment of spasticity with Botulinum Toxin: a double blind study. *Ann Neurol* 1990, **28**:512-515.

Soderberg J. MS and the family system. In: Kalb R, Scheinberg LC, eds. *Multiple sclerosis and the family*. New York: Demos; 1992:1-7.

Spackman AJ, Doulton DC, Roberts MHW, *et al.* Caring at night for people with multiple sclerosis. *Br Med J* 1989, **299**:1433.

Tallis RC, Illis LS, Sedgwick EM. The quantitative assessment of the influence of spinal cord stimulation on motor function in patients with multiple sclerosis. *Int J Rehab Med* 1983, **5**:10-16.

Todd J. Physiotherapy in multiple sclerosis. In: Capildeo R, Maxwell A, eds. *Progress in rehabilitation: multiple sclerosis*. London & Basingstoke: Macmillan Press; 1982: 31-44.

Todd J. Multiple sclerosis–management. In: Downie PA, ed. *Cash's textbook of neurology for physiotherapists, 4th edition*. London: Faber & Faber; 1986: 398-416.

Tourtellotte WW, Booe IM. Multiple sclerosis: the blood-brain barrier and the measurement of *de novo* central nervous system IgG synthesis. *Neurology* 1978, **28**(suppl):76-82.

Weiner HL, Mackin GA, Orav EJ, *et al.* Intermittent cyclophosphamide pulse therapy in progressive multiple sclerosis: Final report of the North East Cooperative Multiple Sclerosis Treatment Group. *Neurology* 1993, **43**:910-918.

Williams G. Disablement and the social context of daily activity. *Int Disabil Stud* 1987, **9**:97-102.

Worthington JA, De Souza LH. The use of clinical measures in the evaluation of neuromuscular stimulation in multiple sclerosis patients. In: Wientholter H, Dichgans J, Mertin J, eds. *Current concepts in multiple sclerosis*. London: Elsevier; 1990:213-218.

Yudkin PL, Ellison GW, Ghezzi A, *et al.* Overview of azathioprine treatment in MS. *Lancet* 1991, **338**:1051-1055.

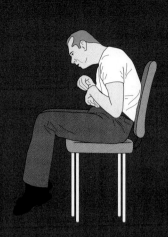

12 PARKINSON'S DISEASE

D Jones &
RB Godwin-Austen

CHAPTER OUTLINE

- Pathology
- Aetiology and epidemiology
- Clinical features
- General management

- Medical management
- Physical management
- Case histories

INTRODUCTION

Parkinson's disease and the 'parkinsonian syndrome' comprise a group of disorders characterised by tremor and disturbance of voluntary movement, posture and balance. Parkinson's disease was first described by James Parkinson in 1817, its pathology was defined about 100 years later, and treatment was revolutionised in the 1960s by the introduction of the drug levodopa.

The parkinsonian syndrome is a group of disorders in which the characteristic symptoms and signs of parkinsonism develop but are secondary to another neurological disease (e.g. encephalitis lethargica, Alzheimer's disease). Thus, whereas Parkinson's disease is a primary degenerative condition occurring in the latter half of life and following a progressive course, the parkinsonian syndrome has a natural history dependent on the cause. The word 'parkinsonism' is used to describe the symptoms and signs, irrespective of the cause of the disease state. Where parkinsonian syndrome is complicated by some generalised degenerative process (e.g. cerebral arteriosclerosis), treatment may be less satisfactory than in the uncomplicated case.

Finally, there is a group of degenerative brain disorders often referred to as Parkinsonism. In these disorders, slowness of movement, rigidity of muscle tone and occasionally tremor may be associated with progressive supranuclear ophthalmoplegia (Steele–Richardson syndrome), or postural hypotension and autonomic dysfunction (multisystem atrophy). These disorders seldom respond well to dopamine agonist (levodopa) treatment.

PATHOLOGY

The symptoms and signs of parkinsonism stem from a disturbance of function in two regions of the basal ganglia—the substantia nigra and the corpus striatum (caudate nucleus and putamen). These central nuclear masses of grey matter contain practically all the dopamine in the human brain (Bannister, 1992). Dopamine is a chemical substance and one of the neurotransmitter amines (like adrenaline and noradrenaline) that transmit electrical impulses from one neurone to the next across the synapse. In parkinsonism there is a specific reduction of dopamine concentration at the synapse. This lack of dopamine results from a degeneration of neurones in Parkinson's disease and the degenerative parkinsonism syndromes (such as Alzheimer's disease), or from focal damage following encephalitis lethargica. In parkinsonism due to phenothiazine drugs there is a chemical block to the action of dopamine.

The mechanism by which this change in neurochemistry causes the symptoms of the disease is complex and poorly understood (Koller, 1992). In the normal situation, a balance of inhibitory and excitatory events in the basal ganglia and motor cortex allows the maintenance of normal posture and movement (see Chapter 2). When this balance is upset, the symptoms and signs of rigidity and involuntary movement supervene, along with abnormalities of posture and associated movement, and slowness of movement. These abnormalities can often be temporarily overcome by voluntary effort (e.g. arm swing when walking) but the automatic subconscious basis of posture and movement is lost.

Parkinson's disease accounts for the great majority of cases of parkinsonism. The cause of the degeneration in the substantia nigra and corpus striatum is unknown but it is a progressive process, often of late onset, with a mean time from onset to death of between 10 and 15 years. Some cases progress more rapidly and in others progression may be so slow that deterioration may be undetectable. In cases of early onset, the rate of progression is often very slow. Furthermore, modern treatment has so improved the prognosis that there is now no overall excess mortality from Parkinson's disease when comparison is made with individuals of the same age.

In the worst cases, increasing immobility leads eventually to weight loss, pressure sores and respiratory complications, which are the usual cause of death.

In parkinsonism secondary to phenothiazine drugs or following encephalitis lethargica (now very rare), involuntary spasms of the eyes (oculogyric crises) may occur. Postencephalitic parkinsonism is often non-progressive and may be associated with widespread brain damage causing behavioural disorder, spastic weakness and visual disturbance.

Features of the parkinsonian syndrome may develop in patients following a single severe head injury or following multiple head injuries (e.g. in boxers). Such cases are generally resistant to drug treatment and, as in those cases where parkinsonism is part of a generalised degenerative process, intellectual impairment commonly occurs and further reduces therapeutic responsiveness.

AETIOLOGY AND EPIDEMIOLOGY

The cause of Parkinson's disease is not known and the treatment is therefore palliative and symptomatic.

The prevalence of Parkinson's disease increases with increasing age. A study of the prevalence of the disease in Scotland quoted 46.6 per 100,000 for ages 40–49, 254 per 100,000 for ages 60–69, and 1924.5 per 100,000 in people aged 80 and over (Mutch et al., 1986). At any one time, 74% of people with Parkinson's disease are aged 70 and over and the mean age at onset is 65.3 years. However, 1 in 7 is diagnosed under the age of 50 (Caird, 1991). In late-onset Parkinson's disease, tremor is often the presenting feature, with rigidity and bradykinesia developing later, whilst in early-onset disease an akinetic–rigid picture predominates throughout (Bostantjopoulou et al., 1991). Depression was found in the same study to be more common with early onset, and higher levels of cognitive impairment in late onset. Early-onset disease is associated with the more frequent occurrence of motor fluctuations and dyskinesias (Pantelatos & Fornadi, 1993).

There is no sex-related difference in prevalence, social class does not appear to affect the incidence, and no convincing geographical differences have been demonstrated. Analysis of mortality data and data from large family studies suggests a genetic component with exposure to a causal environmental agent in early life. For a full review of these aspects the reader is referred to Stern (1990).

CLINICAL FEATURES

There are no diagnostic tests for Parkinson's disease. Diagnosis is made on clinical grounds which involves the recognition of the characteristic symptoms and physical signs. The principles of medical diagnosis are discussed in Chapter 3.

The patient with parkinsonism may present with the characteristic tremor (see Chapter 5) although it is important not to label other forms of tremor 'parkinsonian'. More than 50% of patients with Parkinson's disease do not have any tremor and the presenting symptoms are then much more diverse.

The patient usually attributes the symptoms of the disease to 'old age'. Common presenting symptoms are slowness of walking and disturbance of balance, with occasional falls or difficulty with fine manipulative movements such as dressing or shaving. Pain is a common presenting complaint and patients may attend a physiotherapy department for the treatment of musculoskeletal problems such as frozen shoulder or backache when their symptoms are, in fact, due to parkinsonism. The pain is rapidly relieved by appropriate treatment for their parkinsonism.

Early symptoms of the disease may include difficulty with specific movements such as writing, difficulty in turning over in bed or rising from a low chair, an excessive greasiness of the skin or an unusual tendency to constipation, and an inability to raise the voice or cough effectively. All the symptoms tend to be disproportionately worse when the patient is under stress and this may lead the patient to withdraw socially.

The general slowing up, associated as it often is with an apathy associated with depression, may lead friends and family to conclude that the patient is dementing. While dementia does occur in a significant proportion of people with Parkinson's disease, it is mild in the early stages and seen frequently only in the elderly (see above).

POSTURE

Postural abnormality is common. When standing there is a slight flexion at all joints, leading to the 'simian posture' with the knees and hips slightly flexed, the shoulders rounded and the head held forward (Figure 12.1). The arms may be bent across the trunk. More rarely, the abnormality of posture will be a tendency to lean backward with a rather erect stance.

When sitting, the patient tends to slump in the chair, often sliding sideways, and the head again may fall forward on the chest. The abnormal posture can be voluntarily corrected but only temporarily and with considerable effort and concentration. Assessment of posture is discussed below.

BALANCE AND GAIT

When standing, these patients characteristically have a tendency to topple forwards. They are unable to make the quick compensatory movements to regain balance and so are easily knocked over. When they start to walk there is difficulty in shifting the centre of gravity from one foot to

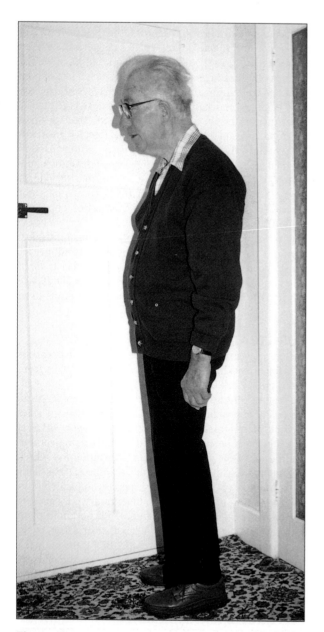

Figure 12.1 Typical posture in a patient with Parkinson's disease. He shows slight flexion at the knees and hips, with rounded shoulders, and holds his head forward.

the other so their paces become short and shuffling. Patients may lean too far forward so that they have to 'chase' their centre of gravity if they are to avoid falling forward, so-called anterpulsion or festination. Retropulsion is a related phenomenon, involving taking several steps backwards after each forward step (Stern, 1990). Wearing low-heeled or flat shoes can exacerbate a tendency to fall backwards, which can be countered by carrying something in front.

There are specific difficulties in initiating the movements of walking and in turning. Sudden interruption of walking (freezing) can occur, especially when obstacles are present. (See 'Physical management' for practical strategies.) The gait of early-onset patients may appear unco-ordinated as a result of drug-induced dyskinesia.

LEARNT AND VOLUNTARY MOVEMENTS

All movements are reduced in range and speed. In walking, the patient tends to take small paces (hypometria) and to walk more slowly (bradykinesia). Speech becomes slower and softer. Handwriting tends to get smaller and after writing a few words slows down and becomes increasingly untidy. Activities such as cutting up food and fastening buttons may become impossible. Repetitive movements such as stirring and polishing are often particularly affected.

In contrast, some complex co-ordinated movements such as driving a car or using a typewriter may be affected relatively little, although performed more slowly than normal (see Chapter 2).

AUTOMATIC MOVEMENTS

These are specifically reduced or lost in Parkinson's disease. The patient blinks infrequently and may have an expressionless 'mask-like' face giving the spurious appearance of stupidity. There are none of the restless associated movements of the hands seen in unaffected people. When walking, the patient does not swing the arms but has them hanging and slightly flexed at the elbow.

Automatic swallowing of saliva is also impaired so that these patients tend to dribble involuntarily, particularly when they sit with the head flexed on the chest. Coughing as an automatic reflex response to clear the airway may be defective and there is therefore a risk of respiratory infection. Unfortunately, current treatment does not restore any of these defects of automatic movement to any significant degree.

RIGIDITY

Muscle tone is increased in parkinsonism but the resistance to passive movement at a joint is uniform throughout the range of movement (ROM) in contrast to spastic hypertonia. Two types of parkinsonian rigidity are described: 'lead pipe', where the resistance is smooth or plastic; and the 'cogwheel', where the resistance is intermittent (see Chapter 5).

Although the rigidity does not account for the poverty of movement which characterises parkinsonism, it undoubtedly contributes to it. Similarly, rigidity plays a part in the cause of the muscle pain already described. Rigidity is usually asymmetrical or even unilateral. It may occasionally affect only one group of muscles to any significant degree, e.g. neck muscles, forearm or thigh muscles, and it increases with nervous tension or in a cold environment.

TREMOR

Like rigidity, tremor is usually asymmetrical or unilateral. It consists of an alternating contraction of opposing muscle groups, causing a rhythmical movement at about 4–6 cycles per second (see Chapter 5). Tremor is usually maximal at the periphery and affects the arm more frequently than the leg.

Tremor is more of an embarrassment to the patient than a disability because it is worst at rest but reduces or disappears with voluntary movement.

GENERAL MANAGEMENT OF PARKINSON'S DISEASE

No treatment has been developed that prevents onset or reliably delays progression of the disease. The management of the patient with parkinsonism must be multidisciplinary and, above all, designed to be appropriate to the individual case. Management of a patient with Parkinson's disease of early onset will take place against a background of different expectations, roles, responsibilities and general health status from that of a patient with late-onset disease (Godwin-Austen, 1984, 1993).

Mutch (1992) suggested that specialist Parkinson's disease clinics, supported by nursing and therapy staff, sharing care with general practitioners, or management via a generic disability service, may best meet the needs of patients. Specialist keyworkers attached to clinics and performing a liaison function have been shown to raise the quality of care (Parkinson's Disease Society, 1994). The core team of medical, nursing and therapy personnel should have ready access to, and good communication with, a wide range of services, including dietetic, continence, counselling, social work, psychology, chiropody and community psychiatric nursing support (Parkinson's Disease Society, 1994).

MEDICAL MANAGEMENT

The main area of medical management is drug therapy; surgical procedures are being used increasingly.

DRUG TREATMENT

Relevant details of the drugs mentioned in this section are given in Chapter 28, particularly in relation to side effects.

The depletion of brain dopamine that occurs in this condition causes a reactive increased production of acetylcholine in the basal ganglia. Treatment is designed, therefore, to replenish the dopamine by administering the dopamine precursor levodopa and to reduce the acetylcholine with anticholinergic drugs such as benzhexol or orphenadrine. Levodopa is usually given in combination with a chemical which prevents its metabolism outside the brain and these combined tablets are marketed in the UK as Sinemet (levodopa plus carbidopa) and Madopar (levodopa plus benserazide).

Levodopa-containing drugs are the most effective treatment for the relief of most of the symptoms and signs, especially the slowness and poverty of voluntary movement that is the main cause of disability. They also relieve rigidity and substantially reduce tremor.

Side effects may be troublesome and vary at different stages. At the start of treatment, nausea and vomiting, postural hypotension and confusional states can occur. Side effects that may appear after months or years of treatment include choreiform involuntary movements (dyskinesia) of the face or limbs, and 'on–off' attacks in which the patient becomes profoundly akinetic and unable to move for periods of 30 minutes to 2 hours. The side effects of both levodopa-containing and anticholinergic types of drug are dose-dependent, disappearing when the dose is reduced.

Anticholinergic drugs, whilst less effective than levodopa, have an additive therapeutic effect with particular benefit to rigidity. Amantadine is sometimes used in the mild case. It probably acts by releasing dopamine in the brain but it is less potent and effective than levodopa. Bromocriptine and pergolide are synthetic compounds that mimic levodopa in all its actions and side effects but have a slightly longer period of action.

Apomorphine is administered subcutaneously by injection and has a mode of action similar to levodopa. Its advantage is that the action is reliable, rapid and lasts about an hour, but side effects are severe (see Chapter 28). Its use is normally confined to patients who suffer short-lived unpredictable 'on–off' attacks (see above).

SURGICAL PROCEDURES

The use of destructive surgical procedures on the thalamus in cases of parkinsonism evolved during the 1950s from the original work by Spiegel et al. (1947).

Tremor continued to be treated by surgical means until the advent of levodopa, which is a more effective and safer method of treatment in most cases. However, surgical treatment has been reintroduced recently using refined techniques. One such technique is pallidotomy which targets precisely the globus pallidus (Laitinen, 1995). This operation may give good results, especially in patients with severe tremor or with severe involuntary movements complicating their medical treatment. Fetal brain implant surgery (Wu et al., 1994) and electrical stimulation treatment of the brain (Limousin et al., 1995) are research techniques which may prove useful in the future. Therapists may become increasingly involved in pre- and post-procedure measurement and treatment.

PHYSICAL MANAGEMENT

Although this section will focus on the physical management of Parkinson's disease, the principles underpin the management of other causes of parkinsonism.

MODELS OF PHYSIOTHERAPY MANAGEMENT

The 'cure' paradigm illustrated in Figure 12.2 was developed for acute conditions and is inappropriate for use in long-term conditions. The current Parkinson's paradigm (Turnbull, 1992) illustrates the prevailing approach employed in the physiotherapeutic management of Parkinson's disease. Referral for therapy takes place, if at all, only when the pharmacological approach begins to fail (Weiner & Singer, 1989). However, in a pilot study of a Neuro Care team model of management in Parkinson's disease, 66% of newly diagnosed patients were experiencing impairments and disabilities requiring medium and high levels of physiotherapy involvement (Oxtoby et al., 1988).

The 'progressive' paradigm aims to maintain optimal function over time by early and continuing targeted therapy. It enables the rehabilitation role, most commonly associated with physiotherapy intervention, to be combined with prevention, support, advice and health education roles (De Souza, 1990).

Principles of Physiotherapeutic Management

Turnbull (1992) identified the principles that should inform physiotherapeutic management programmes in Parkinson's disease (reprinted from Turnbull, 1992, with permission):

- Early implementation of a preventive exercise programme.
- Meaningful assessment to identify treatment priorities and monitor progress.
- Targetted intervention, focusing on areas of deterioration.
- Use of structured programmes based on principles of psychomotor learning to address motor deficits.
- Involvement of patient and carer in decision-making to improve motivation and compliance.
- A forum to identify needs of patients and carers and educate individuals about Parkinson's disease.
- Teaching of handling techniques to carers.

These principles apply to physiotherapy service delivery across the full range of settings from hospital to home. Carers include personnel involved with the patient from a variety of services or agencies.

PHYSIOTHERAPY ASSESSMENT AND TREATMENT PLANNING

The physiotherapy database will include information about the patient's history of Parkinson's disease and other medical conditions, together with details of pharmacological and other medical management. Information about the patient's social background, together with details of other professionals

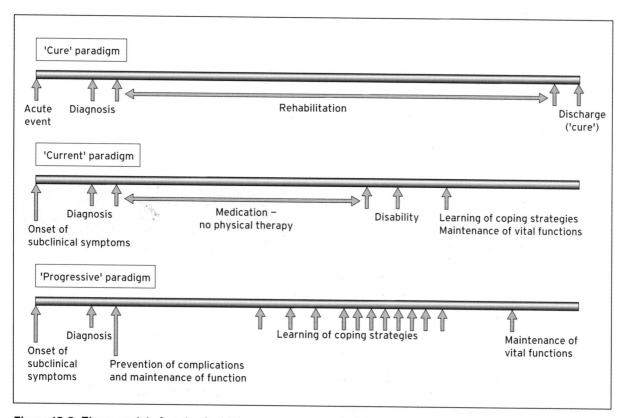

Figure 12.2 Three models for physical therapy management of Parkinson's disease. (Top) The cure model; (centre) the model frequently used; and (bottom) the progressive model. (Redrawn from Turnbull, 1992, with permission.)

and services involved in management will be noted. The assessment will include the carer, e.g. health status and handling strategies, and the home environment. Assessment should take account of possible performance fluctuations and reassessment timed to facilitate comparison of results. The reader is referred to Chapter 4 for further details.

Outcome Measures

Whenever possible, an outcome measure—a 'measurement tool (instrument, questionnaire, rating form, etc.) used to document change in one or more patient characteristics over time' (Cole et al., 1994)—should be incorporated into the assessment process. Outcome measures can be used in both problem-oriented and goal-setting contexts. Physiotherapists need to consider appropriate uniprofessional outcomes and their contribution to multidisciplinary outcomes when working in a team context. Potential outcome measures for the evaluation of motor behaviour are reviewed below at three levels: performance-based functional assessment; impairment assessment; and movement strategy assessment (Shumway-Cook & Woollacott, 1995). The use of quality of life and self-report measures are considered.

Performance-based Functional Assessment

Performance-based functional assessment relates to disability in the World Health Organisation (1980) classification. Wade (1992) recommended that the Barthel Activities of Daily Living (ADL) index is repeated for both best and worst performance to account for fluctuations. In addition, an extended ADL test, 10-metre walk, timing of any specific activity, step-second test, Rivermead Mobility Index, the Nine-hole Peg Test and Self-Assessment Parkinson's Disease Disability Scale (SAPDDS) are recommended (Wade, 1992).

Impairment Assessment

Consideration could be given to the incorporation of selected ratings, e.g. of tremor, rigidity, dyskinesia and 'on–off' fluctuations, from the Motor Examination and Compli- cations of Therapy sections of the Unified Parkinson's Disease Rating Scale (UPDRS; Wade, 1992), into a patient's physiotherapy database.

Mechanical/electronic/video recording of motor impairments is recommended (Wade, 1992). Kinsman (1986) designed a video assessment of Parkinson's disease to include impairment and disability assessment. A diagrammatic grading of standing posture is included in the physiotherapy assessment form for Parkinson's disease (Franklyn, 1986a). Sitting posture should also be graded. Recording of ROM may be appropriate. Postural, righting and protective reflexes may be abnormal (Stern, 1990) and should be assessed.

Wade (1992) suggested that the Short Orientation-Memory-Concentration Test could be used to assess cognitive dysfunction. Details of all outcome measures in sections on 'performance-based functional assessment' and 'impairment assessment', except Kinsman (1986) and Franklyn (1986b), can be found in Wade (1992).

Visual analogue scales could be considered for evaluation of pain and fatigue.

Movement Strategy Assessment

Research into movement strategies used in functional tasks, such as gait, postural control and gross motor skills, should result in the development of clinical assessment tools, as has been the case with gait analysis (Shumway-Cook & Woollacott, 1995). Handford (1993) has reviewed the parameters that have been used to describe abnormalities in parkinsonian gait, which include stride dimensions, time components of the walking cycle, and angular displacements of the head, trunk and upper and lower limbs. These parameters can provide a starting point for the assessment of gait strategy in individual patients.

In the research setting, Kamsma et al. (1994) developed an observation scheme for the analysis of video recordings of people with Parkinson's disease turning in bed and rising from a chair. Discrete movements of the limbs, head, shoulders, trunk and pelvis were identified and their timing noted. This work formed the basis of the design of alternative movement strategies (see Box 12.1). Strategies provided a framework for performance that could be scored for errors and quality of initial and final positioning. A subsequent scoring system recorded intention to execute steps in the strategies, effectiveness of execution and sequencing of steps (Kamsma et al., 1995).

Quality of Life

A 39-item Parkinson's Disease Questionnaire (PDQ-39) has recently been developed and validated; this measures function and wellbeing to gain the patient's assessment of the effect of Parkinson's disease on everyday life (Jenkinson et al., 1995). It is envisaged that the questionnaire could be used to evaluate a range of interventions in Parkinson's disease, including pharmacology, specialist nursing and therapies (Peto et al., 1995). However, its

---

Alternative strategy for a patient turning from lying on the back to lying on the side in a single bed

1. Pull the knees well up

2. Shift the pelvis and the shoulders alternately, moving them laterally to the side of the bed away from the intended direction of turn, creating a free space in the centre

3. Rotate the knees in the intended direction of turn

4. Then rotate the trunk and come to a comfortable position

Box 12.1 Redrawn from Kamsma et al., 1995, with permission of Erlbaum (UK) Taylor & Francis, Hove, UK, and the authors.

validity as a tool to measure the outcome of physiotherapy intervention needs to be established.

Self-report Measures

Consideration should be given to the use of self-report outcome measures and treatment planning tools. Brown *et al.* (1989) found that patients could accurately report levels of disability, regardless of the presence of depression and cognitive impairment. Montgomery & Reynolds (1990) found patients able to self-monitor and report their symptoms in a diary, while Yekutiel (1993) found diaries of falls in the home could aid treatment planning and monitoring.

Assessment Interpretation and Treatment Planning

Shumway-Cook & Woollacott (1995) suggested that a model of disablement can supply a hierarchical framework for ordering the results of assessment and planning treatment. The Schenkman & Butler (1989a) model for the evaluation and treatment of people with neurological dysfunction has been applied to Parkinson's disease. Using the WHO (1980) definitions of impairment and disability, the model differentiates between: impairments that are direct effects of CNS pathology, e.g. rigidity, akinesia; indirect effects of non-nervous system pathology, e.g. postural deformity as a result of musculoskeletal system changes; and composite effects of both, e.g. impaired balance (Schenkman & Butler, 1989b). All impairments are linked to possible resultant disability: physical, e.g. bed mobility; social, e.g. withdrawal; and emotional, e.g. depression (Schenkman & Butler, 1989b). Treatment is directed principally at the indirect effects of the disease on the musculoskeletal system.

Handford (1993) has based a framework for assessment, interpretation and treatment planning in Parkinson's disease on the Schenkman & Butler (1989a) model. Movement, locomotion or postural problems contributing to a functional difficulty are identified and assigned to one of five categories: primary; secondary; combined (related to Schenkman & Butler, 1989a, categories); drug therapy; or other conditions. The influence of the various categories of deficit is assessed and a treatment plan aimed at improving the functional problem is formulated (Handford, 1993).

Whalley Hammell (1994) underlines the importance of addressing the patient's agenda, as opposed to the therapist's, when setting goals. Patient goals in the early stage of Parkinson's disease may relate to continuing in employment (particularly in early-onset disease), maintaining fitness and pursuing leisure interests. In the middle stage, maintaining independence in self-care activities is likely to be important. Later, the ability to remain living at home may be paramount.

PHYSIOTHERAPEUTIC APPROACHES IN PARKINSON'S DISEASE

Homberg (1993) suggested that the design of motor training techniques for people with Parkinson's disease should be based on the known neurophysiology of motor deficit in the condition (Mak & Cole, 1991). Historically, unlike the physiotherapy treatment of stroke, approaches specific to Parkinson's disease have not been developed (Turnbull, 1992). Instead, techniques drawn from a range of approaches, primarily developed in relation to other conditions, are employed. Approaches can be broadly grouped under four headings: biomechanical; neurophysiological; theories of learning; and biopsychosocial. More information on several of the treatment approaches outlined here can be found in Chapter 22.

Biomechanical

This was the basis of the 'traditional approach' prior to the introduction of levodopa (Ball, 1967). Schenkman (1992) uses mechanical and kinesiological principles to address problems of motor control in Parkinson's disease. Techniques such as relaxation, breathing exercises and exercises focusing on ROM, flexibility and movement sequencing are employed. Only if the patient cannot relearn the mechanically favourable movement strategies automatically is conscious control of movement taught (Schenkman, 1992).

Neurophysiological

Proprioceptive neuromuscular facilitation (PNF) techniques have been used in the treatment of Parkinson's disease in an attempt: (1) to diminish rigidity by influencing the fusimotor system and encouraging activity in antagonist muscles, and (2) to improve akinesia by the initiation and facilitation of movement (Irwin-Carruthers, 1971). Chan *et al.* (1993) used a single case study design to assess a largely PNF intervention in parkinsonian gait and recorded a significant increase in step and stride lengths. The concepts elaborated by Bobath and Rood may be employed for the reduction of tone (Schenkman *et al.*, 1989).

Sensory Cueing

The use of visual cues (e.g. marks placed on the floor) and verbal cues (e.g. counting) to improve gait in people with Parkinson's disease has been a feature of physiotherapy programmes over time (Murray, 1956; Irwin-Carruthers, 1971). Bagley *et al.* (1991) and Weissenborn (1993) reported that cueing, in the form of cardboard rods on the floor and verbal instruction to focus on objects above eye level, respectively, brought gait closer to normal but that generalisation to natural environments needed to be evaluated.

Theories of Learning

Conductive education in Parkinson's disease attempts to promote neuropsychological reorganisation through structural intervention in, and practice of, functional movement (Nanton, 1986). Key elements of the approach are: (1) the use of verbal regulation and the creation of rhythmical intention in the accomplishment of motor activities, and (2) the fostering of motivation in a group context under the guidance of a conductor (Nanton, 1986).

Studies by Yekutiel *et al.* (1991) and Kamsma *et al.* (1994, 1995) have drawn on a neuropsychological knowledge base when devising interventions specific to Parkinson's disease. Yekutiel *et al.* (1991) evaluated a home-based programme aimed at improving 'whole body movements' and conscious strategies for accomplishing functional activities. Significant gains were recorded in a laboratory setting in speed of accomplishing everyday mobility tasks. Questions of reinforcement to ensure carry-over remain.

Kamsma *et al.* (1995) devised alternative movement strategies in three skill domains—chair, bed and walking—based on detailed kinesiological analysis related to motor control deficits in Parkinson's disease and neuropsychological knowledge. The logical structure of the strategies, consisting of simple movements performed sequentially at a conscious level, facilitated clear cognitive representation. Mental rehearsal and verbalisation of strategies were encouraged. The essential difference between this approach and that of others in retraining gross motor skills is an emphasis on alternative movements accomplished using preserved abilities as opposed to attempts to reinstate the original movement by practising its constituent parts. Box 12.1 details the strategy for turning from lying on the back to lying on the side in bed. Promising results on the reproducibility and utilisation of the strategies need to be replicated when taught in a clinical as opposed to an experimental setting (Kamsma *et al.*, 1995).

Biopsychosocial

The use of group therapy may be associated with many of the approaches discussed above, most notably conductive education. However, the biopsychosocial approach aims to address physical aspects of the condition in conjunction with psychological and social aspects (Szekely *et al.*, 1982; Gauthier *et al.*, 1987). Often delivered within a multidisciplinary context and including carers in activities, the biopsychosocial approach emphasises motivation, support, education and the sharing of information between people with the condition, their carers and professionals.

PHYSIOTHERAPY INTERVENTION RELATED TO DISEASE STAGE

The characteristic progression of Parkinson's disease symptoms has been described above. Cutson *et al.* (1995) suggested that therapeutic intervention requires a changing emphasis across the early, middle and late stages of the disease. This model will be employed here to examine key issues at each stage.

Assessment and treatment in the environment where everyday activity takes place are likely to increase the relevance of physiotherapeutic input (Banks & Caird, 1989; Banks 1991). Treatment should coincide with periods of maximal drug efficacy, and treatment sessions and home programmes should be monitored for their effect on fatigue levels. Home programme content and level of compliance need regular review, particularly when cognitive deficit is present.

Early Stage

In the early stage of Parkinson's disease the focus is on prevention of musculoskeletal impairments. Informing people with Parkinson's disease and their carers about the condition, and discussing their fears and perceptions, will help to foster positive involvement with a general home exercise programme. This would include ROM, strengthening and endurance exercises, in addition to specific stretches, e.g. Achilles tendon, or positioning indicated as a result of assessment. Relaxation should be incorporated in the programme. Turnbull (1992) details a programme entitled 'HELP' (Helpful Exercises for Living with Parkinson's) run in conjunction with local Parkinson's Disease Society (PDS) branches.

Middle Stage

In the middle stage, techniques to promote ROM, enhance postural awareness and correct musculoskeletal impairment where possible would be continued. Strategies to support motor performance would be introduced as necessary. The booklet *Living with Parkinson's disease* (Franklyn *et al.*, 1982), available from the PDS, contains practical suggestions for overcoming the difficulties experienced at this stage, as well as a basic exercise programme. For example, stabilising the upper arm against the trunk may reduce tremor enough to allow dexterity in the hand. Movement strategies for sitting down in, and rising from, a variety of chairs (including sitting at a table), turning in bed (see Box 12.1) and getting off the floor may need to be explored with individuals and carers. Disturbance of gait and balance control may result in falls. Stopping walking when the pattern deteriorates or freezing starts to occur can help prevent falls. Being aware of upright posture, increasing the distance between the feet, and consciously placing the heel to the ground first (reinforced by saying or thinking 'heel', perhaps prompted by a carer) can improve gait quality. Rocking from side to side, marching on the spot, or stepping back before swinging the foot forward can help initiate movement, as can using a carer's foot to step over. Safe turning is facilitated by walking in a curved as opposed to a sharply angled course. Two-handled wheeled walking aids may prove more functional than walking sticks as loss of axial rotation and flexed posture makes reciprocal movements of the upper and lower limbs difficult to co-ordinate.

Assessment at a specialist Mobility Centre may be appropriate if continued ability to drive is questioned. Information and advice on the full range of local services and statutory benefits should be available. Equipment to support activities such as bathing or showering, dressing and eating may be required. Intervention may need to be tailored to take account of depression and early cognitive impairment.

Late Stage

With respiratory function and swallowing likely to be compromised, chest care is important. Attention to skin care is necessary when nutrition and mobility are compromised. Equipment to support bed mobility and transfers may be required, in addition to attendant-propelled wheelchair use.

As with earlier stages, multidisciplinary teamwork and active involvement of the patient are critical to ensure quality care.

RESEARCH INTO PHYSIOTHERAPY AND PARKINSON'S DISEASE

Although studies have been referred to throughout this chapter, studies of speech, occupational and physiotherapy account for <1% of 400–500 publications annually on the management of Parkinson's disease (Ward, 1992). Studies have employed a wide range of research methodologies, outcome measures, treatment approaches and techniques and, in common with stroke research (Ashburn et al., 1993), there is a lack of confirmation of findings. This situation makes moving towards evidence-based practice difficult.

For example, in relation to methodology, the relevance of controlled cross-over designs, used by Gibberd et al. (1981) to compare 'active' and 'inactive' physiotherapy and by Comella et al. (1994) to compare physical therapy programme and normal activity, has been challenged as inappropriate in rehabilitation where, unlike drug trials, a learning effect is sought (Andrews, 1981). In terms of outcome, studies that show improvement in groups undergoing widely differing exercise regimens (Palmer et al., 1986) have suggested that therapy content may not be important and that more cost-effective ways of improving patient performance might be developed (Weiner & Singer, 1989). For example, Montgomery et al. (1994) report a postal-based health promotion programme but evaluation of such would require a long-term study.

Implications for Clinical Practice

The perceived lack of systematic evaluation of physiotherapy in Parkinson's disease is posing a threat to its purchase in the current health service market (Baker, 1994).

Clinical physiotherapists could add to the physiotherapy knowledge base by using outcome measures, preferably standardised, in their clinical work, possibly in the context of single case design methodology (Lincoln, 1995). In this way, questions that are important to the patient, carer and physiotherapist will be addressed, and the basis of the physiotherapy management of Parkinson's disease will be strengthened.

CASE HISTORIES

CASE HISTORY 1: MR A

Mr A was 67 years old when diagnosed as having Parkinson's disease by his general practitioner. He was referred to a Neuro Care Team for multidisciplinary management. On initial medical assessment he exhibited tremor, rigidity and bradykinesia. His speech was affected and his face was immobile. In discussion with the team's co-ordinator/counsellor immediately following initial medical consultation, Mr A and his wife were able to discuss and receive advice about how best to cope with the diagnosis, uncertainties about prognosis and concerns about driving.

When the Neuro Care Team speech therapist, occupational therapist, and physiotherapist first visited Mr and Mrs A in their home, Mr A was leading an active retirement and was independent in all activities of daily living. He walked about a mile a day. Driving was restricted to short distances. His wife reported that he was increasingly forgetful and tended to get upset easily which was uncharacteristic. General advice was given and a home exercise programme devised, focusing on maintaining mobility and function. Mrs A found she gained benefit from performing the exercises with her husband and her participation helped maintain motivation. Later in the disease course she was taught chest physiotherapy to help her husband remove retained secretions at the back of the throat.

Whilst attending a maintenance speech therapy group 2 years after diagnosis, Mr A reported being woken at night by pain in his left heel, hip and chest. His restlessness was affecting his wife's sleep. Subsequent physiotherapy assessment noted marked dyskinesia. Medical colleagues were consulted about drug dosage, and posture, transfers and gait were reviewed. Mr A was needing help with dressing at all times and assistance with most self-care activities on bad days. Help was given by the team to apply for relevant allowances.

Four and a half years after diagnosis Mr A was experiencing marked 'on–off' fluctuations. His wife reported that he was confused and behaving strangely at times and this greatly concerned her. The support of the co-ordinator/counsellor was important at this time. A review of the medication was undertaken.

CASE HISTORY 2: MR B

Mr B was referred to a Neuro Care Team where he was diagnosed as having Parkinson's disease at 51 years of age. Stiffness, weakness and tremor in his left arm had been attributed to musculoskeletal problems arising from injuries sustained whilst performing heavy manual work. On diagnosis he was experiencing fatigue together with marked problems with functional activities.

Lack of acceptance of the diagnosis meant that Mr B was reluctant to have any early input from the Neuro Care Team therapists. He maintained contact with the co-ordinator/counsellor who was instrumental in involving other team members. Targeted input over time involved courses of speech therapy; occupational therapy advice on balancing rest/relaxation/sleep, continued driving, sleeping downstairs and wheelchair use, and physiotherapy, which included transcutaneous nerve stimulation in an attempt to reduce rib pain (see Chapter 24). Mr B was interested in discussing alternative therapies with the team, such as acupuncture and homoeopathy, and press coverage of approaches such as pallidotomy and neural grafting.

Mr B retired at age 53 which enabled him to manage better physically but reduced his self-esteem. Self-consciousness about his dyskinesia and speech difficulties, plus deteriorating independent mobility, curtailed activities outside the home. He found it hard to tell people about his diagnosis and rejected the suggestion that he carry a card explaining he had Parkinson's disease.

Four years after diagnosis, Mr B's wife's health was deteriorating as a result of stress. Drug therapy was manipulated in an attempt to reduce 'on–off' periods, freezing, violent dyskinesia, and later paranoid tendencies and hallucinations. A Day Centre place was sought. Mr and Mrs B overcame their concerns about meeting others with Parkinson's disease and finally attended a PDS meeting which they found helpful.

Six years after diagnosis, Mr and Mrs B accepted that an attendant-propelled wheelchair would increase outdoor mobility. Mr B had injured his wrists in falls. Consideration was being given to the use of the drug apomorphine, which would be introduced with nurse specialist support.

Acknowledgments

Diana Jones wishes to thank Professor Rowena Plant and Dr Colin Chandler for reading and commenting on the physical management section, and Sue Nightingale (Co-ordinator/Counsellor), Sue Patterson (Occupational Therapist), Ruth Warburton (Physiotherapist) and Helen Hughes (Speech Therapist) of the Romford Neuro Care Team for background to the case histories.

REFERENCES

Andrews, K. Controlled trial of physiotherapy and occupational therapy for Parkinson's disease. [Correspondence] *Br Med J* 1981, **282**:1475.

Ashburn A, *et al*. Physiotherapy in the rehabilitation of stroke: a review. *Clin Rehabil* 1993, **7**:337-345.

Bagley S, *et al*. The effect of visual cues on the gait of independently mobile Parkinson's disease patients. *Physiotherapy* 1991, **77**:415-420.

Baker M. Presidential address. *In European Parkinson's Disease Conference, Glasgow*. Macmillan Magazines; 1994.

Ball JM. Demonstration of the traditional approach in the treatment of a patient with parkinsonism. *Am J Phys Med* 1967, **46**:1034-1036.

Banks MA. Physiotherapy. In: Caird FI, ed. *Rehabilitation in Parkinson's disease*. London: Chapman and Hall; 1991.

Banks MA, Caird FI. Physiotherapy benefits patients with Parkinson's disease. *Clin Rehabil* 1989, **3**:11-16.

Bannister R. Parkinsonism and movement disorders. In: Bannister R, ed. *Brain and Bannister's clinical neurology, 7th edition*. Oxford: Oxford University Press; 1992:632-682.

Bostantjopoulou S, *et al*. Clinical observations in early and late onset Parkinson's disease. *Funct Neurol* 1991, **6**:145-149.

Brown RG, *et al*. Accuracy of self-reported disability in patients with parkinsonism. *Arch Neurol* 1989, **46**:955-959.

Caird FI. Parkinson's disease and its natural history. In: Caird FI, ed. *Rehabilitation in Parkinson's disease*. London: Chapman and Hall; 1991.

Chan J, *et al*. Physiotherapy intervention in parkinsonian gait. *NZ J Physiother* 1993, April.

Cole B, *et al*. *Physical rehabilitation outcome measures*. Toronto: Canadian Physiotherapy Association; 1994.

Comella CL, *et al*. Physical therapy and Parkinson's disease: a controlled trial. *Neurology* 1994, **44**:376-378.

Cutson TM, *et al*. Pharmacological and nonpharmacological interventions in the treatment of Parkinson's disease. *Phys Ther* 1995, **75**:363-373.

De Souza L. *Multiple sclerosis: Approaches to management*. London: Chapman & Hall; 1990.

Franklyn S. User's guide to the physiotherapy assessment form for Parkinson's disease. *Physiotherapy* 1986a, **72**:359-361.

Franklyn S. Introduction to physiotherapy for Parkinson's disease. *Physiotherapy* 1986b, **72**:379-380.

Franklyn S, *et al*. *Living with Parkinson's disease*. London: Parkinson's Disease Society; 1982.

Gauthier L, *et al*. The benefits of group occupational therapy for patients with Parkinson's disease. *Am J Occup Ther* 1987, **41**:360-365.

Gibberd FB, *et al*. Controlled trial of physiotherapy and occupational therapy for Parkinson's disease. *Br Med J* 1981, **282**:1196.

Godwin-Austen RB. *The Parkinson's disease handbook*. London: Sheldon Press; 1984.

Godwin-Austen RB. *Parkinson's disease: a booklet for patients and their families*. London: Parkinson's Disease Society; 1993.

Handford F. Towards a rational basis for physiotherapy in Parkinson's disease. *Baillière's Clin Neurol* 1993, **2** :141-158.

Homberg V. Motor training in the therapy of Parkinson's disease. *Neurology* 1993, **43** (Suppl 6):S45-S46.

Irwin-Carruthers SH. An approach to physiotherapy for the patient with Parkinson's disease. *Physiotherapy* 1971, March:5-7.

Jenkinson C, *et al*. Self-reported functioning and well-being in patients with Parkinson's disease: comparison of the Short-form Health Survey (SF-36) and the Parkinson's Disease Questionnaire (PDQ-39). *Age Ageing* 1995, **24**:505-509.

Kamsma YPT, *et al*. Prevention of early immobility in patients with Parkinson's disease: a cognitive strategy training for turning in bed and rising from a chair. In: Riddoch MJ, Humphreys GW, eds. *Cognitive neuropsychology and cognitive rehabilitation*. Hove: Lawrence Erlbaum Associates Ltd; 1994.

Kamsma YPT, *et al*. Training of compensational strategies for impaired gross motor skills in Parkinson's disease. *Physiother Theory Pract* 1995, **11**:209-229.

Kinsman R. Video assessment of the Parkinson patient. *Physiotherapy* 1986, **72**:386-389.

Koller WC. Handbook of Parkinson's disease. New York: Marcel Dekker; 1992.

Laitinen LV. Pallidotomy for Parkinson's disease. *Neurosurg Clin N Am* 1995, **6**:105-112.

Limousin P, Pollak P, Benazzouz A, *et al*. Effect on parkinsonian signs and symptoms of bilateral subthalamic nucleus stimulation. *Lancet* 1995, **345**:91-95.

Lincoln NB. Research in stroke rehabilitation. In: Harrison MA, ed. *Physiotherapy in stroke management*. Edinburgh: Churchill Livingstone; 1995.

Mak MKY, Cole JH. Movement dysfunction in patients with Parkinson's disease: a literature review. *Aust J Physiother* 1991, **37**:7-17.

Montgomery EB, *et al*. Patient education and health promotion can be effective in Parkinson's disease: a randomised controlled trial. *Am J Med* 1994, **97**:429-435.

Montgomery GK, Reynolds NC. Compliance, reliability, and validity of self-monitoring for physical disturbances of Parkinson's disease. *J Nerv Ment Dis* 1990, **178**:636-641.

Murray W. Parkinson's disease: aspects of functional training. *Phys Ther Rev* 1956, **36**: 587-594.

Mutch WJ. Specialist clinics: a better way to care? *J Neurol Neurosurg Psychiat* 1992, **55**(Suppl):36-40.

Mutch W J, *et al*. Parkinson's disease in a Scottish city. *Br Med J* 1986, **292**:534-536.

Nanton V. Parkinson's disease. In: Cottam PJ, Sutton A, eds. *Conductive education: A system for overcoming motor disorder*. London: Croom Helm Ltd; 1986.

Oxtoby M, *et al*. *A strategy for the management of Parkinson's disease and for the long-term support of patients and their carers*. London: Parkinson's Disease Society; 1988.

Palmer SS, *et al*. Exercise therapy for Parkinson's disease. *Arch Phys Med Rehabil* 1986, **67**:741-745.

Pantelatos A, Fornadi F. Clinical features and medical treatment of Parkinson's disease in patient groups selected in accordance with age at onset. *Adv Neurol* 1993, **60**:690-697.

Parkinson's Disease Society. *Meeting a need?* [Discussion document]. London: Parkinson's Disease Society, 1994.

Peto V, *et al*. The development and validation of a short measure of functioning and well being for individuals with Parkinson's disease. *Qual Life Res* 1995, **4**:241-248.

Schenkman M. Physical therapy intervention for the ambulatory patient. In: Turnbull GI, ed. *Physical therapy management of Parkinson's disease*. New York: Churchill Livingstone; 1992.

Schenkman M, Butler RB. A model for multisystem evaluation, interpretation, and treatment of individuals with neurologic dysfunction. *Phys Ther* 1989a, **69**: 538-547.

Schenkman M, Butler RB. A model for multisystem evaluation treatment of individuals with Parkinson's disease. *Phys Ther* 1989b, **69**:932-943.

Schenkman M, *et al*. Management of individuals with Parkinson's disease: rationale and case studies. *Phys Ther* 1989, **69**:944-955.

Shumway-Cook A, Woollacott M. *Motor control: Theory and practical applications*. Baltimore: Williams & Wilkins; 1995.

Spiegal EA, *et al*. Stereotaxic apparatus for operations on the human brain. *Science* 1947, **100**:349-350.

Stern G, ed. *Parkinson's disease*. London: Chapman & Hall; 1990.

Szekely BC, *et al*. Adjunctive treatment in Parkinson's disease: physical therapy and comprehensive group therapy. *Rehab Lit* 1982, **43**(3-4):72-76.

Turnbull GI, ed. *Physical therapy management of Parkinson's disease*. New York: Churchill Livingstone; 1992.

Wade D. *Measurement in neurological rehabilitation*. Oxford: Oxford University Press; 1992.

Ward C. Rehabilitation in Parkinson's disease. *Rev Clin Gerontol* 1992, **2**:254-268.

Weiner WJ, Singer C. Parkinson's disease and nonpharmacologic treatment programs. *J Am Geriatr Soc* 1989, **37**:359-363.

Weissenborn S. The effect of using a two-step verbal cue to a visual target above eye level on the parkinsonian gait: a case study. *Physiotherapy* 1993, **79**:26-31.

Whalley Hammell KR. Establishing objectives in occupational therapy practice, part 1. *Br J Occup Ther* 1994, **57**:9-14.

World Health Organisation. *International classification of impairments, disabilities and handicaps*. Geneva: World Health Organisation; 1980.

Wu CY, Zhon MD, Bao XF, *et al*. The combined method of transplantation of foetal substantia nigra and stereotacic thalamotomy for Parkinson's disease. *Br J Neurosurg* 1994, **8**:709-716.

Yekutiel MP. Patients' fall records as an aid in designing and assessing therapy in Parkinsonism. *Disabil Rehab* 1993, **15**:189-193.

Yekutiel MP, *et al*. A clinical trial of the re-education of movement in patients with Parkinson's disease. *Clin Rehab* 1991, **5**:207-214.

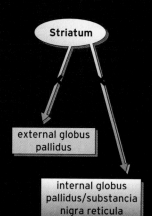

external globus pallidus

internal globus pallidus/substancia nigra reticula

Striatum

13 O Quarrell & B Cook
HUNTINGTON'S DISEASE

CHAPTER OUTLINE

- Prevalence
- Genetics
- Neuropathology
- Signs and symptoms and their general management

- General aspects of management
- Physical management
- Aspects of terminal care

INTRODUCTION

George Huntington may not have been the first to describe this condition but he gave a clear and concise account of the clinical and genetic features in 1872 (Huntington, 1872). In the early literature, the condition was called Huntington's chorea, which denotes emphasis on the most obvious clinical sign. However, not all patients have chorea, so focusing on this one sign may detract from other important aspects. The term Huntington's disease (HD) seems more appropriate and is now widely accepted.

The major features of HD may be considered as a triad of: a movement disorder, often choreic in nature; an affective disturbance; and cognitive impairment. The condition is inherited as an autosomal dominant, so on average half the offspring of an affected person will be similarly affected. The recent identification of the mutation causing HD means that laboratory diagnostic and pre-symptomatic tests are now much easier. Despite this, there is no treatment that will effectively prevent or ameliorate the progressive neurodegeneration. Current treatment is, at best, supportive and symptomatic, requiring input from different professionals at different stages of the disease. Ideally, needs should be anticipated and continuity of care maintained throughout all stages of the disease so that a relationship builds up between professionals, patients and their families.

This chapter will describe the genetic and pathological aspects of the disease before describing the major clinical features and general management. Physical management strategies will be considered under broad categories of early, mid and late stages of the disease. Other useful texts which discuss this condition include Harper (1996) and Ward et al. (1993).

PREVALENCE

There have been a number of studies of the prevalence of HD in different areas of the UK but there is a problem obtaining a picture from a large population (see Harper, 1992, for review). Most UK studies quote the range of 4–10 per 100,000 and most European countries, the USA, Australia and South Africa have also given prevalence rates within this range. Low prevalence has been documented in Finland and Japan. The low prevalence in Finland may indicate that the population has been relatively isolated from the rest of Europe. The low prevalence in Japan cannot be due to poor ascertainment and requires a separate explanation. It is difficult to be sure of prevalence in parts of the world in which there have not been extensive surveys.

Whilst HD may be considered a rare disorder, it should be remembered that the burden will be great for the patient, the immediate carers and the offspring, half of whom will, on average, develop the condition.

GENETICS

Since HD is inherited in an autosomal dominant fashion, a mutation on one copy of a pair of genes is sufficient to cause the disorder. The disease is virtually fully penetrant, implying that provided an individual with the mutation lives long enough he or she will develop the disorder. One anomaly which has not been fully explained is that cases of juvenile onset are much more likely to have inherited the gene from the father.

The gene for HD was localised to chromosome 4 in 1983 (Gusella *et al.*, 1983) but it was not until 10 years later that the mutation was identified (Huntington's Disease Collaborative Research Group, 1993). The gene has been called IT15 and the protein encoded by that gene termed huntingtin. The 3-base pair DNA sequence, CAG, which codes for the amino acid glutamine, is repeated a number of times on the normal gene but there is a marked expansion in the number of repeats on HD genes. The abnormal huntingtin protein can therefore be said to contain an expanded polyglutamine tract.

In most laboratories normal chromosomes have less than 35 repeats, with a modal group of approximately 17, whereas HD chromosomes usually have more than 38 repeats. There may be a small area of overlap between the upper end of the normal range and lower end of the HD range in the region of approximately 36 repeats. The mutation is said to be dynamic in that the number of repeats on the HD gene varies between generations. The increase in the number of repeats is specific for HD and does not occur in patients with Parkinson's disease, schizophrenia or other movement disorders (Kremer *et al.*, 1994; Rubinsztein *et al.*, 1994, 1995).

It is relatively easy to determine the number of CAG repeats from a sample of venous blood. This has made confirmation of diagnosis reliable in the vast majority of cases. It also means that a simple laboratory test is now available for anyone at risk of HD, to determine whether or not they have inherited the mutation. Given that there is no effective treatment to delay or alter the nature of the progressive degeneration, presymptomatic predictive testing should be undertaken in the context of skilled genetic counselling. There is an inverse correlation between the number of CAG repeats and age of onset; the higher the number of repeats, the lower the age of onset. It should be emphasised that 50% of the variability in age of onset is attributed to the number of repeats; this degree of correlation is insufficient to give useful information to an individual who has been identified as having the gene presymptomatically.

Whilst identifying the gene has simplified diagnostic tests and facilitated presymptomatic predictive testing, this was not an end in itself. Cloning the gene was considered an essential prerequisite to understanding the pathophysiology, which is essential if effective treatments are to be developed.

NEUROPATHOLOGY

The most striking neuronal cell loss occurs in the basal ganglia, especially the caudate and putamen nuclei, which together are termed the striatum (see Figures 2.3, 2.4). However, it should be noted that neuronal cell loss occurs in other areas of the brain, including the cortex, particularly layers III, V and VI (Roos, 1986). To emphasise this point, the brain of a patient with HD will be smaller and weigh less than that of an age-matched control.

Perry *et al.* (1973) demonstrated loss of the inhibitory neurotransmitter GABA (gamma amino butyric acid) in the basal ganglia. It has since been shown that there is selective loss of the efferent medium spiny neurones in the striatum, with relative sparing of the large aspiny interneurones. A clear understanding of the neuropathophysiology of HD requires an explanation of how the abnormal huntingtin protein results in late-onset selective neurodegeneration, and also a detailed description of how the cognitive, affective and physical signs and symptoms of the disorder are related to the observed changes within the brain. It is not possible to present such a detailed account of the neuropathophysiology of HD here. However, there is one theory, which may need further modification, to explain the occurrence of chorea early in the course of the disease, whereas bradykinesia and rigidity tend to occur later (Albin *et al.*, 1989; Storey & Beal, 1993).

The striatum receives excitatory neurones from the cortex and has efferent neurones containing the neurotransmitters GABA and substance P or GABA and metencephalin. These neurones project to the internal globus pallidus and substantia nigra via direct and indirect pathways. The pathways damaged in HD are shown in Figure 13.1. Loss of neurones from the indirect pathway results in loss of inhibition of the external globus pallidus, which produces more inhibition of the subthalamus, less stimulation of the internal globus pallidus, less inhibition of the thalamus and overstimulation of the thalamocortical feedback, resulting in chorea.

Loss of neurones from the direct pathway results in increased inhibition of the thalamus, less activity of the thalamocortical feedback, producing bradykinesia and rigidity. The exact distribution of motor signs seen in a patient will, in part, depend on the degree of degeneration between these two pathways. Hedreen & Folstein (1995) have suggested that both pathways degenerate at a similar rate but that excess dopamine from the substantia nigra produces an inhibitory effect on the indirect pathway and a stimulatory effect on the direct pathway, thus giving an apparent appearance of a different rate of degeneration. This theory is consistent with the observation that medical treatment with dopa-blocking drugs or dopa-depleting drugs can modify the physical sign of chorea.

The huntingtin protein is present in a wide variety of neurones (Landwehrmeyer *et al.*, 1995); therefore, it is unclear why a huntingtin protein with an expanded polyglutamine tract should result in selective neuronal degeneration. Recent reports have indicated enhanced

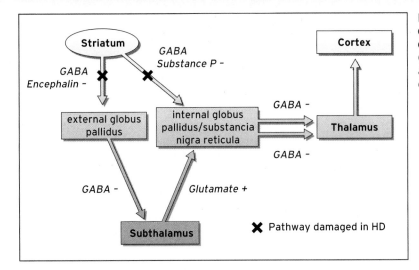

Figure 13.1 Connections of the basal ganglia, showing the pathways damaged in Huntington's disease. (Abreviations: GABA, gamma-aminobutyric acid; HD, Huntington's disease.)

binding to two proteins, Huntington-associated protein 1 and glyceraldehyde 3-phosphate dehydrogenase (Li *et al.*, 1995; Burke *et al.*, 1996). Complete understanding of the pathophysiology of HD will have to await further knowledge of the interactions of huntingtin with other cellular proteins.

A separate line of evidence suggests that selective neurodegeneration results from the effects of an excitotoxin. One of the major causes of the motor signs in HD results from loss of GABAergic neurones in the striatum. The afferent corticostriatal neurones contain the excitatory amino acid glutamate. If excitatory amino acids are allowed to remain in the synapse they can result in cell death. This has led a number of workers to use glutamate analogues as excitatory neurotoxins in the development of animal models of HD (for a review of these experiments see MacMillan & Quarrell, 1996). Although the details remain to be identified, a reasonable hypothesis is that neurones which contain a huntingtin protein, with an expanded polyglutamine tract, have a disturbed metabolism which probably renders them more susceptible to the effects of excitotoxin.

SIGNS AND SYMPTOMS AND THEIR GENERAL MANAGEMENT

Onset of HD is most frequently between the ages of 35 and 55, which is after the usual years of reproduction, although it can develop at almost any age. Onset may occur before the age of 20, which is arbitrarily defined as 'juvenile onset', and may also occur after the age of 60. Patients with juvenile onset tend to have more bradykinesia and rigidity than chorea. Those with onset after the age of 60 appear to have an illness which subjectively appears milder than those with onset in middle age.

The onset of HD is insidious. Patients may present with frank neurological or psychiatric signs and symptoms and either they, or their relatives, have some difficulty in dating the onset. Alternatively, a patient with a family history of HD may present with non-specific complaints of feeling depressed, forgetful or clumsy, and it is difficult to be sure if these features are the onset of HD or have another cause. Under these circumstances it may be prudent to wait a year or so to see if more definite features of HD develop.

MOVEMENT DISORDERS

It has been emphasised that HD patients have a mixture of movement abnormalities, but chorea is seen most frequently. Lakke (1981) defined chorea as 'A state of excessive, spontaneous movement, irregularly timed, randomly distributed and abrupt. Severity may vary from restlessness with mild intermittent exaggeration of gesture, fidgeting movements of the hands, unstable dance-like gait to a continuous flow of disabling violent movements.'

In the early stages of the disease the chorea may be barely perceptible, although those who see HD patients on a regular basis will be aware of the movements even if the patient and his or her relatives are unaware of them. All parts of the body may be affected. As the disease develops, the chorea may become progressively more obvious and then reach a plateau (Folstein *et al.*, 1983). In the later stages of the disease, other movement disorders may become more prominent, such as dystonia, bradykinesia and rigidity (see Chapter 5) which are important features of HD.

Dystonia implies sustained slow muscle contractions that may result in twisting movements of the trunk or abnormal postures of the limbs. This sign may be more obvious in the later stages of the disease. The bradykinesia and rigidity may also worsen as the disease progresses, but early in the course of the disease there may be impairment in the rhythm and speed of rapid alternating movements, e.g. finger taps, movement of the tongue between the corners of the mouth, or alternating pronation and supination of the forearm (Folstein *et al.*, 1986). A useful early sign may be impaired saccadic eye movements; i.e. an impaired ability to flick the eyes from side to side without undue blinks, delay or head movements. As the disease progresses, the patient may become unable to perform this test.

Patients with a very early age of onset, or those in the later stages, may have little in the way of chorea. At one time the phrase 'rigid variant' was used, but this is not a helpful term as patients with rigidity do not truly have a different variety of HD; it is just that one particular movement disorder predominates over another.

Abnormalities of heel-to-toe walking may occur in the early stages but as the disease progresses the gait is wide-based and staggering. Patients with HD do fall; however, it is surprising that falls are not more frequent given the abnormal posture of the trunk and limbs. As the disease progresses, patients may become chair- or bed-bound and require considerable nursing care and physiotherapy. Other aspects of the motor disturbance include dysarthria and dysphagia (see below). Motor disorders in HD were discussed in relation to electrophysiological findings by Yanagisawa (1992).

DYSARTHRIA

The rate and rhythm of speech may be disturbed early in the course of HD (Folstein et al., 1986), progressing to become unintelligible; occasionally patients become mute. Abnormalities in phonation have been noted with the movement abnormality affecting the laryngeal and respiratory muscles (Ramig, 1976). The neuronal loss causes a cognitive impairment (see below) and may disrupt linguistic ability (Gordon & Illes, 1987). A speech and language therapist can advise on methods of communication and provide technological aids (see Chapter 14).

DYSPHAGIA AND CACHEXIA

Dysphagia, particularly for liquids, is a common complaint in middle to late stages of the disease, with abnormalities occurring in all aspects of the swallowing process (Kagel & Leopold, 1992). Indeed, aspiration and choking may ultimately be the cause of death. Advice from a speech and language therapist will help with feeding, and assessment of swallowing problems will indicate the risk of choking.

Advice needs to be given regarding seating the patient in an upright position and encouraging him or her to eat slowly with bite-sized pieces. It is useful to consider whether a dry mouth is a known side effect of any medication prescribed for the patient. As the disease progresses, consideration needs to be given to practical issues such as non-slip plates and utensils with large grips. Carers need to be instructed in the use of the Heimlich manoeuvre. Over time patients may become unable to feed themselves and the dietician may recommend that the texture of the food be altered so that it is soft and smooth (Ramen et al., 1993).

Weight loss is an integral part of the disease process for the majority of patients; the neuropathological aetiology of this is unclear. Patients may be offered high-calorie diets. For some patients with significant cachexia, it may be appropriate to discuss the use of a gastrostomy feeding tube with the affected patient, if possible, and the family. The objective is to provide nourishment and comfort but the decision has to be tempered by a consideration of the

patient's general mobility, ability to communicate and quality of life (Harper, 1996). This subject should be approached before the patient is unable to communicate or take an active part in this decision.

INCONTINENCE

Urinary and faecal incontinence occur in the late stage and may be due to dementia rather than a specific neurological cause. However, in a small study of six patients, Wheeler et al. (1985) found some evidence of detrusor hyper-reflexia. Nursing care involving regular changing and cleaning will help to prevent skin breakdown and pressure sores, as well as maintain dignity.

PSYCHIATRIC FEATURES AND BEHAVIOURAL MANAGEMENT

For many of the carers of HD patients, disturbances of affect (depression, temper tantrums and apathy) and the cognitive impairment may be as difficult to manage as the movement disorder (or more difficult). The management of psychiatric and behavioural problems is discussed in Chapter 27.

Depression is said to be very common in patients with HD and may precede the onset of a variety of neurological disorders. Morris & Scourfield (1996) summarised the prevalence of depression from eight surveys and found rates of 9–44%. There may be difficulties in comparing diagnostic criteria between surveys. However, further surveys have reported high prevalence rates of 39–44% (Folstein et al., 1983; Mindham et al., 1985; Shiwach, 1994). Frank psychosis with schizophrenia-like symptoms is known to occur in HD. Specific psychiatric syndromes or diagnoses should be sought in patients with HD, as they may respond to therapy with tricyclic antidepressants or dopa blockers as appropriate. Onset of psychiatric symptoms before motor problems can cause a patient to be placed in psychiatric care before the diagnosis of HD is made, therefore posing difficulties for obtaining appropriate physical management.

Carers of patients with HD may also complain about apathy, irritability and temper tantrums. Whilst these may not be seen as a problem by the patient, they can pose difficult management problems for the family. In addition, disturbance of sleep patterns may be a particularly difficult management issue for the family. Although behavioural problems are accepted and recognised symptoms of the disease, they may sometimes result from inadequate support and 'crisis management'. Patients may be forced into unfamiliar situations that cause anger, fear and non-compliance. Carers need to learn to deal with outbursts of aggression, and behavioural psychotherapy for the patient may be necessary (Marks, 1986).

The older literature commented on anecdotes of increased libido and abnormal sexual behaviour. Whilst this may occur, it is likely that decreased libido is more common. A systematic study of sexual disorders in HD was conducted by Federoff et al. (1994).

In his original description, George Huntington commented on the tendency to suicide. There is an increased rate of suicide amongst HD patients, mainly occurring around the time of onset or early in the course of the disease, possibly associated with depression (Shoenfeld *et al.*, 1984; Di Maio *et al.*, 1993).

The principles of management of behavioural problems in HD are similar to those in other conditions involving dementia. As mentioned above, support and social care are important so as not to exacerbate the effects of the underlying psychiatric disorder. Specific literature on this area is lacking but case reports give helpful insight (e.g. van der Weyden, 1994).

COGNITIVE IMPAIRMENT

This is the third in the triad of characteristic abnormalities seen in HD. There is general decline in intellectual function during the course of HD but it is qualitatively different from the more global dementia of Alzheimer's disease, as aphasia, agnosia and apraxia are not prominent features (for a review see Brandt, 1991). Patients with either Alzheimer's disease or HD have been compared over the course of the two disorders using brief tests of mental state: the mini-mental state exam or the dementia rating scale, and different cognitive profiles obtained (Brandt *et al.*, 1988; Rosser & Hodges, 1994; Paulsen *et al.*, 1995). This supports the concept of qualitative differences in the nature of cognitive impairment in a disease which mainly affects the cortex, as in Alzheimer's, and a disorder which affects the subcortex (basal ganglia), as in HD. Patients with HD have difficulty with concentration (especially if there are distractions), forward planning and cognitive flexibility. These deficits in executive function may contribute to the behavioural problems seen in HD.

Despite slowness of thinking and dysarthria, it should be remembered that the patient retains the ability to comprehend throughout most of the course of the illness. Therefore, care should be taken when talking about patients in their presence.

DURATION OF ILLNESS

The average duration of illness is difficult to estimate. Whilst the age of death may be recorded accurately, the age of onset is of necessity inexact. There is considerable variation of the duration of the disease from patient to patient but estimates from a number of studies have varied between an average of 10 and 17 years (Harper, 1996). Our experience would suggest that the average is towards the higher end of that range. The average duration is similar for HD of juvenile and adult onset; those with a late age of onset have a lower duration, perhaps because of other unrelated causes of death (Harper, 1996; Roos *et al.*, 1993).

SECONDARY COMPLICATIONS

Complications that may occur are shown in Table 13.1. All these complications will give rise to pain or discomfort and therefore result in diminished performance. In order to correct or control these complications, more input is required from the physiotherapist and there is also an increased care load on all clinical staff. Continuous physical management is therefore necessary to reduce the risk of these complications (see below).

GENERAL ASPECTS OF MANAGEMENT

Given the slowly progressive nature of the disease, the wide spread in age of onset and the variations in relative importance of motor, cognitive and affective dysfunction between individual patients, it is difficult to describe a comprehensive management suitable for all patients. At best some general guidance may be attempted. A useful overview of management which contains many practical suggestions has been given by Ramen *et al.* (1993).

THE MULTIDISCIPLINARY TEAM (MDT)

The complexity of physical, social and behavioural aspects of HD require considerable efforts from all professionals involved to achieve appropriate management of the patient and family. The secondary complications listed in Table 13.1 indicate the range of disciplines needed to care for the HD patient. The main disciplines include social work, dietetics, speech therapy, medicine, physiotherapy, occupational therapy, psychology and nursing.

The roles of the team members overlap in places and the degree of input required varies for the different stages of the

Symptoms and secondary complications in Huntington's disease	
Symptoms	**Complications**
Choreiform movements	Asymmetry Injury Loss of range Loss of function
Rigidity	Loss of range Immobility Contracture/deformity Pain
Spasms	Exaggerated head and neck movements Pain at end-of-range movements
Speech abnormalities	Communication breakdown
Swallowing problems	Aspiration Chest infections
Weight loss	Infections Pressure problems Poor healing of injury Fatigue General debilitation
Incontinence	Discomfort Indignity

Table 13.1 Symptoms and secondary complications in Huntington's disease.

disease. For example, the speech therapist will help with speech and swallowing problems in the middle stage to cope with current problems and also prepare the patient and team for the late stage when communication aids may need to be provided. The physiotherapy input (see 'Physical management') essentially concerns maintenance of function in the early/middle stages, safety and prevention of secondary complications in the middle stage and management of complications to minimise discomfort in the terminal stage. The social worker is the key person at every stage to co-ordinate services and ensure that respite care, transition into residential care and other milestones are managed with minimal trauma to the patient and family. This involves liaison with funding authorities and the different support services. Forward planning is essential; deterioration can occur, so placement must be available and the MDT must be able to respond when help is needed.

MEDICAL MANAGEMENT

There is no pharmacological treatment which will reverse the underlying neurodegenerative process. In the past there has been a tendency to treat the movement disorder using dopamine-blocking or dopamine-depleting drugs. There are problems with focusing therapy on the physical sign of chorea. First, this may not be the most important problem experienced by the patient and family; depression, irritability, aggression or apathy may be more difficult problems. Secondly, since the movement disorder is a mixture of chorea, bradykinesia and dystonia, treating chorea alone may make the bradykinesia, dystonia and apathy worse. Chorea may be the focus of pharmacological treatment if it is of large amplitude or causing distress to the patient; otherwise the focus of pharmacological management should be on depression and irritability. A complaint by some patients and their carers is that after a diagnosis has been made, nothing specific is done for years. General practitioners and hospital clinics have a role in being generally supportive to families over a prolonged period of time.

GENETIC COUNSELLING

The genetic counselling clinic has a role to play in supporting the family, especially the extended family, due to the implications of this inherited disease (Harper, 1996). Some members of the family may seek predictive testing and, depending on the outcome, may need support for some time afterwards.

'SOCIAL' MANAGEMENT

In the early stages of the disease the movement disorder and the intellectual decline may be minimal, enabling the patient to continue in employment for some time. As the disease progresses, a social worker may advise on disability payments. The principal carer will need help, support and an opportunity to take a break, even if that involves someone else looking after the patient for a few hours per week.

Many of the behavioural problems of the patient are difficult to manage but, where possible, practical solutions should be considered to provide a safe and calm environment. Given the selective cognitive deficits, a non-confrontational approach should be adopted, with a routine established if possible.

Patients with HD do fall; therefore physiotherapists and occupational therapists have a role in suggesting modifications to the home, such as the provision of additional handrails so as to maintain mobility and independence with reduced risk.

The carer may need advice on the management of incontinence, following the exclusion of a urinary tract infection. Practical advice may focus on regular toileting, depending on mobility, or the use of incontinence pads.

Respite Care

As the disease progresses further, the degree of physical dependence will increase so that the social worker has a role in organising home help and, depending on the degree of co-operation of the patient, respite care. Placement into residential care in the later stages is made easier if periods of respite have been taken in the same establishment. Such periods prior to admission enable the patient and family to become familiar with the environment and make the transition less traumatic. They may also avoid 'crisis placement' for terminal care, a situation which is far from satisfactory.

Support in the Community

In the later stages of the disease, over half of patients need residential care. The main reasons are the inability of the family to cope, often because of unreasonable behaviour, or because patients who are living alone are unable to manage and home conditions may become too unkempt. Patients may become a danger and health hazard to themselves and to others.

Local authority services can be very important in enabling the affected person to remain in the community for as long as possible. The support and quality of care will depend on the resources of the authority and the co-operation of the patient. The MDT should be involved at this stage to provide the best package of care.

PHYSICAL MANAGEMENT

As the patient progresses through the stages of the disease, careful management can ease the impact of change by anticipating the patients' needs before each functional loss occurs.

The physical management of HD is similar to that of motor neurone disease (see Chapter 14) but certain features of HD due to the movement disorders require specific attention.

PRINCIPLES OF PHYSIOTHERAPY

At present there is no means of allaying the progression of the disease but physiotherapy can be valuable in preventing secondary complications and maintaining independence for as long as possible. Principles of physiotherapy are based on clinical experience since research into this area of HD is lacking.

The specific approaches to treatment and techniques used are not discussed in detail here but can be found in Chapters 22 & 24, respectively. In the early and middle stages, physiotherapy aims to maintain balance and mobility, and in the middle to late stages to achieve optimal positioning and comfort. Mobility aids may be prescribed where appropriate. The physiotherapist can also teach the patient relaxation techniques and instruct carers in movement and handling techniques. Literature on physiotherapy for patients with HD is sparce but an exercise programme was suggested by Peacock (1987).

Early, middle and late management stage are not definite categories into which signs and symptoms can be easily placed or for which time scales can be given. This is due to the variability of the disease in different patients.

Early Stage

This is the time from diagnosis to the stage of decreasing independence. Active physiotherapy is not necessary at this stage but it is beneficial to make contact with the patient and family and encourage the patient to participate in his or her own management. The benefits of functional activity, and how to identify any postural changes, can be explained. The physiotherapist can give advice at this stage on stretching exercises to prevent contracture and deformity from soft tissue shortening (see Chapter 25).

HD can have such a devastating effect on the patient and the family that the postural problems may be considered insignificant and ignored. Physical problems can therefore become established and escape notice until they cause functional disability.

Middle Stage

At this stage, the patient still has some independence and is usually managed in his or her own home. The main aims of physiotherapy are to maintain functional ability and prevent contractures and deformity. The disorder of posture, balance and movement is apparent and manifests itself with increased chorea, dystonia, a weaving gait and bradykinesia (see Chapter 5). These contribute to a decline in functional activity which can result in apathy. This may defeat any attempt at physical intervention; support of the family and care team may be the only possibility. Physiotherapists and occupational therapists can advise on equipment and furniture, and health and safety issues, particularly those relating to moving and handling.

Continuous assessment and re-evaluation of the physical ability of the patient, which can change quite dramatically, is important to maintain a safe environment for both patient and carers. An occupational therapist may provide adaptions to the home to help with safety, e.g. stair rails, poles for transferring in and out of the bath.

Many people mistakenly presume that involuntary movements and walking will maintain range of movement. With such a bizarre disorder of posture, balance and movement, (in spite of the activity) there is malalignment of body segments and patients lose the ability to rotate. Alignment and rotation are essential for postural control and efficient movement and functional ability. Specific exercises are required to maintain ROM (see Chapters 24 & 25).

Preventive care is beneficial and a routine of physical management must be devised and be practical and cost-effective. The overall approach to treatment is to help the patient to organise and regulate his or her movements in order to function more effectively and to have the opportunity to remain independent for as long as possible. In this intermediate stage, a daily physiotherapy programme that is useful for identifying problems before they become too established might include prone lying for 20 minutes, exercise to maintain ROM, walking for endurance, and posture control (see below). The physical management in the middle stage of HD was discussed by Imbriglio (1992).

Late Stage

As the disease progresses, specially adapted padded chairs may need to be suggested to control posture whilst seated and to minimise damage from the effects of chorea or progressive dystonia. Further progression of the disease may mean that wheelchairs have to be considered if the patient is to be taken for an appreciable distance outside the home. In the later stages of the disease, chorea may be less troublesome but stiffness and dystonia more marked. These symptoms may predominate throughout the course of the disease in those patients with an early onset. Patients are at risk of developing the complications listed in Table 13.1. Physical management at this stage is aimed at aiding nursing care and comfort. It has been suggested that treatment of specific disabilities may not be effective and that a general programme may be more appropriate (Mason *et al.*, 1991).

ASSESSMENT

There are a number of rating scales which have been used to quantify clinical aspects of HD; a useful, simple and practical one is the functional disability scale of Shoulson & Fahn (1979). Examples of functional and motor assessment forms were described by Imbriglio (1992).

The principles of physiotherapy assessment are discussed in Chapter 4; the main aspects applicable to HD include assessment of co-ordination, mobility, functional abilities and safety in activities of daily living.

MAINTAINING JOINT RANGE AND MOBILITY

Physiotherapy plays an important part in maintaining movement and mobility. The bizarre movements that patients may have, contribute to asymmetry and the development of preferred postures. This may lead to secondary complications such as deformities and contractures, which will cause seating and management problems.

Positioning and posture should be controlled at all times, i.e. lying, sitting and standing. Standing frames, standing risers and tilt-tables may be useful in the later stage when the patient is no longer able to stand. Posture in sitting and lying is discussed below.

Prone Lying and Stretching Exercises

Prone lying should be encouraged as part of a daily routine, e.g. 20 minutes each day, to help maintain ROM and is particularly useful for identifying any asymmetry or preferred postural pattern.

Full-range movements of all joints can be incorporated into daily activities such as dressing or, if preferred, a suitable programme of self-assisted exercises (see Chapter 25). In the later stages, passive/assisted and passive stretching will be required to maintain joint ROM.

A variety of techniques may be used to reduce rigidity and facilitate movement and functional activity: trunk mobilisations, proprioceptive neuromuscular facilitation (PNF), joint proximation, gym ball activities, and relaxation techniques. Details of these techniques are discussed in Chapter 24.

Walking and Functional Activities

Walking should be encouraged to maintain stamina and ability for as long as possible. The tendency is to offer too much support, thus inhibiting locomotion and denying the patient the opportunity to walk (Gardham, 1982). Walking may become physically impossible or too dangerous for the patient and the carers. Whatever the reason, a multidisciplinary decision must be made which includes the patient and carers. The quality of the gait can be analysed and abnormalities identified and modified if possible.

Many HD patients are severely disabled, largely due to disuse. Skilled handling can facilitate efficient movement and enable the patient to participate actively and thus become more independent. Functional activity is the most effective way of maximising remaining ability.

Head control is important, as stability of the head is vital for communication, eating, visual fixation, manual activities, and all activities requiring balance, including walking. The patient should be encouraged to look at what he or she is doing, and practice eye–hand co-ordination activities.

All functional activities involve patterns of movement and have an element of rotation, which plays an important role in postural adjustment and normal postural activity. Rotation is vital for balance and activities should include rotation of the trunk.

Patients can be stimulated through exercise, sport and the provision of an element of competition for those who need it. Hydrotherapy can provide recreation and enjoyment (see Chapter 24). Gym group activities can include skittles, balloon badminton, archery and throwing games.

Experience has shown that regular activities such as hydrotherapy and gym groups are looked forward to, and that with familiarity and regularity participation is increased. This is also the case with music therapy and occupational therapy and reinforces the reasoning behind many claims that the majority of patients are cognitively aware, in spite of their dementia and inability to communicate.

Transfers

Independent transfers should be maintained for as long as possible. Standing transfers may require only one person to facilitate movement. The two-person lift is now discouraged, particularly in patients with low muscle tone, as it can be injurious to their shoulders due to lack of stability around the joint. In some cases it is safe only with a third person assisting with either a 'bottom catch' or a 'bottom lift'. Transfers may be assisted by means of equipment, and hoists are a necessity in the later stages for some people. The type of hoist and sling must be assessed for each individual patient.

SAFETY

In all stages of the disease it is a great challenge to everyone concerned to match the needs of the patient with health and safety needs. Many patients apparently have no fear and seem unaware of danger, and this can put themselves and their carers at risk. Many of the minor injuries that are sustained can be caused by restraining devices that are provided in the interest of safety. Special seating and beds are discussed below. A balance must be found between function, freedom, risk, challenge and health and safety.

Carers may be at risk from injury when managing the patient, so advice on moving and handling using an ergonomic approach is essential. The European Community Directive (1992) looks at the task, the patient, the environment and the carer's ability.

Carers need to be informed about the disease and need support from appropriate people to help them to cope with the patient's personality changes and bizarre behaviour.

POSTURE AND SEATING

Awareness of posture and signs of developing abnormalities must be taught in the early stages and include posture in standing, sitting and lying. Posture and special seating for neurological patients were discussed in detail by Pope (1996).

Positioning in the Early and Middle Stages

Posture and seating should be addressed in the early stage and a suitable seating regimen for everyday activities agreed upon, e.g. a comfortable easy chair for some activities and a change of chair for sitting at a table. Long periods of poor positioning or habitual postures may lead to deformity and reduced ability and independence later on, so seating needs to be monitored from the outset of HD.

The choice of chair aims to achieve the optimal position to suit the individual person's needs, and adaptations will be necessary as disability increases.

Symmetry of posture and movement should be sought, as this helps the patient to organise himself or herself and provides a more natural position from which to initiate movement.

Special Seating in the Middle to Late Stages

When it is no longer possible or safe to walk independently, a wheelchair may be appropriate, though not always acceptable, for some patients. On the whole, the standard wheelchair is adequate and patients may be able to propel themselves with their arms or 'paddle' with their feet. Trays and footplates are not always appropriate or desirable; the floor can act as a stable footrest and the chair can be parked at a table for mealtimes or reading. While patients are still reasonably able, functional independence is of vital importance.

If a patient is seated in a chair for several hours each day, a firm base is essential as well as an appropriate seat cushion, and a pelvic strap. Extra padding may be needed to protect patients from knocks. Because of the progression of the disease and the nature of the symptoms, it is unlikely that a powered wheelchair would be appropriate; there may, however, be exceptions to this.

If wheelchairs are not acceptable to the patient, ordinary upright chairs or suitable armchairs can be adequate and maintain normality for as long as postural stability allows.

When the movements become so exaggerated that the patient is endangering himself or herself, then it is time for some other form of seating (see 'Special seating systems' in Chapter 8; and Pope, 1996).

Patients with high tone and rigidity will need a very supportive seating system. This could be a recliner chair with adaptations, or a more custom-made system such as a full matrix support system (see Chapter 8). There are many chairs on the market which can be used as the support base for the special seating systems, e.g. the Kirton chair that was developed for the HD patient. Some of the special chairs on the market can provide safety but they do nothing to maintain function or ability.

Because of the variation in range and velocity of movement, it is not ethical or possible to provide physical restraint against such movements; restraint may be more injurious than actually falling out of the chair.

Positioning in Bed in the Middle and Late Stages

Special beds, 'log' rolls, 'T' rolls and bed wedges can help maintain alignment and stability of posture, but obviously uncontrolled movements will limit their effectiveness. Positioning strategies are also discussed elsewhere in relation to patients with brain injury (Chapter 8) and motor neurone disease (Chapter 14).

The choreiform movements place the patient at risk of injury and falling out of bed. Net beds may be chosen for safety reasons since they conform to the body and spread the load, thus reducing pressure; the patient can be turned without handling, thereby reducing injury to carers, and the bed does not have to be made. The disadvantages of these hammock-like net beds are:

- They maintain a flexed unfunctional posture.
- They are difficult for transfers.
- It is not possibe to sit the patient up.
- There is no stability for functional movement.
- It is difficult to protect the sides without awkward gaps.
- The patient's fingers can get caught in the netting.
- The patient is deprived of human contact.
- The patient is not able to use equipment which promotes stability and alignment.

Net beds provide a supposedly safe enviroment but should be used only as a last resort as they increase disability.

Profile beds can provide some stability and enable the patient to have changes of position, i.e. sit up in bed. They have good cot sides which can be protected by cushions and have air-filled mattresses. The bed can be used with 'log' rolls, 'T' rolls and bed wedges, though ideally these are better placed on a firm mattress.

If a patient's movements are so violent that he or she is damaged by hitting the cot sides, even when padded, it may be appropriate to place a mattress on the floor. A pelvic strap may have to be used to maintain safety.

ASPECTS OF TERMINAL CARE

Management in the terminal stage of the illness involves keeping the patient as comfortable as possible and supporting the relatives. A paper defining palliative care and describing the care and ethical issues involved was published by the American Acadamy of Neurology Ethics and Humanities Subcommittee in 1996. This is also a very difficult time for the care team who have come to know the patient and family. Imbriglio (1992) discussed the importance of support between team members. Terminal care, which is similar to that for motor neurone disease (Chapter 14), aims to allow the patient to die with dignity and minimal discomfort.

REFERENCES

Albin RL, Young AB, Penny JB, *et al*. The functional anatomy of basal ganglia disorder. *Trends Neurosci* 1989, **12**:366-375.

American Academy of Neurology Ethics and Humanities Subcommittee. Palliative care in neurology. *Neurology* 1996, **46**:870-872.

Brandt J. Cognitive impairments in Huntington's disease: insight into the neuropsychology of the striatum. In: Boller F, Grofman J, eds. *Handbook of Neuropsychology, vol 5*. Amsterdam: Elsevier; 1991:241-263.

Brandt J, Folstein SE, Folstein MF. Differential cognitive impairment in Alzheimer's disease and Huntington's disease. *Ann Neurol* 1988, **23**:555-561.

Burke JR, Enghild JJ, Martin ME, *et al*. Huntingtin and DRPLA proteins selectively interact with the enzyme GAPDH. *Nature Medicine* 1996, **2**:347-350.

Di Maio L, Squitieri F, Napolitano G, *et al*. Suicide risk in Huntington's disease. *J Med Genet* 1993, **30**:293-295.

European Community Directive. *Manual Handling Operations Regulations*. London: Health and Safety Executive; 1992.

Federoff JP, Peyser C, Franz ML, *et al*. Sexual disorders in Huntington's disease. *J Neuropsych* 1994, **6**:147-153.

Folstein SE, Jensen B, Leigh RJ, *et al*. The measurement of abnormal movement: methods developed for Huntington's disease. *Neurobehav Toxicol Teratol* 1983, **5**:605-609.

Folstein SE, Leigh RJ, Parhad IM, *et al*. The diagnosis of Huntington's disease. *Neurology* 1986, **36**:1279-1283.

Gardham F. *On nursing Huntington's disease*. London: Huntington's Disease Association; 1982:28-30.

Gordon WP, Illes J. Neurolinguistic characteristics of language production in Huntington's disease: a preliminary report. *Brain Lang* 1987, **31**:1-10.

Gusella JF, Wexler NS, Conneally PM, *et al*. A polymorphic DNA marker genetically linked to Huntington's disease. *Nature* 1983, **306**:234-238.

Harper PS. The epidemiology of Huntington's disease. *Hum Genet* 1992, **89**:365-376.

Harper PS. *Huntington's disease, 2nd edition*. London: WB Saunders; 1996.

Hedreen JC, Folstein SE. Early loss of neostriatal neurones in Huntington's disease. *J Neuropath Exp Neurol* 1995, **54**:105-120.

Huntington G. On chorea. *Medical and Surgical Reporter* 1872, **26**:317-321. [Republished in *Adv Neurol* 1973, **1**:33-35].

Huntington's Disease Collaborative Research Group. A novel gene containing a trinucleotide repeat that is expanded and unstable on Huntington's disease chromosomes. *Cell* 1993, **72**:971-983.

Imbriglio S. Huntington's disease at mid-stage. *Clin Manage* 1992, **12**:63-72.

Kagel MC, Leopold NA. Dysphagia in Huntington's disease: a 16 year perspective. *Dysphagia* 1992, **7**:106-114.

Kremer B, Goldberg P, Andrew SE, *et al*. A worldwide study of the Huntington's disease mutation. *New Engl J Med* 1994, **330**:1401-1406.

Lakke PWF. Classification of extrapyramidal disorders. Proposal for an international classification and glossary of terms. *J Neurol Sci* 1981, **51**:313-327.

Landwehrmeyer GB, McNeil SM, Dure LS, *et al*. Huntington's disease gene: regional and cellular expression in brain of normal and affected individuals. *Ann Neurol* 1995, **37**:218-230.

Li X-J, Li SH, Sharp AH, *et al*. A huntingtin-associated protein enriched in brain with implications for pathology. *Nature* 1995, **378**:398-402.

MacMillan JC, Quarrell OWJ. The neurobiology of Huntington's disease. In: Harper PS, ed. *Huntington's disease, 2nd edition*. London: WB Saunders; 1996:317-358.

Marks IM. Behavioural psychotherapy: *Maudsley pocket book of clinical management*. Bristol: Wright; 1986.

Mason J, Andrews K, Wilson E. Late stage Huntington's disease - effect of treating specific disabilities. *Br J Occ Ther* 1991, **54**:4-7.

Mindham RHS, Steele C, Folstein MF, *et al*. A comparison of the frequency of major affective disorder in Huntington's disease in a case series and in families. *Psychol Med* 1985, **13**:537-542.

Morris M, Scourfield J. Psychiatric aspects of Huntington's disease. In: Harper PS, ed. *Huntington's disease, 2nd edition*. London: WB Saunders; 1996:73-122.

Paulsen JS, Butters N, Sadek JR, *et al*. Distinct cognitive profiles of cortical and subcortical dementia in advanced illness. *Neurology* 1995, **45**:951-956.

Peacock IW. A physical therapy program for Huntington's disease patients. *Clin Manage* 1987, **7**:22-23,34.

Perry TL, Hansen S, Kloster M. Huntington's chorea: deficiency of gamma-aminobutyric acid in brain. *New Engl J Med* 1973, **288**:337-342.

Pope PM. A model for evaluation of input in relation to outcome in severely brain damaged patients. *Physiotherapy* 1988, **74**:647-650.

Pope PM. Postural management and special seating. In: Edwards S, ed. *Neurological physiotherapy: a problem solving approach*. London: Churchill Livingstone; 1996:135-160.

Ramig LA. Acoustic analyses of phonation in patients with Huntington's disease. *Ann Otol Rhinol Laryngol* 1976, **95**:288-293.

Ramen NG, Peyser CE, Folstein SE. A physicians guide to the management of Huntington's disease. London: Huntington's Disease Association; 1993.

Roos RAC. Neuropathology of Huntington's chorea. In: Vinken PJ, Klawans HL, eds. *Extrapyramidal disorders*. Amsterdam: Elsevier Science; 1986:315-326. (Handbook of Clinical Neurology, vol 5).

Roos RAC, Hermans J, Vegter-van der Vlis M, *et al*. Duration of illness in Huntington's disease is not related to age of onset. *J Neurol Neurosurg Psychiat* 1993, **56**:98-100.

Rosser AE, Hodges JR. The dementia rating scale in Alzheimer's disease, Huntington's disease and progressive supranuclear palsy. *J Neurol* 1994, **241**:531-536.

Rubinsztein DC, Leggo J, Goodbarn S, *et al*. Study of the Huntington's disease (HD) gene CAG repeats in schizophrenic patients shows overlap of the normal and HD affected ranges but absence of correlation with schizophrenia. *J Med Genet* 1994, **31**:690-695.

Rubinsztein DC, Leggo J, Goodbarn S, *et al*. Normal CAG and CGG repeats in the Huntington's disease gene of Parkinson's disease patients. *Am J Med Genet* (Neuropsychiatric genetics) 1995, **60**:109-110.

Shiwach R. Psychopathology in Huntington's disease patients. *Acta Psychiatr Scand* 1994, **90**:241-246.

Shoenfeld M, Myers RH, Cupples LA, *et al*. Increased rate of suicide among patients with Huntington's disease. *J Neurol Neurosurg Psychiat* 1984, **47**:1283-1287.

Shoulson I, Fahn S. Huntington's disease: clinical care and evaluation. *Neurology* 1979, **29**:1-3.

Storey E, Beal MF. Neurochemical substrates of rigidity and chorea in Huntington's disease. *Brain* 1993, **116**:1201-1206.

van der Weyden RS. Caring for a patient with Huntington's disease. *Nurs Times* 1994, **90**:33-35.

Ward C, Dennis N, McMillan T. Huntington's disease. In: Greenwood R, Barnes MP, McMillan TM, *et al*., eds. *Neurological rehabilitation*. London: Churchill Livingstone: 1993:505-516.

Wheeler JS, Sax DS, Krane RJ, *et al*. Vesico-urethral function in Huntington's chorea. *Br J Neurol* 1985, **57**:63-66.

Yanagisawa N. The spectrum of motor disorders in Huntington's disease. *Clin Neurol Neurosurg* 1992, **94**(Suppl):S182-S184.

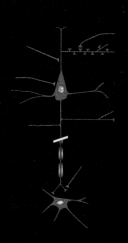

14

B O'Gorman & D Oliver

DISORDERS OF NERVE I: MOTOR NEURONE DISEASE

CHAPTER OUTLINE

- Genetics and prevalence
- Clinical presentation
- Diagnosis
- Symptoms and their control

- Physical management
- Psychosocial aspects
- Terminal management
- Case history

INTRODUCTION

Motor neurone disease (MND) is characterised by the progressive degeneration of: anterior horn cells of the spinal cord, causing lower motor neurone lesions; the corticospinal tracts, causing upper motor neurone lesions: and certain motor nuclei of the brainstem, leading to bulbar palsy.

The aetiology of the disease is unknown, although many theories for its cause have been suggested. About 5% of the patients have a familial form; they often present earlier in life and with the spinal form of the disease (Figlewicz & Rouleau, 1994). As with other degenerative neurological disorders (e.g. Huntington's disease, see Chapter 13), the impact on the family can be devastating and care must take into account the needs of the family as well as the patient.

GENETICS AND PREVALENCE

Recently, in a small number of families with the familial form of the disease, a mutation of the superoxide dismutase (SOD) gene has been found and it was suggested that the disease may be due to an excess of free radicals within nerve cells (Rosen et al., 1993). If the SOD gene is abnormal, the free radicals are not removed and the cell is damaged and may die.

The prevalence is 1 per 12,000 (MND Association, see 'Associations and Support Groups') and there is a slightly higher occurrence in males. It is a disease of later middle

life, most patients being between 50 and 70 years, although younger people may be affected.

The mean duration of survival from the onset of symptoms, without ventilatory support, is 3 years, although some patients live for much longer. In one large study, the overall 5-year survival rate was 40% (Rosen, 1978). However, the survival depended on the age of the patient, being 60% for patients less than 50 years and only 31% for patients over 50 years; the presence of bulbar symptoms reduced the 5-year survival rate to 14%.

CLINICAL PRESENTATION

The clinical presentation tends to be insidious and depends on the part of the CNS affected. If lower motor neurone degeneration is predominant, the main features are of weakness, wasting and fasciculation of the muscles supplied by the nerves undergoing degeneration. Upper motor neurone degeneration also leads to weakness and often to muscle wasting but the muscles become spastic (see Table 14.1). Due to plasticity, involving enlargement of surviving motoneurones, up to 50% of mononeurones can be lost before weakness becomes apparent (see Chapter 6).

Three main forms of the disease are recognised: amyotrophic lateral sclerosis (ALS); progressive bulbar palsy; and progressive muscular atrophy.

Lesions in motor neurone disease and their related symptoms		
Site of lesion	**Type of lesion**	**Symptoms**
	Upper motor neurone lesion — Pseudobulbar palsy	Tongue-spastic no fasciculation Speech-spastic and explosive dysarthria Dysphagia Increased reflexes Emotional lability and decreased control of expression
Medulla	Upper and lower motor neurone lesions	Dysarthria Dysphagia Wasting of tongue Jaw jerk increased
	Lower motor neurone lesion — Bulbar palsy	Tongue-shrunken, wrinkled, fasciculation Speech-slurred Dysphagia Paralysis of diaphragm
Corticospinal tracts	Upper motor neurone lesion	Spastic weakness Stiffness Increased reflexes Extensor plantar responses
Anterior horn cells	Lower motor neurone lesion	Flaccid weakness Muscle wasting Muscle fasciculation

Table 14.1 Lesions in motor neurone disease and their related symptoms. (Data from Oliver, 1994, with permission.)

AMYOTROPHIC LATERAL SCLEROSIS

ALS accounts for about 66% of all patients with MND and is commoner in older men. There are both lower motor neurone changes, such as muscle fasciculation, weakness and flaccidity, together with upper motor neurone changes, such as spasticity and weakness. There may also be a mixture of bulbar signs, including dysarthria and dysphagia, and emotional lability.

Most commonly ALS first affects the hands, with symptoms of clumsiness and weakness and evidence of wasting of the thenar eminences. The shoulders may also be affected early in the disease. If there is bulbar involvement the tongue becomes wasted and fasciculates, and speech and swallowing are affected because of muscle weakness.

PROGRESSIVE BULBAR PALSY

About 25% of patients with MND present with progressive bulbar palsy, which affects the bulbar region and causes dysarthria and dysphagia. When lower motor neurones are affected, the tongue is atrophied, fasciculates and has reduced mobility, and there is nasal speech and dysphagia. If the upper motor neurones are affected, the tongue is spastic and causes dysarthria. Emotional lability may occur, with only a

small or no obvious stimulus. Although the limbs may be affected little early in the disease, as it progresses there may be weakness of the arms and legs (Tandan, 1994).

PROGRESSIVE MUSCULAR ATROPHY

About 10% of patients with MND present with progressive muscular atrophy; it develops earlier in life, affecting predominantly men under 50 years. Initially, only the lower motoneurones are affected and there is wasting and weakness of the arms. There may be progression to the legs, but bulbar involvement is rare until late in the disease. The rate of progression is slower than in the other forms and the majority of patients live more than 5 years, often more than 10 years.

Although these three main forms of the disease are described, many patients present, or develop, a mixed picture of symptoms and signs. Every patient is different and the development of the disease varies greatly. The sphincter control of bladder and bowels is rarely affected. Mental deterioration and dementia are found in less than 5% of patients (Tandan, 1994), although anxiety and depression, understandably associated with a progressive, seriously disabling disease, may be seen.

DIAGNOSIS

The clinical diagnosis is confirmed by electromyography (EMG). The motor neurone conduction velocity is normal until late in the disease. The motor action potentials are of increased amplitude and duration, but are reduced in number, whereas the sensory action potential is normal. On mechanical stimulation of the needle, fibrillation and fasciculation potentials are seen (Schwartz & Swash, 1995).

Other investigations may be necessary to exclude other conditions leading to muscle wasting and bulbar palsy, such as syringomyelia or cervical spondylosis (Swash & Schwartz, 1995).

SYMPTOMS AND THEIR CONTROL

Control of the following problems involves the multidisciplinary team (MDT); the specific role of the physiotherapist is elaborated in 'Physical management'. Drug treatments mentioned are covered in detail in Chapter 28.

PAIN

About 50–60% of patients with MND complain of pain (O'Brien et al., 1992), although sensory nerves are not affected. Pain may be musculoskeletal or due to muscle cramp or skin pressure.

Musculoskeletal pain may occur in joints with restricted movements and altered muscle tone. Non-steroidal anti-inflammatory drugs may be of help, and intra-articular injection of steroids and local anaesthetic may also be helpful, especially if a shoulder is very painful.

Pain from muscle cramps due to immobility may occur early in the disease and can be eased by diazepam or quinine sulphate at night.

Pain can occur from pressure on the skin, as the patient is less able to move. Careful positioning and regular turning may help relieve pain and are necessary to prevent pressure sores. Often an opioid analgesic may be the most effective treatment for pain.

DYSPNOEA

The dysfunction of respiratory muscles caused dyspnoea in 47% of the patients in one series (O'Brien et al., 1992). A calm and confident approach is necessary as dyspnoea may be exacerbated by anxiety. Careful positioning is important, especially of the neck when there is neck weakness, and the body and shoulder girdle need to be stabilised to ease breathing. Morphine, or other opioids, may reduce the feelings of breathlessness. Antibiotics may be considered if there is evidence of infection in the early states of the disease (Oliver, 1993).

An episode of acute breathlessness may be treated effectively by an injection of an opioid (such as diamorphine) with hyoscine, to reduce secretions and act as a sedative and an amnesic (Oliver, 1994).

Opioid analgesics, when used in carefully selected doses, effectively control distressing symptoms such as pain, dyspnoea, restlessness and cough. In a series of patients in a hospice, 89% of patients received parenteral opioids that were effective in controlling acute breathlessness or choking and the symptoms of terminal illness (O'Brien et al., 1992).

DYSPHAGIA

Impaired swallowing is a troublesome symptom in over 75% of patients, and is due to involvement of the motor nuclei of the medulla. There is not only muscle weakness but spasticity and inco-ordination. Careful, slow feeding is essential and semi-solids may be taken more easily than liquids. Favourite beverages (from tea to whisky) can be given as ice cubes.

Dribbling salivation can be controlled by hyoscine, as atropine tablets, sublingually, or as a transdermal patch. Choking and respiratory distress is a great fear of patients but if the symptoms are well controlled it is rarely a cause of death. Only one patient died in a choking attack in two large series (Saunders et al., 1981; O'Brien et al., 1992) and no evidence of obstruction of the respiratory tract was found on autopsy (O'Brien et al., 1992). By careful positioning of the patient and by controlling salivation, choking attacks may be prevented. In a choking attack, diamorphine (to reduce the cough reflex and lessen anxiety) and hyoscine (to dry up secretions, relax smooth muscles and act as an amnesic) may be given as an injection.

If feeding becomes more difficult and the patient becomes very tired during meals, he or she may start to lose weight. The advice of a speech and language therapist and a dietitian will then be necessary. Alternative enteral feeding systems may be necessary to supplement or replace the oral diet. Nasogastric feeding is unpleasant and unsightly and may increase the oropharyngeal secretions (Scott & Austin, 1994). A percutaneous endoscopic gastrostomy (PEG) may be very helpful in maintaining nutritional status. The PEG tube is inserted under local anaesthesia and sedation in a relatively simple procedure (Rawlings & Allison, 1994).

DYSARTHRIA

Difficulties with speech are experienced by 80% of patients with MND and on admission to a hospice 36% had no intelligible speech (O'Brien et al., 1992). Great patience and concentration are necessary to understand the patient. An ice cube may be rubbed around the lips to help stimulate the facial muscles and aid speech. Assessment by a speech and language therapist will allow the most to be made of the remaining speech, and carers may spend much time aiding communication. Aids for writing and typing may be helpful and very sensitive switches allow a patient with minimal movement to summon help, thus aiding confidence. Communication aids are discussed further below.

SORE EYES

Eye blinking may be reduced as a result of muscle weakness and the eyes may then become sore and secondarily infected. Lubricating eye drops are helpful and antibiotic eye drops may be necessary if infection occurs.

CONSTIPATION

Any patient who is inactive, debilitated and taking a low-roughage diet may become constipated. If the abdominal muscles weaken it may be difficult to raise the intra-abdominal pressure sufficiently to open the bowels. A regular aperient prevents this but local rectal measures such as suppositories, enemas or manual evacuation may become necessary in some patients.

INSOMNIA

Insomnia may be due to insecurity, fear and pain, and was reported in 48% of patients admitted to a hospice (O'Brien *et al.*, 1992). Attention to detail and regular positioning will aid confidence and, therefore, sleep. A sensitive switch that allows the patient to call for help may enable him or her to relax and sleep at night. Sedatives, antidepressants and opioid analgesics should also be considered (Chapter 28).

TIREDNESS

Activity should be encouraged but not so as to overextend the patient, as tiredness is a common symptom. Patients should be encouraged to pace their activities, incorporating periods of rest into their daily routines. Corticosteroids may aid appetite and increase the feeling of wellbeing, but if they are used for long periods weakness may be increased and other side effects encountered.

PRESSURE SORES

Pressure sores are uncommon, as sensation is retained. Prevention by regular turning and the use of pressure-relieving cushions and mattresses is important (see 'Comfort and positioning'). The treatment of established sores is by the preferred methods of the nursing team.

URINARY PROBLEMS

Weakness of the abdominal wall musculature may lead to urinary retention in some patients but urinary incontinence is always due to other pathological processes, e.g. benign prostatic hypertrophy in men. Urinary catheterisation may be necessary in some cases for the convenience of nursing care.

PHYSICAL MANAGEMENT

The physical management will depend on the physical symptoms present as well as the rate of progression, which may be gained from the history. It is important that the onset of the symptoms is known rather than the date of diagnosis, as it is from the onset that the rate of deterioration of the disease can be gauged.

There are no clearly defined 'stages' of progression in MND and patients do not follow a set pattern. The distribution of weakness and clinical course of the condition are variable, so that management must be specific to the individual, but general guidelines to rehabilitation can be given (Burford & Pentland, 1985).

EARLY STAGE

Physical management may involve:
- Assessment of motor power and joint range of movement (ROM).
- Assessment of chest function.
- Assessment of functional abilities.
- Provision of aids to daily living (ADL).
- Instruction in 'how to exercise' to carer and patient.
- Information on caring agencies, e.g. MND Association.
- Support for patient and carer.

LATER STAGE

Physical management may involve:
- Reassessment of motor power.
- Reassessment of joint ROM, introduction of passive stretches.
- Pain relief measures, e.g. ultrasound, ice, radiant heat, acupuncture (see Chapter 24).
- Reassessment of chest function.
- Reassessment of functional abilities.
- Assessment of ADL and update if necessary.
- Update on 'how to exercise', addressing particular areas of need.
- Advice on manual handling for all transfers into and out of cars.
- Support for patient and carer.

TERMINAL STAGE

Physical management may involve:
- General reassessment of physical and functional abilities.
- Aim to influence exercise and overall management.
- Reassessment and provision of ADL if applicable and advice on withdrawal of ADL.
- Advice to patient, carer and professionals on positioning.
- Advice to carers and professionals on chest management and the implications of deterioration.

GENERAL ASPECTS OF PROGRESSION

Some patients experience a rapid decline in their abilities with continual losses—at times weekly. Others will have a slow decline and not notice much loss over a period of months. If the early presentation is of weakness in one foot or one hand, referral to an out-patient physiotherapy department to teach exercises and possibly provide a splint such as an ankle–foot orthosis (AFO) will help. Ideally, review appointments should be set up to monitor abilities, power and any early signs of joint stiffness.

If bulbar signs present first, with dysphasia or dysphagia becoming an escalating early problem, referral to a speech and language therapist will be the first priority. If speech is severely affected, an alternative means of communication will be needed (Unsworth, 1994; Langton Hewer, 1995).

Eventually the general weakness is so profound as to confine the patient to bed or a wheelchair. Many may need admission to a unit caring for the terminally ill or chronically sick, but some families manage to the end in the patient's own home. The overall aim of physical management is the maintenance of independence, however small. The physiotherapist can do much to help in this aspect, and as a member of the team looking after such patients will learn that lines of demarcation between disciplines become blurred. Much of the physiotherapist's role involves teaching and advising the other team members as well as the patient and family.

Support may be forthcoming if there is an MND Care Team in the patient's area. These teams are multidisciplinary and are often based in a Care and Research Centre or neurology unit. The MDT is able to facilitate the co-ordination of the care provided by all the professionals and carers in the community.

EXERCISE AND STRETCHING

On the first treatment or home assessment visit, an assessment chart is completed which covers a detailed assessment of the physical ability of the entire body in terms of both ROM and muscle power (e.g. using the Oxford scale). A functional assessment covers everything from general comfort through to specific problems at home and comments from the carer will also be of value. Any aspect of this detailed assessment can then be referred to and updated by the physiotherapist and the MDT (see Chapter 4).

The weakened muscles cannot be strengthened but the joints should be kept free from stiffness. If the patient's joints do become stiff, then normal daily activities will become a problem and associated with pain. Research has shown that benefits in terms of improved pain-free joint range and muscle length can be demonstrated, and in some cases maintained over long periods with the involvement of physiotherapist or 'trained carers' (Brooke & Steiner, 1989).

Regular exercise is necessary to maintain muscle elasticity, prevent stiffness and maximise muscle power for as long as possible. If a patient with MND has a period of enforced immobility, for whatever reason, it is seldom possible to regain any independence and mobility that has been lost. It is important to make a differential diagnosis to ascertain whether 'limb stiffness' is due to joint stiffness, muscle inelasticity or indeed predisposing factors such as osteoarthritis, as the physical management and medication are different depending on the cause.

Whether patients are affected with an upper motor neurone lesion resulting in spasticity, or a lower motor neurone lesion resulting in flaccidity, or a combination of both, regular exercise is necessary. Spasticity in the legs can be used when standing the patient, and the use of muscle relaxant drugs needs to be carefully monitored as they can decrease this spasm and, therefore, its usefulness.

The patient should be encouraged to move his or her limbs actively throughout the day in as full a range as possible, using either free active exercises or self-assisted active exercises. All limbs affected need to be exercised, together with the head, neck and chest. Once taught, a carer can help the patient perform the exercises, or, if necessary, carry out passive movements. When the muscles are still able to contract but are weak, assisted active exercise should be used. Some patients suffer from overwhelming fatigue throughout the disease and exercise may make them feel worse. It is important to ensure that energy is conserved for the activities of daily living and not wasted in exercising muscles (Brooke & Steiner, 1989). Passive exercises are indicated when the limbs cannot be moved at all by the patient (see Chapter 25).

RESPIRATORY CARE

An attempt should be made to maintain chest expansion by deep breathing, and diaphragmatic breathing should be taught. Some patients are prone to cough if swallowing saliva and liquids is difficult. They may also develop a cough due to a cold or to inhaled food, and the cough may be ineffective due to weakness. Occasionally, gentle shaking of the thorax on expiration, pressure on the abdomen from a hand, or bending the patient forward so as to increase the intra-abdominal pressure, may aid coughing and clearing of secretions ('assisted coughing'). Other techniques to assist respiration and coughing, such as the 'active cycle of breathing' technique and the forced expiratory technique (FET; Hough, 1991) are not appropriate in this condition since the majority of patients cannot cough effectively or even huff.

Postural drainage is not used as it is too traumatic for these patients. Similarly, aspiration of secretions is rarely used, or seldom justified. Accumulation of secretions in the base of the lungs causes relatively little discomfort. However, if mucus is in the upper areas of the lungs or bronchi it can be extremely distressing since the main airways become obstructed. At this stage, hyoscine helps to dry secretions whilst at the same time sedating the patient, so alleviating the distress. In a choking attack the patient must not be left alone; if the attack does not subside naturally, diamorphine and hyoscine can be given. The injection causes sedation and retrograde amnesia; when the patient awakes there is often little or no recollection of the severity of the attack.

The physiotherapist should inform the MDT of any reduction in a patient's chest expansion, as this is often a sign of the rate of deterioration of the disease. Morning headaches due to a high level of carbon dioxide at night are often another sign of deterioration. Many patients do not die from a chest infection but from respiratory failure when they merely cease to breathe. The family needs to be fully informed of a failing chest expansion and the implications of this, in order that they are as prepared as possible. If the family and team members have not been told of this deterioration, it can be an untoward shock.

WEAKNESS

Progressive muscle wasting leads to increasing weakness. Careful positioning and nursing are necessary, in conjunction with physiotherapy, to prevent deformity and maintain possible movement. Particular attention to the support of the neck is essential if the neck muscles are weak. See 'Comfort and positioning'.

MUSCLE STIFFNESS

The discomfort of stiffened spastic muscles may be reduced by careful positioning. Muscle relaxant drugs such as diazepam, baclofen or dantrolene may be useful, but the side effects encountered reduce their usefulness (Chapter 28). The dose of muscle relaxant may need to be carefully adjusted to allow a balance between spasticity and flaccidity, as relief of spasticity may seem to the patient to be merely increased weakness. Massage or aromatherapy may assist muscle relaxation.

MOBILITY

It is important to maintain the patient's ability to walk or stand for as long as possible. Careful thought must always be given before keeping a patient in bed. If a patient is unable to stand from sitting unaided, but can still walk, then a chair with an electric seat raise will overcome this problem.

To assist walking, human support can be used; sometimes a stick is sufficient, and occasionally a tetrapod or Rollator walking aid is helpful. If the patient is only just able to walk, the surface on which walking is attempted should be considered—it is easier to walk on linoleum or cork flooring than on carpet.

If the patient is unable to walk, standing with the aid of several helpers in order to 'stretch' the whole body, especially the hips and lower back, should be considered. When walking becomes an exercise rather than a means of getting about, a wheelchair should be considered. A self-propelling model might be possible; if not, an electric wheelchair will give the patient some independence.

COMFORT AND POSITIONING

It is extremely difficult to make patients with MND comfortable and the combined resources of the nursing and physiotherapy staff are needed to achieve even some degree of comfort. Families often develop the knack and should be consulted.

Positioning is of prime importance. As the patient's trunk, head and limbs become weaker and emaciated, due to reduced muscle bulk, it becomes increasingly difficult to maintain the upright position. This applies whether the patient is standing, sitting in a wheelchair or sitting in bed. It is not sufficient to place more and more pillows behind and around the patient. At all times, whether in bed or being reclined in an armchair or a reclining wheelchair, gravity and its action on the body must be considered.

In order to minimise the effect of gravity on the body, the patient should be reclined back from the vertical at the hips. By doing this, either in bed or in a reclining wheelchair or armchair, the line of gravity will then pass in front of the head and neck through the thorax. A further advantage to the patient from being placed in this position is the relief of pressure of the thorax on the abdomen. This allows the diaphragm to work more efficiently and so aid breathing, which is often restricted due to involvement of the intercostal muscles with resulting decrease in vital capacity.

Sheepskins can be used, with some form of cushion or a foam wedge on which to sit, in conjunction with a small neck or support pillow. Special seating systems to support the patient may be required and are discussed in Chapter 8.

AIDS TO DAILY LIVING

An assessment of these aids will be needed, but often they are not accepted readily by the patient, who feels that they are a sign of deterioration. For patients with marked bulbar signs, hot plates and heated food dishes make slow eating more palatable. Anti-slip table mats and thickened handles on cutlery, pens and toothbrushes aid independence.

Call systems sensitive to light touch can be operated by head, hands or feet, enabling the patient to signal for help. Anti-slip floor mats and the Rototurn aid transfers, and the use of Velcro and zip fasteners will help dressing. Various communication aids including POSSUM will need to be considered, often being used for environmental control as well as communication (Unsworth, 1994; Langton Hewer, 1995). If patients spend time alone, the provision of an 'alarm-call system' may be needed.

A variety of communication systems is available; some connect to the telephone and can 'speak' recorded phrases, including emergency messages, activated by pressing buttons on a keypad. Some also have a memory capacity which allows the speech-impaired person to answer an incoming telephone call by using recorded phrases instead of speech. Telephone answer machines may allow those with impaired speech to receive messages, the response being made by family or carer. Fax machines can also facilitate communication.

The Royal National Institution for Deaf People operates 'Typetalk', which allows a person with speech difficulties to type in a message; a trained operator then speaks the message to the caller, who is then able to reply. The service operates all day every day (see 'Associations and Support Groups').

ORTHOSES

Lively or rigid splints and lightweight orthoses can be of use but careful assessment of their value must be made frequently. AFOs are particularly useful in the early stages of foot drop in order to assist safe mobility. As the condition progresses it may well be necessary to consider below-the-knee callipers, especially if the patient is being cared for at home and transfers need to be maintained safely.

As has been explained, positioning and inclination back from the vertical so that gravity acts differently on the body are the primary factors in supporting the head and trunk, using small pillows attached to the chair or wheelchair. If this fails, or if the patient is able to maintain mobility, collars are sometimes helpful in an attempt to support a drooping head. A soft collar may help. Sometimes a collar cut from block foam to act as a wedge on which the chin can rest may help. There are now two specially designed rigid head supports available: one is the 'Headmaster Collar' and the other is the 'MND Association Mary Marlborough Lodge' collar. These support the head whilst allowing a small amount of anteroposterior movement, and are open at the front so that the throat is not compressed. In extreme cases, a head support that fits over the patient's head like a crash helmet, and is then attached to the bed or wheelchair, may help.

PSYCHOSOCIAL ASPECTS

The emotional and spiritual needs of the patient and family require attention, and counselling is part of the care given by all team members.

EMOTIONAL PROBLEMS

The moods of patients seriously disabled by a progressive illness will vary. Moreover, communication and the expression of emotion may be restricted by dysarthria, and, due to reduced facial movements, the control of expression may be lost and lead to an inability to control laughing or tears. These changes may frighten both the patient and the family and it is important to stress the physiological causes, and that there is no mental deterioration in the illness so that patients are not treated as if they are of reduced intelligence.

Every person will have his or her own particular fears and concerns. It is essential to allow patients the opportunity to share these concerns with members of the caring team and to address them if possible. Fears may be of the disease itself, of the future, of disability and dependence, or of death and dying.

Anxiety may be reduced by a calm and confident approach from the caring team and by careful control of the other symptoms. Sedatives may be helpful, and in an emergency situation of severe panic an injection will promptly control the anxiety.

It is often very difficult to differentiate a depressive illness from the natural sadness of a severely disabled patient. Careful listening and explanation are important and antidepressants may be helpful.

FAMILY CARE

The family of someone with MND will face their own challenges and fears. They may fear the disease, or the future deterioration, or the death of the patient. These fears need to be shared and, if possible, the patient and the family should be able to be open and share their concerns together. There may also be the need to discuss the sexual needs of the patient and spouse. Although the disease may not affect sexual drive, the disability will affect performance. Help and advice on movement and sexual positions, or the consideration of other ways of expressing sexuality, such as mutual masturbation, may be necessary.

There may also be wider family issues. If there are young children, the help of a social worker may be very helpful in talking with the children about their understanding and fears of the disease. There may also be financial issues to be addressed.

Listening to, and supporting, the family is essential to management. The family needs to be closely involved in the care of the patient and in the formulation of any plans for care.

SPIRITUAL ASPECTS

Many people with a serious illness may start to think about the more profound aspects of life, even if they are not 'religious'. There are no easy answers to these questions, such as 'Why me?', but listening and sharing the concerns may be very helpful. Local religious leaders may be of help.

COUNSELLING

The patient may seek more knowledge or advice about the condition from the physiotherapist. As part of the MDT, the physiotherapist must feel able to seek help from the appropriate person to suit the patient's needs. When the physiotherapist provides the relevant information, he or she must ensure that not only the family and patient receive it but also the rest of the team. One must not give too much information at one session, or too soon, as it may not be absorbed.

The physiotherapist needs to be aware of the process of grief and loss, not only for a life that is coming to an end, but for the ongoing losses that the patient and indeed the family are experiencing (McAteer, 1990; Oliver, 1995). 'Physiotherapists can, and must be prepared to, step out of their more traditional role as purely physical therapists and be available to offer their patients, not only physical treatment, but a counselling relationship as well' (McAteer, 1989).

The multidisciplinary approach is vitally important, not only for the ongoing support of the professional carers but in order that management problems are addressed as early as possible. O'Gorman & O'Brien (1990) stated:

'...care of the patient may become difficult because natural preferences occur for different team members and their way of working. With continuing losses it is understandable that the patient may feel insecure, angry and become demanding in his/her behaviour. These problems have the potential of splitting the team. It could become necessary to address these problems with team members and the patient, to define boundaries.'

Ted Holden, an in-patient at St Christopher's Hospice for nearly 6 years, wrote (Holden, 1980):

'Obviously and naturally my wife's visits have the greatest impact, but our very closeness means that we can more easily hurt each other and so we do have our problems, but we keep trying and considering the strains and tensions we manage pretty well. I believe that the main problem is simply to expect too much. One spends hours in eager anticipation which creates an oversensitive reaction to anything which falls short of expectation. The disappointment leads to poor communication and misunderstanding and as one realises that the mood is set and one is fully aware of the fundamental stupidity of it all, frustration, anger and remorse ensure that there is little prospect of recovery. What is sad is that you can do nothing until the next meeting which can be a long, long time. It needs the skill of the interdisciplinary team to attempt to stay alongside such feelings...'

A patient's view was also given by Henke (1980).

Not all patients with MND will be found in special units, and the physiotherapist may not have the back-up of a committed team. In such instances, the therapist must apply the principles which are outlined not only in this chapter but throughout this book. Continual assessment is necessary as MND follows no rules and what suits one patient may be useless for another. Individual gadgets, aids and appliances are essential.

At times, a 'family meeting' to include family, appropriate professionals (not necessarily the whole team) and/or the patient will help to discuss problems, ongoing care and overall management. As many members of the family as appropriate should be included so that issues can be discussed with everybody hearing the same information at the same time. This minimises misinterpretation of the facts. The physiotherapist can play a useful part in such meetings.

TERMINAL MANAGEMENT

As the patient deteriorates, there is an even greater need to ensure that the symptoms are well controlled and the patient and family are supported. The final deterioration may be short; of the hospice patients studied, 40% deteriorated over a period of <12 hours (O'Brien et al., 1992). The commonest course of the disease is development of a respiratory infection with increased secretions and increasing respiratory distress (if untreated), and death from respiratory failure. A smaller proportion of patients have acute respiratory failure, with a sudden deterioration in respiration and death occurring within minutes.

Anticipation of any potential problems is essential. It is important to ensure that all the team caring for the patient are aware of the changes and that medication is easily available for any emergency. Oral medication may be possible until close to death, but if swallowing deteriorates parenteral medication may be necessary. The Motor Neurone Disease Association has developed the Breathing Space Programme to help patients at this time. The Breathing Space Kit is a box containing the necessary injections for use in emergency, together with a leaflet on their use. The patient and family can discuss the use of the Kit with their own doctor, who can then prescribe the medication so that it is immediately available at home if there is an episode of pain, breathlessness or choking.

Terminal care and respite care are discussed further in Ellershaw (1993), Ellershaw et al. (1993) and Hicks & Corcoran (1993). With careful symptom control and support of the patient and family, patients are able to die peacefully.

The Motor Neurone Disease Association

The MND Association acts as a support and information service as well as funding research. It publishes a number of leaflets, for the patient and the family as well as for professionals involved in care. Regional support groups for patients and carers are available throughout the UK. There is also a 24-hour help line and the Association is able to loan equipment (see 'Associations and Support Groups').

CASE HISTORY

Mr G was a 74-year-old married man who had noticed weakness of his left arm while doing DIY in December 1994. The diagnosis of MND was made in May 1995 and he was first visited at home by a doctor and physiotherapist from the hospice in September 1995.

A full assessment showed a very disabled person whose wife was finding the situation very difficult. The power in Mr G's arms ranged from 0 to 2 on the Oxford Scale, the best strength being in the right elbow. All joint movements were restricted by pain. The legs were also weak; the left hip flexors had only a flicker of movement but the right leg was stronger. There was some oedema of the right hand and lower legs. He required assistance from two people to stand and walking was impossible. Chest expansion was reduced and he needed help for all personal care, feeding, transfers and even wiping his nose. He was unable to change his position in bed at night. He had received only limited help from a physiotherapist, occupational therapist and speech therapist early after diagnosis. His main carer was his 75-year-old wife who was 'desperate'. The District Nurse visited weekly and carers came twice a day to help him out of and into bed.

It was agreed that he would be admitted to the hospice for 2 weeks for respite care and assessment. A reclining wheelchair was provided and a regular programme of active and passive movements started as a daily exercise regimen to mobilise joints and maximise ability. A page turner allowed him to read unassisted. He talked about his deterioration and manner of death with the physiotherapist during one of these treatments. After a meeting of the family it was decided that he would remain at the hospice.

A lumbar cushion and head support cushion were necessary in the wheelchair and a non-slip mat prevented his feet slipping from the foot rests. As he tended to fall forwards it was suggested that the wheelchair should be reclined further but he refused this. By October the chair was reclined twice a day for rest periods, but as it was difficult to drink and eat in the reclined position, it could not be reclined for longer. Throughout this time he continued to have regular physiotherapy with a regular exercise programme.

Joint pain was a problem, so a non-steroidal anti-inflammatory drug was commenced. This helped initially but the pain became more pronounced and on 19th October morphine elixir 2.5 mg was started at night. After further difficult nights, morphine sulphate modified release tablets were started at night. The nights improved but he continued to deteriorate, and swallowing and speech became more difficult. The exercise programme continued.

By 6th December a hoist was tried as this would soon be necessary to move him but he did not like it. His voice was very weak and there was severe oedema of the legs and Tubigrip bandages were used. On 13th December his chest expansion was very poor and morphine was increased due to increasing pain. He continued to deteriorate: his speech was very difficult to understand and chest expansion was hardly perceptible; the accessory muscles of respiration were being used. On 6th January a communication chart was supplied. He was tearful at times. However, the exercise programme continued.

On 9th January 1996 the physiotherapist was asked by the nursing staff for help as Mr G could not transfer due to his knees giving way. After discussion with Mr G, he agreed reluctantly to the use of the hoist, as he preferred to be in the chair. He was unable to swallow and said he was not hungry and did not feel the need to eat. His wife needed increasing support and was seen by a social worker.

On 11th January he was very weak but still insisted on getting up and having exercises. He eventually returned to bed. He was only able to take a little fluid by syringe. A subcutaneous infusion, using a syringe driver, was used for analgesia. Mr G died peacefully during the night.

This case history illustrates the rapid decline in power and function, and the many measures needed to assist in comfort and positioning. It also shows the involvement of the physiotherapist in the daily management of a person with advancing MND and how one patient was committed to his daily exercise regimen.

REFERENCES

Brooke A, Steiner TJ. Physiotherapy in the management of patients with motor neurone disease. Report to the Motor Neurone Disease Association (personal communication) 1989.

Burford K, Pentland B. Management of motor neurone disease: the physiotherapist's role. *Physiotherapy* 1985, **71**:402-404.

Ellershaw J. Motor neurone disease, Part 1. *Pall Care Today* 1993, II(II):25-26.

Ellershaw J, Deeson A, O'Gorman B. Motor neurone disease, Part 2. *Pall Care Today* 1993, II(IV): 52-53.

Figlewicz DA, Rouleau GA. Familial disease. In: Williams AC, ed. *Motor neuron disease*. London: Chapman & Hall; 1994:427-450.

Henke E. Motor neurone disease - a patient's view. *Br Med J* 1980, **4**:765-766.

Hicks F, Corcoran G. Should hospices offer respite admissions to patients with motor neurone disease? *Pall Med* 1993, **7**:145-150.

Holden T. Patiently speaking. *Nurs Times* 1980, **76**:1035-1036.

Hough A. *Physiotherapy in respiratory care*. London: Chapman & Hall; 1991.

Langton Hewer R. The management of motor neurone disease. In: Leigh PN, Swash M, eds. *Motor neurone disease: biology and management*. London: Springer Verlag; 1995:391-393.

McAteer MF. Some aspects of grief in physiotherapy. *Physiotherapy* 1989, **75**;55-58.

McAteer MF. Reactions to terminal illness. *Physiotherapy* 1990, 76:9-12.

O'Brien T, Kelly M, Saunders C. Motor neurone disease - a hospice perspective. *Br Med J* 1992, **304**:471-473.

O'Gorman B, O'Brien T. Motor neurone disease. In: Saunders C, ed. *Hospice and palliative care: An interdisciplinary approach*. London: Edward Arnold; 1990:41-45.

Oliver D. Ethical issues in palliative care - an overview. *Pall Med* 1993, **7**(Suppl 2):15-20.

Oliver D. *Motor neurone disease, 2nd edition*. Exeter: Royal College of General Practitioners; 1994.

Oliver D. *Motor neurone disease: A family affair*. London: Sheldon Press; 1995.

Rawlings JK, Allison SP. Nutritional support. In: Williams AC, ed. *Motor neurone disease*. London: Chapman & Hall; 1994:265-279.

Rosen AD. Amyotrophic lateral sclerosis. *Arch Neurol* 1978, **35**:638-642.

Rosen DR, Siddique T, Patterson D, *et al.* Mutations in Cu/Zn superoxide dismutase gene are associated with familial amyotrophic lateral sclerosis. *Nature* 1993, **362**:59-62.

Saunders C, Walsh TD, Smith M. Hospice care in motor neurone disease. In: Saunders C, Summers DH, Teller N, eds. *Hospice: The living idea*. London: Edward Arnold; 1981:126-147.

Schwartz MS, Swash M. Neurophysiological changes in motor neurone disease. In: Leigh PN, Swash M, eds. *Motor neurone disease: biology and management*. London: Springer Verlag; 1995:331-344.

Scott AG, Austin HE. Nasogastric feeding in the management of severe dysphagia in motor neurone disease. *Pall Med* 1994, **8**:45-49.

Summers DH. The caring team in motor neurone disease. In: Saunders C, Summers DH, Teller N, eds. *Hospice: The living idea*. London: Edward Arnold; 1981:148-155.

Swash M, Schwartz MS. Motor neurone disease: the clinical syndrome. In: Leigh PN, Swash M, eds. *Motor neurone disease: biology and management*. London: Springer Verlag; 1995:1-17.

Tandan R. Clinical features and differential diagnosis of classical motor neurone disease. In: Williams AC, ed. *Motor neurone disease*. London: Chapman & Hall; 1994:3-27.

Unsworth J. Coping with the disability of established disease. In: Williams AC, ed. *Motor neurone disease*. London: Chapman & Hall; 1994:231-234.

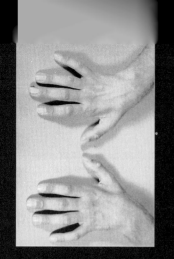

15 J Nicklin

DISORDERS OF NERVE II: POLYNEUROPATHIES

CHAPTER OUTLINE

- Pathological processes affecting peripheral nerves
- Classification of polyneuropathies
- Assessment and diagnostic investigations
- Treatment
- Case History

INTRODUCTION

The term polyneuropathies refers to the group of disorders where the peripheral nerves are affected by one or more pathological process, resulting in motor, sensory, and/or autonomic symptoms. Generally these symptoms are diffuse, symmetrical and predominantly distal. Muscle weakness may be confined distally or may be more extensive in chronic cases. The range of sensory symptoms covers the spectrum from complete loss of sensation to mild tingling to unbearable painful dysaesthesia.

Autonomic dysfunction, such as disturbances of blood pressure, can be present in some of the polyneuropathies, e.g. diabetic neuropathy. Most neuropathies are slowly progressive, the deterioration occurring in a step-wise fashion, or as a continuous downward progression.

For the physiotherapist, patients with a polyneuropathy present a challenge best managed using a problem-solving approach. In this chapter, the range of polyneuropathies will be described and a case presentation given to illustrate some of the issues confronted in these conditions. Mononeuropathies and neuropathies due to trauma are not included. The anatomy and neurophysiology of the neurone has been described in Chapter 1.

PATHOLOGICAL PROCESSES AFFECTING PERIPHERAL NERVES

Pathological processes affecting the peripheral nerves are defined according to which structures are involved: the axon (axonopathy); the Schwann cell that produces the myelin sheath (myelinopathy); or the nerve cell body (neuronopathy).

AXONOPATHIES

Interruption to the axon results in axonopathy. All metabolic processes occur in the cell body, which supports the axon, and if axonal transport of nutrition fails the axon dies back from the distal end. Surviving axons will conduct at a normal rate but, because of the reduced number, will be less effective in producing a muscle contraction. Early loss of the ankle jerk is seen because the longest, large-diameter fibres, such as those to the leg muscles of the posterior compartment, are the most vulnerable to axonopathy. This process underlies most metabolic and hereditary neuropathies and leads to long-term disability. Regeneration is slow, at 2–3 mm per day (Schaumburg *et al.*, 1992).

MYELINOPATHIES

When the Schwann cell that produces myelin is damaged, nerve conduction is slowed. Normally the impulse is conducted by jumping from node to node (saltatory conduction), which is extremely fast. The internodes (area between nodes) become longer where myelin has been destroyed and the impulse is conducted comparatively slowly along this part of the nerve fibre. If several adjacent segments of nerve become demyelinated, the effect is magnified and this can result in complete block of nerve conduction in that particular axon (Hopkins, 1993). This leads to the clinical manifestations of weakness and fatigue. Remyelin-ation can occur, producing shorter sections of myelination.

NEURONOPATHIES

Once the cell body is damaged, recovery is unlikely. Either the sensory or motor nerves can be affected. Motor neurone disease is one example of a neuronopathy (see Chapter 14).

Once the nerve is affected by one of the above processes, it is at greater risk of entrapment or pressure. Severe disability may predispose to prolonged pressure, e.g. at the fibula head, but entrapment neuropathies occur despite adequate cushioning, suggesting other processes (de Jager & Minderhoud, 1991). Focal neuropathies (see Table 15.1) affecting one nerve may be replicated in several nerves over time and come to resemble a polyneuropathy. This picture is seen where ischaemia occurs to the nerve, as in polyarteritis.

CLASSIFICATION OF POLYNEUROPATHIES

The neuropathies are broadly divided into acquired and inherited types. Many of the named neuropathies are rare and will not be discussed in great detail in this chapter. However, the principles of assessment and treatment remain the same. For greater detail, consult the definitive reference book by Dyck & Thomas (1993).

ACQUIRED NEUROPATHIES

Table 15.1 shows the classification of acquired neuropathies, which may be generalised or focal.

Metabolic Neuropathies

The peripheral nerves are vulnerable to disorders affecting their metabolism and this gives rise to the largest group of neuropathies.

Diabetic Neuropathy

This is the commonest form of neuropathy in developed countries and is becoming more common with an increase in the ageing population and hence in the prevalence of diabetes (Mitchell, 1991). The prevalence of neuropathy rises from 7.5% at diagnosis of diabetes to 50% after 25 years (Pirart, 1978). The patterns of neuropathy seen are distal symmetrical sensory neuropathy and proximal motor neuropathy.

Distal symmetrical sensory neuropathy—This is the most common presentation, producing weakness and sensory impairment in the feet. These sensory symptoms range from numbness to an aching pain. The discomfort is often worse at night (Thomas & Thomlinson, 1993). Occasionally, the loss of joint positional sense can be severe, leading to sensory ataxia. Loss of deep pain sense and ischaemia increase the risk of chronic foot ulceration. Weakness of intrinsic foot muscles produces changes in foot alignment and distribution of pressure when weight-bearing. Diabetic ulcers can be prevented with careful checking of the skin and attention to footwear. Where necessary, footwear may need to be individually tailored to prevent pressure (see 'Orthoses').

Proximal motor neuropathy—This is seen predominantly in elderly diabetics. The weakness and wasting are asymmetrical and affect most often the iliopsoas, quadriceps and hip adductor muscles. Pain can be severe, especially at

Classification of acquired neuropathies	
Symmetrical generalised neuropathies	
Metabolic:	Diabetes In renal disease In alcoholism Vitamin deficiencies
Inflammatory:	Guillain-Barré syndrome (acute) Chronic Inflammatory Demyelinating Polyneuropathy
Drug/Toxin-induced:	Antineoplastic Antirheumatic n-Hexane Acrylamide Tri-orthocresyl Phosphate
Associated with malignant disease:	Carcinoma of the breast, lung, colon
Associated with monoclonal disease:	Paraproteinaemias
Infection:	Leprosy HIV Diphtheria
Focal or multifocal neuropathies	
Collagen vascular disease:	Polyarteritis nodosa Systemic lupus erythematosus Rheumatoid arthritis

Table 15.1 Classification of acquired neuropathies.

night. Recovery normally follows better control of the diabetes but may take months and may not be complete. Pain is the most distressing symptom for the patient. Drugs such as phenytoin and antidepressants have been used with varying success (Thomas & Thomlinson, 1993).

Renal Disease

A symmetrical distal motor and sensory neuropathy that affects the legs more than the arms is associated with chronic renal failure. Uraemic patients often complain of 'restless legs', i.e. their legs are continuously moving and uncomfortable in bed. Dialysis or transplantation causes the neuropathy to stabilise or improve (Hopkins, 1993).

Alcoholism

Neuropathy can occur as a result of long-term alcohol abuse. Weakness of the lower limbs progresses from the feet proximally but can usually be detected in all the lower limb muscles to a variable degree. Muscle pain (myalgia) and unpleasant dysaesthesiae are common. The major reason for the neuropathy is thought to be nutritional deficiencies, and possibly the effect of alcohol on the nerve (Asbury & Bird, 1992). However, Monforte et al. (1995) demonstrated a significant correlation between the total time a patient had been drinking excessively and the presence of a neuropathy, and no correlation with nutritional status. The risk of an autonomic neuropathy also increased with duration of alcoholism, leading to changes in heart responses to exercise. Ataxia is seen in people with chronic alcoholism but this can be attributed to specific cerebellar damage as much as to sensory loss (Thompson & Day, 1993).

Vitamin Deficiencies

Neuropathies can appear with a poorly balanced diet without starvation. Nutritional deficiency in western countries is seen in some forms of dieting, malabsorption and anorexia nervosa. In the Third World, nutritional polyneuropathy is commonly a result of dietary deprivation. Beriberi is one example still common in countries where people live mainly on a diet of highly milled rice. This is due to the specific lack of thiamine in the diet.

The motor sensory neuropathy starts distally but progresses to affect more proximal musculature. Cardiac involvement is common. It is often difficult to define exactly which vitamins are lacking in the diet. Treatment generally consists of multivitamin supplements in a balanced diet (Windebank, 1993). Foot drop may persist for many months following initiation of treatment (Schaumburg et al., 1992).

Inflammatory Demyelinating Polyneuropathies

Demyelination is the primary pathological process in this group. Axonal degeneration can be a feature and if it occurs it results in the more serious clinical manifestations sometimes seen in Guillain–Barré syndrome (Feasby, 1992). There are two forms of these neuropathies, one acute and the other chronic. Both are considered autoimmune disorders.

Acute Inflammatory Demyelinating Polyneuropathy: Guillain-Barré Syndrome

The prevalence of Guillain–Barré syndrome (GBS) has been reported as 0.5–4.0 per 100,000 (Sridharan et al., 1993). Most commonly leg weakness is noted first (Ropper et al., 1991). Often this progresses proximally and can involve all muscle groups including those of the upper limb, trunk and face.

Many patients will have experienced a respiratory tract or gastric infection in the weeks preceding muscle weakness. Immunisation and surgery have also been cited as precipitating factors (Hartung et al., 1995). In order to be classified as GBS, the time from onset to peak disability (i.e. nadir) should be <4 weeks. Studies have shown that 50% of patients will reach nadir within 2 weeks (Asbury & Cornblath, 1990).

Some patients become fully paralysed at the height of the illness. Nearly 50% of patients have facial weakness. Frequently the bulbar muscle groups are affected sufficiently to require nasogastric feeding to avoid aspiration. Paralysis of the respiratory muscles, causing the vital capacity to fall to <15 mm/kg, occurs in 30% of patients. Elective ventilation is indicated in this situation (Ng et al., 1995). Autonomic dysfunction occurs in some more severe cases and can lead to sudden unexpected mortalities, normally because of cardiac arrhythmias (McLeod, 1992).

GBS is predominantly a motor neuropathy but 42–75% of patients have some alteration in sensation (Pentland & Donald, 1994). Winer et al. (1988) found that joint positional sense was absent in the toes of 52% of patients. Pain is a frequent feature that appears very early in the disorder (Asbury, 1990). It has been postulated that the inflamed and tightened neural structures that occur in the acute stage may be the source of the pain (Simionato et al., 1988). During recovery, it is suggested that pain may be due to abnormal forces on joints, poorly protected by weakened muscles (Pentland & Donald, 1994).

Recovery generally begins within a month of nadir and has the potential to be complete, provided secondary omplications, such as contractures, are avoided. However, a percentage of patients with GBS do not make a full recovery. deJager & Minderhoud (1991) found that 37% of patients with GBS could not perform at the same physical level as prior to their illness at least 2 years after the nadir.

Periarticular contractures are one major cause of residual disability but there are few studies of their incidence, cause and prevention (Soryal et al., 1992). Physiotherapy is noted as important to prevent contractures (Ropper et al. 1991; Soryal et al., 1992) but this has not been researched. A case history of a GBS patient is given at the end of this chapter.

The Miller Fisher syndrome is a variant of GBS. The classic features are ataxia, ophthalmoplegia (causing double vision) and areflexia (Berlit & Rakicky, 1992). Diplopia and ataxia are the commonest first symptoms. Severe weakness is less common in Miller Fisher syndrome but when evident it may mask the ataxia.

Chronic Inflammatory Demyelinating Polyneuropathy (CIDP)

This chronic form of polneuropathy occurs mainly in the fifth or sixth decade of life. Sensory loss is more apparent in CIDP than in GBS. It is also differentiated from GBS by a longer time course to nadir, >4 weeks, developing over longer time periods in the majority of cases. Most patients have foot drop severe enough to require ankle–foot orthoses (AFOs). Fine hand control and grip may also be impaired. Autonomic dysfunction is uncommon (McLeod, 1992). Most cases are slowly progressive but some follow a relapsing–remitting course (Albers & Kelly, 1989); patients tend to have a more favourable prognosis if in the latter group (Ropper et al., 1991). Most will remain able to walk with aids but a few become dependent on a wheelchair.

Toxin- or Drug-Induced Polyneuropathies

There are many industrial and agricultural chemicals which can produce neuropathies. Adhesives and their solvents can cause an axonal neuropathy which may be seen in industrial or agricultural workers and in solvent-abusers.

Adulterated rapeseed oil caused a notorious epidemic of peripheral neuropathy in Spain in 1981. Ingestion of the oil resulted in severe axonopathy, and there were a number of deaths (Schaumburg et al., 1992). Organophosphates used in agriculture have been implicated in cases of peripheral neuropathies. The effect of a toxin does not arrest once the cause is removed; rather, the symptoms progress over weeks or months due to continuing axonal degeneration (Schaumburg et al., 1992). Because the damage is generally axonal, the symptoms are often severe and only partially reversible.

Drug groups that are known to carry the risk of neuropathic side effects include antirheumatic, antineoplastic, antimicrobial and anticonvulsant medication. Ceasing the drug has variable results.

Neuropathies Associated with Malignant Disease

Compression and infiltration of nerve roots by neoplasms is common. Less frequently, polyneuropathies may occur as a remote effect of carcinoma of the lung, stomach or breast (Schaumburg et al., 1992). Sensory symptoms predominate, with motor symptoms developing much later. The features can appear between 6 months and 3 years prior to the detection of a tumour. Tumours of the peripheral nerve do occur, the majority of which are benign. In schwannomas (tumours arising from the Schwann cell), pain is always the predominant feature. Sensory or motor loss is rarely seen.

Neuropathies Associated with Monoclonal Disease

γ-globulins are plasma proteins associated with antibody activity in the immune system. In paraproteinaemias, excessive amounts of γ-globulins are present in the blood, often associated with reduced immune activity. They act to attack the myelin sheath (Albers & Kelly, 1989). IgM is the most common γ-globulin; excess IgM produces a mixed sensorimotor neuropathy which appears in the sixth decade or later in life. Tremor and ataxia are frequently seen. These are distressing symptoms, which greatly affect hand function, particularly as tremor is worse on activity. Other γ-globulins present in neuropathies are IgG and IgA.

Neuropathies Associated with Infection and Infestation

Neuropathy occurs with infections of the nervous system, and can involve both sensory and motor nerves.

Leprosy

Leprosy is the most common cause of peripheral neuropathy in the world and is caused by infection with *Mycobacterium leprae* (Hopkins, 1993). Sensory loss is a cardinal feature. Nerves become enlarged in response to invasion by bacteria and eventually, in addition to widespread sensory loss, motor loss becomes evident. Weakness of the intrinsic hand muscles is often noted first.

Human Immunodeficiency Virus (HIV)

A distal symmetrical polyneuropathy is detectable in over a third of patients infected with HIV who have developed acquired immune deficiency syndrome (AIDS). Most complain of a burning sensation in their feet, particularly at night (Simpson & Olney, 1992). A motor neuropathy is also seen and can look like GBS (Schaumburg et al. 1992). A multidisciplinary approach to managing this patient group is recommended (McClure, 1993).

Neuropathies Associated with Collagen Vascular Disease

Single or multifocal ischaemia of nerves may follow occlusion of small blood vessels to the nerves. The symptoms—pain, loss of strength and sensation—occur suddenly. Repeated episodes lead to a symmetrical and predominantly distal polyneuropathy. Two thirds of all patients with polyarteritis will develop a mononeuropathy that may proceed as detailed above (Schaumburg et al., 1992). In rheumatoid arthritis, compression neuropathies are common. A mild sensory polyneuropathy is sometimes seen. Systemic lupus erythematosus (SLE) may be associated with neuropathy of variable presentation.

INHERITED NEUROPATHIES

The inherited neuropathies are listed in Table 15.2 and the metabolic abnormality, where known, is given.

Hereditary Motor and Sensory Neuropathy

This is also known as Charcot–Marie–Tooth disease or Peroneal Muscular Atrophy. Most hereditary motor and sensory neuropathies (HMSNs) are inherited in an autosomal dominant fashion. The abnormal gene is located on chromosome 17 and the disorder results from a duplication of part of it. The most common forms are: type I, a predominantly demyelinating form; and type II, an axonal disorder. The symptoms are similar for the two forms but

Classification of inherited neuropathies	
Unknown metabolic defect	**Known metabolic deficit**
Hereditary motor sensory neuropathy:	Porphyria
Type I (Charcot-Marie-Tooth disease)	
Type II	Refsum disease
Type III (Dejerine-Sottas)	Leucodystrophy
Hereditary sensory neuropathy:	
Types I–IV	
Amyloidoses	

Table 15.2 Classification of inherited neuropathies.

they generally appear at a younger age in type I (Harding, 1993).

Initial symptoms are pes cavus, loss of tendon reflexes, and clumsiness of gait. This clumsiness is partly due to increasing weakness of the muscles in the peroneal compartment and sensory changes in the feet (also seen in the hands). This muscle imbalance leads to the characteristic high stepping gait and increasing foot deformities seen in this group. If sensory loss is severe, patients rely on visual information for regulation of postural control. When standing, they show more postural sway in the fore–aft direction than normal, which is due to distal weakness and deformities affecting the ankle strategy of controlling sway (Geurts et al., 1992). The lower leg takes on a stalk-like appearance because of peroneal wasting. Cramps and paraesthesiae are common early symptoms. The combination of deformity of the foot and changes in sensation predisposes patients with HMSN to tissue damage, which may lead to ulceration.

Surgical intervention to correct the deformity of high arches and/or very flexed toes with hyperextension of the metatarsophalangeal joints includes arthrodesis. However, early and appropriate provision of orthoses may make surgery unnecessary. Generally, patients with HMSN remain walking, albeit with orthoses and aids such as sticks. In some patients, particularly with type II HMSN, the disorder is more progressive and wheelchairs are needed.

The diaphragm is involved in some cases. Vital capacity should be measured in lying and sitting and will be much lower in the reclining position where the diaphragm is involved. Other symptoms may include orthopnoea, morning headaches and general fatigue. These need to be investigated further because nocturnal ventilatory support may be necessary to alleviate the symptoms (Hardie et al., 1990).

With the discovery of the genetic defect in these types of neuropathies, genetic counselling is possible and very important. Prenatal testing is available in some specialist centres but its use remains controversial.

Hereditary Sensory Neuropathy

Hereditary sensory neuropathies are inherited in a dominant fashion and affect the sensory nerves. Trophic changes occur in the hands and feet and may lead to severe ulcers and loss of digits. In another form, there is additional loss of unmyelinated fibres that produces insensitivity to pain. There may also be involvement of the autonomic system and this condition is termed sensory autonomic neuropathy.

Other Forms of Inherited Neuropathy

Most other forms are very rare. In acute episodes of porphyria, a proximal motor neuropathy appears with rapid wasting of affected muscle groups; the neuropathy can be severe enough to warrant ventilation.

ASSESSMENT AND DIAGNOSTIC INVESTIGATIONS

Principles of clinical examination by the neurologist and physiotherapist are described in Chapters 3 & 4. Features of assessment that are particularly important for the polyneuropathies are discussed below.

ELECTROPHYSIOLOGICAL TESTS

Electromyography (EMG) is important for differentiating between a demyelinating and an axonal process. The effect of an axonopathy is permanent because of the greater difficulty in repair of the axon. The presence of axonal changes in GBS is considered a poor prognostic indicator, although there are cases that confound this axiom (Feasby, 1994).

GENETIC TESTING AND COUNSELLING

Genes for the inherited neuropathies can be identified by DNA (deoxyribonucleic acid) testing (Harding, 1995). Once a patient is shown to have the gene, counselling can be offered and the implications for other family members discussed. Prenatal testing can identify a fetus at risk of developing an inherited neuropathy and give the parents

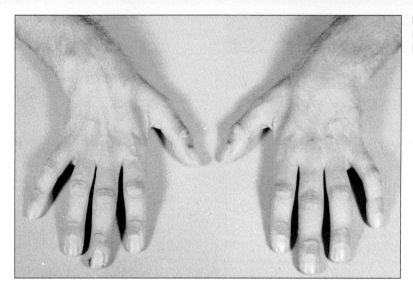

Figure 15.1 Typical wasting of small hand muscles as seen in chronic neuropathies.

the option of termination. However, testing does not predict the severity of the neuropathy as an adult, and approximately 20% of patients will be asymptomatic.

OBSERVATION

Analysis of movement, and observation of the condition and shape of muscle contours, is essential as part of the problem-solving approach. Wasting of the intrinsic hand muscles may be noted (Figure 15.1), leading to clumsiness in gripping a cup or difficulty manipulating small items such as bottle tops. If the patient displays this kind of functional difficulty, the therapist should also consider what role sensory changes play in the problem.

Muscle imbalance will lead to shortening of unopposed muscle groups (Mann & Missirian, 1988). The intrinsic foot and the anterior leg compartment musculature are most commonly affected and foot deformities may result.

GAIT ASSESSMENT

Distal weakness, more marked in the dorsiflexors than the plantaflexors, will lead to a tendency to trip and a compensatory high stepping gait. As the quadriceps muscles weaken, hyperextension occurs at the knees to produce a rigid structure when weight-bearing . Proximal muscle weakness, especially in the hip abductors, gives rise to a positive Trendelenberg sign in more severely affected patients. Gait analysis laboratories, pressure transducers coupled with EMG, and video recordings (Mueller *et al.*, 1994) are all useful for analysing movement and for objective comparison over time. However, little research has been published on the neuropathic gait.

MUSCLE STRENGTH TESTING

Grading strength 0–5, using an ordinal scale such as the Medical Research Council (MRC) scale, is inadequate (see Chapter 4). Whilst this semiquantitative scale will give a global clinical picture, it does not allow for accurate comparisons over time. Measurement is recommended using

an interval scale such as that produced by isokinetic or isometric equipment (see Chapter 4). These approaches are sensitive enough to detect changes where the strength may not change in grade on the manual testing scale, although improving or deteriorating. This is particularly relevant for muscles measuring Grade 4. For instance, 90% of the range of muscle strength available in the biceps muscle falls in Grade 4 (Munsat, 1990). Change is not recorded in the most relevant part of the range if one relies solely on the MRC scale. A hand-held myometer has been shown to be sensitive and reliable in assessing neuropathies (Wiles *et al.*, 1990), in particular GBS (Bohannon & Dubuc, 1984; Karni *et al.*, 1984). Positions for testing, commands and techniques must be standardised. Some authors have pointed out the need for frequent testing of inter-examiner reliability and have shown that one examiner performing repeated tests is more desirable than having several different examiners (Lennon & Ashburn, 1993).

Weakness of the hand muscles can best be assessed and monitored using a grip dynamometer. This is often a very sensitive measure in the distal motor neuropathies. Reference values are available for many muscle groups, including hand grip and pinch grip (Wiles *et al.*, 1990; van de Ploeg *et al.*, 1991). This allows the degree of weakness to be compared to the normal range and expressed as a percentage of the lower limit of normal. The most sensitive measure of strength change is achieved if the assessment method mirrors the type of exercise used in a regimen, e.g. measurements of isokinetically gained strength should be made using an isokinetic device.

FATIGUE TESTING

There is a subgroup of patients with neuropathies who have difficulties with fatigue. The fatigue may be of a global nature, i.e. getting tired writing letters or walking distances; there is also a more specific variety that affects the actual contraction of a muscle. Timed tests give the best indication of endurance and are most appropriate to physiotherapy practice (Cook & Glass, 1987). These are discussed under 'Functional assessment' and in Chapter 4. However, endurance tests are dependent on motivation, and feedback is essential.

Fatigue diaries are a good way of analysing more generalised fatigue where over-work is suspected. The patient is asked to keep a diary documenting activities and length of time performing each one. In addition, symptoms of fatigue are noted. The diary may then be analysed, to try and develop a structure to the patient's activities that prevents severe fatigue, but does not lead to the opposite problem of weakness from disuse by cutting out all activity that causes any degree of fatigue.

SENSORY TESTING

Although subjective sensory testing is unreliable, it is important to note the extent and distribution of sensory loss or impairment. Some attempts have been made to devise grading scales which combine motor and sensory changes, but they have not yet been validated (Dellon, 1993).

FUNCTIONAL ASSESSMENT

In the majority of neuropathies functional changes are subtle and gradual, such that a very sensitive objective measure is required. Appropriate timed tests are a useful indicator of change (Moxley, 1990), particularly up and down a standardised set of stairs or a timed 10-metre (Watson & Wilson, 1992) or 30-metre walk (Nicklin, unpublished data). The longer distance is preferred because it is only over this extended walk that change is shown, probably due to fatigue (Cook & Glass, 1987). In the case of GBS, the possible changes in performance cover many varied areas, e.g. ability to breath independently through to ability to run. A performance indicator must be employed that can demonstrate these large changes but also capture more subtle changes (Karni *et al.*, 1984). Dyck *et al.* (1995) used ability to rise from a chair and standing on heels in their study of diabetic neuropathy.

Whilst the use of an outcome measure involving function is both desirable and necessary to assess disability, the therapist must be aware that changes in the score may occur as a result of compensation as opposed to changes in strength, and that a change in sensation may have a significant effect, particularly on fine hand function. Another factor may be increasing body weight, particularly affecting activities such as rising from the floor or climbing stairs.

TREATMENT

A multidisciplinary problem-solving approach is recommended in the management of disability in order to maximise function, and an example of this approach is illustrated in the case history below. A proposed structure for a problem-solving approach is given in relation to stroke in Chapter 7. Where a problem-solving approach is taken, many members of the MDT may be involved. However, it must be recognised that the number of health workers involved in a patient's care may be bewildering. For this reason, the use of a key-worker system is recommended to improve communication and reduce anxiety.

PRINCIPLES OF PHYSIOTHERAPY INTERVENTION

A scientific basis for much of physiotherapy in this specialty has not been demonstrated and there is a paucity of research in this field. Therapy can be management of problems that cannot be reversed or treatment where improvement is possible, but should always address specific problems identified during assessment.

Acute Neuropathies

Important aspects of physical management in acute neuropathies include: prevention of contractures; control of pain; and respiratory care.

Stretching to Prevent Contractures

Neuropathy may result in severe disability whereby the patient is bed-bound. Prevention of contractures and musculoskeletal stiffness is a priority if maximum potential is to be achieved. When muscles are not stretched adequately but are left in a shortened position, structural changes, involving loss of sarcomeres, occur and compromise potential recovery (see Chapter 25). The therapist should ensure that all structures, including the nervous system, are moved through their full range. Adverse neural tension (ANT) signs can occur if neural tissues are not stretched and this concept is discussed in Chapter 23. Wherever possible, the patient should be encouraged to join in with the movement and use what is still available. Using a continuous passive motion machine has been suggested (Mays, 1990) as a means to maintain ROM. Tightening of the posterior crural muscle group develops rapidly. This is nearly always preventable in neuropathy. In the bed-bound patient, foot drop splints should be provided and gentle stretches performed. More able patients should be taught self stretches in a weight-bearing position.

Positioning

Truncal weakness can cause the patient to lie with scapulae retracted, unless a wedge is positioned under the thoracic region as well as the head and shoulders. The pelvis should be supported in a position of posterior tilt with the hip flexors stretched, to prevent shortening. Positioning by nurses and physiotherapists can help prevent pressure neuropathies, e.g. at the medial epicondyle or fibula head (Watson & Wilson, 1989), though these can occur spontaneously.

Pain

The therapist should be aware of the existence of pain and liaise with the medical team to provide effective management (see Chapter 26). Pain is an early symptom in acute neuropathy such as GBS (Ropper *et al.*, 1991) but has never been satisfactorily explained. Many patients demonstrate pain from adverse neural tension (see Chapter 23). Some therapists, including Freeman (1992), have suggested that the reason why patients with acute GBS enjoy large-amplitude mid-range movements is because of their pain-relieving properties. This accords with the findings of Butler who gives two examples of mobilising the nervous system in GBS (Butler, 1991). In other neuropathies, massage and ice packs have been found to be helpful.

Respiratory Care
In some instances the patient may be ventilated and the role of the physiotherapist is to help prevent atelectasis when breathing is compromised (Smith & Ball, 1998).

Where the autonomic system is affected, disturbed blood pressure is of particular relevance to the physiotherapist, especially when using suction (Ng et al. 1995) or when attempting early sitting (Ropper et al., 1991). It is therefore essential to monitor vulnerable patients.

Chronic Neuropathies
The role of the physiotherapist is largely one of management in chronic cases. Early referrals are important to advise on activities to maintain ambulation and prevent avoidable complications such as foot deformities (see also 'Orthoses').

Strengthening Exercises
Historically, there has always been a wariness of giving muscle strengthening exercises to patients with neuromuscular diseases. This arose out of several anecdotal papers (e.g. Bennett & Knowlton, 1958). More recently there have been papers supporting the use of exercise to improve strength or endurance (Aitkens et al., 1993; Lindeman et al., 1995; Rutland & Shields, 1997). Kilmer et al. (1994) found that high-resistance exercise was no better than low-resistance exercise for strengthening muscle and there was some evidence of damage when tested eccentrically. Most research on exercise in neuromuscular disorders has used a heterogeneous group and it is difficult to generalise results to specific polyneuropathies (Aitkens et al., 1993; Milner Brown et al., 1988).

Some authors have suggested concentrating on exercising the hip and knee, not the more severely affected distal muscle groups, in order to compensate and produce a more stable gait pattern (Mueller et al., 1994). The addition of an AFO would also increase stability by allowing the development of plantarflexor movement, despite very weak muscles, as well as preventing tripping. Compliance with an exercise regimen is variable and improvement is often gradual. A successful adjunct to face-to-face sessions with the physiotherapist is an exercise diary for recording both changing symptoms and amount and quality of exercise (Lindeman et al., 1995). Of particular relevance is the noting of abnormally prolonged muscle ache following exercise, or sudden loss of functional ability. This may indicate damage from overuse. These symptoms should be noted and exercise modified to allow recovery.

The effect of exercise should be explained to the patient, including the possibility that the rate of deterioration may be reduced or recovery hastened but without affecting the underlying disorder (Cowan et al., 1993).

The degree of weakness will have an effect on the final outcome. Where muscles are severely weakened, below 10% of the lower limit of normal for that group, the chance of strengthening is slim and exercise could cause further damage to the motor unit (Milner Brown & Miller, 1988).

Anecdotally, patients have been known to lose strength permanently following a bout of unaccustomed exercise such as decorating a room. In contrast, someone with a stable neuropathy may become less active, perhaps due to surgery, and then lose a former ability to perform an everyday function, primarily due to disuse and resulting weakness. Whenever the neuropathic patient becomes bed-bound, for whatever reason, physiotherapy is essential to facilitate functional recovery. Atrophy following disuse is preventable by specific exercises for identified muscle groups.

Where weakness is severe, it may be necessary to explore ways of maximising function through compensatory techniques. Generally, those with the slower progressive disorders develop strategies for themselves.

Other Techniques
Ice, massage and vibration are suggested as means to diminish painful chronic sensory neuropathies, particularly in patients with HIV infection. Transcutaneous electrical nerve stimulation may also be helpful. These treatment techniques are discussed in Chapter 24.

FUNCTIONAL AND MOBILITY AIDS
Equipment used to aid function and mobility includes a range of orthoses and wheelchairs.

Orthoses
Where there is an abnormal gait pattern, mainly due to weakness of the dorsiflexors and/or the intrinsic muscles of the feet, the use of orthoses should be considered. Often, by the time a patient is referred to the physiotherapist or orthotist, foot deformities have become irreversible and insoles are necessary to allow the foot to sit comfortably in a standard shoe and to redistribute the weight across the total surface of the sole. Custom-made shoes may be necessary. In the first instance, insoles should be tried prior to using AFOs (Edwards & Charlton, 1996). Where foot drop exists, the option of a lightweight polypropylene splint should be discussed with the patient. Ready-made AFOs can be experimented with first to establish their usefulness. The permanent orthosis should mould to the calf and support the foot at 90 degrees, extending as far as the toes. Where there is poor fit around the leg, there is the risk of chafing and skin damage, and the splint will also be less effective at maintaining the foot at 90 degrees. Unless the forefoot is supported, the long flexors will be able to tighten where they are unopposed and may become contracted.

It is essential to discuss skin care with the patient. Many of those requiring splints will have sensory problems and there is always a risk of pressure areas developing. The patient should take responsibility for daily vigilance of the state of his or her skin. Where there is progressive weakness, muscle wasting will also occur and will lead to the need for remoulding of the splint. The use of any orthoses is an emotive subject and women, in particular, may not like their appearance. Careful explanation and, where possible, video recording of the improved gait attained whilst wearing a splint may help guide the patient's decision. However, there are disadvantages to wearing bilateral AFOs, such as negotiating stairs, and these should be considered when assessing the patient (Edwards & Charlton, 1996).

Hand function is often compromised through weakness or paralysis of intrinsic muscles of the thumb and fingers. The patient notices particular difficulties with the pincer grip. The introduction of a simple thumb opposition splint may allow a patient to produce legible writing for a longer time, or to grip a cup or knife. However, the difficulties of fitting and using a splint must be weighed against the benefits derived from wearing one. Where the thenar eminence becomes severely weak and wasted, a night splint cast in a functional position will help prevent severe contracture.

Wheelchairs

In a minority of cases the neuropathy progresses to render the patient dependent on a wheelchair. Assessment by specialists in posture and seating will lead to provision of appropriate wheelchairs (see Chapter 8). In the early stages of rehabilitating a patient with GBS, a reclining wheelchair is valuable to help cope with possible fluctuations in blood pressure and to allow gradual accommodation to the upright position.

DRUG THERAPY

For the majority of the inflammatory and immune-based neuropathies, the mainstay of drug therapy is steroids and immunosuppressants. Deviations from this have already been mentioned above, as have drugs for pain management (see also Chapters 26 & 28). Immunosuppressants, such as azathioprine, carry the risk of neoplasms but are effective in combination with prednisolone.

PLASMAPHERESIS AND IMMUNOGLOBULIN THERAPY

There are two treatments used for polyneuropathies which have a likely immunological basis. Plasmapheresis (plasma exchange) is an invasive technique whereby the patient's plasma is removed from the blood and treated to remove the antibodies attacking the myelin sheath, before being replaced (Hartung *et al.*, 1995). Several controlled trials have demonstrated the benefits of plasma exchange, particularly in GBS where recovery time was shown to be shortened (Winer *et al.*, 1988).

Immunoglobulin therapy is an alternative to plasmapheresis. The patient is given a booster of immunoglobulin over a period of 1–5 days. In pure motor GBS this has been shown to be possibly more effective in reducing recovery time (Visser *et al.*, 1995). A percentage of patients with CIDP respond to immunoglobulin therapy (van-Doorn,

1994) but the effect gradually fades and patients require repeated treatments to maintain functional level and prevent significant deterioration.

CASE HISTORY: A PATIENT WITH GUILLAIN-BARRÉ SYNDROME

A 31-year-old woman was admitted with a 3-day history of increasing weakness in the legs and paraesthesiae in the hands and feet, following an upper respiratory tract infection. A provisional diagnosis of GBS was made. The problems identified were:

Impairments
1. Generalised motor impairment.
2. Impaired respiratory function.
3. Pain.
4. Reduced distal sensation.
5. Autonomic disturbance.

Disabilities
6. Difficulty in swallowing.
7. Dependent for activities of daily living.
8. Inability to communicate effectively.
9. Anxiety.

The time course for these events is illustrated in Figure 15.2; nadir was reached at 12 days.

A multidisciplinary plan was agreed to address the above problems, and was modified as new problems appeared and others became inactive. At all stages, the patient was encouraged to be fully involved in the planning. Short-term realistic goals with functional significance were used to motivate the patient and provide structure to the problem-solving process. This approach enabled rehabilitation to continue throughout 24 hours with the support of the nurses. Management of each of the problems is discussed below.

1. Generalised Motor Impairment

The motor impairment was the primary cause of problems 2, 6, 7 and 8. Where weakness was profound, especially at nadir, only passive movements were possible. Stretches were included to mobilise the nervous tissue, as well as the muscles and supportive tissues. The nurses and physiotherapist positioned the patient to prevent shortening of muscles and relieve pressure areas, using wedges.

Together, the occupational therapist and physiotherapist made splints to support the feet in a plantigrade position and the hands in flexion at the metacarpophalangeal joints, with abduction of the thumb.

As muscle power began to recover, assisted active movements were performed by the physiotherapist with the patient. Encouragement was given to concentrate on the feeling of movement and join in as possible. Where an imbalance of returning muscle strength around a joint was identified, the physiotherapist encouraged the patient to relax the dominant group and facilitated the weaker group (see Chapter 23, 'Muscle imbalance').

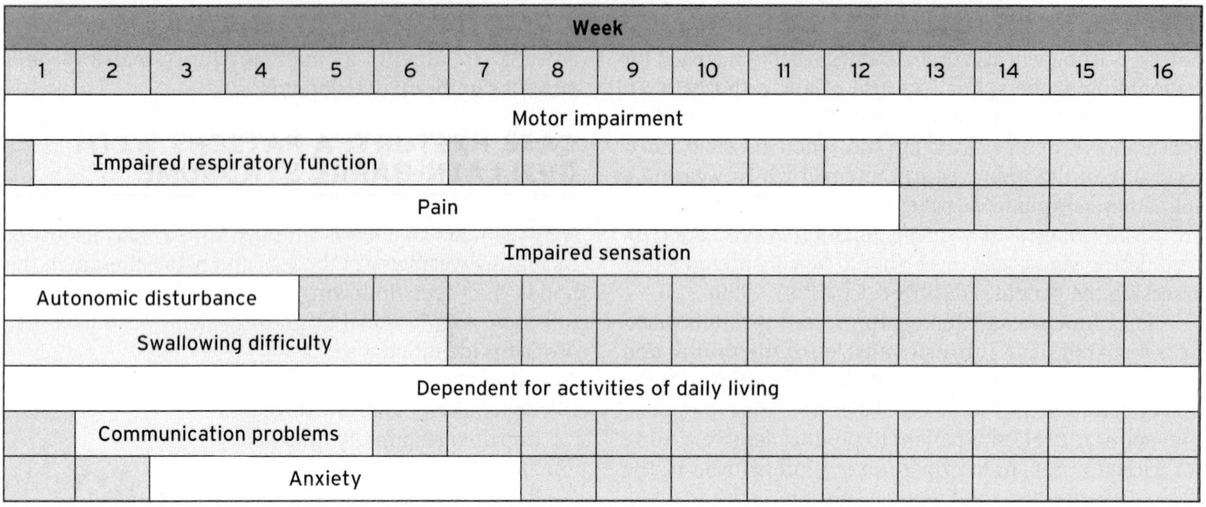

Week															
1	2	3	4	5	6	7	8	9	10	11	12	13	14	15	16
Motor impairment															
	Impaired respiratory function														
Pain															
Impaired sensation															
Autonomic disturbance															
	Swallowing difficulty														
Dependent for activities of daily living															
	Communication problems														
		Anxiety													

Figure 15.2 Time course of problems presenting in a patient with Guillain-Barré syndrome over a 16-week period. The case history of this patient is described in the text.

As soon as some recovery occurred in the trunk muscles (3 weeks after onset), while still ventilated, the patient worked on trunk control in sitting, to improve endurance in postural muscles and truncal alignment. Antigravity muscles were strengthened in standing, initially requiring two physiotherapists. Later, backslabs were used to support the lower limbs in extension. To supplement rehabilitation sessions, a regimen of low-resistance strengthening exercises for the elbow extensors, hip extensors/abductors and quadriceps muscles was used by the patient. Relatives were involved in helping the patient perform her exercises.

As trunk and pelvic control was gained, the emphasis shifted to improving lower limb power and co-ordination. Knee control was refined standing at a table and then the patient progressed to practising control of the weight-bearing leg when stepping. Muscle strength was monitored using a hand-held myometer. At the patient's weakest, recordings could be obtained only in the neck side flexors and right elbow pronators. Demonstrating objective strength improvements during the first 3 weeks, when the patient could not perform any activity, was encouraging for her.

2. Impaired Respiratory Function

Following admission, respiratory status was monitored regularly. Forced Vital Capacity (FVC) readings dropped rapidly because of respiratory muscle weakness, necessitating intubation and ventilation. Nurses and physiotherapists provided appropriate respiratory care, ensuring blood pressure was monitored when using suction. Ventilation was necessary for 4 weeks, after which the patient was gradually weaned off the ventilator.

3. Pain

Pain appeared as an early symptom. The physiotherapists and nurses positioned the patient to alleviate discomfort as far as possible, e.g. the 'frog position' (legs flexed, abducted and laterally rotated over a pillow, taking care to avoid pressure to the common peroneal nerve; see Figure 9.3). Massage of affected muscles and large-amplitude passive movements gave temporary relief but medication was required, particularly at night. Later, increasing pain and the resulting disturbance to sleep limited more active physiotherapy. Treatment had to be co-ordinated with effective analgesia. Pain remained the limiting factor for rehabilitation during the acute phase.

4. Reduced Distal Sensation

Impaired sensation occurred in a glove–stocking distribution, and there was impairment of joint position sense below the knees. This reduction in sensation caused considerable difficulties with positioning the feet on initial standing and walking (10 weeks after onset). Air-cast splints were used to increase sensory input and mirrors provided visual feedback. Stairs were particularly difficult. Two weeks working on compensatory strategies enabled the patient to be safely discharged to her two-storey house.

5. Autonomic Disturbance

Tachycardia and profound sweating occurred each time the patient was moved from lying to sitting (however slowly) during the first 3 weeks. Gradual adjustment to the upright position was one of the goals set by nurses and physiotherapists. Use of a reclining chair and a tilt-table allowed graded movement into the upright position. At all times, blood pressure and cardiac trace were monitored.

6. Difficulty in Swallowing (Dysphagia)

A nasogastric tube was inserted following assessment by the speech therapist which demonstrated a poor ability to swallow that placed the patient at risk of aspiration. Nurses and a dietitian monitored her nutritional intake. Five weeks later, the patient was able to commence a soft diet under the guidance of the speech therapist. Concurrently, the physiotherapist worked with the patient on an effective cough to prevent aspiration.

7. Dependent for Activities of Daily Living

The interaction of impairments led to dependency in all aspects of care. Throughout rehabilitation, functional goals were set. This allowed the patient to 'measure' her improvement in terms of regaining useful activities rather than gradual improvement of an impairment. The patient's sudden loss of functional independence and dignity was handled sensitively by all team members. Wherever possible, remaining functional ability was maximised by assisting the patient rather than taking over the task, e.g. allowing time for the patient to initiate rolling and then assisting as directed by the patient.

Wheelchair assessment occurred whilst the patient was still being ventilated. This allowed the patient to regain a more normal view of the world as well as being an adjunct to coping with autonomic disturbance (see above). As some recovery began, the physiotherapist aimed to improve trunk control so that the patient had a stable base of support to perform activities of daily living. Once achieved, movements over the base of support were incorporated. Sitting to standing from a high plinth allowed work on pelvic and trunk control (essential for gait) and enabled the patient to transfer independently. The physiotherapist and occupational therapist worked together to improve posture and hand control to regain independence in feeding.

Independence in the wheelchair was achieved by week 8, as a result of better trunk and hand control. Backslabs were made to allow the patient to practise standing when knee control was still poor. Stepping became possible after 10 weeks but air-cast splints were essential to prevent inversion of the ankle. Gait re-education progressed over the next 4 weeks. Crutches were used initially, progressing to two sticks and finally one stick.

8. Inability to Communicate Effectively

Intubation and ventilation prevented speaking and increasing weakness hindered gesturing. At nadir, communication was only possible using eye blinks. At all times staff would make every effort to understand the patient and in turn spend time talking to her. The speech therapist provided a communication aid which was used for 5 weeks until bulbar muscles recovered.

9. Anxiety

The patient's anxiety increased the longer she remained on the ventilator. Close relatives also needed to be reassured about the prognosis. A visitor from the GBS Support Group with personal experience of GBS was helpful in allaying both the patient's and relatives' fears (see 'Associations and Support Groups'). Five weeks after onset, the patient started becoming agitated if her daily routine was disturbed. Maximum effort was made to adhere to a timetable drawn up with the patient.

At Discharge

Sixteen weeks after admission most problems had resolved and the patient was discharged. The remaining problems were:

Impairments
1. Weakness of specific muscle groups, e.g. the dorsi-flexors bilaterally, right elbow extensors, left thenar eminence and the quadriceps.
2. Reduced proprioception below the knees, right worse than left.

Disabilities
3. Requiring one stick and an air-cast splint on the right ankle to walk.
4. Requiring bath aids and grab rail (fitted in the home before discharge) to bathe independently.

The patient was discharged with a scheme of exercises to strengthen the major groups which still fell below the normal range. A home exercise programme was drawn up with the patient to further her recovery. Arrangements were made for continuing physiotherapy in the community.

The problems encountered by this patient are typical of those in GBS, although the time scale can vary. The wide range, and constantly changing nature of the problems, highlights the need for an integrated and co-ordinated multidisciplinary intervention for the successful management of this syndrome.

REFERENCES

Aitkens SG, McCory MA, Kilmer DD, et al. Moderate resistance exercise program: its effect in slowly progressive neuromuscular disease. Arch Phys Med Rehab 1993, **74**:711-715.

Albers JW, Kelly JJ. Acquired inflammatory demyelinating polyneuropathies: clinical and electrodiagnostic features. Muscle Nerve 1989, **12**:435-451.

Asbury AK. Pain in generalised neuropathies. In: Fields HL, ed. Pain syndromes in neurology. London: Butterworth; 1990:131-141.

Asbury AK, Bird SJ. Disorders of peripheral nerve. In: Asbury AK, McKhann GM, McDonald IW, eds. Diseases of the nervous system: clinical neurobiology, 2nd edition. Philadephia: WB Saunders; 1992:252-269.

Asbury AK, Cornblath DR. Assessment of current diagnostic criteria for Guillain-Barré syndrome. Ann Neurol 1990, **27** (suppl):21-24.

Bennett RL, Knowlton GC. Overwork weakness in partially denervated skeletal muscle. Clin Orthop 1958, **12**:22-29.

Berlit P, Rakicky J. The Miller Fisher Syndrome: review of the literature. *J Clin Neuro-Ophthalmol* 1992, **12**:57-63.

Bohannon RW, Dubuc WE. Documentation of the resolution of weakness in a patient with Guillain-Barré Syndrome: a case report. *Phys Ther* 1984, **64**:1388-1389.

Butler DS. *Mobilisation of the nervous system*. Melbourne: Churchill Livingstone; 1991.

Cook JD, Glass DS. Strength evaluation in neuromuscular disease. *Neurol Clin* 1987, **5**:101-123.

Cowan J, Greenwood R, Fletcher N. Disorders of peripheral nerve. In: Greenwood R, Barnes MP, McMillan TM, *et al*. eds. *Neurological rehabilitation*. Edinburgh: Churchill Livingstone; 1993:607-613.

deJager AEJ, Minderhoud JM. Residual signs in severe Guillain-Barré syndrome. *J Neurol Sci* 1991, **104**:151-156.

Dellon AL. A numerical grading scale for peripheral nerve function. *J Hand Ther* 1993, **6**:152-160.

Dyck PJ, Litchy WJ, Lehman KA, *et al*. Variables influencing neuropathic endpoints. *Neurology* 1995, **45**:1115-1121.

Dyck PJ, Thomas PK. *Peripheral neuropathy, 3rd edition*. Philadelphia: WB Saunders; 1993.

Edwards S, Charlton P. Splinting and the use of orthoses in the management of patients with neurological disorders. In: Edwards S, ed. *Neurological physiotherapy: a problem solving approach*. London: Churchill Livingstone; 1996:161-188.

Feasby TE. Inflammatory demyelinating polyneuropathies. In: Dyck PJ, ed. *Neurologic Clinics: Peripheral Neuropathy: New Concepts and Treatments, Vol 10 No.3*. Philadelphia: WB Saunders; 1992.

Feasby TE. Axonal Guillain-Barré Syndrome. *Muscle Nerve* 1994, **17**:678-679.

Freeman J. Clinical notes of physiotherapy management of the patient with Guillain-Barré syndrome. *Synapse* 1992, April.

Geurts ACH, Mulder TW, Neinhuis B, *et al*. Postural organisation in patients with hereditary motor and sensory neuropathy. *Arch Phys Med Rehab* 1992, **73**:569-572.

Hardie R, Harding AE, Hirsch N, *et al*. Diaphragmatic weakness in hereditary motor and sensory neuropathy. *J Neurol Neurosurg Psychiat* 1990, **53**:348-350.

Harding AE. *Hereditary motor and sensory neuropathies (HMSN)*. London: Muscular Dystrophy Group of Great Britain and Northern Ireland; 1993. (Fact Sheet HE2).

Harding AE. From the syndrome of Charcot, Marie and Tooth to disorders of peripheral myelin proteins. *Brain* 1995, **118**:809-818.

Hartung HP, Pollard JD, Harvey GK. Immunopathogenesis and treatment of the Guillain-Barré Syndrome. Part II. *Muscle Nerve* 1995, **18**:154-164.

Hopkins A. *Clinical neurology: a modern approach*. Oxford: Oxford University Press; 1993.

Karni Y, Archdeacon L, Mills KR, *et al*. Clinical assessment and physiotherapy in Guillain-Barré Syndrome. *Physiotherapy* 1984, **70**:288-292.

Kilmer DD, McCory MA, Wright NC, *et al*. The effect of a high resistance exercise program in slowly progressive neuromuscular disease. *Arch Phys Med Rehab* 1994, **75**:560-563.

Lennon SM, Ashburn A. Use of myometry in the assessment of neuropathic weakness: testing for reliability in clinical practice. *Clin Rehab* 1993, **7**:125-133.

Lindeman E, Leffers P, Spaans F, *et al*. Strength training in patients with myotonic dystrophy and hereditary motor and sensory neuropathy: a randomised clinical trial. *Arch Phys Med Rehab* 1995, **76**:612-620.

Mann RA, Missirian J. Pathophysiology of Charcot-Marie-Tooth disease. *Clin Orthop* 1988, **234**:221-228.

Mays ML. Incorporating continuous passive motion in the rehabilitation of a patient with Guillain-Barré syndrome. *Am J Occup Ther* 1990, **44**:750-753.

McClure J. The role of physiotherapy in HIV and AIDS. *Physiotherapy* 1993, **79**:388-393.

McLeod JG. Autonomic dysfunction in peripheral nerve disease. In: Bannister R, Mathias C, eds. *Autonomic failure, 3rd edition*. Oxford: Oxford Medical Publications; 1992:659-681.

Milner-Brown HS, Miller RG. Muscle strengthening through high-resistance weight training in patients with neuromuscular disorders. *Arch Phys Med Rehab* 1988, **69**:14-19.

Mitchell S. Neuropathies. *Rev Clin Gerontol* 1991, **1**:347-357.

Monforte R, Estruch R, Valls-Sole J, *et al*. Autonomic and peripheral neuropathies in patients with chronic alcoholism. *Arch Neurol* 1995, **52**:45-51.

Moxley RT. Functional Testing. *Muscle Nerve* 1990, **13**:26-29.

Mueller MJ, Minor SD, Sahrmann SA, *et al*. Difference in gait characteristics of patients with diabetes and peripheral neuropathy compared with age-matched controls. *Phys Ther* 1994, **74**:299-308.

Munsat TL. Clinical trials in neuromuscular disease. *Muscle Nerve* 1990, **13**:3-6.

Ng KPP, Howard RS, Fish DR, *et al*. Management and outcome of severe Guillain-Barré syndrome. *Q J Med* 1995, **88**:243-250.

Pentland B, Donald SM. Pain in Guillain-Barré syndrome: a clinical review. *Pain* 1994, **59**:159-164.

Pirart J. Diabetes mellitus and its degenerative complications: a prospective study of 4,400 patients observed between 1947 and 1973. *Diabet Care* 1978, **1**:168-188.

Ropper AH, Wijdicks EFM, Truax BT. *Guillain-Barré syndrome*. Philadelphia: FA Davis; 1991.

Rutland JL, Shields RK. The effects of a home exercise program on impairment and health – related quality of life in persons with chronic peripheral neuropathies. *Phys Ther* 1997, **77**:1026-1039.

Schaumburg HH, Berger AR, Thomas PK. *Disorders of peripheral nerves, 2nd edition*. Philadelphia: FA Davis; 1992.

Simionato R, Stiller K, Butler D. Neural tension signs in Guillain-Barré syndrome: two case reports. *Aust J Physiother* 1988, **34**:257-259.

Simpson DM, Olney RK. Peripheral neuropathies associated with human immunodeficiency virus infection. In: Dyck PJ, ed. *Neurologic Clinics: Peripheral Neuropathy: New Concepts and Treatments Vol 10 no.3*. Philadelphia: WB Saunders; 1992:685-711.

Smith M, Ball V. *Cardiovascular/Respiratory Physiotherapy*. London: Mosby; 1998. In progress.

Soryal I, Sinclair E, Hornby J, *et al*. Impaired joint mobility in Guillain-Barré syndrome: a primary or a secondary phenomenon? *J Neurol Neurosurg Psychiat* 1992, **55**:1014-1017.

Sridharan GV, Tallis RC, Gautam PC. Guillain-Barré syndrome in the elderly. *Gerontology* 1993, **39**:170-175.

Thomas PK, Thomlinson DR. Diabetic and hypoglycaemic neuropathy. In: Dyck PJ, Thomas PK, eds. *Peripheral neuropathy, 3rd edition*. Philadelphia: WB Saunders; 1993:1219-1250.

Thompson PD, Day BL. The anatomy and physiology of cerebellar disease. *Adv Neurol* 1993, **61**:15-30.

van de Ploeg RJO, Fidler V, Oosterhuis HJGH. Handheld myometry: reference values. *J Neurol Neurosurg Psychiat* 1991, **54**:244-247.

van-Doom PA. Intravenous immunoglobulin treatment in patients with chronic inflammatory demyelinating polyneuropathy. *J Neurol Neurosurg Psychiat* 1994, **57** (suppl):38-42.

Visser LH, Van-der-Meche FG, Van-doorn PA, *et al*. Guillain-Barré syndrome without sensory loss (acute motor neuropathy): a sub group with specific clinical diagnostic and laboratory features. *Brain* 1995, **118**:841-847.

Watson GR, Wilson FM. Guillain-Barré syndrome: an update. *N Z J Physiother* 1989, **17**:17-24.

Wiles CM, Karni Y, Nicklin J. Laboratory testing of muscle function in the management of neuromuscular disease. *J Neurol Neurosurg Psychiat* 1990, **53**:384-387.

Windebank AJ. Polyneuropathy due to nutritional deficit and alcoholism. In: Dyck PJ, Thomas PK, eds. *Peripheral neuropathy, 3rd edition*. Philadelphia: WB Saunders; 1993:1310-1321.

Winer JB, Hughes RAC, Osmond C. A prospective study of acute idiopathic neuropathy, clinical features and their prognostic value. *J Neurol Neurosurg Psychiat* 1988, **51**:605-612.

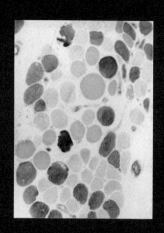

16

I Fahal, RHT Edwards & N Thompson

DISORDERS OF MUSCLE

CHAPTER OUTLINE

- **General issues in neuromuscular disorders**
- **Muscle disorders and their clinical features**

- **Physical management of neuromuscular disorders**

INTRODUCTION

Disorders of muscle due to neuromuscular disease may be inherited or acquired; the age of onset of symptoms tends to be characteristic for the different disorders. Disorders of childhood onset, such as Duchenne muscular dystrophy (DMD), are discussed in Chapter 21, but it is stressed here that these should not be seen only as paediatric conditions. As patients survive for longer times, more are presenting for physiotherapy as adults and knowledge of this condition tends to be poor amongst non-paediatric physiotherapists.

This chapter describes muscle disorders which mainly present in adulthood, though some of them can occur earlier. An overview of the disorders is given so that the physiotherapist is aware of the different diagnoses, as these can influence overall management. For a comprehensive text on muscle disorders the reader is referred to Walton *et al.* (1994).

The principles of physical management of muscle disorders are discussed in general in this chapter and in more detail in Chapter 21. This arrangement is to avoid repetition and to show the continuum of management from childhood to adulthood. Where special consideration is required for a particular disorder, due to specific clinical features, these are discussed where relevant in both chapters.

GENERAL ISSUES IN NEUROMUSCULAR DISORDERS

The neuromuscular diseases are individually rare inherited or acquired conditions which lead to significant physical disability and, in a number of cases, to early death. Together the neuromuscular diseases cause a significant amount of disability in the community. An estimate of the total number of persons so disabled in the European Union was 210,600 in May 1990 (Poortman, 1990). This represents a major economic challenge to meet the individual patient's needs and the costs of enablement to facilitate life in the community (Martin *et al.*, 1988).

CLASSIFICATION AND DIAGNOSTIC INVESTIGATIONS

Neuromuscular disorders may be inherited or acquired disorders. They can be classified according to the site of the defect in the motor unit (Table 16.1); those that are inherited can be classified by genetic defect (Mastaglia & Laing, 1996) as shown for the muscular dystrophies in Table 16.2. Motor neurone disease (MND) involves both lower and upper motorneurones and is discussed in Chapter 14.

Acquired disorders include inflammatory myopathies from viral or bacterial infection and drugs, and endocrine myopathies. Other drug-induced muscle disorders include myalgia, forms of myotonia and mitochondrial myopathy, and steroid myopathy from corticosteroids (Mastaglia & Laing, 1996). Toxic myopathy can result from alcoholism.

Investigations for differential diagnosis involve electromyography (EMG), muscle biopsy and biochemical

Classification of neuromuscular diseases according to the site of defect in the motor unit	
Site of defect	**Diagnosis**
Anterior horn cell	Spinal muscular atrophy (proximal & distal) Poliomyelitis Motor neurone disease*
Nerve fibre	Peroneal muscular atrophies Inflammatory polyradiculoneuropathies Toxic myopathy Metabolic myopathy Guillain-Barré syndrome
Neuromuscular junction	Myasthenia gravis Lambert Eaton syndrome Botulism
Muscle fibre	Muscular dystrophies Congenital myopathies, e.g. central core disease Mitochondrial myopathies Glycogen storage diseases affecting muscle (e.g. phosphorylase deficiency, acid maltase deficiency & phosphofructokinase deficiency) Disorders of lipid metabolism (carnitine deficiencies & carnitine palmityltransferase deficiencies) Inflammatory myopathies (polymyositis & dermatomyositis) Endocrine myopathies (hyper- & hypothyroidism)

* Motor neurone disease involves not only the motor unit but also upper motoneurones (see Chapter 14)

Table 16.1 Classification of neuromuscular diseases according to the site of defect in the motor unit.

studies of blood for enzyme activity and molecular diagnosis using gene probes. The serum concentration of creatine kinase (CK) is the most reliable biochemical indicator of muscle disease but this is not conclusive evidence and diagnosis requires confirmation by other means. The degree of raised CK varies in different disorders. Clinical investigations are discussed in Chapter 21 in relation to muscular dystrophies, and in Chapter 3 in general. Mastaglia & Laing (1996) reviewed genetic testing as well as other investigations in muscle disorders.

IMPAIRMENT, DISABILITY AND HANDICAP

In general, the neuromuscular diseases illustrate very well the World Health Organisation's classification into Impairment, Disability and Handicap (see 'Preface') with the attendant therapeutic challenges (Edwards, 1989).

Impairment is in virtually all cases muscle wasting, due either to a central loss of motor units (e.g. spinal muscular atrophy) or to a muscular cause (e.g. muscular dystrophy). The consequence of the wasting, causing loss of the cross-sectional area of the muscle, is weakness.

Disability involves biomechanical factors such as the

extent to which the effectiveness of muscular contraction to perform everyday tasks may be influenced by excessive weight, contractures or lever length. Locomotor disability is a cause of loss of walking ability and difficulties with feeding. Loss of strength of the respiratory muscles becomes a major factor, determining life expectancy, not only because of loss of respiratory function (vital capacity) but because of possible sleep-related respiratory disorders such as sleep apnoea (Smith et al., 1991).

Handicap is a psychosocial issue. Patients with neuromuscular diseases are not 'ill' but they are disabled. Their ability to have a full life depends very much on the extent to which they can be so enabled by physical disability aids, availability of carers, education, and modern computer-based technology. A positive attitude on the part of the patient and supportive attitudes of more able-bodied members of society, coupled with a commitment to facilitate mobility, access, and employment opportunities, become paramount issues.

GENETICS

Major advances have been made in identifying the genetic mutations and defective proteins involved in neuromuscular

Classification of some of the muscular dystrophies in relation to the genetic defect

Inheritance	Locus	Gene	Diagnosis	Onset
X-linked				
short arm of X chromosome	Xp21.1	Dystrophin	Duchenne dystrophy	3-5 years
	Xp21.2	Dystrophin	Becker dystrophy	Childhood
long arm of X chromosome	Xq28	Emerin	Emery-Dreifuss	Childhood
Autosomal recessive				
	Various	Various	Scapulohumeral Limb girdle 5 types 2A-E	Any age Early adult life
	6q2	Merosin	Congenital LAMA 2	Hypotonia at birth
	9q31-q33		Fukuyama	
Autosomal dominant	4q35		Fascioscapulohumeral Scapuloperoneal	Any age 2nd-5th decade
	5q22-q34		Limb girdle 1A LGMD 1B	Early adult life Early adult life
	14q11.2-q13		Oculopharyngeal	Adulthood
	14q		Distal	Adulthood
	Chromosome 19	Myotonin protein kinase	Myotonic dystrophy	Adulthood usually but can be congenital

N.B. Genetic information continues to emerge for different disorders. Further genes and loci may have been identified since constructing this table, so the current scientific literature should be consulted.

Table 16.2 Classification of some of the muscular dystrophies in relation to the genetic defect.

diseases (Mastaglia & Laing, 1996). This has led to a significant role for genetic counselling with regard to possible transmission of the disorder to offspring or in relation to other family members. For the patient himself or herself, the precise genetic detail becomes of less importance than the specific effects of the disease on lifestyle. What is increasingly recognised is the fact that even with a specific genotype there are great differences in the phenotype, i.e. the clinical features and extent of impairment, disability and handicap. This may in part be affected by other genetic factors but it must also be recognised that the extent to which the patient has been looked after and maintained free from deformity, and how weight has been controlled, may be important determining factors.

PRINCIPLES OF MANAGEMENT

Whilst there is a great deal of research interest in seeking a successful treatment for patients with neuromuscular diseases, it must also be recognised that it is likely that only those who are free of secondary complications (e.g. contractures and spinal deformity) are likely to derive the greatest benefit from such treatment when it becomes available. A basic philosophy in the management of patients with

neuromuscular diseases is that, as Irwin Siegel said in his book for children with neuromuscular diseases, *Everybody's different; nobody's perfect* (Siegel, 1982). Whilst these diseases are at present incurable, they are not untreatable and considerable benefit can be seen when there is close attention to detail in the day-to-day management of the patient. Orthopaedic surgery has a certain amount to offer, particularly in relation to correction of certain deformities, e.g. toe walking, but here consideration must be given to the biomechanical consequences, and to spinal stabilisation (e.g. by the Luque procedure). These procedures appear to have an influence on the quality of life and may facilitate wheelchair posture and ease of nursing care.

The principles of the management of neuromuscular diseases come from the recognition of the patient's needs, depending on the degree of impairment, disability or handicap, rather than a specific diagnosis. However, knowledge of the different disorders and their diagnostic features and progression is important, particularly in those which involve very specific problems. Therefore the management of patients with neuromuscular diseases and their families is best dealt with through an integrated multidisciplinary approach (medical, clinical genetics, physiotherapy,

The course of neuromuscular disease		
Problem	**Components**	**Management options**
Early		
Impairment	Suspicion Diagnosis Prognosis Genetic risks	Accurate diagnosis Encouragement/support Personal responsibility Counselling
Disability	Muscle weakness Walking difficulties Risks of falling Loss of ambulation	Orthoses Weight control Corrective surgery
Handicap	Employment problems Mobility Sexual relations	Education Expert advice Counselling Patient support groups
Late	Loss of independence Respiratory problems	Sheltered accommodation Helpers Confidence in local medical support
	The final illness Bereavement	Counselling Family support group Voluntary work on behalf of others

Table 16.3 The course of neuromuscular disease. Some milestones for the patient and family.

paediatrics, orthopaedics, dietetics, orthotics, occupational therapy), taking into account the important psychological milestones (Table 16.3).

MUSCLE DISORDERS AND THEIR CLINICAL FEATURES

Disorders which predominantly manifest in adulthood are discussed here and those which present in childhood are discussed in Chapter 21.

FASCIOSCAPULOHUMERAL MUSCULAR DYSTROPHY

This is a disease inherited in an autosomal dominant fashion. It has a prevalence of 1.5–3 per 100,000 in the UK (Emery, 1991) and estimated prevalence of 1.5–2.5 per 100,000 in Europe and North America (Emery, 1991; Lunt & Harper, 1991). Both sexes are affected equally.

This genetic disorder is found on chromosome 4q35 (Wijmenga et al., 1991). The age at onset, degree of severity and course of the disease are more variable than in many other neuromuscular diseases. Within a family it may range from someone who has minimal facial weakness (a failure to whistle effectively is a characteristic finding) with slow progression and normal lifespan, to a condition which has a more marked progression of lower limb

weakness and can cause very severe disability early in life. The most important physical feature is that of failure to raise the outstretched arms, a procedure which causes marked winging of the scapulae.

The term facioscapulohumeral implies weakness of much of the face, shoulder girdle, and proximal arm muscles. Shoulder girdle weakness is often asymmetrical and scapular winging or shoulder 'terracing' on abduction of the arms reflects weakness of the serratus anterior, trapezius and rhomboid muscles. Later the biceps and triceps muscles are affected. The deltoids are preserved in 50% of cases (Bunch & Siegel, 1993) but even if the deltoids are not involved the muscles lose their mechanical advantage due to lack of shoulder girdle stability, causing limitation of active abduction and flexion. The patient may compensate surprisingly well, using trick movements to raise the hand above shoulder level, but can be more obviously compromised if the activity involves lifting objects of any weight. Foot drop may occur early in the disease due to peroneal and anterior tibial muscle weakness. Leg muscle weakness may eventually progress to loss of ambulation. The heart and intellect are not affected. Life expectancy may be normal but is usually reduced. Confirmation of diagnosis usually requires EMG and muscle biopsy, and CK is often normal or only slightly elevated.

General Management

No specific treatment is yet available for fascioscapulo-humeral muscular dystrophy. Ankle–foot orthoses are helpful for foot drop. Thoracoscapular fusion may be effective in managing patients with scapular winging, provided a functional deltoid is retained. Some improvement in both shoulder range of movement (ROM) and appearance can be achieved and this is most beneficial for patients whose occupation specifically requires the ability to sustain flexion and abduction. However, this approach should be considered very carefully since complications include pneomothorax, pleural effusion, atelactasis, fracture of the scapula and pseudoarthrosis (Letournel *et al.*, 1990).

MYOTONIC DYSTROPHY

Myotonic dystrophy is an autosomal dominant multisystem disease, characterised by muscle weakness and slowed relaxation after contraction. The prevalence is 5 per 100,000 (Harper, 1989) and the gene defect is located on chromosome 19 (Friedrich *et al.*, 1987). Recognition of the disease is important, not only because it can be a major cause of physical disability but also because it is associated with cardiac arrhythmias (Anonymous, 1992), respiratory problems and the risks of anaesthesia (Moore & Moore, 1987). Features of the disease include intellectual impairment, hypersomnia, cardiomyopathy and conduction defects, cataracts, prefrontal balding (mainly in men), gonadal atrophy, respiratory failure and gastrointestinal disease.

Weakness begins insidiously in adolescence and progresses slowly and symmetrically, involving the distal muscles more than the proximal. The muscles first affected are the facial muscles with ptosis, masticatory, sternomastoid, forearm and lower leg muscles. Myotonia is demonstrable by asking the patient to clench his or her fist and then let go quickly. The EMG findings show spontaneous activity due to the instability of the muscle cell membrane. The classic 'dive bomber' effect, which can be heard through the loudspeaker, is characteristic and occurs when movement of the EMG needle causes high-frequency discharges, which first increase in amplitude and then rapidly decrease (Fawcett & Barwick, 1994).

General Management

Education, monitoring and avoidance of complications remain the cornerstone in the management of patients with myotonic dystrophy. Cardiac arrhythmias are the most serious complication. Permanent cardiac pacing may sometimes be required. Anaesthesia and surgery need special attention as patients are at risk with general anaesthesia. Several drugs can be used to relieve the myotonia but this symptom is less troublesome than the weakness, and drug therapy is complex as safety is limited by the associated cardiac problems.

MYOTONIA CONGENITA

This condition can cause inconvenient muscular cramps or difficulties with relaxation that can impede fine movements. It is not, however, a disabling condition and is not progressive. There is some weakness but in general the condition causes no major problem during life. The person who described the condition, which has come to be known as Thomsen's disease (Thomsen, 1876), was from a large family whose members led essentially normal lives.

General Management

As for myotonic dystrophy, education is an important aspect of the management of myotonia congenita.

LIMB GIRDLE MUSCULAR DYSTROPHIES

Limb girdle muscular dystrophies are a group of disorders characterised by the predominance of weakness in the limb girdle muscles, with sparing of the facial muscles. They begin in the second or third decade of life and can be inherited in an autosomal recessive or dominant manner; seven varieties of genetic defect have been identified (Mastaglia & Laing, 1996). The sexes are affected equally. The onset of weakness can be in muscles of the shoulder girdle or the pelvic girdle. Wasting and weakness may become widespread in the limbs and severe disability usually results within 20 years of onset. CK is usually increased and EMG helps in distinguishing neurogenic and inflammatory causes for the syndrome.

General Management

As with other disabling neuromuscular diseases, patients with limb girdle syndromes require both medical treatment and support. Attention to the consequences of immobility is required. Oedema, obesity, constipation and gastrointestinal problems, bone loss and pressure sores are all preventable and most are treatable.

MITOCHONDRIAL MYOPATHIES

These are rare myopathies with a wide range of clinical presentation from mild extraocular weakness to severe fatal infantile myopathies. The first mitochondrial DNA mutations were discovered in 1988 and the classification of different types can be seen in Mastaglia & Laing (1996). The disorder may be confined to the muscles, causing weakness, or may present in a variety of clinical settings, e.g. dementia, convulsions, ataxia, stroke-like episodes, extrapyramidal syndromes, deafness and peripheral neuropathy. Muscle biopsy reveals the characteristic feature—'ragged red fibres'—due to accumulation of mitochondria at the periphery of the muscle fibres. Onset can occur at any age and management depends on presenting symptoms and their severity.

GLYCOGEN STORAGE DISEASES

McArdle's disease is the most important member of this group of metabolic myopathies. It is due to deficiency of myophosphorylase, leading to impaired utilisation of muscle glucose. Muscle pain and cramps on exercise are the cardinal symptoms. Myoglobinuria (giving the urine a reddish 'bloody' appearance), severe enough to cause renal failure, can develop on severe exercise. Muscle biopsy findings, raised CK and lack of rise in venous lactate during an ischaemic exercise test help in diagnosis, and recently a DNA test has been established (Bartram *et al.*, 1993). Strenuous anaerobic exercise should therefore be avoided to prevent muscle damage and potentially fatal renal failure. Light, regular exercise is appropriate, paying attention to fatigue. A similar syndrome to this is phosphofructokinase deficiency, which causes muscle pain and cramps.

A glycogen storage disease that causes progressive muscle weakness is acid maltase deficiency. The infantile and childhood forms are fatal in early life. The adult form involves progressive muscle weakness and respiratory problems, which can be managed with nocturnal ventilation.

MYASTHENIA GRAVIS

Myasthenia gravis is a disorder of the neuromuscular junction. It is characterised by weakness and fatiguability of proximal limb, ocular and bulbar muscles. It is twice as common in women as in men and can occur at any age. Fatiguability is a constant feature and weakness of the extraocular muscles is the first manifestation of the disease in about 60% of patients. Other features of the disease are dysarthria, dysphagia and difficulties with mastication, and respiratory difficulties may occur. The disease is confirmed by the Tensilon test. Edrophonium, an anticholinesterase, is injected as a bolus; in a positive test, improvement of weakness occurs within seconds and lasts for 2–3 minutes. Antibodies to the serum acetylcholine receptor are present in about 90% of patients. Oral anticholinesterases are used in the treatment of this condition but they do not cure the disease.

INFLAMMATORY MYOPATHIES

Dermatomyositis occurs in two main age groups: the young (juvenile dermatomyositis; Carpenter *et al.*, 1976); and the older age group, in which there may be a significant correlation with malignancy (Callen, 1988). The disease is characterised by skin changes and muscle weakness. Polymyositis is an inflammatory disease of muscle of unknown cause that may be very acute and life-threatening, less acute, or chronic and disabling, due to slow progressive loss of muscle. In the past there was some confusion between late-stage inflammatory muscle disease and one of the muscular dystrophies because all such diseases tend to end up as loss of muscle with replacement by fat and/or fibrous tissue.

Polymyositis refers to a group of acquired, inflammatory myopathies. Proximal muscle weakness, leading to difficulty in rising from a chair, climbing stairs or lifting, is the cardinal feature. Muscles ache and are sometimes tender. Serum CK is raised and EMG reveals myopathic changes. Muscle biopsy shows an inflammatory infiltrate and necrosis.

A number of bacterial, viral and parasitic organisms can cause inflammatory myopathies but these are rare in the UK.

ENDOCRINE MYOPATHIES

Endocrine disorders, such as hypothyroidism, hyperparathyroidism and osteomalacia, can cause muscle weakness and pain. Medical treatment of the endocrine disorder relieves the muscular symptoms but patients may require physical management while symptoms are uncontrolled.

PHYSICAL MANAGEMENT OF NEUROMUSCULAR DISORDERS

Physical management is aimed at preventing deformity from contractures, respiratory complications and pressure sores, as well as maintaining function and mobility for as long as possible. Assessment is not required as regularly in adults as it is in children, but contact should be maintained with a physiotherapist and care team.

Management depends on the presenting signs and symptoms as well as the prognosis, and a multidisciplinary problem-solving approach is preferable. To avoid repetition, the principles of physical management are discussed in Chapter 21. Specific aspects of management in fascioscapulohumeral muscular dystrophy and myotonic syndromes are discussed below.

FASCIOSCAPULOHUMERAL DYSTROPHY

Postoperative management after scapular fixation requires the shoulder to be managed in a shoulder spica, with the arm abducted in the salute position, for 2–3 months. Isometric deltoid exercises should be encouraged with the spica cast in place. The likely occurrence of some muscle atrophy from disuse during the period of immobilisation, over and above any dystrophic process, implies that those with mild to moderate, rather than severe, weakness are more likely to benefit from surgical intervention. All parties need to be clear that the patient will be able to cope with this both practically and psychologically. Bunch & Siegel (1993) reported one patient who was so self-conscious in the shoulder spica he refused to leave his home and subsequently lost the abililty to climb the stairs due to exacerbation of weakness.

Despite the name given to this condition, it is important not to overlook trunk and lower extremity involvement. Pelvic girdle weakness, and specifically hip extensor weakness, may give rise to a compensatory lordosis. This is sometimes so severe that the sacrum assumes a horizontal plane and it can lead to back pain and spondylosis that may jeopardise the patient's ambulatory status. Targetting strengthening exercises to the hip and trunk extensors should be considered before this stage is reached. A flexible spinal support may relieve the back symptoms without destroying the necessary functional lordosis, although the two are difficult to reconcile. The therapist should be vigilant for the development of hip flexor contractures which would exacerbate the problem.

MYOTONIC SYNDROMES

Prevention of contractures due to muscle weakness are managed as in other muscle disorders (see Chapter 21). The myotonia, which is less of a problem than weakness, can be overcome by utilising the 'warm-up' effect (Cooper *et al.*, 1988). Prior to an activity, the patient contracts the muscles several times, so that relaxation in between the contractions becomes faster and the contractions themselves become stronger. This enables the activity to be carried out more effectively. Examples include strategies which patients may have worked out for themselves, such as chewing gum before an interview so that speech is fluent, arm exercises prior to playing golf, or opening and closing the fist prior to a handshake. Appropriate strategies could be worked out for different functional activities.

CONCLUSION

While awaiting a successful cure for patients with neuromuscular diseases, it must be recognised that they are not untreatable and considerable benefit can be seen when there is close attention to detail in the day-to-day management of the patient. Physiotherapy, as part of an integrated multidisciplinary management approach, has a major contribution to offer, particularly in relation to preserving posture, physical fitness and muscle strength, and preventing contractures.

Acknowledgements
Support from the Muscular Dystrophy Group of Great Britain and Northern Ireland is gratefully acknowledged.

REFERENCES

[Anonymous] The heart in myotonic dystrophy. *Lancet* 1992, **339**:528-529 [Editorial].

Bartram C, Clague J, Edwards RHT, Beynon R. McArdle's disease: a nonsense mutation in exon 1 of the muscle phosphorylase gene explains some but not all cases. *Hum Mol Genet* 1993, **2**:1291-1293.

Bunch WH, Siegel IM. Scapulothoracic arthrodesis in Fascioscapulohumeral Muscular Dystrophy. *J Bone Joint Surg* 1993, **75A**:372-376.

Callen JP. Malignancy in polymyositis/dermatomyositis. *Clin Dermat* 1988, **2**:55-63.

Carpenter S, Karpati G, Rothman S, *et al.* The childhood type of dermatomyositis. *Neurology* 1976, **26**:92.

Cooper RG, Stokes MJ, Edwards RHT. Physiological characterisation of the 'warm up' effect of activity in patients with myotonic dystrophy. *J Neurol Neurosurg Psych* 1988, **51**:1134-1141.

Edwards RHT. Management of muscular dystrophy in adults. *Br Med Bull* 1989, **45**:802-818.

Emery AEH. Population frequencies of inherited neuromuscular diseases – a world survey. *Neuromusc Dis* 1991, **1**:19-29.

Fawcett PRW, Barwick DD. The clinical neurophysiology of neuromuscular disease. In: Walton JN, Karpati G, Hilton-Jones D, eds. *Disorders of voluntary muscle, 6th edition*. Edinburgh: Churchill Livingstone; 1994:1033-1104.

Friedrich U, Brunner H, Smeets D, *et al.* Three points linkage analysis employing C3 and 19cen markers assign the myotonic dystrophy gene to 19q. *Hum Genet* 1987, **75**:291-293.

Harper PS. *Myotonic dystrophy, 2nd edition*. Philadelphia: WB Saunders; 1989.

Letournel E, Fardeau M, Lytle JO, *et al.* Scapulothoracic arthrodesis for patients who have Fascioscapulhumeral Muscular Dystrophy. *J Bone Joint Surg* 1990, **72A**:78-84.

Lunt PW, Harper PS. Genetic counselling in fascioscapulohumeral muscular dystrophy. *J Med Genet* 1991, **28**:655-664.

Martin J, Meltzer H, Eliot D. *Office of Population Censuses and Surveys (OPCS): Survey of disability in Great Britain: Report 1: The prevalence of disability among adults*. London: HMSO; 1988.

Mastaglia FL, Laing NG. Investigation of muscle disease. *J Neurol Neurosurg Psych* 1996, **60**:256-274.

Moore JK, Moore AP. Postoperative complications of dystrophia myotonica. *Anaesthesia* 1987, **42**:529-533.

Poortman YS. *Respiratory insufficiency in neuromuscular diseases: Report of an international workshop*. Arnhem: EAMDA publications; 1990.

Siegel IM. *Everybody's different, nobody's perfect*. London: Muscular Dystrophy Group of Great Britain; 1982:1-13.

Smith PEM, Edwards RHT, Calverley PMA. Mechanisms of sleep-disordered breathing in chronic neuromuscular disease: implications for management. *Q J Med* 1991, **296**: 961-973.

Thomsen J. Tonische krampfe in willkurlich beweglichen muskeln in folge von erebter psychischer disposition (ataxia muscularis). *Archiv Psychiatr Neurenkrankheiten* 1976, **6**:702.

Walton JN, Karpati G, Hilton-Jones D. *Disorders of voluntary muscle, 6th edition*. Edinburgh: Churchill Livingstone; 1994.

Wijmenga C, Padberg GW, Moerer P, *et al.* Mapping of fascioscapulohumeral gene to chromosome 4q35-qter by multipoint linkage analysis and *in situ* hybridization. *Genomics* 1991, **9**:570-575.

SECTION 3

LIFETIME DISORDERS OF CHILDHOOD ONSET

Neurology (newr-ol-je): The section of medicine that deals with the study and treatment of diseases of the nervous system.

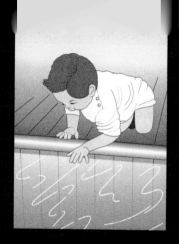

17

C deSousa & H Rattue

GENERAL INTRODUCTION TO PAEDIATRIC NEUROLOGY

CHAPTER OUTLINE

NEUROLOGICAL DISORDERS OF CHILDHOOD

There is a continuum of neurological illness from infancy to adulthood. Most disorders that occur in adults also occur in children—this includes common adult disorders such as stroke, multiple sclerosis and Parkinson's disease. The prevalence of these disorders in childhood is often much less than in adults and prevalence also varies in children of different ages. There may be different underlying causes for some disorders that also occur in adults: cerebrovascular disease in children is seldom due to atherosclerosis; the most frequently encountered childhood cause of bacterial meningitis is *Haemophilus influenzae,* which is a less common pathogen in older people; and cerebral tumours in children occur more commonly in the posterior fossa than at other sites, unlike in adults.

A pathological process, such as cerebral ischaemia or demyelination, may exert a very different effect on the developing nervous system compared to its effect in the fully mature individual. The developing nervous system is at risk from any process that permanently alters development at critical stages, as occurs with congenital infections such as rubella or cytomegalovirus. Despite this, the plasticity of the infant brain often means that extensive recovery of function can take place following surgery, ischaemia or damage to one cerebral hemisphere (see Chapter 6).

Neurological disorders are a major cause of illness in childhood (Kurtz & Stanley, 1995). Approximately 7% of all children have some form of moderate handicap and 0.7% have a severe handicap; there is neurological dysfunction in a high proportion of such children. One fifth of children admitted to hospital have a neurological problem, either as their principal complaint or in association with it. Three categories of neurological disorder predominate in children: cerebral palsy, epilepsy and complex mental handicap. Each of these categories includes individual disorders with a variety of aetiologies and outcomes, and many affected individuals will suffer from more than one of these. The prevalences of these and some other neurological disorders are given in Table 17.1. The prevalence of some of these neurological disorders of childhood is changing with time. There is an increase in the prevalence of cerebral palsy (see Chapter 19) and cerebral tumours. There is a decrease in the prevalence of neural tube defects (Chapter 20), epilepsy, serious head injury and *Haemophilus meningitis*. Some of these changes are due to changing medical practice, but the reasons for others are not well understood.

Many of the neurological disorders of childhood are congenital and occur because of maldevelopment of the nervous system or as a result of adverse factors during pregnancy and birth. Many genetic disorders give rise to neurological dysfunction from birth but others, such as Duchenne muscular dystrophy (Chapter 21) or some inborn errors of metabolism, do not manifest symptoms for months or years. Acquired neurological disorders of childhood include important treatable and sometimes preventable conditions such as central nervous system (CNS) infection (particularly in infancy), serious head injury (most commonly in older children and teenagers) and brain tumours (in all age groups). In some disorders there is considerable improvement during childhood, but many neurological disorders arising in childhood have implications for later life. It is important for therapists who treat adults with disorders of childhood onset to be familiar with how these conditions present in childhood.

PHYSIOTHERAPY FOR CHILDREN WITH NEUROLOGICAL DISORDERS

All aspects of the management of childhood neurological illness require familiarity with normal development (Chapter 18) and the ability to work effectively and sympathetically with children and families. The child is an integral part of a family. The parents of the child newly diagnosed as having a neurological disorder undergo a period of adaptation which is not dissimilar to a grief response. There may be denial, anger and sadness at the loss of the child they expected. The assessment and treatment of such a child will require the therapist to balance the expectations of parents with the abilities and requirements of the child.

Table 17.1 Prevalence of neurological disorders in childhood.

Prevalence of neurological disorders in childhood	
Neurological disorder	**Prevalence**
Epilepsy	8 per 1000
Complex mental handicap	5 per 1000
Cerebral palsy	2 per 1000
Duchenne muscular dystrophy	3 per 10,000 boys
Spina bifida	6 per 10,000
Hydrocephalus	5 per 10,000
All neurodegenerative disorders	5 per 10,000
Meningitis	4 per 10,000 per year (incidence)
Neurofibromatosis	3 per 10,000
Rett syndrome	1 per 10,000 girls
CNS tumours	0.5 per 10,000

Table constructed from various sources cited in the text and reflecting worldwide prevalence. Values for some disorders are changing with time.

It is important to be able to engage and communicate with children, some of whom have severe cognitive, communication and behavioural problems. Therapy techniques need to be adapted to children of different ages, and active participation is difficult to obtain in the younger child. Medical and physical management must be integrated into the whole life of the child, including education, play, and family and social life. Parents and carers should be made to feel involved in the assessment and treatment of the child. Parents are often the best therapists the child has. The therapist and the family achieve the best for the child by sharing their skills and by developing a working relationship in which each is sensitive to the other's needs. Some families like to be very involved in the child's care whilst others require support to feel confident in their abilities with the child. It is important that the therapist assesses the individual child's and family's needs and plans intervention that is appropriate to that particular situation. There will be some children with neurological disorders for whom physiotherapy is not appropriate or in whom therapy should be postponed or discontinued temporarily for a variety of reasons.

ASPECTS OF PHYSIOTHERAPY MANAGEMENT

There are four aspects to the work of physiotherapy in children with neurological disorders. The first is the assessment of the child's abilities and difficulties, to define whether a problem exists and what the nature of the problem is. This assessment may also be part of the medical diagnosis of underlying causes. The second aspect is the treatment of the child to enhance function, improve quality of life and alter outcome in the face of neurological deficits. The third is the measurement of change in function with time, which is necessary in order to evaluate the effects of intervention and to plan further treatment. The fourth aspect is the involvement of the physiotherapist in linking specialist knowledge about the child's physical development to the overall treatment of the child, including other aspects of development (cognitive, communication, social and emotional).

THE MULTIDISCIPLINARY TEAM (MDT)

The child with a neurological disorder may have differing areas of need and will benefit from an holistic approach to treatment. The physiotherapist works as part of the MDT. There are many examples of problems which can be dealt with most effectively by professionals from different backgrounds working together. These include the feeding disorders of children with motor handicaps, which can be addressed by a 'feeding disorders team' comprising a speech therapist, physiotherapist and dietitian; and the 'clumsy' school-age child who can be helped by a joint approach from occupational and physiotherapy. The physiotherapist is also a key member of the multidisciplinary assessment team of the child with suspected neurodevelopmental abnormalities; and of the team planning orthopaedic and non-surgical treatments for children with gait and postural disorders.

ASSESSMENT AND OBSERVING CHANGE

The assessment of children with static or progressive neurological disorders can be difficult, especially in the early stages. It is always important to listen carefully to what parents are describing, as in many cases such a description is more valuable than a 'hands on' assessment with an uncooperative child. The observation of children at play, in the home or at school, is invaluable. The process of assessment needs to make allowance for many factors which can influence the individual's performance. These include: cultural and family norms; the effects of prematurity; coexisting systemic disease in infancy (cardiac, renal or gastro-intestinal) that may cause significant changes in function; and the effects of drugs such as antiepileptics. Regression, or the loss of previously acquired skills, is a hallmark of degenerative disorders of the CNS, such as metachromatic leucodystrophy. At an early stage, however, there will be only a slowdown in the acquisition of skills, which is then followed by plateauing and eventually a loss of skills. Loss of function is also sometimes seen in children with non-progressive disorders. The child with a congenital spastic hemiplegia, for instance, may develop increasing gait abnormality in later childhood due to progressive shortening of the Achilles tendon in the absence of progression of the underlying neurological disorder.

TRANSITION FROM PAEDIATRIC TO ADULT SERVICES

The time of transition from children's services to the adult services can be unsettling for the adolescent with a neurological disorder as well as for the family. It may come at a time of upheaval in the life of a young person who is seeking greater independence in the face of continuing neurological handicaps. One way to facilitate a smooth transition from paediatric to adult services is for therapists from both services to meet, jointly with patients, in order to plan in advance for the move from one service to another. This often provides an opportunity to review the objectives, goals and methods of therapy.

CHROMOSOMAL DISORDERS AND RECOGNISABLE PATTERNS OF MALFORMATION

Chromosomal disorders are caused by an abnormality in an individual's complement of chromosomes. The normal situation is to possess 23 pairs of chromosomes, of which one pair are sex chromosomes (two X chromosomes in females and an X and a Y in males). Individuals with Down's syndrome have an additional chromosome 21, with most having a total of 47 chromosomes. This disorder occurs in approximately 1 in 800 births and is more common with advancing maternal age (Jones, 1988). Children with Down's syndrome have an increased likelihood of a variety of congenital abnormalities, including cardiac malformations, intestinal atresias and cataracts. The intellectual development of children with Down's syndrome is slower than normal and the average IQ is around 50. Other specific neurological problems include hypotonia, an increased incidence of epilepsy and the occurrence of dementia from 40 years onwards in many individuals.

Physiotherapy alone or as part of a multidisciplinary programme has been used in the management of children with Down's syndrome. There is evidence for improvement in motor skills, particularly following early intervention programmes that include a series of individualised therapy objectives (Harris, 1981; Connolly et al., 1984). Physiotherapy includes management of low muscle tone (see Chapter 25) and strategies to improve strength, coordination, general fitness and functional activities. Many children with Down's syndrome have asymptomatic atlantoaxial instability and around 1% are at increased risk of atlantoaxial subluxation, which may cause quadriplegia. Cervical spine radiographs are not carried out routinely in children with Down's syndrome, but should be taken if there is head tilt or the emergence of neurological signs, or if participation in tumbling or contact sports is planned (Chaudry et al., 1987).

Other trisomies include Edward's syndrome (trisomy 18) and Pattau's syndrome (trisomy 13), both of which cause profound retardation and usually death in early infancy.

Some chromosomal anomalies can be detected only by high-resolution chromosomal studies or by analysis of dioxyribonucleic acid (DNA). Prader–Willi syndrome, for instance, is due to a deletion of part of chromosome 15. Most affected infants are extremely hypotonic in the neonatal period, often with marked feeding difficulties that require tube feeding. Later they have excessive appetites and obesity, short stature, and moderate learning difficulties. Because of the hypotonia there is an increased risk of scoliosis in early infancy and the role of physiotherapy includes providing advice about positioning and seating to promote good postures and reduce the risk of deformity developing.

MALFORMATIONS OF THE CNS

The development of the CNS in the fetus and embryo is a complex process and it is not surprising that abnormalities may occur at any stage (Chapter 18). Malformations that result from such abnormal development are an important cause of neurological illness in childhood (Aicardi, 1992). Between one third and a half of all infants who die in the first year of life have a serious CNS malformation. The survivors may have a range of neurological disorders including motor deficits, mental retardation, epilepsy and impairments of the special senses.

In those malformations that arise before about 20 weeks of gestation there is usually a disturbance of CNS morphology (Table 17.2). This is a time of intense change in the structure of the nervous system, including neural tube closure (by 29 days), formation of the forebrain and diencephalon (by 6 weeks) and migration of cortical neurones (by 20 weeks). Abnormal development may occur because of a faulty genetic code (e.g. in Miller-Dieker syndrome in

which there is a deletion of chromosome 17 and lissencephaly) or there may be external abnormalities that interfere with CNS development. Well recognised causes include: fetal infections (such as rubella, which causes microcephaly, and cytomegalovirus, which can cause abnormal neuronal migration); drugs (such as sodium valproate, which can cause spina bifida); and drug abuse (alcohol causing microcephaly and 'crack' cocaine causing early vascular destruction). No cause can be identified in about two thirds of children with CNS malformations of early onset.

By about 20 weeks of gestation all the major components of the nervous system are in place and most malformations arising after this time do so because of destructive processes. One example is periventricular leucomalacia, in which there is destruction of white matter adjacent to the lateral ventricles of the brain. This usually arises between 20 and 30 weeks of gestation, and is the neuropathological change seen most often in children with diplegic cerebral palsy who were born prematurely.

The physiotherapeutic needs of children with cerebral malformations depend upon the nature of the motor and other neurodevelopmental deficits as well as other individual and family factors. This group includes some children with the most severe impairments. Although the malformations themselves are not progressive, there is a high morbidity and mortality related to intercurrent infection, epilepsy and feeding disorders. In many cases, malformations of the nervous system coexist with abnormalities of other organ systems, including congenital heart disease and limb abnormalities. It is important to be aware of these when these children are undergoing physiotherapy.

NEUROCUTANEOUS SYNDROMES

The neurocutaneous syndromes are a group of disorders in which abnormalities of the skin and brain coexist (Gomez, 1987). Both the skin and the nervous system are derived from the ectodermal layer of the developing embryo. Many of these disorders are genetic and arise because of faulty chromosomal regulation of cell growth and proliferation. Other body organs may also be involved.

NEUROFIBROMATOSIS TYPE 1 (VON RECKLINGHAUSEN DISEASE)

This is the commonest neurocutaneous syndrome with a prevalence of around 1 in 3000 of the population (Huson et al., 1988). It is inherited as an autosomal dominant trait, with affected individuals having a 50% chance of passing on the condition to their children. About a third of cases are new mutations. The skin abnormalities are multiple café-au-lait patches, axillary freckles and firm subcutaneous neurofibromas. The most frequent neurological abnormalities are mild learning difficulties, attention deficit disorders and poor co-ordination. There is an increased risk of developing CNS tumours, especially gliomas of the optic pathway. Although many children with neurofibromatosis type 1 will not need physiotherapy, some will benefit from therapy if they have motor

Some important malformations of the central nervous system

Malformation	Description	Clinical features
Cerebral malformations		
Microcephaly	Abnormally small brain	Usually learning difficulties, may also have motor deficits
Lissencephaly	Smooth brain without normal central gyri	Severe learning difficulties, epilepsy, hypotonia and pyramidal motor deficits
Hydrocephalus	Enlargement of cerebral ventricles due to impaired CSF drainage	May be normal; often specific learning deficits and language disorders
Holoprosencephaly	Undivided forebrain, often with fused lateral ventricles	Severe learning difficulties, midline facial clefts, hypopituitarism
Porencephaly	Destructive change in one cerebral hemisphere	Often hemiplegia; may have epilepsy, learning difficulties and hemianopia
Cerebellar malformations		
Cerebellar hypoplasia	Maldevelopment of cerebellar hemispheres or vermis	Ataxia, hypotonia, disordered eye movements
Dandy Walker syndrome	Posterior fossa cyst and cerebellar vermis hypoplasia	Symptoms of hydrocephalus and may have learning difficulties
Chiari malformation	Cerebellar tonsils project through foramen magnum	Type I–rarely symptomatic Type II–occurs with spina bifida
Neural tube defects		
Encephalocele	Skull defect with protrusion of meninges with or without brain	Anterior: meningitis, CSF leak Posterior: high mortality and disability
Myelomenigocele	Vertebral defect with exposed meninges and spinal cord	Paraplegia, neuropathic bowel and bladder, hydrocephalus
Spina bifida occulta	Maldevelopment of lower spinal cord and vertebrae covered by skin	Progressive unilateral foot deformity and weakness, neuropathic bladder

Table 17.2 **Some important malformations of the central nervous system (CNS).** (Abbreviation: CSF, cerebrospinal fluid).

deficits resulting from brain tumours, spinal cord and root compression or bony deformity of the limbs.

TUBEROUS SCLEROSIS

Tuberous sclerosis is also inherited in a dominant fashion but it is both rarer (1 in 10,000) and more severe than neurofibromatosis. The skin changes include hypopigmented skin patches and red papules (angiofibromata) over the nose and cheeks. The neurological abnormalities include epilepsy in 80% and learning difficulties (which may be severe) in 50%. Motor deficits are not common. Brain scans demonstrate tubers, which are benign growths in the cortex. Cerebral tumours can also occur and may cause hydrocephalus.

STURGE-WEBER SYNDROME

This is another, rarer neurocutaneous syndrome that is frequently associated with motor deficits. These children have a 'port wine' haemangioma over the upper face, in the area innervated by the first division of the trigeminal nerve. They may have congenital glaucoma. They also have an angioma on the meninges on one or both sides of the brain, usually extending over the occipital cortex. Although most such children are normal at birth, many have debilitating focal epileptic seizures and a progressive hemiplegia, often together with progressively more apparent learning difficulties. Physiotherapy is often required for the hemiplegia and associated abnormalities.

GENETIC METABOLIC AND NEURODEGENERATIVE DISORDERS

There are a large number of individually rare genetic metabolic disorders that cause neurological symptoms in childhood (Holton, 1994). Some important disorders are listed in Table 17.3. Some may cause symptoms from birth, for instance phenylketonuria and hypothyroidism. Others may not present until after months or years of normal development, as occurs with some of the leucodystrophies. Some may cause intermittently severe symptoms such as coma, ataxia and seizures, as occurs in children with organic acidaemias. In others there is a progressive deterioration in motor and cognitive abilities, resulting eventually in death, as occurs with the gangliosidoses. Specific and effective treatments are available for some disorders. In phenylketonuria and hypothyroidism, screening for the defect at birth allows treatment to be commenced immediately and minimises the risk of neurological sequelae. Even in those disorders for which a specific treatment is not available it is important to make a diagnosis. Most of these disorders are inherited in an autosomal recessive fashion with a 1 in 4 risk of siblings being affected. Prenatal diagnosis can be offered to many couples (by chorionic villous biopsy), allowing for the termination of an affected fetus at an early stage of the pregnancy.

There are some disorders of childhood that share features in common with these neurometabolic disorders, but for which no cause is known. One such disorder is Rett syndrome, which occurs in 1 in 10,000 girls and is one of the most important causes of progressive neurological handicap in girls (Hagberg, 1993). Girls with Rett syndrome appear normal or only slightly slow in their development until 6–18 months of age. At around this time they undergo a period of regression in development, followed by many years of almost developmental standstill. At the same time new features appear, including stereotyped hand-wringing movements, tachypnoea and breath-holding, progressive gait apraxia, scoliosis and epilepsy. Ambulation is usually lost and feeding difficulties are often severe. Despite these considerable difficulties most girls survive into adulthood. Physiotherapy has an important part to play in the management of girls with Rett syndrome. It is important that the therapist is familiar with the natural history and particular features of this singular disorder. The maintenance of optimum function and prevention of deformity is very difficult in the face of a

Important genetic, metabolic and degenerative disorders of childhood

Group of disorders	Examples	Clinical symptoms
Amino acidurias	Phenylketonuria*	Microcephaly, severe learning difficulties, quadriplegia and epilepsy
Organic acidurias	Glutaric aciduria	Encephalopathy, dystonia, seizures
Leucodystrophies	Metachromatic leucodystrophy	Progressive spasticity, ataxia and peripheral neuropathy
Batten's disease	Juvenile Batten's disease	Progressive visual impairment, seizures and dementia
Mucopolysaccharidoses	Hurler's syndrome	Coarse features, learning difficulties, kyphosis
Gangliosidoses	Tay-Sachs disease	Dementia and progressive spasticity and blindness in infancy
Hypothyroidism	Congenital hypothyroidism*	Learning difficulties ('cretinism')
Copper metabolism	Wilson's disease*	Progressive dystonia, ataxia and behavioural changes in adolescence
Mitochondrial disorders	MELAS	Encephalopathy, lactic acidosis and stroke-like episodes

*These disorders can be treated successfully

Table 17.3 Important genetic, metabolic and degenerative disorders of childhood.

changing series of neurodevelopmental abnormalities, often combined with periods of agitation and misery on the part of these girls. Important aspects include the provision of adequate aids to seating and mobility, as well as surveillance and early intervention for the scoliosis which is common in this condition.

CNS INFECTION AND INFLAMMATORY DISORDERS IN CHILDHOOD

Infections of the CNS are amongst the most frequent causes of injury to this system in childhood. The likelihood of permanent sequelae following CNS infections is related to the age of the child, the site of infection, the nature of the organism, the rapidity with which effective treatments are commenced, and the need for intensive care support. Most children with viral meningitis due to an organism such as the mumps virus make an excellent recovery, whereas viral encephalitis due to herpes virus often leads to permanent sequelae including seizures, hemiparesis and memory impairments. Bacterial meningitis due to *Haemophilus influenzae* is largely preventable by immunisation and much less likely to cause permanent damage than is tuberculous meningitis, which often causes hydrocephalus, cranial nerve palsies, hemiparesis and visual loss. If recognised and treated early, a cerebral abscess resulting from extension from sinus infection often has a very good outcome. However, the neonate who develops abscesses as a result of infection with an organism such as Citrobacter is often left with severe damage, resulting in quadriplegia, seizures and blindness.

Physiotherapy for children with such infections may start during the period of hospital treatment, at which stage it may still be difficult to predict the eventual outcome. Early interventions are intended to prevent deformity and encourage rehabilitation. Regular review and assessment are necessary to monitor how the child is recovering function.

The amount and type of physiotherapy input can be reviewed regularly as the child's recovery indicates, and in response to each family's needs.

Some viruses may cause chronic CNS infection, resulting in relentlessly progressive and severe neurological disorders. Measles virus causes subacute sclerosing panencephalitis in about 1 in 100,000 infected children, with an onset of symptoms 5–15 years after the original infection. Neurological deficits include myoclonus, dementia and dystonia, with death occurring within months to years from onset.

The human immunodeficiency virus (HIV) is neurotropic and frequently causes neurological symptoms in affected children (Epstein *et al.*, 1986). These include a slowing in the acquisition of developmental skills followed by a loss of previously acquired milestones. A progressive paraparesis is common. Opportunistic CNS infections in children with acquired immune deficiency syndrome (AIDS) may cause severe sequelae.

HEAD INJURY IN CHILDHOOD

Head injury becomes an increasingly important cause of neurological morbidity or death as children get older, especially boys. Serious head injury in older children is usually the result of accidents outside the home. Certain children are more vulnerable, including those from poorer homes or living in deprived areas, as well as those with pre-existing behavioural or neurodevelopmental problems. When rehabilitating a child following a head injury, it is important to know about problems that were present before the accident.

Non-accidental head injury occurs especially in children less than 1 year of age (Krugman *et al.*, 1993). Parents or other carers are the usual perpetrators. They may themselves have been the victims of violent abuse in childhood. Some children, including those with pre-existing neurological handicaps, are more at risk of being abused. The mechanism of injury includes shaking ('infantile whiplash injury'), blows to the head or throwing the child against a hard surface. Injury is often repeated and associated with other evidence of abuse including fractures of the limbs and ribs. Intracranial injury includes subdural haematomas (often of differing ages) with contusion of the underlying brain (Figure 17.1). There may be more widespread brain injury than at first suspected, with shearing injuries of the white matter of the brain. Retinal haemorrhages are a frequent finding. Surgical treatment may be required for the subdural haemorrhage. Over half these children have

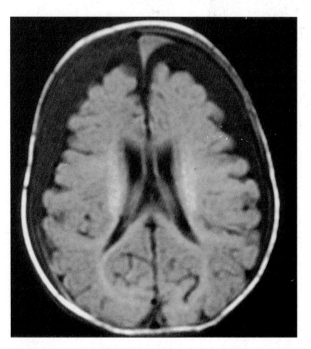

Figure 17.1 Subdural haemorrhage in non-accidental injury. Magnetic resonance (MR) brain scan (T1 weighted) shows bilateral subdural collections with layering of the fluid, suggesting haemorrhage on two or three separate occasions.

permanent neurological handicaps including hemiplegia or quadriplegia, seizures and visual impairments.

The physiotherapist will often be involved from an early stage in the management of a child who has suffered a head injury (see Chapter 8). Early involvement will include the maintenance of good respiratory function, whilst ensuring that the techniques used have no detrimental effects on the injured brain. During the acute stages it is important to maintain the range of movement in all joints. Splinting is often necessary to maintain good joint position, although this will depend upon the nature of the underlying neurological deficit. The rehabilitation of the child with a serious head injury involves close working with parents, nursing staff, doctors, speech therapists, occupational therapists, psychologists and school teachers (Scott-Jump *et al.*, 1992). Reintegration into schooling and the successful provision of support from community-based professionals (including physiotherapists and doctors) are essential following severe head injuries.

CNS TUMOURS IN CHILDHOOD

Brain tumours are the commonest solid tumours of childhood and second only to leukaemia as a cause of malignancy in this age group (Deutsch, 1990). Certain types of brain tumour are more common in children than in adults (Table 17.4), particularly medulloblastomas (primitive neuroectodermal tumours; Figure 17.2) and craniopharyngiomas, whereas secondary brain tumours are rarer. About half of brain tumours in children arise in the posterior fossa, a much higher rate than in adults. Presenting symptoms include progressive ataxia (in children with posterior fossa tumours), headaches due to raised intracranial pressure, seizures due to some tumours of the cerebral hemispheres and cranial nerve palsies due to brainstem tumours.

Most brain tumours are treated by surgery and in many cases the outcome correlates most closely with the extent of surgical resection. Surgery can sometimes produce deficits where none existed previously, in an attempt at radical treatment of a potentially fatal tumour such as a

Table 17.4 Tumours of the central nervous system (CNS) in childhood.

Tumours of the central nervous system in childhood

Site	Type	Frequency (%)
Brain		
Cerebral hemispheres	Glioma	20
	Ependymoma	3
	Primitive neuroectodermal tumour	5
	Meningioma	2
	Pineal germinomas and teratomas	4
	Choroid plexus papilloma	1
Pituitary region	Craniopharyngioma	7
	Pituitary adenoma	2
Cerebellum	Medulloblastoma	20
	Astrocytoma	17
	Ependymoma	5
Brainstem	Glioma	7
	Other types	7
		100
Spinal cord		
Extradural	Neuroblastoma	40
	Rhabdomyosarcoma	
	Histiocytosis X	
Intradural and extramedullary	Meningioma	25
	Schwannoma	
Intradural and intramedullary	Astrocytoma	35
	Ependymoma	
		100

medulloblastoma. Malignant and partially resected tumours are often treated with radiotherapy, sometimes in combination with chemotherapy to reduce the chance of relapse (Deutsch, 1990). These treatments, especially radiotherapy, can also produce neurological deficits. Radiotherapy particularly affects the growing brain, causing intellectual loss and occasionally more severe neurological disorders such as radionecrosis. For this reason radiotherapy is not now given to children under 3 years of age.

The outcomes of treatment depend upon the site and type of tumour. The worst prognosis is in children with brainstem gliomas, <20% of whom will be alive 5 years after treatment. The best prognosis is in children with benign gliomas, >80% of whom survive for longer than 5 years (Duffner *et al.*, 1986).

Spinal cord tumours are much less common than brain tumours (Table 17.4). They are often diagnosed very late, with intervals of sometimes months or even years between the onset of symptoms and diagnosis. This is because the significance of changes in gait or sphincter control and the onset of back pain may be overlooked, especially in young children. Diagnosis by MR imaging is much more rapid and less invasive than myelography, which was used in the past. Treatment of these tumours is with surgery, radiotherapy and chemotherapy; again, a high risk exists of worsening neurological deficits with treatment.

Children with brain and spinal tumours have a high incidence of motor deficits, especially ataxia and hemiplegia with brain tumours and paraplegia with spinal tumours. Some of these may worsen with time, either as a result of tumour progression or as a side effect of treatment. They require skilled physiotherapy from a person who understands the nature of the underlying disorder, the often long drawn-out treatment that may be necessary and the impact on the child and family.

CEREBROVASCULAR DISORDERS IN CHILDHOOD

Stroke occurs much less commonly in children than in adults (see Chapter 7), affecting 1 child in 40,000 per year. About half of childhood strokes are due to haemorrhage (subarachnoid and/or intracerebral) and half to ischaemia (Table 17.5; Riela & Roach, 1993). Most haemorrhages are from arteriovenous malformations. Aneurysms affect the vertebrobasilar circulation more often in children than in adults. In 15% of cases no cause is found for cerebral haemorrhage. Most ischaemic strokes occur during or following infections, including meningitis. Atherosclerosis is very unusual in young children.

Children, and especially young infants, can recover impressively following strokes. In part this may be due to plasticity of the nervous system which is particularly evident in the developing brain (Chapter 6). A good example is the transference of language function from the dominant to the non-dominant hemisphere that occurs during the recovery from middle cerebral artery infarction (Figure 17.3) in early childhood.

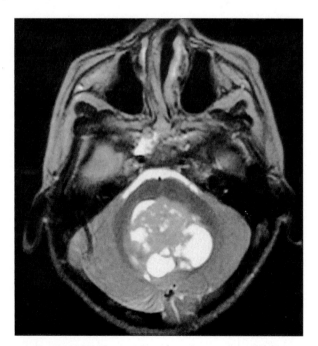

Figure 17.2 Medulloblastoma. MR brain scan (T2 weighted) shows a large mixed solid and cystic mass arising from the middle of the cerebellum.

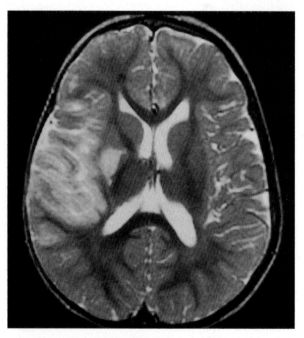

Figure 17.3 Middle cerebral artery infarction. MR brain scan (T2 weighted) shows a signal change in the distribution of the right middle cerebral artery (left side of image) as a result of ischaemia and reperfusion.

Table 17. 5 Causes of stroke in childhood.

Causes of stroke in childhood	
Type	Cause
Haemorrhagic (50%)	Arteriovenous malformation Aneurysm Unidentified
Ischaemic (50%) Thrombotic	Postinfectious (e.g. chickenpox, bacterial meningitis) Sickle cell disease Hypercoagulation (e.g. Protein C deficiency) Moyamoya disease Cerebral vasculitis (e.g. lupus) Metabolic (e.g. homocystinuria) Migraine
Embolic	Endocarditis Myocarditis Congenital heart disease Dissecting aneurysm

PERIPHERAL NERVE INJURIES

Nerve injuries are discussed in detail in Chapter 10, but obstetric brachial plexus injuries deserve special mention here. These occur in 1 in 4000 births and are associated with shoulder dystocia in two thirds of cases and with breech delivery in a further 15% (Rossi *et al.*, 1982). Most are Erb's palsies involving the C5 and C6 roots of the brachial plexus and only rarely is there involvement of C8 and T1. Around 75% recover, although recovery may take many months and can continue for some years. Nerve grafting is indicated for the most severe lesions (Laurent & Lee, 1994). The failure to develop active elbow flexion in the affected limb by 3–6 months of age may be one indicator of poor outcome in a lesion, and grafting should be considered.

SPINOCEREBELLAR DEGENERATIONS AND HEREDITARY ATAXIAS

Congenital ataxia may be due to structural abnormalities of developing cerebellum, principally affecting either the cerebellar hemispheres or vermis (Aicardi, 1992). Some of these disorders are genetic, for instance Joubert syndrome, an autosomal recessive disorder in which, in addition to the ataxia, there are learning difficulties, retinal abnormalities and abnormalities of respiratory pattern.

Acquired ataxia in childhood may be due to progressive disorders (Table 17.6). As well as structural lesions, such as cerebellar tumours, there are genetic disorders. Friedreich's ataxia is inherited as an autosomal recessive disorder and has its onset usually between 5 and 15 years. As well as a progressive ataxia, affected people develop pes cavus and scoliosis. Cardiomyopathy and diabetes mellitus are other frequent findings. Most patients lose the ability to walk by about 15 years after the onset of symptoms.

Ataxia telangiectasia is another disorder inherited in an autosomal recessive fashion with its onset in early childhood. Affected children have an increased susceptibilty to sinopulmonary infections and their skin is excessively sensitive to exposure to sunlight. They have a tendency to develop malignancies, especially leukaemias and lymphomas, from adolescence onwards. In neither of these disorders is dementia a feature.

CHILDREN WHO RAISE CONCERNS

Most children acquire motor developmental milestones in a predictable pattern and at similar ages. When children deviate from these it may serve as a warning that there is a significant underlying disorder. For instance, the boy who does not walk until after 18 months of age could have Duchenne muscular dystrophy (see Chapter 21). However, there are some children who have an unusual pattern of early motor development for which no cause can be found. In some cases this may be a familial pattern. An example is children who 'bottom-shuffle' rather than crawl and who often do not walk independently until well after their first birthday and often closer to their second.

HYPOTONIA

Hypotonia in infancy may be due to neuromuscular disorders or to central causes (including neurological disorders, chromosomal abnormalities and metabolic disorders). There are some children who are hypotonic in infancy in the absence of discernible underlying disease and who can be markedly delayed in their early motor development, but with normal acquisition of other developmental skills. After infancy many such children often have little residual abnormality, if any. The term benign congenital hypotonia has been applied to this group, which probably includes

Important causes of progressive ataxia in childhood	
Group of disorders	Examples
Structural lesions	Cerebellar tumour
Parainfectious and paraneoplastic	Dancing eye syndrome
Demyelinating	Multiple sclerosis
DNA repair abnormalities	Ataxia telangiectasia
Metabolic diseases	Wilson's disease
Spinocerebellar degenerations	Friedreich's ataxia

Table 17.6 **Important causes of progressive ataxia in childhood.**

more than one cause for this striking variation in early development. A similar group of children often have a familial tendency to joint hypermobility, in the absence of a definable disorder of connective tissue, and many of them are also often delayed in their early gross motor development. Hypotonia and other abnormalities of tone and movement are discussed in Chapters 5 & 25.

The role of physiotherapy includes the assessment of such children and the differentiation of patterns which are normal variants from those due to underlying disease. This requires familiarity with the range of normal development (Chapter 18).

THE 'CLUMSY' CHILD

There is a further group of children who present to the medical and therapy services with increasing frequency. These are children with the label of 'clumsiness'. The description covers a variety of different problems. Some children demonstrate particular difficulties with acquisition of fine motor skills such as pencil skills, using utensils and tying laces or doing up buttons. Others have greater difficulties with tasks requiring good hand–eye co-ordination and balance, such as ball throwing or learning to ride a bicycle. Some children have problems in several of these areas, others in only a few. What they have in common is the absence of definable neurological deficits, such as ataxia, spasticity or dystonia. Often there is a family history of a parent or sibling with similar difficulties. Many such clumsy children suffer from poor self-esteem. They can be helped by occupational therapists and physiotherapists to learn strategies to overcome areas of particular difficulty (Schoemaker *et al.*, 1994). The majority grow up to be normal adults, often choosing in their adolescent years to shun physical activities which they find hard to succeed at. A number of descriptions have been applied to these children, including 'minimal brain damage', 'dyspraxia' and 'cerebral palsy'. None of these terms is accurate for all of this group and 'motor learning disorders' is the preferred term (see Chapter 19).

NON-ORGANIC NEUROLOGICAL DISORDERS IN CHILDHOOD

Some children adopt a 'sick' role as a means of avoiding intolerable life situations. Such illness behaviour is not often seen in children under 10 years of age but occurs with increasing frequency in young teenagers. The presenting problem may be an abnormal gait, a paralysed limb, or pain or sensory loss in one part of the body. The onset is often after a minor illness or accident, for which the child may have received medical attention. The symptom frequently causes the child to withdraw from normal activities and absence from school can be prolonged, despite attempts at encouraging a return.

Many of these children have had some personal experience of illness, either in themselves or in a close relative. One or other parent may have experienced a similar period of illness in the past. The parents, or one parent, will often closely identify with the child and may find it very difficult to accept that there is not a serious illness underlying the symptoms. Health professionals may unwittingly collude in perpetuating the child's symptoms by expressing concern and uncertainty about an undiagnosed disease process. Children may be referred from one specialist to another for opinions and tests which serve only to reinforce the worry the child has about his or her own health. Many of these children are academically or athletically very able, sometimes setting themselves very high standards that they may find hard to achieve. Others may be the victims of bullying at school or of physical or sexual abuse at home. In our experience, many children presenting with 'chronic fatigue syndrome' and some with 'reflex sympathetic dystrophy' are indistinguishable from this group with non-organic neurological disorders.

These children need an assessment of their condition which reaches a definite conclusion, and this can then be confidently and sympathetically discussed with the child and parents. This is followed by a goal-oriented rehabilitation programme. It is important that there is good teamwork between the disciplines involved, as opportunity exists to play professionals off against one another. Physiotherapy has a key role in the physical rehabilitation of these children, but therapists will often need the support of doctors and psychologists if they are going to succeed. It can be helpful to have a child draw up his or her own list of goals for a coming week, which can then be renegotiated each week on an ongoing basis. It is important to reintegrate the child into education, beginning for instance with the hospital school and gradually building up to a return to full-time school. If there are underlying issues within the home or school these also need to be tackled, usually by child psychiatrists or clinical psychologists working with the whole family.

MEASURING OUTCOMES

Some parents will express satisfaction with the care and interest that is shown in their child's condition. They may feel more confident and in control of the situation when there is someone to guide them as to how to manage their child's physical problems. Others may embark on a search for new therapies for their child, often in the belief that what is readily available is never enough and that exceptional treatments exist that may unlock their child's potential. Sometimes they are right and some children will benefit from forms of therapy which are more intensive or use novel techniques. Too often, however, this search for novel remedies or additional therapy places undue emphasis on the motor disorder at the expense of education, play, emotional and social development. It can also distort the care that other children in the family receive (which may already be considerably affected by having a sibling with a neurological disorder).

Any form of therapy requires evaluation. However, assessing the effectiveness of interventions can be particularly difficult when working with children with neurological disorders. It requires validated measures, which are responsive to clinically important functional change. Unfortunately there are too few such measures designed for this purpose in children with neurological disorders (Rosenbaum *et al.*, 1990) and some are mentioned in Chapter 4. Although there have been a number of studies which have sought to evaluate physiotherapy for children with neurological disorders such as cerebral palsy, it is difficult not to make the focus of such studies a too narrow set of goals (Sommerfeld *et al.*, 1981). Some assessments used in adults (see Chapter 4) may be applicable to children but require evaluation and perhaps modification. Some simple practical measures can be used, such as ROM, photography and video recording, to monitor changes in functional abilities and deformity.

Change in motor function is not the only clinical change that requires evaluation. The goals of a therapy programme should also include patient comfort, prevention of deformity, integration into schooling, ability to participate in leisure activities and family satisfaction. Measures of quality of life are also lacking but developments are being made in this area (see Chapter 27).

IMPORTANT MOTOR DISORDERS IN CHILDHOOD

The remaining chapters of this section, on disorders of childhood onset, deal with the most common motor disorders in which physiotherapy plays an important role. These include the cerebral palsies (Chapter 19), neural tube defects such as spina bifida (Chapter 20) and muscle disorders, including the muscular dystrophies and spinal muscular atrophy (Chapter 21). As mentioned previously, an understanding of normal development is essential when treating children with such disorders and this topic is outlined in Chapter 18. With more children surviving further into adulthood with these disorders, the need for those involved in adult services to understand these conditions is stressed throughout the subsequent chapters.

REFERENCES

Aicardi J. *Diseases of the nervous system in childhood*. Oxford: MacKeith Press/Blackwell Scientific Publications; 1992.

Chaudry V, Sturgeon C, Gates AJ, *et al.* Symptomatic atlantoaxial dislocation in Down's syndrome. *Ann Neurol* 1987, **21**:606-609.

Connolly B, Morgan S, Russell F. Evaluation of children with Down syndrome who participated in an early intervention program. *Phys Ther* 1984, **64**:151-155.

Deutsch M. *Management of childhood brain tumours*. Boston: Kluwer; 1990.

Duffner PK, Cohen ME, Myers MH, *et al.* Survival of children with brain tumours: SEER program 1973-1980. *Neurology* 1986, **36**:597-601.

Epstein LG, Sharer LR, Oleske JM, *et al.* Neurologic manifestations of human immunodeficiency virus infection in children. *Paediatrics* 1986, **78**:678-687.

Gomez MG. *Neurocutaneous diseases - a practical approach*. Boston: Butterworth; 1987.

Hagberg B. *Rett Syndrome - clinical and biological aspects*. London: MacKeith Press; 1993. (Clinics in developmental medicine, No. 127).

Harris SR. Effects of neurodevelopmental therapy on motor performance of infants with Down's syndrome. *Dev Med Child Neurol* 1981, **23**:477-483.

Holton J. *The inherited metabolic diseases*. London: Churchill Livingstone; 1994.

Huson SM, Harper PS, Compston DAS. Von Recklinghausen neurofibromatosis: a clinical and population study in south-east Wales. *Brain* 1988, **111**:1355-1381.

Jones KL. *Recognisable patterns of human malformation*. Philadelphia: WB Saunders; 1988.

Krugman RD, Bays JA, Chadwick DL, *et al.* Shaken baby syndrome: inflicted cerebral trauma. Committee on child abuse and neglect. *Paediatrics* 1993, **92**:872-875.

Kurtz Z, Stanley F. Epidemiology. In: Harvey D, Miles M, Smyth D, eds. *Community child health and paediatrics*. Oxford: Butterworth Heinemann; 1995:3-22.

Laurent JP, Lee RT. Birth-related upper brachial plexus injuries in infants: operative and non-operative approaches. *J Child Neurol* 1994, **9**:111-117.

Riela AR, Roach ES. Etiology of stroke in children. *J Child Neurol* 1993, **8**:201-220.

Rosenbaum PL, Russell DJ, Cadman DT, *et al.* Issues in measuring change in motor function in children with cerebral palsy - a special communication. *Phys Ther* 1990, **70**:125-131.

Rossi LN, Vassella F, Mumenthaler M. Obstetrical lesions of the brachial plexus. Natural history in 34 personal cases. *Eur Neurol* 1982, **21**:1-7.

Schoemaker MM, Hijlkema MGJ, Kalverboer AF. Physiotherapy for clumsy children: an evaluation study. *Dev Med Child Neurol* 1994, **36**:143-155.

Scott-Jump R, Marlow N, Seddon N, *et al.* Rehabilitation and outcome after severe head injury. *Arch Dis Child* 1992, **67**:222-226.

Sommerfeld D, Fraser B, Hensinger RN. Evaluation of physical therapy service for severely mentally impaired students with cerebral palsy. *Phys Ther* 1981, **61**:338-344.

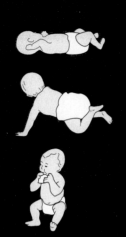

18   E Green

DEVELOPMENTAL NEUROLOGY

CHAPTER OUTLINE

- **Prenatal development of the brain and spinal cord**
- **Postnatal development**
- **Postnatal landmarks in the development of postural control, reflexes, balance and movement**

- **Theories of sensorimotor skill development**
- **Development of vision**
- **Development of hearing**
- **Landmarks of intellectual development**

PRENATAL DEVELOPMENT OF THE BRAIN AND SPINAL CORD

The brain develops from a single cell into a very complex structure containing billions of neurones. This chapter describes the developmental aspect of brain development. The brain's life cycle can be studied in greater detail in Thompson (1993).

STRUCTURAL DEVELOPMENT

There are many unanswered questions about how the human brain develops its precise, detailed and extremely complicated neuronal circuits. The answers will probably be found at the level of individual nerve cells (neurones) and their interactions, their processes of growth and migration, as well as the physical or chemical events responsible for those processes.

Induction

Induction is the general principle believed to underlie the development of the nervous system. Neurones are first formed from the embryo's outer ectodermal layer, similar to the cells of the epidermis covering the outer body surface. They are formed by interaction with the cells beneath them, which will become the vertebral column and other

tissues constituting the mesoderm. Before the ectodermal cells interact with the mesodermal cells, the epidermal cells can become either nerve cells or skin cells. It is presumed that the mesodermal cells release a substance that causes certain ectodermal cells to change into neurones.

Neural Plate and Neural Tube

About 3 weeks after conception, the neural plate is formed by a thickening of the ectodermal cells on the dorsal surface of the embryo (Figure 18.1A). This is the start of the process called neurulation, in which the first phase of neural tube formation occurs with the development of a neural groove with a neural fold along each side. By the end of the third week the neural folds have begun to fuse with one another, so converting the neural groove into a neural tube (Figure 18.1B,C). This is the forerunner of the brain and spinal cord.

Neural Crests

Neuroectodermal cells not incorporated into the tube form neural crests running dorsolaterally along each side of the neural tube (Figure 18.1C). From the neural crests are derived: the dorsal root ganglia of spinal nerves, some of the neurones in sensory ganglia of cranial nerves, autonomic ganglia, the non-neuronal cells (neuroglia) of the peripheral nerves, and the secretory nerves of the adrenal medulla. Others differentiate into cells of non-neural tissue, such as the melanocytes of the skin and some of the bones, muscles and other structures of the head that are of dermal origin. The target tissues determine the fate of the neural crest cells, though it is not yet clear how. This stage of migration is practically complete by 24 weeks after conception. It is thought that the time of migration of different cells is controlled by the neurones losing their capacity to synthesise deoxyribonucleic acid (DNA) and therefore ceasing to divide and form new cells.

Neuroblasts–Precursors of Neurones

The first population of cells produced in the neural tube are neuroblasts, the precursors of neurones. The number of neuroblasts formed in the neural tube far exceeds the number of neurones in the adult brain and spinal cord. Outgrowth of axons and dendrites from the cells occurs and neuroblasts that fail to make synaptic connections die as part of the normal course of development (see Chapter 6, 'Plasticity'). This happens particularly in the spinal cord. As the developing neurones send out axons, the basic form of the grey matter (cell bodies) and white matter (axons) of the spinal cord develops (Figure 18.1D).

Formation of the Brain

Growth and differentiation is greatest at the end of the neural tube where the brain develops; the rest of the neural tube becomes the spinal cord. Three distinct regions are formed at the end of the fourth week: the forebrain; the midbrain; and the hindbrain. Within each of these three regions and within the embryonic spinal cord, neuroblasts multiply and migrate to form the characteristic structures of the brain as aggregates of neurones. These neurones send their axons in fibre tracts to other brain regions and also receive synaptic input from axons migrating from other brain regions. The forebrain and the hindbrain both divide further during the fifth week to form a structure with five regions. During this expansion, the neural tube takes on a number of flexures, or bends, to accommodate its length within the skull. The parts of the brain derived from the five regions are shown in Figure 18.2. The development of the human brain in stages from 25 days until birth can be seen in Figure 18.3.

Neuronal and Synapse Production

Myelination and transmitter production take place in parallel to the axonal growth and synapse formation, and continue postnatally. The structural layers of the cerebral cortex are completed during the last months of pregnancy and the first postnatal months. Synapse production and network formation continue to a considerable extent through the first years of life. At the end of the first year synapse density is greatest, decreasing to adult densities at about 7 years of age. The reduction in the number of neurones seems to be an active, genetically determined process.

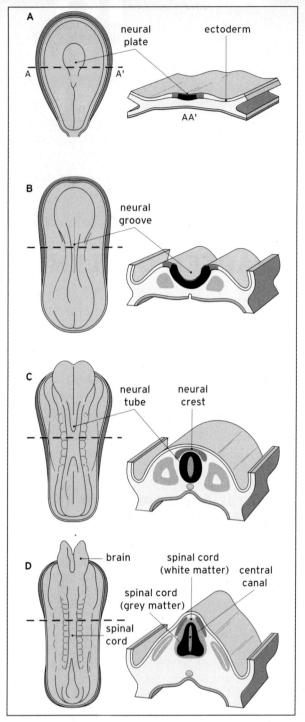

Figure 18.1 Early development of the human nervous system. Drawings on the left are external views; cross-sections are shown on the right. (A) Neural cells develop from ectoderm (skin-to-be) cells to form the neural plate. (B) The plate folds in to form the neural groove. (C) Further folding inwards forms the neural tube. (D) As the developing neurones send out axons, the basic form of the grey matter (cell bodies) and white matter (axons) of the spinal cord develops.

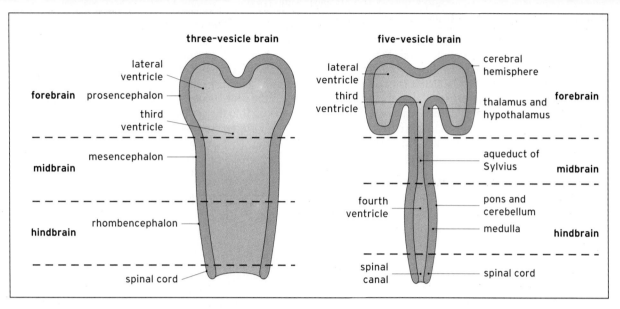

Figure 18.2 Development of the human brain from three vesicles (A) to five vesicles (B).

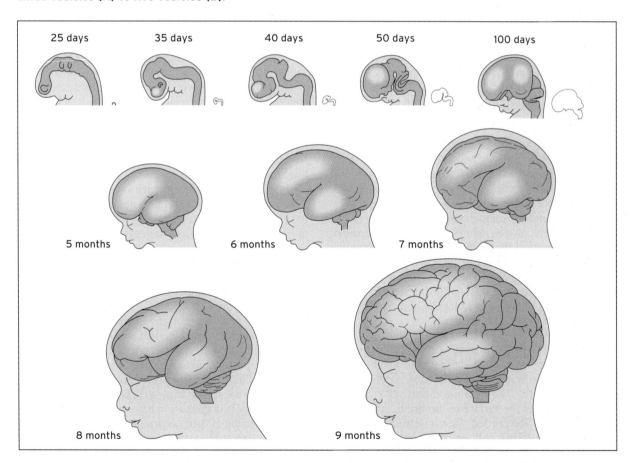

Figure 18.3 Development of the human brain in stages from 25 days until birth. The drawings from 5-9 months are about one-third life size. Those from 25-100 days are much enlarged. The actual sizes are shown to the right of each (note the little speck at 25 days). The three major parts of the brain—forebrain, midbrain and hindbrain—begin as swellings in the neural tube. As the human brain grows, the cerebral hemispheres (forebrain) expand enormously and cover most of the rest of the brain.

217

DEVELOPMENT OF THE SPINAL CORD

As the brain is developing, there is a parallel development of spinal cord structures and of the connections between them. Spinal cord neurones form two discrete regions of grey matter, which become the posterior (sensory) and the anterior (motor) regions respectively. Some motoneurones in the anterior horn send their axons to innervate the sympathetic ganglia, part of the autonomic nervous system. In the peripheral nervous system the neural crest cells migrate along pathways which do not have organised glial structures.

MECHANISMS OF BRAIN DEVELOPMENT

The three different ways that the specific pathways and patterns of connections are 'hard-wired' in the brain are: chemical signals; cell and terminal competition; and fibre-guided cell movements.

Chemical Signals or Trophic Growth

Chemical gradients of some substances encourage the growth of the axon in a particular direction and to a particular set of target cells. Nerve growth factor (NGF) was the first chemical signal to be discovered by Levi-Montalcini & Hamburger in 1951 (Levi-Montalcini, 1982) and it is specific to the neurones of the sympathetic ganglia. Injection of NGF into chickens triggers a large increase in cell division in the sympathetic ganglia (Thompson, 1993). Several other growth factors have been identified and offer some hope of repair of brain damage in the future.

Cell Competition and Death

Neuronal death is probably regulated by competition for trophic substances released by the target tissue. An example of this is in the innervation of skeletal muscle fibres. Initially a motoneurone connects with several muscle fibres by sending out motor axons, usually several to one muscle fibre. As development proceeds, the terminal branches of most of the motor axons retract so that one motoneurone comes to dominate a given muscle fibre completely (see Chapter 6). The process of retraction and cell loss appears to be general in the development of the nervous system, allowing modification of the anatomical organisation of synaptic connections.

Fibre-guided Cell Movement

Fibre-guided cell movement is thought to result from a growing neurone sending out a fibre alongside radially oriented glial cells. The neurone eventually reaches a boundary, such as the surface of the brain, and cannot grow any further. The cell body then travels up the fibre to the boundary. Glial cell proliferation starts very early in pregnancy and continues through the postnatal years.

DEVELOPMENT OF THE CEREBRAL CORTEX

The cerebral cortex begins as one layer a few cells thick, known as the germinal zone. As the cells proliferate, some stop dividing and move up to another layer. From here, some cells move up to form the next layer and so on, forming a columnar organisation superimposed on the horizontally arranged cellular layers. A particular type of neurone (subplate neurone) lies under the developing cortex in the white matter. The subplate neurones send their axons up into the cortex and appear to be physiologically active, forming synapses with the developing neurones in the cortex. They may play an important role in the guidance of the growth of the cortical neurones and the incoming fibres which die out as the cortex becomes established.

PLASTICITY IN DEVELOPMENT

Experience also plays an important part in the ultimate growth and fine tuning of the neural circuits in the brain. The role of experience is discussed further below in 'Innate versus learned behaviour' and plasticity is discussed in detail in Chapter 6.

TIMES OF VULNERABILITY TO DAMAGE

The central nervous system (CNS) is most vulnerable to damage during periods of rapid change, for example when the constituents of the neural networks are being formed. Teratogenic substances (i.e. those which produce physical defects in the developing embryo), such as drugs, are particularly damaging during the early weeks of pregnancy. The anticonvulsant medication, sodium valproate, can cause neural tube defects if taken in the third week after conception, during neurulation. Viruses such as hepatitis B and rubella, as well as irradiation, have their most damaging effects during neuronal proliferation in the first trimester of pregnancy. Maternal alcoholism appears to have a teratogenic effect at, and following, the second and third months of gestation.

Infections with organisms such as cytomegalovirus and *Toxoplasma* may damage the neural developmental processes over a much longer time interval, sometimes throughout pregnancy. Cytomegalovirus transmission through the placenta has most clinical effect during the first two trimesters of pregnancy, whereas toxoplasmosis is most devastating in early pregnancy even though the protection against maternofetal transmission is also greatest at that time.

The placenta has a protective effect and some damage to the developing nervous system may occur from maternal or fetal metabolic disease when the protection has ended after birth. Migration failures, which are thought to be responsible for some types of epilepsy and dyslexia, occur during the second trimester (Touwen, 1995).

Disturbances of circulation have varying effects according to the timing of their occurrence. Reduced blood flow carries the risk of impairing the blood supply to the fetus, especially to the most metabolically active parts of the nervous system. These areas are notably the germinal matrix around the central canal and ventricles during the phase of cell proliferation and initial migration, and, at later fetal ages, those areas to which the cells have migrated and where axonal and synapse formation are taking place, such as the cortex and basal ganglia. Hypoxic and ischaemic episodes have different effects depending on the stage of neural development. In young preterm babies, periventricular leucomalacia (softening of the white matter) and haemorrhage result, with cortical and basal ganglia involvement in term babies.

FUNCTIONAL DEVELOPMENT OF THE NERVOUS SYSTEM *IN UTERO*

The first signs of movement *in utero* have been picked up by ultrasound scanning at about 7–8 weeks after conception, with a fast increase in the repertoire of movement. By 20 weeks of gestation, all types of movement seen in the term fetus are present. They consist of well organised and complex patterns, with no craniocaudal or proximal–distal sequence in the development of these types of subcortically mediated movements (Prechtl, 1984).

The time of the first discernible fetal movements coincides with the time of direct contact between the motoneurones and muscle fibres and the afferent and efferent cells in the spinal cord. However, the wide range of movement develops before the time of most of the major morphological processes in the brain, suggesting that the immature brain can still generate active motor patterns in spite of limited structural development. It is likely that the increase of structural development of the brain allows the quality of the movement to develop postnatally.

POSTNATAL DEVELOPMENT

Changes that occur postnatally include maturation of the CNS, and the development of learning and perception.

PHYSIOLOGICAL MATURATION OF THE CNS

Maturation of the CNS involves myelination and changes in synaptic density. These occur at different rates in the different areas of the brain.

Myelination and Regional Brain Maturation

The rate of myelination varies with both site and age. Some neural tracts are myelinated early and rapidly, others early and slowly. In general, those which function first tend to be myelinated first and those with long phases of myelination are particularly at risk of damage. Myelination begins earliest in the lower brainstem and spinal cord, starting in mid-gestation, and there is heavy myelination here by birth. Myelination reaches the cerebral hemispheres by birth and cortical myelination shows an anatomical sequence. It begins in the sensorimotor systems, followed by the secondary cortical areas. It occurs last in the frontal, parietal and temporal association cortex and myelination of the association fibres continues throughout adulthood. Myelination principally affects the speed of transmission (see Chapter 1) and therefore cannot be taken as a direct marker of functional significance. Some myelination is not complete until adolescence.

Synaptic density in the striate cortex (an early maturing sensory region) is maximal at about 8 months of age, whereas that in the prefrontal cortex (one of the latest maturing regions) is maximal at about 2 years of age. In both areas, synaptic density declines during the first decade to reach adult values during adolescence. Total brain size reaches adult values at about 2 years of age but specific patterning of synapses presumably occurs later, leading to emerging psychological processes. Induction of brain structure also occurs by experience (see below).

INNATE VERSUS LEARNED BEHAVIOUR

The double influence of experience and learning on one hand, and of biological inheritance on the other, has led to the argument called the 'nature–nurture controversy'. The focus of the argument is the extent to which human behaviour is determined by genetic inheritance and how much it can be modified by experience.

Whenever skills and habits are acquired, whether these are manipulative, motor, intellectual or social, learning takes place.

Innate Learning

Knowledge of biological or innate inheritance has increased greatly over the past century. Mendel discovered that, for simple physical traits such as eye colour, there are statistically valid relationships between the traits of the parents and those of their offspring.

Later biological and chemical research has identified chromosomes with genes carrying genetic information occupying specific sites on the chromosomes. The term genotype is used to describe this genetic inheritance. The term phenotype describes the characteristics the person displays. Genetic inheritance is increasingly proving to be complex as the interactions of the different genes become more fully understood. For example, it is now known that some genes may alter the effect of other genes.

Learning through Experience

Even if the genetic material is laid down without mishap, experience by the individual has been shown to be necessary to ensure that the appropriate neuronal architecture develops. The most researched example of this is in the growth and development of the visual system. Wiesel & Hubel's experiments on the developing visual system of kittens in the early 1960s led to the concept that a clear visual stimulus is necessary for normal physiological and morphological development of previously immature visual pathways and that there is a critical period of time during which this development can take place. Kittens who had one eye occluded from birth to the age of 3 months showed histological evidence of small shrunken cells in the lateral geniculate body, the part of the visual pathway which should have been receiving stimulation from the occluded eye. Kittens who had one eye occluded from birth for only 2 months produced similar but less severe histological changes. No changes were seen at all in adult cats deprived of vision. A similar picture has been found in experiments on other animals.

Movement of the eyes during this critical period has also been found to be essential to enable the development of cells in the visual cortex that will give information about orientation. Immobilisation of all movements of the animal apart from those of the eyes does not impair neurones in the visual cortex becoming selective for orientation (Buisseret *et al.*, 1978). However, if the eye movements are prevented, even selectively, there is a corresponding effect on the development of the visual cortex. The visual experience necessary for the development of the visual cortex includes information about eye movements and head movements (Gary-Bobo *et al.*, 1986). It is likely that children developing with impairment of kinaesthetic sensation and limitation of eye movements consequently develop an impairment of the structural formation of the visual cortex.

DEVELOPMENT OF PERCEPTION

Perception involves visual and spatial aspects that are obviously related.

Development of Visual Perception

The neuroanatomy of the eye and the visual system is described in Thompson (1993). The optic nerve transmits information to the various parts of the brain where analysis of visual sensations occurs. When a person moves through the environment or the environment moves relative to the person, a moving pattern of light falls on the retina. The resulting 'optical flow field' provides useful information about the person's movement as well as the three-dimensional layers of the scene. Sensitivity to optic flow develops early in life.

Bower (1977), in experiments with young babies, some only a few days old, has shown that visual events such as the sight of an object looming up and appearing to be on a path to hit the person ('hit path') are just as likely to be interpreted by the baby as they would by an adult. The baby moves its head back and raises its arms as if to defend itself against an impending contact.

The role of visual proprioception (feedback) in the development of postural stability in normal infancy has been studied using a moving-room technique. Lee & Aronson (1974) found that in standing infants, when the end of the room moved away from or towards them, balance was lost in a direction specific to the movement of the room. Butterworth & Hicks (1977) replicated the experiment on two groups of infants. The first group could both sit and stand unsupported whilst the second group could sit unsupported but could not stand. The proprioceptive effect of vision influenced both sitting and standing postures. In another study the role of postural experience on the proprioceptive effects of vision was examined (Butterworth & Cicchetti, 1978). A group of infants who could both sit and stand were compared with a group who were only able to sit. It was found that the effect of partial visual feedback was greatest in the first 3 months after acquiring the ability to sit or stand and declined thereafter. This was true for normal babies and for those with motor delay such as Down's syndrome. The same effect is seen when adults stand on a narrow beam inside a moving room. They can fall off the beam even after the walls shift by as little as 1 or 2 cm.

Gibson & Walk (1960) performed the 'visual cliff' experiment in which visual cues for the height of the cliff were achieved by a texture change and parallax (Figure 18.4). Babies aged 8 months were allowed to crawl over a flat surface that appeared to have a deep step or 'cliff' in the floor surface. The babies, and the young of other species, avoided the deep side of the cliff. The same effect was seen in rats reared in the dark, suggesting that the tendency to avoid the cliff is independent of experience.

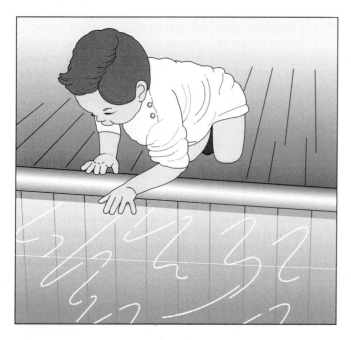

Figure 18.4 The visual cliff: the baby will not cross a drop, despite a strong glass cover.

Perception of Space: Learned or Innate?

In learned perception, the retina transfers information about space in a two-dimensional form to the brain. The brain, however, is able to convert that to a three-dimensional experience by associating aspects of visual experience simultaneously with previous experiences giving direct spatial knowledge. An example of this inference using experience can be seen in Figure 18.5. In (A) the brain suggests that the square is nearer since it appears to be in front of the circle; in (B) the brain suggests that the pencil is nearer because of the familiar relative sizes of a pencil and a van; and in (C), the line grid suggests that the triangle is further away.

Innate perception of space is achieved by a combination of convergence of the eyes, accommodation and stereopsis. As each eye sees the world from a slightly different angle, there are minute differences between right and left retinal images.

Link between Appreciation of Spatial Relations and Mobility

Benson & Uzgiris (1985) demonstrated a relationship between appreciation of spatial relations and infants' mobility. The infants were placed behind a plastic barrier

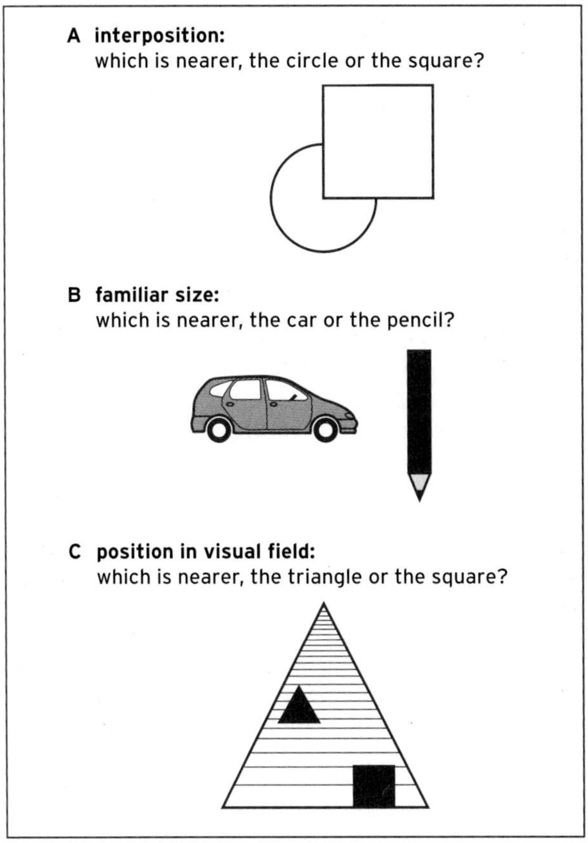

Figure 18.5 Distance cues in perception.
(A) Interposition. (B) Familiar size. (C) Position in visual field.

and then watched someone place a toy under one of two tablecloths. The infants were then allowed to walk or crawl round, or were carried if immobile. It was found that those who were carried round were not as successful at retrieving the object as those who crawled or walked.

POSTNATAL LANDMARKS IN THE DEVELOPMENT OF POSTURAL CONTROL, REFLEXES, BALANCE AND MOVEMENT

Classically, children's development has been viewed from a neurological perspective, particularly looking at the changing neurological reflexes during the first year of life. However, there are changes also in the relative positions of the bony structures of the body, such as the pelvis and shoulder girdle, which play an important role in the child's increasing developmental ability.

NEUROLOGICAL PERSPECTIVE/ REFLEXES AND RESPONSES

Detailed neurological observations of children during the first 2 years of life have led to a number of classic studies (Andre-Thomas & Saint-Anne Dargassies, 1960; Prechtl & Beintema, 1964; Touwen, 1976; Prechtl, 1977). Brazelton (1973) provided further information about the newborn infant, particularly from a behavioural perspective.

Neonatal or 'Primitive' Reflexes

These are present even in babies with a severe neurological abnormality, but asymmetry, absence of a response at the normal stage and persistence of the response after the normal stage are all important neurological signs. The term 'primitive reflex' was coined during a period when it was thought that all infant behaviour resulted from reflex function of the brain rather than from cortically controlled voluntary activity. However, evidence of early function such as perceptual function, and of individual movement patterns in the fetus that do not change much during the course of gestation, has discounted this notion of solely reflex activity. There are striking similarities between prenatal and postnatal patterns of movement, the only differences being in the quality of movement, probably because of the increased influence of gravity after birth. There is a noticeable continuum of neural function from prenatal to postnatal life (Prechtl, 1984).

Reflexes and responses remain a useful part of neurological examination of infants and will be discussed below. Assessment of muscle tone is also very important, exaggerated or marked hypotonia suggesting abnormality (see Chapter 5). Interpretation of most of these tests requires experience and the presence of abnormality should not rely on one negative test result. Further evidence from other neurological tests is required to substantiate abnormality.

Moro Response

This is usually elicited by allowing the baby's head to fall backwards by about $10°$ when supported in the supine position, particularly behind the chest and head. The response is abduction of the shoulders and arms and extension of the elbows followed by the 'embrace' adduction and flexion of the arms. The legs extend and flex during the sequence. The Moro response is well developed in the newborn infant and gradually disappears during the first 4 months of life.

Palmar Grasp
With the child lying supine, a finger put transversely across the palm elicits a strong sustained flexion of the fingers for several seconds. This grasp reflex normally lasts for the first 2 months of life.

Plantar Grasp
Stimulation of the plantar surface of the root of the toes elicits active flexion. A clear developmental range of expression for this sign has not been found.

Rooting Response
Both corners of the child's mouth are stroked in turn. The response consists of a head turn towards the side which has been stroked, together with mouth opening and apparent reaching with the lips. It is seen before feeding in babies up to 6 months of age.

Sucking Response
The index finger is placed in the child's mouth with the finger pad uppermost. A normal sucking response is a strong sustained sucking action. The sucking response is variable and inconsistent.

Walking Response
The child is held in a standing position with chin and head well supported. A normal response is discernable steps, with knee and hip flexion. The response has usually disappeared by about 4–6 weeks of age.

Asymmetric Tonic Neck Response (ATNR)
In this response, when the child's head is turned to the side, the arm and leg extend on that side and flex on the opposite side. Although this posture is seen in normal babies up to the age of about 3 months, an ATNR is not seen as an obligatory response in neurologically normal babies.

Forward Parachute Reaction
This appears at about 7 months and consists of extension of the arms and hands with spreading and slight hyperextension of the fingers when the child is held in the prone position and moved downwards towards the ground. It is an important test as it demonstrates asymmetry of function well, and its absence at the appropriate age suggests abnormality.

Downward Parachute Reaction
This also appears at about 7 months and consists of extension of the legs and feet as the child is lowered in an upright position towards the ground.

Sideways Saving Reaction
Tilting the child sideways whilst in a sitting position elicits an arm movement to that side. The reaction starts at about 7 months and should always be present by 15 months.

DEVELOPMENT OF EARLY POSTURAL CONTROL
Modern models of motor development are based on systems theory (see below and Chapter 22) and take account of the fact that emergent motor behaviour depends on the organism, the environment and the motor task involved. An outline of the developmental changes of movement of the trunk, head and limbs, as well as of the changes in load bearing, biomechanics and function, provides a useful model on which to base assessment of early postural control and more information than assessment of neurological responses alone. The latter are also unreliable, being dependent particularly on the state of the child (e.g. relaxed, anxious) and the environment. Levels of postural ability in the supine and prone positions, and of sitting ability, are described in full in Green et al. (1995) and in summary in Figures 18.6, 18.7 and 18.8. The child progresses from an asymmetric non-conforming position, through a symmetrical fairly static position, to a variety of mobile, active and voluntary positions.

Development of Lying Ability
This is shown in Figure 18.6 for supine and Figure 18.7 for prone ability. At levels 1 and 2, the child lies asymmetrically with the pelvis posteriorly tilted and shoulder girdle retracted. In supine the pelvis, trunk, shoulder girdle and head are all load bearing, although very momentarily at level 1. Dissociation of head movement from the trunk and pelvic movement is very difficult, causing an inability to move the head without concomitant pelvic movement. In the prone position, the posterior pelvic tilt prevents load bearing through the pelvis and most of the load bearing is through the upper trunk and head, making lifting of the head very difficult.

Progression to levels 3 and 4 results in a symmetrical posture as the shoulder girdle becomes more protracted and the pelvis more anteriorly tilted. Load bearing in the supine position is through the shoulder girdle and pelvis. In the prone position it is through the abdomen and thighs, with hands or arms used to prop the upper trunk. This increase in girdle control allows dissociation of movement between the upper and lower trunk and the beginning of arm movement independent from that of the trunk. The ability to vary the position of the pelvis and shoulder girdle begins at level 4.

When the child reaches levels 5 and 6, no predominant positions are displayed. A full range of movement in the shoulder girdle and the pelvis allows the child to adopt a variety of positions. As this is achieved, the child can move in the position, such as pivoting or moving backwards, as well as into and out of the lying position.

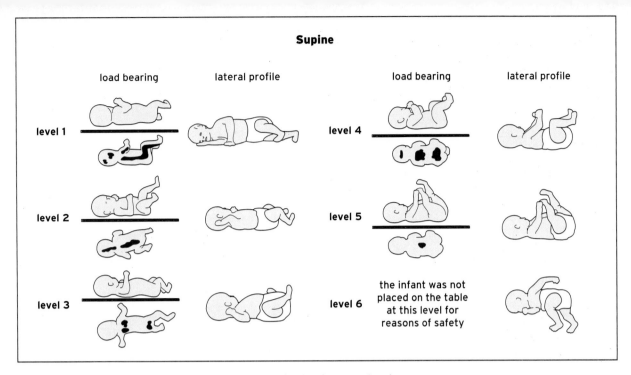

Figure 18.6 Levels of supine lying ability. For reflected images showing load bearing, the child was placed on a clear acrylic-topped table with a mirror angled at 45° beneath it. (Redrawn from Green *et al.*, 1995, with permission.)

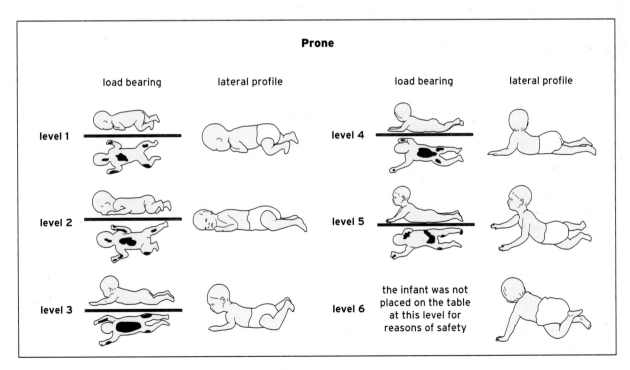

Figure 18.7 Levels of prone lying ability. For reflected images showing load bearing, the child was placed on a clear acrylic-topped table with a mirror angled at 45° beneath it. (Redrawn from Green *et al.*, 1995, with permission.)

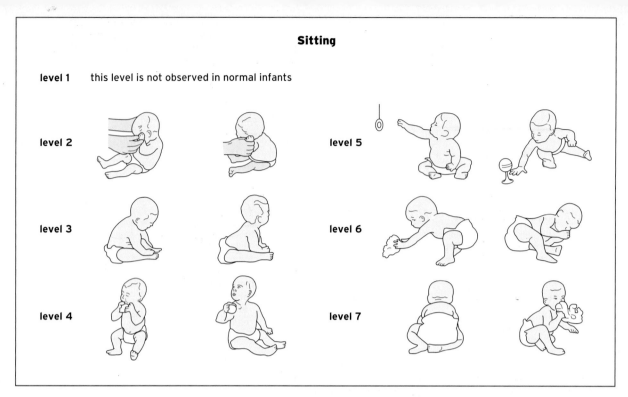

Figure 18.8 Levels of sitting ability. (Redrawn from Green *et al.*, 1995, with permission.)

Age ranges for the different levels of ability are not available but level 3 is usually achieved soon after 6 weeks, with level 6 starting at about 4 months, and present in all infants with normal development by 15 months.

Development of Sitting Ability

Levels of sitting ability are shown in Figure 18.8. From early infancy (level 1 lying ability) a child can be supported in a sitting position as well as anchoring his or her bottom when pulled to a sitting position. Anchoring means that the child can bear weight through the pelvis sufficiently to enable the trunk to be brought forwards over it and to be maintained upright (level 2 sitting ability). The lateral profile at this level has a rounded spinal curvature with a posteriorly tilted pelvis and the shoulders maintained forwards over the sitting base in order to balance.

Independent sitting is achieved only after the child is able to tilt the pelvis anteriorly and protract the shoulder girdle and, when lying, to transfer weight efficiently and longitudinally (level 4 lying ability). This begins at about 6 months of age. In sitting the child has adequate pelvic and shoulder girdle stability to bear weight through the ischial tuberosities and through the arms in a forward prop position (level 3 sitting ability).

As the child masters the ability to shift weight laterally when lying (level 5 lying ability), he or she becomes able to move outside the area of the sitting base and to continue to maintain balance (level 5 sitting ability). The ability to counterpoise laterally is seen before the ability to recover sitting balance when the trunk weight is behind the sitting base.

As the interplay between pelvic and upper trunk stability and movement becomes efficient, the child gains increasing ability to transfer weight in an upright position. He or she becomes efficient at counterpoising in a variety of sitting postures, including long sitting, eventually gaining control of movement between sitting and lying, and movement from the prone position to sitting in a variety of ways.

Development of Reach and Hand Function

There is a close relationship between the development of postural control and the development of independent arm and hand movement. At level 3 lying ability the child starts to have unilateral hand grasp and to be able to take toys to the mouth. By level 4 lying ability, increased protraction of the shoulder girdle enables midline play above the chest with the hands together. Level 5 lying ability means a full range of pelvic movement, allowing efficient limb movements with prehensile feet. Hand play is well established at this stage. All children reach level 4 lying ability before level 3 sitting ability, the start of independent sitting when the child can sit momentarily, often using the hands for support. By level 4 sitting ability, the arms can be raised to shoulder height and by level 5 the child can reach sideways outside the base of support and recover balance.

There is a developmental progression in the arc of movement as a child reaches for an object, in both lateral

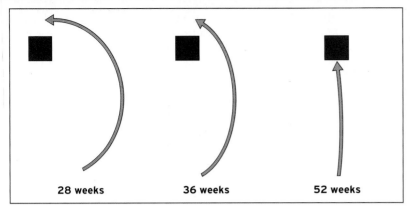

Figure 18.9 Developmental progression in arc of movement taken by a child when reaching for an object.

28 weeks   36 weeks   52 weeks

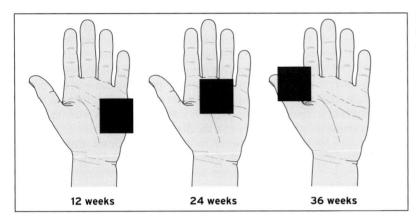

Figure 18.10 Developmental changes in the position of a grasped cube on the palm of the hand.

12 weeks   24 weeks   36 weeks

and vertical deviation (Figure 18.9), and a progression in the position of the object grasped (distally and radially) with respect to the palm (Figure 18.10).

Development of Standing

There is a similar developmental sequence in the standing posture which is currently under evaluation. During the prestanding levels of ability, the infant is able to make either no or minimal movements against gravity. During the levels of supported early standing, the height of support needed changes from waist height to shoulder height as the level of ability improves. This change coincides with an increase in controlled weight shift and leg movements. At low levels of standing ability, the standing base is narrow, with weight bearing taken particularly through tiptoes. At higher levels of ability, the standing base widens, using flattened feet, before narrowing again later as standing balance improves. The appearance of standing with support shows a wide range of variation from 9 to 18 months. The median age for standing free is about 15 months of age.

DEVELOPMENT OF MORE COMPLEX MOTOR SKILLS

Once an independent standing posture is achieved, it becomes increasingly necessary to assess the way that a motor skill is performed, i.e. a qualitative assessment rather than simply whether it is performed, which is a quantitative score. Standardised measures of motor ability

are listed in Chapter 19. Noller & Ingrisano (1984) suggest that it is important to measure both the emergence and achievement of a motor skill. These may vary in different skills both in time interval and in performance pattern. For example, the ability to stand up from the floor without support shows emergence at 12–17 months with achievement by 18–23 months. However, standing up from the floor without trunk rotation is likely to be achieved only between 66 and 71 months. Walking with arms at low guard has a much quicker development, with emergence at 12–17 months and achievement at 18–23 months.

THEORIES OF SENSORIMOTOR SKILL DEVELOPMENT

Some of the theories outlined here relate to theories of motor control discussed in Chapters 2 & 22.

NEUROMATURATIONAL MODEL

This is the traditional model of motor development (e.g. Gesell & Armatruda, 1947) and provides the framework for many therapeutic techniques. Neuromaturational theory proposes that changes in gross motor skills during infancy result solely from the neurological maturation of the CNS. Increased myelination of the CNS is accompanied by concurrent inhibition of the lower subcortical nuclei of the brain by the higher functioning cerebral cortex. This is seen as the organisational centre for controlled movement, with the instructions for the emergence of motor skills encoded in the brain and little influence from the environment. Piper & Darrah (1994) challenge the assumptions of this model, which was influenced by the early embryologists demonstrating that the embryo developed in a symmetrical manner, beginning in cephalocaudal and proximal–distal directions.

CENTRAL EXECUTIVE

The development and execution of movements are entirely dependent on commands from a 'central executive' in the brain (situation unspecified).

OPEN-LOOP MODEL

Input from the environment, such as environmental conditions and posture, passes to a central process or programme that arranges the output as movement.

CLOSED-LOOP MODEL

This has a feedback loop in addition to the arrangement noted under the open-loop model. There are a number of feedback loops proposed according to the model, such as sensory feedback and kinaesthesis. Laszlo & Bairstow (1985) explain this model in greater detail.

DYNAMIC SYSTEMS THEORY

Rather than considering functional activity as simply the result of a set of neural commands generated hierarchically as part of a motor programme, the dynamic systems theory of motor activity involves many subsystems. Systems theory arises from the natural sciences, where it was observed that when elements of a system work together, certain behaviours or properties emerge that cannot be predicted from the elements separately. A new behaviour is constructed that is dependent on input from all the parts of the system. This is called 'emergent behaviour' (Thelen et al., 1987; Shepherd & Carr, 1991).

DEVELOPMENT OF VISION

Detailed information about the development of vision is given in Grounds (1996). From birth, babies are capable of searching out detail, thus ensuring that the visual system develops satisfactorily. Cortical awakening generally occurs between 3 and 6 months postnatally. It is shortly after that period that any restricted input to one eye causes reduction of acuity to begin. Colour vision is normal by about 2 months. Visual acuity and contrast sensitivity have a long time scale of development, taking up to 6–12 years to become truly adult-like. Infants' eyes tend to be long-sighted for some months but appear short-sighted because of the lack of cortical development.

DEVELOPMENT OF HEARING

Babies should have normal levels of hearing from birth, although this may not be easy to demonstrate (Yeates, 1980). Early hearing responses are measured by the child becoming still on hearing a sound. Once head and upper trunk control has started to develop, the child is able to turn towards a sound at the level of the ear. Localisation of a sound above and below the ear is present by about 1 year.

LANDMARKS OF INTELLECTUAL DEVELOPMENT

Important aspects of the intellectual development of the child are outlined below. Further details can be found in Illingworth (1983) and Eysenck (1984).

LEARNING AND MEMORY

The simplest forms of learning, habituation and sensitisation are non-associative. Habituation is simply a decrease in a response to a stimulus with repeated stimulation. Sensitis-ation is an increase in a response to a stimulus as a result of stimulation. A human presented with a sudden loud sound usually jumps but if the sound is repeated with no other consequence, jumping will cease at the sound (habituation). If, however, a painful shock is given just before the loud sound, jumping will be greater than after a sound without a shock (sensitisation).

Associative learning is a very broad category that includes much of learning, such as learning to be afraid, learning a foreign language and learning the piano. It involves the formation of associations amongst stimuli and/or responses or movement sequences. It is generally divided into classical and operant conditioning or learning.

In classical conditioning, a reflex response is conditioned so that it may be elicited by a new stimulus. Pavlov's experiments showed that a dog's salivation at the sight of food could be conditioned to occur at the sound of a bell if this was rung just before, or as, the food was presented. Eventually the dog salivated at the sound of the bell.

In operant conditioning, the animal's own behaviour plays a part in what happens. The behaviour is instrumental in obtaining a particular outcome and therefore in the learning process itself. The subject's behaviour can lead to either the gain or the loss of something, e.g. a rat receives food each time it presses a lever.

Positive reinforcement refers to the gain of something after a particular response is made, e.g. food being given to the rat. Negative reinforcement occurs if there is loss of something unpleasant once a particular response is made, such as an electric shock stopping when a lever is pressed. The hypothalamus, the amygdala and the cerebellum appear to be the parts of the brain where the memory traces are formed.

Visual Learning

There are two visual memory systems in the monkey brain and this is also assumed to be the case in the human brain. One of these systems extends from the primary visual cortex in the occipital lobe through visual association areas to the temporal lobe. The other projects from the primary visual cortex to the parietal cortex.

Memory and the Hippocampus

Studies on humans, particularly those with damage to brain structures, have identified at least three different types of long-term memory formation: declarative (learning what); procedural (skill or learning how) and implicit (memory without awareness). Declarative and procedural memory are based in the hippocampus; the brain circuits for implicit memory are not yet known.

Mechanisms of Long-Term Memory Storage

There is overwhelming evidence that experience results in structural changes at synapses (Chapter 6). This is particularly true of experience early in life. A wide variety of early experiences cause an increase in the extent of the dendritic branching in output neurones, especially in the cortex.

Human Memory Sequence

After an initial sensory information storage stage, the memory passes through a temporary storage stage (short-term memory) before transfer to long-term storage. Children's memory ability increases up to about the age of 18 years, with a particular increase of memory ability at around 7 years.

LANGUAGE ACQUISITION

Babies are born as competent, active beings capable of complex, organised behavioural sequences. Initially communications are expressed non-verbally, then by co-ordinating behaviour with vocalisation and, finally, verbal expression. Communication is the exchange of thought and messages by speech, signals or writing. Language is the basis of communication and may be verbal or non-verbal.

Non-verbal Communication

Early in life a baby can signal by crying, smiling, vocalising and chuckling and can show orientation by watching and listening. Smiling is elicited by human voices during the first month and by faces by 3 months. Crying has identifiable characteristics for causes such as hunger and pain. Over the first 2–3 months, babies show a gradual increase in their ability to interact with other people.

Co-ordination of Behaviour with Vocalisation

Vocalisations start from the age of 7–8 weeks and progress into babbling at around 4 months. Neither vocalisation nor babbling is dependent on adequate hearing. By 4 months, babies can associate the tape-recorded speech of a parent with the appropriate parent. Babies lead communication at this stage, timing their movements and attention in a way that supports and strengthens the interaction. By 6 months, awareness of strangers begins.

Verbal Communication

By 9 months babies use more complex vocalisations and early words. Children learn the meaning of words by associating them with objects but further development of language depends on simultaneously increasing cognitive skills. From the age of 9 months, babies develop knowledge that objects and events still exist when not being directly seen or experienced, of cause and effect and of yes/no understanding. This development of both spoken language and comprehension takes time to develop, comprehension often preceding speech by some months. For example, around the age of 18 months, a baby can often indicate the parts of the body such as the nose and mouth, not only on him- or herself but also on a doll of reasonable size. Naming of the body parts comes much later.

Situational Understanding

Between 8 and 12 months the child understands familiar phrases as part of a sequence of events without the individual words having meaning.

Symbolic Understanding

Approximate age levels for the levels of symbolic understanding are shown in Table 18.1.

Levels of symbolic understanding during a child's development	
Concrete objects Understanding is shown by using objects appropriately, i.e. brushes hair with a hairbrush	12-18 months
Object representation Understanding of representational objects, e.g. in Wendy house play Small doll play and use of miniature toys, e.g. dolls' house furniture and dolls	18-21 months
Picture by name Understanding of two-dimensional representation	18-24 months
Picture by function	24-30 months
Matching symbol to symbol Matching small toys to non-identical pictures	24-30 months
Meaningful symbol	36-42 months
Alphabet/abstract symbol	4-5 years

Table 18.1 Levels of symbolic understanding during a child's development.

COGNITIVE DEVELOPMENT

Piaget organised the growth of a child's mind into four periods (Piaget, 1967). In the sensorimotor period the child is preoccupied with co-ordinating his or her sensory and motor abilities (birth to 2 years). During the preoperational period (2–6 years), perception and language are the dominant areas of development. In the concrete operational period (7–11 years) the child acquires the ability to think intuitively, and during the period of formal operations (12 years plus) the ability to think logically and to understand the scientific method.

PERSONAL, SOCIAL AND EMOTIONAL DEVELOPMENT

The basic biological drives of a young infant change into the complex goals of childhood such as achievement and curiosity. Parents also influence their children, both through the genes passed to their offspring and through the family atmosphere in which the child grows. The first major social interactions occur within the family but after about 6 years of age both peers and educators come to exert increasingly more control over the child's social behaviour.

NUTRITIONAL NEEDS OF THE DEVELOPING CNS

The infant's developing brain has high nutritional needs. An increasing body of research is clarifying the essential fatty acids that are necessary, particularly for the formation of myelin (Brown, 1995). Brain lipids in the human infant are known to change according to dietary lipid intake and there are concerns that fatty acid deficiency may be partly related to the failure of myelination seen in some types of cerebral palsy. Myelin produced by inadequate means may be unstable and responsible for demyelination in later life. It is also known that certain nutritional deficiencies, such as that of folate, cause neural tube defects. Deficiency of iodine causes mental impairment and diplegia, and the role of zinc deficiency is under investigation.

REFERENCES

Andre-Thomas YC, Saint-Anne Dargassies S. *The neurological examination of the infant.* London: William Heinemann Medical Books Ltd; 1960. (Keith RC, Polani PE, Clayton-Jones E, eds. Spastics International Medical Publications. Clinics in Developmental Medicine, No. 1).

Benson JB, Uzgiris IC. Effect of self-initiated locomotion on infant search activity. *Dev Psychol* 1985, **21**:923-931.

Bower TGR. *The perceptual world of the child.* London: Fontana; 1977.

Brazelton TB. *Neonatal behavioural assessment scale, 2nd edition.* London: William Heinemann Medical Books Ltd; 1973. (Spastics International Medical Publications. Clinics in Developmental Medicine, No. 88).

Brown JK. Food for thought. *Dev Med Child Neurol* 1995, **37**:189-190.

Buisseret P, Gary-Bobo E, Imbert M. Ocular motility and recovery of orientation properties of visual cortical neurones in dark-reared kittens. *Nature (London),* 1978, **272**:816-817.

Butterworth G, Cicchetti D. Visual calibration of posture in normal and motor retarded Down's Syndrome infants. *Perception* 1978, **7**:513-525.

Butterworth G, Hicks L. Visual proprioception and postural stability in infancy. A developmental study. *Perception* 1977, **6**:255-262.

Cowan WM. The development of the brain. In: *The brain (a Scientific American book).* San Francisco: WH Freeman & Co.; 1979:298.

Eysenck MW. Cognitive development. In: *A handbook of cognitive psychology.* London: Lawrence Erlbaum Assoc.; 1984:231-245.

Gary-Bobo E, Milleret C, Buisseret P. Role of eye movements in the developmental processes of orientation selectivity in the kitten's visual cortex. *Vision Res* 1986, **26**:557-567.

Gesell A, Armatruda C. *Developmental diagnosis, 2nd edition.* New York: Harper & Row; 1947.

Gibson EJ, Walk PD. The 'visual cliff'. *Sci Am* 1960, **202**:64.

Green EM, Mulcahy CM, Pountney TE. An investigation into the development of early postural control. *Dev Med Child Neurol* 1995, **37**:437-448.

Grounds A. Child visual development. In: Barnard S, Edgar D, eds. *Pediatric eye care.* Oxford: Blackwell Science Ltd; 1996:43-74.

Illingworth RS. *The development of the young child, normal and abnormal, 8th edition.* Edinburgh: Churchill Livingstone; 1983.

Introduction to Psychology Unit 5, Milton Keynes: Open University Press; 1981:34.

Laszlo JI, Bairstow PJ. *Perceptual-motor behaviour: Developmental assessment and therapy.* London: Holt, Rinehart & Winston; 1985.

Lee DN, Aronson E. Visual proprioceptive control of standing in human infants. *Percep Psychophys* 1974, **15**:529-532.

Levi-Montalcini R. Developmental neurobiology and the natural history of nerve growth factor. *Ann Rev Neurosci* 1982, **5**:341-362.

Noller K, Ingrisano D. Cross-sectional study of gross and fine motor development: Birth to 6 years of age. *Phys Ther* 1984, **64**:308-316.

Piaget J. *The child's conception of the world.* Totowa, NJ: Littlefield, Adams; 1967.

Piper MC, Darrah J. *Motor assessment of the developing infant.* Philadelphia: WB Saunders; 1994.

Prechtl HFR. *The neurological development of the full term newborn infant, 2nd edition.* London: William Heinemann Medical Books; 1977. (Spastics International Medical Publications. Clinics in Developmental Medicine, No. 63).

Prechtl HFR. *Continuity of neural functions from prenatal to postnatal life.* London: Spastics International Medical Publications; 1984. (Clinics in Developmental Medicine, No. 94).

Prechtl HFR, Beintema DJ. *The neurological development of the full term newborn infant.* London: William Heinemann Medical Books; 1964. (Spastics International Medical Publications. Clinics in Developmental Medicine, No. 12).

Shepherd R, Carr J. An emergent or dynamical systems view of movement dysfunction. *Aust J Physio* 1991, **37**:4-5,17.

Thelen E, Kelso JAS, Fogel A. Self-organising systems and motor development. *Dev Rev* 1987, **7**:39-65.

Thompson RF. *The brain, 2nd edition.* New York: WH Freeman & Co.; 1993.

Touwen B. *Neurological development in infancy.* London: William Heinemann Medical Books; 1976. (Spastics International Medical Publications. Clinics in Developmental Medicine, No. 58).

Touwen B. Development of the central nervous system. In: Harvey D, Miles M, Smyth D, eds. *Community child health.* Oxford: Butterworth Heinemann; 1995:396-400.

Yeates S. *The development of hearing.* Lancaster: MTP Press; 1980. (Studies in Developmental Paediatrics, No. 2).

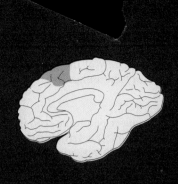

19

N Hare, S Durham & E Green

THE CEREBRAL PALSIES AND MOTOR LEARNING DISORDERS

CHAPTER OUTLINE

- Cerebral palsies
- Motor learning disorders

- Physical management of motor dysfunction

INTRODUCTION

In 1862, Little described spastic diplegia resulting from birth asphyxia and brain damage. However, Sigmund Freud suggested that 'infantile cerebral paralysis' was caused by prenatal abnormalities, birth asphyxia being a marker for, rather than a cause of, brain dysfunction (Pellegrino, 1995). Little's views were accepted until the last 25 years during which epidemiological studies have refuted the causation of cerebral palsy by birth trauma and asphyxia. Also, greater understanding of genetic and other constitutional disorders has led to a change in the 'brain damage' model. This had been applied to a wide range of developmental disabilities ranging from cerebral palsy to mental retardation, learning disabilities and attention deficit hyperactivity disorder. Although there was little proof of actual brain damage, there was an assumption that a milder degree of birth asphyxia or other brain-damaging event had resulted in a milder form of impairment.

Cerebral palsy is now more commonly used as a description of the disability suffered due to an unspecified deficit rather than of the impairment itself (see Preface for the WHO Classification of impairment, disability and handicap, 1980). A similar situation occurs with the less severe motor impairments seen as part of a generalised neurological dysfunction such as in disorders of learning, motor control and attention. These are now classified in the Diagnostic and Statistical Manual of Mental Disorders (American Psychiatric Association, 1994) by descriptions of observable behaviour rather than by aetiology.

The lifestyle and opportunities available to people with cerebral palsy have improved remarkably and many adults live independent, though supported, lives and contribute to society through employment and further education. Children with cerebral palsy have a right to mainstream education; they are accepted by their peers, included in holidays and outings, and can take part in competitive games. Advances in technology have also made a significant contribution, particularly in the area of communication.

CEREBRAL PALSY

The clinical manifestations and general management are now discussed, and physical management is dealt with later, together with that for motor learning disorders.

DEFINITION AND DIAGNOSIS

Cerebral palsy is an umbrella term encompassing a wide range of different causative factors and describing an evolving disorder of motor function secondary to a non-progressive pathology of the immature brain. A definition by the World Commission for Cerebral Palsy in 1988 was: 'a persistent but not unchanging disorder of posture and movement, caused by damage to the developing nervous system, before or during birth or in the early months of infancy' (see Griffiths & Clegg, 1988).

A diagnosis of cerebral palsy should not be made unless the motor disorder is obvious in comparison to other findings such as developmental delay. This excludes most children with clumsiness and also children with a severe degree of mental retardation and motor signs such as mild spasticity or mild hypotonia.

EPIDEMIOLOGY

Mutch *et al.* (1992) reported on a number of international meetings devoted to the epidemiology of cerebral palsy. There have been consistent reports of recent rises in the prevalence amongst live births of cerebral palsy and of its severity, particularly amongst preterm infants. The rises can be accounted for largely by improvements in survival rate, since the incidence of low birthweight and the birthweight-specific prevalence rates of cerebral palsy amongst birthweights of 2500 g or more seem to be remaining largely stable. Data are documented from Great Britain, Western Australia and Sweden, showing a consistent trend from low to high cerebral palsy rates as birthweight falls. Within countries in the low-birthweight populations there is a trend to higher rates of cerebral palsy as mortality falls. The birthweight-specific prevalence of cerebral palsy in the highest weight group seems to remain stable within each population, despite falling mortality levels.

AETIOLOGY AND PATHOGENESIS

Rosenbloom (1995) reviewed the aetiology and pathogenesis of cerebral palsy. The different types of cerebral palsy will now be described briefly.

Tetraplegic Cerebral Palsy

The tetraplegic or quadraplegic syndrome is seen in both preterm and term infants. Preterm infants who are tetraplegic often have an accompanying posthaemorrhagic hydrocephalus. Causes are a wide number of pathologies such as intrauterine infections, malformations, fetal encephalopathies and perinatal hypoxic ischaemic encephalopathy. A genetically determined disorder should always be considered when there is no history of a significant perinatal abnormality.

The tetraplegic group are the most severely affected, unable to acquire and retain abilities in lying, sitting or standing without training, instruction and ongoing management. Abnormalities in muscle tone are pronounced, and in later years fixed deformity of limbs and body, resulting from immobility and persistent spasticity, is not uncommon. Patients often have difficulty with speech and communication.

Diplegic Cerebral Palsy

The diplegic syndromes are seen characteristically in children born prematurely with haemorrhagic infarction of the periventricular areas of the brain. The underlying mechanisms are thought to be periventricular leucomalacia and periventricular haemorrhagic venous infarction. These are seen in the increasing number of infants who survive in spite of being born very prematurely. Diplegia does not show a correlation with birth asphyxia.

The diplegic group have use of their hands and arms, readily acquire sitting balance, and have most difficulty with standing and walking. They have a characteristic flexed/adducted gait which is likely ... growth spurts, a tendency to deform... usually no problem with speech or comm...

Hemiplegic Cerebral Palsy

Hemiplegia is the second commonest syndrome seen in infants born preterm and the commonest in term infants. Hemiplegia in preterm infants has a non-specific association with birth problems whilst term hemiplegia most commonly results from events early in the third trimester of pregnancy involving poor blood supply. Malformations and infarction of the area of the brain perfused by the middle cerebral artery are other causes.

Children with hemiplegia are an able, self sufficient group, achieving standing and walking by 2–3 years at the latest. They tend to reject the affected side and to lead and lean towards the unaffected side. If not given appropriate and ongoing advice from an early age, asymmetry persists and can result in unnecessary limitation, discomfort and deformity as adults.

Dyskinetic Cerebral Palsy

This includes those with fluctuating dystonia as well as those with involuntary choreoathetoid movements. It has a close association with obvious perinatal adversities such as severe but short-lived birth asphyxia, although often only a mild or moderate hypoxic ischaemic encephalopathy. Basal ganglia pathology appears to be the basis of the dyskinesis which is typically of the dystonic type with preservation of the primitive neonatal reflex patterns (see Chapter 18). Severe and prolonged birth asphyxia can also lead to both cortical, subcortical and basal ganglia damage, resulting in a mixed clinical picture.

The choreoathetoid form of dyskinetic cerebral palsy is now rare since the prevention of bilirubin encephalopathy. Previously untreated high levels of bilirubin neonatally led to basal ganglia damage. Despite the rarity of athetosis in infants now, there are a significant number of adults with athetoid cerebral palsy. The condition is misleading because of the severity of its presentation. This includes facial grimacing, involuntary movement, impairment of hearing and speech, and absence of postural control leading to severe spasticity and deformity in later life. The ability of this group to understand, their desire for communication and their motivation to do something about their condition should not be underestimated or overlooked.

Congenital Ataxias

Most congenital ataxias have a prenatal origin that is often genetic, although acquired haemorrhagic cerebellar lesions have been described. Imaging of the brain in the familial variety may show developmental abnormalities, especially of the vermis of the cerebellum.

DIAGNOSIS AND THE ROLE OF INVESTIGATIONS

Neonatal examination is vital, especially if the infant is premature or has been exposed to events which are known to hold risks for young infants, such as feeding or respiratory problems. Dubowitz (1988) described the common findings in the examination of infants who are small for their gestational age, those who survive significant intraventricular bleeding, the evolving picture seen in periventricular leucomalacia and the clinical stages of hypoxic ischaemic encephalopathy.

Clinical signs of concern are: altered consciousness, such as irritability or decreased alertness; persistent generalised disturbance of tone; seizures; feeding difficulties; and persistent asymmetries of posture and movement. Infants displaying some of these signs neonatally must have skilled and repeated examinations as the child develops, so that signs of cerebral palsy may be picked up as early as possible and appropriate help initiated. The clinical examinations must include measurement of head growth, visual and auditory behaviour, consideration of seizures, and examination of muscle tone and movement.

Since cerebral palsy is an umbrella term encompassing a wide range of different causative factors, the part played by investigative procedures will vary from child to child. For some with a clear history of the probable cause, no invasive investigations may be indicated or at least until the child is old enough to manage these without general anaesthesia. Other children may require chromosomal analysis if a genetic disorder is suspected or the child's appearance is dysmorphic (not normal in appearance). If there is concern that the motor disorder is showing progressive deterioration or that there are no explanatory factors in the child's history, neuroimaging and biochemical tests are indicated.

MEDICAL TREATMENT OF THE MOTOR DISORDER

Various medical treatments may be required and are mentioned briefly below.

Drug Treatments

Medications are used to attenuate the motor disorder, e.g. by reducing muscle tone or excess movements to aid management and improve function. Those most commonly used in children are baclofen (for spasticity), benzhexol, benztropine and levodopa derivatives (for other problems of tone). Botulinum toxin intramuscular injections have been found to be of help in the treatment of cerebral palsy (Cosgrove *et al.*, 1994). Information on these drugs can be found in Chapter 28.

Neurosurgery

Selective dorsal rhizotomy—partial sectioning of the lumbosacral dorsal rootlets of the spinal cord—is a treatment for spasticity, but used less in the UK than in North America (McLaughlin *et al.*, 1994).

Orthopaedic Management

Musculoskeletal problems are common in cerebral palsy, especially when there is associated spasticity. Increasing postural deformity during rapid growth is probably the most important factor determining the loss of physical ability in many children. The spine, hips and feet are at particular risk of structural deformity.

Scrutton (1989) reviewed the early management of the hip, listed a number of important lessons to be learnt in this area and noted that the most important factor in hip stability is the age of pulling to stand. It is imperative that children with tetraplegia are given experience of standing as soon as possible. Cornell (1995) also reviewed the hip in cerebral palsy and gave definitions of terms used in proximal femoral anatomy, reviewed the current state of knowledge of the development of the hip and the pathogenesis of subluxation and dislocation of the hip in cerebral palsy.

Kyphoscoliosis is the most common and serious structural change in the spine of people with cerebral palsy and is most frequent and severe in those with asymmetrical stereotyped postures and those unable to walk.

Orthopaedic surgery, when indicated, needs to be part of the overall programme of physical management. A thorough preoperative assessment of abilities and muscle strength and provision for a period of immobilisation followed by rehabilitation must be included. Surgery may be either bony (osteotomy) or muscular (muscle/tendon lengthening or transfer). The correction of severe scoliosis to prevent further deterioration and improve comfort and ease of management has met with some success (Hallet, 1992). Surgical intervention is of most immediate benefit to older patients, and when used as a corrective rather than a preventive measure.

TREATMENT OF ASSOCIATED MEDICAL CONDITIONS

There are several conditions that can occur with cerebral palsy and require specific management.

Epilepsy

Epilepsy occurs frequently in children with cerebral palsy, with a higher incidence in children with tetraplegia and a lower incidence in those with dyskinesia and spastic diplegia, especially preterm infants. Cerebral palsy associated with epilepsy is more likely to be accompanied by sensory handicap and cognitive impairment. Seizures are not thought to cause damage to the brain unless they are prolonged. Infantile spasms present in the first year of life, occurring most often in babies with brain damage, and are often accompanied by developmental regression, particularly in cognitive and visual development. Aicardi (1990) offered a full review of epilepsy in cerebral palsy. It is not necessarily a long-term condition in these children and treatment with anticonvulsant therapy such as carbamazepine or sodium valproate is usually effective. Surgical treatment is now an option for intractable seizures.

Feeding Difficulties

These are common in severe physical handicap. Reilly & Skuse (1992) reported on the characteristics and management of feeding problems of young children with cerebral palsy. Generally, stature and weight seem to be related to the level of disability, with gross inco-ordination of chewing and swallowing leading to poor nutritional intake and becoming more common as the level of disability increases. Hiatus hernia and gastro-oesophageal reflux, with consequent ulceration, bleeding and anaemia, may occur, as well as silent aspiration of stomach contents into the lungs, causing repeated respiratory infections or wheezing. Hypoxaemia during oral feeding has been documented. Some children with cerebral palsy expend excessive amounts of energy either in athetoid movement or in spasm. Management of the nutritional problems in cerebral palsy must be directed towards diagnosis. Treatment of gastro-oesophageal reflux is with surgery or medication, therapy to improve oral skills, positioning for eating and boosted nutrition, either orally or through a gastrostomy. Multidisciplinary assessment of feeding, together with videofluoroscopy, has been found to be very useful.

Visual Impairments

These are common in children with cerebral palsy. The prevalence of strabismus (squint) in normal children is about 6% but rises to 15–60% in children with cerebral palsy (Duckman, 1987). There is a similarly high prevalence of other visual problems such as significant refractive errors, amblyopia, accommodative insufficiency, oculomotor dysfunction, pathology and visual perceptual dysfunction. Structural abnormalities of the visual pathways have been demonstrated. Such central visual disturbance is not always permanent as partial recovery is possible. Children with athetosis have been found to have fewer visual–perceptual disorders than children with spasticity, with those with bilateral spasticity presenting the highest incidence.

Hearing Impairment

Hearing impairment is now rare in cerebral palsy, although it used to be a common finding in those with a severe dyskinetic disorder caused by high neonatal bilirubin levels. Children with cerebral palsy are just as likely as other children to have middle ear problems and conductive deafness. Children with neurological problems due to intrauterine infection or to neonatal meningitis are at high risk of a sensory hearing deficit.

Sensation

Sensory disorder is an integral part of cerebral palsy and has been demonstrated by evaluating two-point discrimination in children with different types of cerebral palsy (Lesney et al., 1993). Yekutiel et al. (1994) confirmed a high prevalence of sensory deficit in the hands of children with cerebral palsy.

MOTOR LEARNING DISORDERS

In the introduction to this chapter, the early 'brain damage' model of motor impairment was discussed. Early terminology used to describe children with less severe motor problems but with associated learning problems reflected this assumption, e.g. brain damage, organic brain dysfunction, minimal cerebral dysfunction (MCD). These have been replaced by a number of other more descriptive terms such as 'the clumsy child' or by terms suggesting the presumed

aetiology of the condition, such as perceptual motor dysfunction, sensory motor deficit, motor organisational problems, developmental co-ordination disorder, motor learning problems, sensory and sensorimotor integration problems, developmental co-ordination disorder and disorder of attention, motor and perception (DAMP). Developmental dyspraxia is another term used generally for this group of children. The term motor learning problems will be used in this chapter.

EPIDEMIOLOGY AND NATURAL HISTORY

In Sweden, a number of short, intermediate and long-term follow-up studies of population-based groups of children with and without DAMP, diagnosed at 6–7 years of age, confirmed the long-term chronic nature of these difficulties (Gillberg, 1989). In a longitudinal study of a cohort of Dutch children, the frequency of minor neurological dysfunction amongst all the children rose with increasing age, but especially so for a group which had been found to be neurologically impaired neonatally (Lunsing et al., 1992). The same authors studied behavioural and cognitive development at 12 years of age in children with and without minor neurological dysfunction (Soorani-Lunsing et al., 1993). Fine manipulative disability related significantly to problems of cognition and behaviour; co-ordination problems related to cognitive problems; and hypotonia and dyskinesia to behavioural problems, the former more than the latter. Losse et al. (1991) re-examined a group of children who had been shown to be clumsy at the age of 6 years. At 16 years they continued to have substantial motor difficulties as well as a variety of educational, social and emotional problems.

DIFFERENTIAL DIAGNOSIS

The majority of children in this group do not have a medical diagnosis and their problems are thought to be constitutional, often genetically based, in origin. A large number of potential diagnoses must be excluded by medical examination before a diagnosis of motor learning difficulties is made by exclusion. Some important ones include: cerebral palsy, neuromuscular diseases such as early Duchenne muscular dystrophy, epilepsy, congenital hypothyroidism, and hydrocephalus.

POSSIBLE AETIOLOGIES OF MOTOR LEARNING PROBLEMS

1. Prenatal, natal or postnatal neurological damage. This remains a possibility in some children who may have been born prematurely or had a history of adverse perinatal events.
2. A dysfunctional neurological state, the pathogenesis of which is not clear but there is often an inherited factor. Deprivation of the normal sensory experience in childhood, e.g. catarrhal deafness, visual problems, lack of binocular vision or biological variation, has been postulated. The possibility of impaired kinaesthetic sensitivity led to a number of studies with conflicting results (Bairstow & Laszlo, 1981; Hulme et al., 1982; Elliott et al., 1988).

CLINICAL SIGNS

Gubbay's 1975 seminal book *The clumsy child* advocated the use of a battery of eight tests of motor proficiency as an adjunct to conventional neurological examination because the latter does not demonstrate the difficulties a child may have with motor tasks needed for daily living activities. Normal referenced tests of motor ability have now superseded simple tests of motor proficiency. Neurological testing can be expanded, however, by testing for 'soft' neurological signs. These are signs which do not necessarily indicate an abnormality of the central nervous system (CNS).

A wide range of different neurological items have been classified as soft neurological signs. These include developmental signs, and signs of abnormality, which have been listed by Tupper (1986). Examples of developmental soft signs are: associated movements; difficulty with building tasks; inability to catch a ball; and gait and speech problems. Soft signs of abnormality include: astereognosis; auditory–visual integration difficulties; choreiform movements; diffuse electroencephalographic (EEG) abnormalities; increased or decreased muscle tone; and significant inco-ordination.

Tupper (1987) summarised the lack of clear definitions, precision and reliability relating to soft signs. Nevertheless, soft signs are often associated with conditions involving the CNS. Rutter *et al.* (1970) concluded: 'A very high number of minor neurological signs makes it likely that the child has some kind of neurological disorder, but a moderate number of minor signs is quite compatible with normality.'

It is important to measure not merely the emergence of a motor skill (Noller & Ingrisano, 1984) but also its achievement. There is a difference between the ability to perform a task and the ability to perform a skill, skill meaning a practised ability or expertise. Children with motor learning difficulties have problems with the organisation of the movement and therefore may be able to perform part of what is required, e.g. a particular hand movement in isolation, but not a planned complex movement.

SYMPTOMATOLOGY

Symptoms experienced by children with motor learning difficulties vary from child to child but may include: inefficient body awareness and control; specific learning difficulties; perceptual disorders; 'soft' neurological signs; language dysfunction; hyperactivity; attentional problems; and emotional lability.

The 'clumsy' group are usually referred for treatment at about the age of 7, when problems involving number shape, writing and reading become identified at school. Physically, they appear inco-ordinate although able to stand and walk, with poor posture and lower-than-normal muscle tone. Occasionally, they are asymmetrical or adopt a toe/heel, flexed gait similar to that in diplegia. They may be withdrawn, lethargic children, reluctant to participate in activities, or, conversely, hyperactive, destructive children possibly with behavioural problems.

Their difficulties are thought to be due to confusion in the response to, and interpretation of, stimuli. For instance, they may have problems with depth perception and therefore a fear of heights; they resist or avoid tactile stimulation and have difficulty with identification of body parts or the whole body in space.

PHYSICAL MANAGEMENT OF MOTOR DYSFUNCTION

The focus of this section will be on the cerebral palsies but the principles are also applicable to other motor disorders, including the motor learning disorders described above. Both groups vary in clinical presentation and degree of severity, and the age at which diagnosis and subsequent referral is made. However, they both benefit from assessment and physical intervention to alleviate problems and educate carers, regardless of diagnosis. Both groups of disorders also persist throughout life, with the presentation changing but the underlying pathology probably remaining the same.

The aim of this section is to enable the physiotherapist to identify physical difficulties, the need for intervention or possible further referral, at any age, and to suggest guidelines for investigation and programme planning. Knowledge of motor development (Chapter 18) and normal motor control (Chapter 2) is essential for assessment, management and intervention.

DISORDER OF POSTURE AND MOVEMENT

The quality and quantity of movement observed is dependent upon the efficiency of posture. Disorder of posture and movement can be defined as the lack of ability of the body to cope effectively with the effects of gravity, and to relate to the earth's surface through the base of support. As a result, ability, mobility, comfort and the shape of the body are compromised and replaced by limitation of movement, inefficiency of posture and postural adjustment, discomfort and deformity (Hare, 1990).

In patients with lifetime motor disorders, there is no experience of normal movement or development to draw upon, and it is almost impossible to predict outcomes on a long-term basis. However, the damaged nervous system is motivated to change and develop. It is influenced by, and will respond to, stimulation (see Chapter 6, 'Plasticity'), hence the need for early evaluation and therapy intervention, even before diagnosis is confirmed.

CLINICAL PRESENTATION, PROBLEMS AND SOLUTIONS

Six age groups of patients with cerebral palsy have been selected in order to discuss their clinical presentation and the problems likely to arise, and to suggest solutions to these. The problems, with suggested solutions, are summarised in Table 19.1.

Many factors influence change, e.g. growth, which has a considerable effect on the normally developing body and can have a disastrous effect on a patient's level of performance.

Problems and solutions in the physical management of cerebral palsy

Age group	Problem	Solution
The infant and young child (0–2 years)	Anxiety, concern, frustration of parents	Explain order and process of development, identify positive achievements and attributes, explain method and findings of assessment
	Difficulties with holding, cuddling, positioning the baby	Suggest and demonstrate positions in lying, when holding, feeding, cuddling the baby; encourage parents to handle and play with the baby; refer to speech therapist for feeding advice if necessary
	Delay in developmental cycle	Explain development is an ongoing process, dependent on practice and repetition; encourage communication between parents and their child, advise them that the baby's ability to signal and respond may be delayed and to give him or her time
The toddler, preschool child (2–5 years)	Ongoing difficulties, parents become more aware of limitations ahead	Point out progress to date, repeat explanation and relevance of programme, goals, share and answer queries and problems
	Noticeable 'gap' in performance, lagging behind peers	Careful selection of aids and appliances to help bridge the gap; involve speech and occupational therapists for advice and opinion if not already involved
	Asymmetry of posture, hazard of deformity	Meticulous assessment and record of this, explain implications to parents; review strategies to counteract these tendencies, involve parents in monitoring procedures
	Enquiry into other methods of treatment, search for further opinions	Revision of procedures to date and their relevance, discussion on various approaches; accept parents' need for reassurance
The schoolchild (5–10 years)	Lack of knowledge, understanding of neurological conditions and apprehension of school staff	Give time to head teacher, staff, care assistants, to answer queries and concerns, suggesting alternatives, ways of coping with child's difficulties. Emphasise ability, and need for balance between maximum participation in school activities and time necessary for specific input
	Difficulties with mobility, furniture, etc.	Discuss provision of ramps, use of walking aids, wheelchairs, adaptations to chairs and tables in the classroom
	Inability to take part in competition, rough and tumble of the playground	Emphasise child's other positive qualities, set realistic goals and activities, suggest development of other interests, hobbies
	Growth, postural changes, effect on ability levels	Record changes, make thorough assessments at least once a term, consider effect of these changes in the long term
	Lack of time, tiredness, disinclination to carry out programmes at school and home	Revise and reduce programmes to essential minimum, attempt to create a balance between the dual importance of education and the child's physical needs

Growth is most intense between the ages of 0 and 3 in both boys and girls, from 8 to 15 in girls and from 10 to 18 in boys (Buckler, 1990). Care must be taken at these times to identify and maintain levels of ability and avoid, if possible, orthopaedic surgery to muscles, postponing such procedures until the growth period is over.

Measurements of the growth process in children and adolescents, i.e. sitting height, overall (standing) height and leg length, are particularly useful when evaluating gait and potential for walking. Measurement is difficult to obtain in standing and sitting, and may be carried out in a supine lying position, using a calibrated surface.

The Infant and Young Child: 0-2 years

The early presentation of a baby with suspected neurological damage may be either restlessness and over-reaction to stimulus or unresponsiveness and difficulty to rouse. A most significant sign is the concern of the parent, who is

Problems and solutions in the physical management of cerebral palsy (Continued)		
Age group	Problem	Solution
The adolescent (10-18 years)	Deterioration in upright ability and mobility, and posture in other positions	Accurate monitoring of changes and consequences to levels of independence; substitute aids and assistance where necessary; record effect on levels of postural competence in lying, sitting and standing
	Fatigue, lack of concentration	Reassessment of working situations particularly sitting posture; suggest further adaptations; refer again for occupational therapy advice
	Concern, distress of parents and patient at obvious and often rapid deterioration	Reassure them that this is a passing phase, stress importance of maintaining abilities in lying, sitting and standing; assess regularly, plan evaluation of situation at end of growth period, possible referral to orthopaedic surgeon for an opinion
	Changes due to growth	Monitor weight gain, measure sitting height, standing height, length of arms and legs; encourage other activities such as swimming
The young adult (18-35 years)	Rejection of physiotherapy advice and regimens	Respect this bid for freedom! Substitute other forms of exercise, possible use of a gymnasium; agree on a date for evaluation
	Need for independence in lifestyle, possible rejection of home and home values	Evaluate abilities and difficulties, recommend minimal maintenance programme if appropriate, suggest aids to further mobility, refer to orthopaedic consultant for management of deformity, discomfort
The older adult (35+ years)	Poor health, later difficulties associated with ageing	Treat and manage as appropriate; knowledge of ageing process and expected lifespan is an asset
	Social difficulties due to overburdening of carer; death of parents	Take immediate action, reassess and refer to social services, other relevant bodies. The impact of such a crisis situation can be reduced by realistic forward planning in earlier years

Table 19.1 Problems and solutions in the physical management of cerebral palsy.

aware that something is interfering with development and is becoming increasingly frustrated and upset. He or she will talk about difficulties with positioning and holding the baby (e.g. 'He isn't a cuddly baby'), the child's difficulty in responding to him or her, and possibly problems with feeding. It is advisable to see such babies at the following ages during the first year: 6 weeks; 3 months; 6 months; and 1 year. If possible, a programme of advice and treatment should be started immediately (Table 19.1).

Apart from handling and observation of the child, it is helpful to place him or her in supine and prone lying positions and to observe attempts to adjust the position. The traction test, when the child is brought to the sitting position from supine lying, is also of significance. The head will lag in the very young child but failure to fix the bottom without help during the manoeuvre suggests a delay in the development of postural control that, if allowed to persist, causes considerable difficulty in physical management in later life.

Six months can be regarded as the watershed of the first year of development. Having mastered abilities in lying, the child is now progressing towards independent sitting and, in time, standing (see Chapter 18). Failure to demonstrate either abilities on lying or independent sitting at 6 months will certainly contribute to confirmation of a neurological problem. Care must be taken to detect early signs of visual or hearing defects in the first year, either in the child's behaviour or in the interaction between parent and child. Suspicious signs should be reported to the consultant concerned without delay.

Children with mild cases of hemiplegia may be referred for the first time at the age of 9 months to a year. The extra effort required to balance and walk results in the characteristic asymmetry of this condition. An observant parent and/or physiotherapist should note signs of postural asymmetry and take steps to counteract it. The first year in the life of a child, who may well be handicapped in the long-term, is particularly stressful for the parents who struggle to understand and come to terms with the reality of the situation. It is very often impossible to give positive answers to their questions. Measures which help parents to gain perspective and manage the situation are: careful, repeated explanation of the process of physical development from lying, to sitting, to standing; practical suggestions in answer to their queries; and a programme of exercise and handling, with realistic and shared goals.

The Toddler and Preschool Child: 2–5 years

The period of rapid change continues. At the age of 5 years the child has an established personality and should be physically and emotionally prepared for school life. Parents may want to seek alternate opinions, explanations and methods of treatment—a difficult situation for the therapist to handle. This tendency to leave no stone unturned has to be accepted by professionals as the parents' right, and understood in the context of their anxiety. Extra activities, such as the local play group or nursery, are to be encouraged and prove helpful for both parents and child.

In contrast to their normal peers, the lack of movement and ability to get themselves around is characteristic of children with difficulty at this age. They remain in the pushchair or on the parent's lap, or are placed on the floor. Some may be progressing satisfactorily, albeit slowly, towards upright mobility; others may be unable to sit without help or to move without falling. Their difficulties can cause them to be withdrawn or overdemanding in their behaviour. Neurological signs, if present, will be exaggerated on movement and attempts to move. Balance may be precarious, and they may demonstrate extreme fear of upright positions. It is unlikely that deformity will have become established at this early stage, but the tendencies towards asymmetrical posturing must be noted, both when the child is still and on attempted movement.

It is wise to alert parents to these tendencies in posture as early as possible and to instruct them in observation of the trunk and spine in horizontal and vertical positions. The hip joints should also be checked from an early age for limitation of movement, particularly of abduction and external rotation, and the parents instructed in this procedure.

The Schoolchild: 5–10 years

Body changes of growth and weight, although discrete in this age group, can affect ability and mobility levels. More able children with greater choice of movement cope well during this period, and as a result are included in activities, often despite their instability. Those with less ability, who are slow and more compromised in the upright position, find it increasingly difficult to keep up and become disillusioned. Other roles and activities should be identified for these children to help build morale and minimise the sense of failure. Particular areas that should be carefully monitored for change and possible deterioration are the sitting posture, the feet and the use of hands.

Physical prowess and competition with age peers predominate amongst this age group, and can cause distress amongst children with handicaps. The challenges of the school environment are considerable: getting from one class room to another; negotiating stairs; keeping up with the others at changing times; carrying books and dinner trays; and the rough and tumble of the playground. Children with difficulties need support, preferably given by a care assistant who will become the mainstay of the physiotherapy programme at school. Abilities learnt in previous years must be maintained and developed.

The need for programmes of exercise and management must be explained and fully accepted by the school staff, and the space, time and personnel allocated to carry out these activities. Parents should be encouraged to continue their involvement and responsibility towards exercise programmes, despite the increasingly busy time schedules and school life.

The Adolescent: 10–18 years

The increasing dominance of education during this period is further compounded by the preparation for, and taking of, exams. However, it is also the major growth period, leading to physical changes in height, weight, limb length and girth that have a dramatic and often disastrous effect on the young person's ability and self-esteem. Hormonal changes further disturb the equilibrium! The ability to stand and walk is particularly affected, causing concern, disappointment and disillusionment for all concerned. Young people, previously able to walk independently or with aids, 'sink' into an increasingly flexed standing position and gradually lose the ability to straighten themselves up against gravity. It is becoming widely accepted in orthopaedic circles that surgery at this time is inadvisable. The rapid changes in weight and height continue until 15 years in girls and 18 years in boys. A possible explanation for this deterioration is that the body has difficulty adjusting to these major changes in the body, rather in the same way that an able walker will experience difficulty carrying a heavy object (Hare, 1992).

The Young Adult: 18-35 years

Adulthood is the threshold to independence, and freedom from the onerous regularity and need for constant monitoring in childhood. Patients should be encouraged to take stock of their physical situation and its implications for their lifestyle and independence. Quite understandably, many patients reject physiotherapy and physiotherapists altogether. This can be beneficial to both parties, giving the opportunity to evaluate further the situation, the achievements made and programmes used. The period of growth and maximum change is over; emphasis at this point should be on coming to terms with limitations, whether mild or severe and maintaining an active lifestyle as far as possible. Responsibility for their physical condition should now rest with the patients, although review and advice should be available if requested. The more disabled may have fixed deformity of the limbs or spine and this can give rise to discomfort, pain and difficulty with daily activities such as dressing and personal hygiene. Further deterioration must be prevented.

An orthopaedic opinion and often intervention can be very helpful at this age. If the physiotherapy programme, and particularly the explanation given and reasons for the measures taken, has been successful during the past years, the patient should be able to assess himself or herself and the potential for change. Continued support must be available to enable a physical activity programme to be implemented and monitored, as well as independence maintained. Several services may be required for optimal employment, housing and social goals to be achieved.

A study conducted on individuals with cerebral palsy between 1951 and 1974 found that prediction of long-term functional outcome was pessimistic when compared with actual outcome (O'Grady et al., 1995). This suggests that future capabilities should be assessed more optimistically.

The Older Adult: 35+ years

Increasing fatigue is characteristic of people with cerebral palsy and is probably due to a lifetime of constant struggle to maintain efficient levels of posture and movement. As the individual grows, and through stages of maturity as an adult, the ratio of body weight to muscle tissue alters. Slow inevitable deterioration takes place, resulting in the loss of ability, functional activities and comfort in positions. In later life, as ease of movement and mobility decline, so individuals become prone to chest infections and other conditions associated with ageing.

Inevitably, the load on the carers increases; they too are ageing, resulting in some cases in a breakdown in their way of life. A common dilemma arises on the death of parents who have been the sole carers for their disabled son or daughter.

STRATEGIES FOR INTERVENTION

Effective management requires careful assessment, treatment and management planning and evaluation of treatment outcome. Assessment and outcome measures to evaluate treatments are lacking in neurological physiotherapy and some of the methods used for adults (see Chapter 4) are not appropriate for children.

Assessment Methods

Some published scales of motor function have been adapted or developed for children (Chapter 4). The Test of Motor Impairment (TOMI) measures performance of daily-life motor skills such as static and dynamic balance, ball skills and fine motor skills. It has both qualitative and quantitative measures and provides normal values for children aged 5 to 11+ (Stott et al., 1984). The functional motor assessment scale (FMAS) was revised and shown to be reliable and valid for assessing gross motor skills in children with cerebral palsy (Vermeer et al., 1995). The Gross Motor Function Measure has been used to assess the effectiveness of physiotherapy (e.g. Bower et al., 1996).

The ABC General Motor Co-ordination Test has two sections, one measuring fine motor functioning and one measuring co-ordination of the whole body. It is useful for children between 6 and 9 years and has age-related normal values (Wiegersma et al., 1988). Others include the Sensory Integration and Praxis Tests (SIPT; Ayres, 1989) and the Developmental Test of Visual-Motor Integration (Beery, 1982). Fairgrieve (1989) compared standard tests used to identify children with motor learning problems.

General Principles of Assessment

Some general principles that can be used independently of diagnostic categories are now proposed as follows: to place the patient in, or ask him or her to assume, positions of lying, sitting and standing ; within each position to observe and record the quality and quantity of movement, symmetry or asymmetry of posture (Pountney et al., 1990); to observe ease or apprehension, confidence or fear; and to investigate the adequacy of the body–supporting surface relationship. An outline for assessment is given in Box 19.1. Details of assessment can be found in the literature cited and some aspects of assessing child development are discussed in Chapter 18.

Box 19.1 A suggested guide to assessment of long-term disability. This should be completed at the first appointment and repeated at appropriate intervals. The guide may be used in part or as a whole.

The following levels of ability are helpful when screening performance in lying, sitting and standing:

5. Able to assume the position.
4. Able to move out of the position (by altering the base of the position).
3. Able to move within the position (without altering the base).
2. Able to maintain the position (without movement).
1. Able to conform (the body) to the supporting surface, when the position is assumed or when the body is placed.
0. Unable to conform to the supporting surface.

Levels 1 and 2 are essential to the retraining of postural disorder, although below the level where function is possible (Hare, 1990). Details of a strategy suggested for the investigation of the disorder of posture and movement are described by Hare (1993).

Management Programme

Management of cerebral palsy is described in several texts (Scrutton 1984; Golding et al., 1986; Griffiths & Clegg, 1988). The management programme consists of guidelines and practical suggestions for the carer to use on a daily basis. The programme will involve the multidisciplinary team (MDT) and can include: suggestions for carrying, lifting and moving the patient; suggestions for positioning to improve comfort and function; methods of feeding, dressing and toiletting; the application and use of orthoses and switches to aid independence and communication; and recommendations for other activities such as swimming and horse riding. The use of aids and adaptations is essential to the successful management of the adult and younger patient with severe disability and must be considered.

Evaluation of Treatment Outcome

Several strategies for the evaluation of clinical work are currently used (see Chapter 4). Some outcome measures include time spent in clinical or clerical contact, others the cost of time spent, equipment and travel. To overcome the problem of 'discharge outcomes' that are not relevant to long-term disability, a system of regular review, once a term for children and once a year for adults, is suggested. Some outcome scales were mentioned above. Bower et al. (1996) found that measurable goals were strongly associated with increased motor skill after physiotherapy.

TREATMENT APPROACHES AND METHODS

Five main concepts of treatment are currently in use for cerebral palsy and motor learning disorders in the UK. These are: the Bobath approach; conductive education; sensory integration therapy; the Hare approach; and the Vojta technique. The first two are discussed in Chapter 22 and specifically for children in Scrutton (1984). Treatment in these patients is largely unevaluated.

A study that evaluated different intensities of physiotherapy in cerebral palsy used the eclectic approach, with physiotherapists selecting the most appropriate methods from the different approaches for each individual child (Bower et al., 1996). Intensive physiotherapy produced a slightly greater, but not significantly different, increase in motor skill than conventional amounts of therapy.

Bobath Approach

The Bobath approach suggests that treatment methods should be flexible and adaptive to the varying needs of the individual, and that programmes should be carried over into the context of daily life. Assessment is guided by the patient's reaction to handling by the physiotherapist. The objective of treatment is to encourage the patient to take control of his or her movement, through techniques of inhibition and facilitation. Treatment of the young child should commence as soon as signs of abnormal tonus and movement patterns become apparent (Bobath & Bobath, 1984).

Conductive Education

Conductive education is used in an increasing number of schools and clinics in the UK. It is a systematic approach in which the patient is actively engaged in his or her own learning, aimed at the development of 'ortho-function', a self-directed, spontaneous approach to problem solving. The patient takes part in a group, led by a conductor (see Chapter 22). Skills introduced and learnt in the group situation are practised throughout the day as part of the activities of daily living. The system is applicable to other conditions and can be used with adults as well as children (Hari & Tilemans, 1984; Scrutton, 1984). Conductive education for children with cerebral palsy has been reviewed at the Birmingham Institute (Bairstow et al., 1993).

Sensory Integration Therapy

Sensory integration therapy was designed primarily for children with cerebral dysfunction, but adults and children with learning difficulties also appear to benefit from this approach. The objective of the concept is to organise sensory input for use, relieving the overt signs of inco-ordination.

Work concentrates on the proprioceptive, tactile and vestibular systems and the equipment used relates to these. The therapist needs to have sound knowledge of the development of sensory processing and be able to make an informed assessment on the analysis of the patient's deficits. Parental or carer instruction and co-operation are essential to support the treatment programme. This treatment approach is discussed by Watter & Bullock (1989), Bundy & Fisher (1991) and Kaplan et al. (1993).

Hare Approach

The Hare approach is based on the hypothesis that overt neurological signs are unreliable as a basis for assessment and treatment planning; instead, the focus is the underlying disorder of posture and movement. A system for the analysis of posture and movement within the context of gravity and the supporting surface ('the human sandwich factor') is described. A classification and levels of ability are identified, based on fundamental postural skills. Assessment is made in positions of lying, sitting and standing, with particular attention to the trunk–body part–supporting surface relationship in each position. Instruction and partnership with the carer are emphasised; the therapist aims to reduce his or her input through building confidence and expertise. Techniques of treatment include the use of arm and leg gaiters, the application of below-knee plaster boots, and the use of aids and adapted furniture as appropriate. The assessment process can be used independently of the treatment method; both are applicable to all ages of patient and most diagnostic categories. Successful outcomes are recognised in increased vocabulary of movement, control of discomfort and the threat of deformity, ease of handling and management, and quality of physical performance (Hare, 1990, 1993; Pope, 1990; Durham & Eve, 1993).

Vojta Technique

The Vojta technique is based on the concept of reflex locomotion and the hypotheses that the 'total movement pattern' develops as a result of stimulation of the periphery (body parts) and that the postural disorder observed in the affected newborn is similar to that of the child with cerebral palsy. Treatment is carried out in supine and prone lying positions, fixed points are identified and stimuli given to the movements of reflex locomotion, with maximal resistance. It is suitable for infants and young children only and treatment ceases after 1 year if no change is apparent. Parents are instructed in the technique. The most successful outcomes are said to occur in infants and in 'pending' rather than 'established' cerebral palsy (Vojta, 1984).

Choice of Treatment Approaches

Attempts to evaluate one treatment approach against another have met with little success (Palmer et al., 1988; Mayo, 1991; Bower & McLellan, 1994). Greater success has resulted from evaluation of parent compliance (Law & King, 1993; Unwin & Sheppard, 1995). Another useful method of evaluation is the single case study design (Riddoch, 1991), which incorporates goal setting, method description, a time span and outcome evaluation. Allen & Donald (1995) summarised some of the research in this area.

No one treatment approach is advocated and the physiotherapist should keep up to date with different approaches, particularly as research to evaluate them produces evidence of effectiveness. Each patient should be assessed as an individual and knowledge from different approaches applied to the needs of each patient.

Treatment programmes should be initiated by the physiotherapist, and may be carried out by the carer, following instruction. The physiotherapy programme should be precise and focus on basic problems of postural deficit.

Seating Systems and Management of Posture

Conservative measures in terms of furniture design and provision, and seating systems for care and handling of the severely disabled with multiple problems, have greatly advanced during recent years (Pope, 1996). Several methods of assessment that stress the importance of the analysis of postural abilities and limitations, the management of deformity, and the possibilities for improvement are now available (Mulcahey et al., 1988; Pope, 1990, 1992, 1996; Green et al., 1992; Pope et al., 1994). Posture and seating are discussed in Chapters 8 & 25.

Management of Muscle Tone

The problem of managing abnormal tone, particularly spasticity, is discussed in Chapter 25. Some of the treatment approaches discussed above, and in Chapter 22, involve strategies to control spastic patterns, as do methods of handling, positioning and providing seating systems. Details of methods for reducing and measuring spasticity can be found in Chapters 24 & 25.

THE ROLE OF THE PHYSIOTHERAPIST IN THE MULTIDISCIPLINARY TEAM

The major responsibility of the physiotherapist working with long-term disability is the analysis, interpretation and resolution of physical difficulties resulting from the original impairment. By virtue of his or her training and understanding of movement and balance, the physiotherapist is often the focus for advice on the treatment and management of physical disability.

The Team Member

The MDT is likely to be composed of three parts: the immediate team; the support team; and the medical team. The immediate team consists of those with direct 'hands-on' contact with the patient and includes the physiotherapist, occupational therapist, speech therapist, the carer and the patient. The physiotherapist should plan and support intervention programmes, in order to reduce the frequency and intensity of input as the knowledge and confidence of other members increases.

The support team consists of professionals in education, social services and housing, and orthotists and engineers. In-service training for care staff and managers and information leaflets can contribute to good working relationships.

The role of the medical team in the early years is to confirm diagnosis and monitor change, and then throughout life to act as a reference for health concerns, changes in the familiar clinical picture, and further referral. The medical team may include a paediatrician, a neurologist, a general practitioner, an orthopaedic surgeon and, ideally, a consultant for the adults. At the time of writing, there is a shortfall in medical coverage for school-leavers and adults.

The Individual Professional

As an individual and professional, the physiotherapist should be able to: devise and use a repeatable form of assessment; plan and execute long- and short-term programmes of intervention; measure outcomes of those interventions; share, explain and communicate knowledge, opinions and findings; monitor change; and examine treatment approaches critically using all available evidence.

Relationship With The Carer

The carer is essential to the carrying out of the physiotherapy treatment and management plan. The well trained carer can be relied upon to carry out individual treatment regimens, possibly on a daily basis, to support management programmes, and to observe and monitor change for the better or worse. The relationship between physiotherapist and carer is of great importance and is built on trust, adequate support and training.

CONCLUSION

The person with cerebral palsy or motor learning disorder has the right of access to assessment and advice throughout life. Ongoing management and support programmes are essential to minimise deterioration and the negative effect this has on quality of life, as well as financial and other resources. The range of motor learning disorders is wide and some can be mild, with the child growing to lead a normal adult life. Intervention must be based upon careful, observant assessment, the sharing of findings, and realistic agreed expectations of the patient, carer and therapist. Clinical experience of all ages and severity will strengthen confidence and knowledge and enable the therapist to better influence the management of patients throughout their lives.

Acknowledgements

Noreen Hare would like to thank Mrs Lynn Allen for her time and skill in preparation of the text; the editor, Professor Maria Stokes, for her availability and positive encouragement; and the countless children, their parents, and adults with disability who have taught me all I know.

REFERENCES

Aicardi J. Epilepsy in brain injured children. *Dev Med Child Neurol* 1990, **32**:191-202.

Allen S, Donald M. The effect of occupational therapy on the motor proficiency of children with motor/learning difficulties: a pilot study. *Br J Occup Ther* 1995, **58**:385-391.

American Psychiatric Association. *Diagnostic and statistical manual of mental disorders, 4th edition.* Washington DC: Americal Psychiatric Association; 1994.

Ayres AJ. *Sensory integration and Praxis tests.* Los Angeles: Western Psychological Corporation; 1989.

Bairstow P, Cochrane R, Hur J. *Evaluation of conductive education for children with cerebral palsy. Final report (Parts I and II).* London: HMSO; 1993.

Bairstow PJ, Laszlo JI. Kinaesthetic sensitivity to passive movements in children and adults, and its relationship to motor development and motor control. *Dev Med Child Neurol* 1981, **23**:606-616.

Beery K. *Revised administration, scoring and teaching manual for the developmental test of visual-motor integration (VMI).* Chicago: Follet Publishing; 1982.

Bobath B, Bobath K. The neuro developmental treatment. In: Scrutton D, ed. *Management of the motor disorders of children with cerebral palsy.* London: Spastics International Medical Publications; 1984:6-18.

Bower E, McLellan DL. Evaluating therapy in cerebral palsy. *Child Health Care Dev* 1994, **20**:409-419.

Bower E, McLellan DL, Arney J, et al. A randomised controlled trial of different intensities of physiotherapy and different goal-setting procedures in 44 children with cerebral palsy. *Dev Med Child Neurol* 1996, **38**:226-237.

Buckler J. *A longitudinal study of adolescent growth*. London: Springer Verlag; 1990.

Bundy A, Fisher AG. *Sensory integration theory and practice*. Philadelphia: Davies and Co; 1991.

Cornell MS. The hip in cerebral palsy. *Dev Med Child Neurol* 1995, **37**:3-18.

Cosgrove AP, et al. Botulinum toxin in the management of the lower limb in cerebral palsy. *Dev Med Child Neurol* 1994, **36**:386-396.

Dubowitz LMS. Clinical assessment of the infant nervous system. In: Levene MI, Bennett MJ, Punt J, eds. *Fetal and neonatal neurology and neurosurgery*. Edinburgh: Churchill Livingstone; 1988:41-58.

Duckman RH. Vision therapy for the child with cerebral palsy. *J Am Optom Assoc* 1987, **58**:28-35.

Durham S, Eve L. Application of the physical ability scale to able children with motor impairment. In: Hare N, ed. *The physical ability scale and variants*. London: Hare Association for Physical Ability; 1993:59-67.

Elliott JM, et al. Development of kinaesthetic sensitivity and motor performance in children. *Dev Med Child Neurol* 1988, **30**:80-92.

Fairgrieve E. Alternative means of assessment: a comparison of standardised tests identifying minimal cerebral dysfunction. *Br J Occup Ther* 1989: **52**:88-92.

Gillberg C. Children with preschool minor neurodevelopmental disorders, IV. *Dev Med Child Neurol* 1989, **31**:14-24.

Golding R, et al. *The caring person's guide to handling the severely multiply handicapped*. Basingstoke & London: MacMillan Education; 1986.

Green EM, et al. *Postural management, theory and practice*. Birmingham: Active Design Ltd; 1992.

Griffiths M, Clegg M. *Cerebral palsy: problems and practice*. London: Souvenir Press; 1988.

Gubbay SS. *The clumsy child*. New York: Saunders; 1975.

Hallet R. Evaluation of physical ability in scoliosis surgery. In: Hare N, ed. *The trunk*. London: Hare Association for Physical Ability; 1992:41-55.

Hare N. The analysis and measurement of physical abiltiy. In: Hare N, ed. *What the hare tortoise*. London: Hare Association for Physical Ability; 1990:2-27.

Hare N. The paradox. In: Hare N, ed. *The trunk*. London: Hare Association for Physical Ability; 1992:11-20.

Hare N. The physical ability scale. In: Hare N, ed. *The physical ability scale and variants*. London: Hare Association for Physical Ability; 1993:7-25.

Hari M, Tilemans T. Conductive education. In: Scrutton D, ed. *Management of the motor disorders of children with cerebral palsy*. London: Spastics International Medical Publications; 1984:19-35.

Hulme C, et al. Visual, kinaesthetic and crossmodal judgements of length by normal and clumsy chidren. *Dev Med Child Neurol* 1982, **24**:461-471.

Kaplan BJ, Polatajko HJ, Wilson BN, Faris PD. Re-examination of sensory integration treatment: a combination of two efficacy studies. *J Learn Dis* 1993, **26**:342-344.

Law M, King G. Parent compliance with therapeutic interventions for children with cerebral palsy. *Dev Med Child Neurol* 1993, **35**:983-990.

Lesney I, et al. Sensory disorders in cerebral palsy: two point discrimination. *Dev Med Child Neurol* 1993, **35**:402-405.

Losse A, et al. Clumsiness in children - do they grow out of it? A 10 year followup study. *Dev Med Child Neurol* 1991, **33**:55-68.

Lunsing RJ, et al. Minor neurological dysfunction from birth to 12 years. I: Increase during late school-age. *Dev Med Child Neurol* 1992, **34**:399-403.

Mayo NE. The effect of physical therapy for children with motor delay and cerebral palsy: a randomised clinical trial. *Am J Phys Med Rehab* 1991, **70**:258-267.

McLaughlin JF, et al. The role of selective dorsal rhizotomy in cerebral palsy: critical evaluation of a prospective clinical series. *Dev Med Child Neurol* 1994, **36**:755-769.

Mulchahey CM, et al. Adaptive seating for motor handicap. *Physiotherapy* 1988, **74**:531-536.

Mutch L, et al. Cerebral palsy epidemiology: where are we now and where are we going? *Dev Med Child Neurol* 1992, **34**:547-555.

Noller K, Ingrisano D. Cross sectional study of gross and fine motor development. Birth to 6 years of age. *Phys Ther* 1984, **64**:308-316.

O'Grady RS, Crain LS, Kohn J. The prediction of long-term functional outcomes of children with cerebral palsy. *Dev Med Child Neurol* 1995, **37**:997-1005.

Palmer FB, et al. The effects of physiotherapy on cerebral palsy, a controlled trial in infants with spastic diplegia. *N Engl J Med* 1988, **318**:803-808.

Pellegrino L. Cerebral palsy: a paradigm for developmental disabilities. *Dev Med Child Neurol* 1995, **37**:834-839.

Pope PM. The management of people with severe disability. In: Hare N, ed. *What the hare tortoise*. London: Hare Association for Physical Ability; 1990:28-45.

Pope PM. Management of the physical condition in cases of severe disability. *Physiotherapy* 1992, **12**:896-903.

Pope PM. Postural management and special seating. In: Edwards S, ed. *Neurological physiotherapy: a problem solving approach*. London: Churchill Livingstone; 1996:135-160.

Pope PM, Bowes CE, Booth E. Postural control in sitting. The SAM system: Evaluation of use over three years. *Dev Med Child Neurol* 1994, **36**:241-252.

Pountney TE, et al. Early development of postural control. *Physiotherapy* 1990, **76**:799-802.

Reilly S, Skuse D. Characteristics and management of feeding problems of young children with cerebral palsy. *Dev Med Child Neurol* 1992, **34**:379-388.

Riddoch J. Evaluation of practice: the single case study approach. *Physiother Pract* 1991, **7**:3-11.

Rosenbloom L. Diagnosis and management of cerebral palsy. *Arch Dis Child* 1995, **72**:350-354.

Rutter M, Graham P, Yule W. *A neuropsychiatric study in childhood*. London: Heinemann; 1970.

Scrutton D. *Management of the motor disorders of children with cerebral palsy*. London: Spastics International Medical Publications; 1984.

Scrutton D. The early management of hips in cerebral palsy. *Dev Med Child Neurol* 1989, **31**:108-116.

Soorani-Lunsing RJ, et al. Is minor neurological dysfunction at 12 years related to behaviour and cognition? *Dev Med Child Neurol* 1993, **35**:321-330.

Stott DH, Moyes FA, Henderson SE. *The Henderson revision of the Test of Motor Impairment*. San Antonio, Texas: Psychological Corporation; 1984.

Tupper DE. Neuropsychological screening and soft signs. In: Obrzut JE, Hynd GW, eds. *Child neuropsychology. Vol 2: Clinical practice*. Orlando, Florida: Academic Press; 1986:50-151.

Tupper DE. *Soft neurological signs*. Orlando, Florida: Grune & Stratton; 1987:1-16.

Unwin J, Shepphard L. Parent satisfaction with the minimal motor dysfunction unit: a survey. *Aust J Physiother* 1995, **41**:197-202.

Vermeer A, Kruithof H, van Zoggel B. The 'functional motor assessment scale' for children with cerebral palsy. *J Rehab Sci* 1995, **8**:94-98.

Vojta V. The basic elements of treatment according to Vojta. In: Scrutton, D, ed. *Management of the motor disorders of children with cerebral palsy*. London: Spastics International Medical Publications; 1984:75-85.

Watter P, Bullock MI. A physiotherapy directed school based group management programme for children with mild motor and co-ordination problems. *N Z J Physiother* 1989, **17**:19-23.

Wiegersma PH, van de Velde A, Reysoo HP, van Wieringen EHC, Kunnen ES, Wiegersma PA. *ABC, Test voor de algemene bewegings-co-ordinatie (General Motor Co-ordination Test)*. Lisse: Swets & Zeitlinger; 1988.

Yekutiel M, Jariwala M, Stretch P. Sensory deficit in the hands of children with cerebral palsy: a new look at assessment and prevalence. *Dev Med Child Neurol* 1994, **36**:619-624.

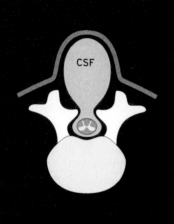

20 T Pountney & G McCarthy

NEURAL TUBE DEFECTS: SPINA BIFIDA AND HYDROCEPHALUS

CHAPTER OUTLINE

- Mechanism of neural tube defects (NTDs)
- Genetic aspects of NTDs
- Prevalence of NTDs
- Management of the spinal lesion after birth
- Hydrocephalus

- Mechanisms of associated neurological problems
- Spinal level of the lesion in spina bifida
- Physical management
- Case history

INTRODUCTION

Neural tube defects (NTDs) are a group of developmental abnormalities in which the neural tube fails to fuse somewhere along its length from the spinal cord to the brain (McCarthy, 1992). Spina bifida is the commonest NTD, where the lesion occurs in the spine. Hydrocephalus commonly occurs in association with spina bifida and is the condition where excess cerebrospinal fluid (CSF) circulates in and around the brain. This chapter describes the different NTDs and then focuses on the management of patients with spina bifida.

MECHANISM OF NEURAL TUBE DEFECTS (NTDs)

The neural tube develops from the neural plate early in embryonic development. Fusion normally occurs smoothly so that only the ends of the tube remain open. This means that the central canal remains in communication with the amniotic fluid. The upper (head) end of the tube develops into the brain and the lower end into the spinal cord (see Chapter 18). The lower end of the cord normally closes at 26 days of embryonic life (Levene, 1988).

The tube can fail to fuse anywhere along its length but this occurs most commonly at the lower end (McCarthy et al., 1992). The vertebrae develop from ectodermal tissue and normally close over the cord at 11 weeks of embryonic life. In spina bifida there may be associated abnormality of the skin, bone, meninges and neural tissue. If only skin, bone and dura meninges are involved, a meningocele occurs (Figure 20.1A). This is relatively uncommon and may be associated with hair or a naevus. In spina bifida cystica the skin, dura and spinal cord are involved, and this is termed a myelomeningocele (Figure 20.1B); this occurs in 80% of spina bifida lesions. When the neural tissue of the spinal cord is displaced and exposed on the surface of the lesion, the term rachischeisis is used (Figure 20.1C). In some cases the defect of the spinal cord and vertebrae may be covered by skin and hidden from sight, producing spina bifida occulta which is a more minor abnormality.

At a higher level in the neural tube, the posterior part of the brain may fail to develop and fuse normally, producing an encephalocele. Of these lesions, 75–80% occur in the occipital region; however, lesions can be anterior, including over the bridge of the nose. If the whole of the anterior aspect of the neural tube fails to develop, anencephaly occurs, when there is complete absence of the cerebral

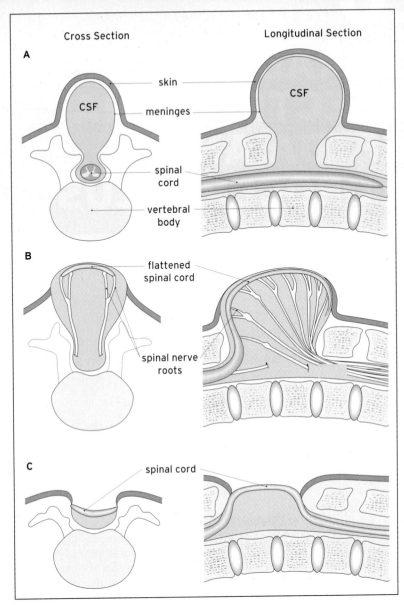

Cross Section   Longitudinal Section

A

skin

CSF   CSF

meninges

spinal cord

vertebral body

B

flattened spinal cord

spinal nerve roots

C

spinal cord

Figure 20.1 Types of spinal lesion in spina bifida. (A) Meningocele: no neural tissue outside the vertebral canal. (B) Myelomeningocele: neural tissue and nerve roots may be outside the vertebral canal. There may be fatty tissue or a bony spur present. (C) Rachischeisis: there is no sac, and the neural tissue lies open on the surface as a flattened plaque. (Redrawn from McCarthy, 1992, with permission.)

hemispheres; this is incompatible with life after birth.

It is possible for both major and subtle abnormalities of the central nervous system (CNS) to accompany the spinal manifestations of spina bifida. The commonest problem is hydrocephalus, caused by obstruction of the outflow of CSF from the cerebral ventricles through the narrow canal or aqueduct, or the small exit foramina that allow the passage of CSF to the surface of the brain (Figure 20.2).

Another common problem is the Arnold–Chiari abnormality, in which the brainstem and cerebellar vermis are herniated through the foramen magnum. This can be associated with cysts, or dilation of the central canal of the spinal cord, syringomyelia, which may present with neurological abnormalities affecting swallowing, phonation, and power and sensation in the arms.

GENETIC ASPECTS OF NTDs

There is known to be a genetic element to the occurrence of NTDs, with a risk of recurrence of spina bifida of 1 in 20 following the birth of a first affected child. The risk of recurrence increases to around 1 in 10 if a second affected child is born. Thereafter, risk increases to 1 in 4. There is known to be a racial bias in the occurrence of NTDs. The Welsh and Irish have a higher incidence than the English, and Europeans a higher incidence than Asians.

PREVALENCE OF NTDs

In the UK the prevalence of NTDs has been falling steadily over the past 30 years. Since it was unclear what part prenatal screening played in the reduced prevalence, a survey

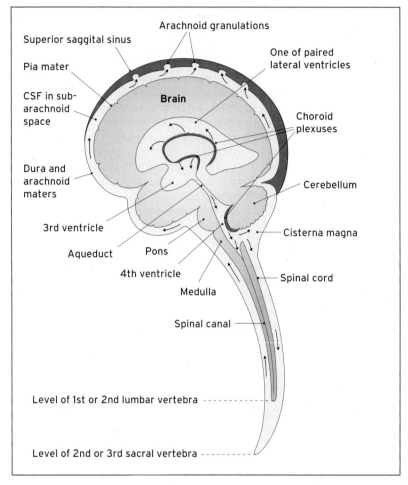

Figure 20.2 Cerebrospinal fluid (CSF) pathways. CSF is made by the choroid plexus in the lateral ventricles and flows through the 3rd ventricle, aqueduct, 4th ventricle and, via the foramina of Magendie and Lushka and basal cisterns, over the surface of the brain, where it is absorbed by the arachnoid granulations. It also passes through the cisterna magna and spinal canal to circulate around the spinal cord. (Redrawn from McCarthy, 1992, with permission.)

Table 20.1 The incidence of anencephaly and spina bifida in Great Britain. Data from the Office of Population Censuses and Surveys. (OPCS, 1995.)

The incidence of anencephaly and spina bifida in Great Britain

Rate/1000 births	1972	1982	1992
Anencephaly	1.47	0.26	0.05
Spina bifida	1.88	0.81	0.12

was carried out to clarify the position in relation to practice in 1985 (Cuckle *et al.*, 1989). The available information in 1985 showed only 36% of the decline in prevalence of spina bifida could be accounted for by terminations of pregnancy. It was concluded that an NTD Register should be set up to monitor the situation accurately. Figures from the Office of Population Censuses and Surveys (OPCS, 1995) show a continuing decline in Great Britain (Table 20.1).

In the mid-1970s, next to Ireland, Great Britain had the highest birth prevalence of NTDs in the world; now it has one of the lowest rates. Prenatal screening and diagnosis have been largely responsible for this but do not give the whole answer.

Folic acid has been shown to have a beneficial effect in preventing the occurrence of NTDs in a population of women at risk of producing further affected babies. An intake of folic acid of 4 mg/day before conception and for the first 3 months of pregnancy was sufficient to reduce the risk of recurrence of NTDs if there was a history of NTDs in the parents or first-degree relatives (Expert Advisory Group, 1992). Wald & Bower (1995) argued for the fortification of flour with folic acid. It is suggested that an increased intake of folic acid by the population in Great Britain of 0.4 mg/day could be sufficient to reduce the incidence of NTDs by approximately 1000 per year.

MANAGEMENT OF THE SPINAL LESION AFTER BIRTH

The neonate with open spina bifida needs to be assessed carefully after birth but it is not necessary to rush into rapid surgical intervention. Experience has shown that full assessment of the neurological, orthopaedic and medical problems should be carried out, together with social and emotional aspects of the family. The parents should be fully involved with decision making, including when not to treat babies with severe problems (Charney, 1990).

The higher the neural lesion and hence the level of paralysis, the worse the prognosis for morbidity and mortality. If severe hydrocephalus is present at birth, or marked spinal deformity or additional birth injury, the outlook is poor. Active surgical treatment of myelomeningocele consists of closure of the lesion on the first or second day of life. The sac is opened, the neural placode mobilised, and the dura then closed over the placode to form a watertight cover that is then covered by skin. Early closure reduces the risk of infection but the back can be covered by a sterile moist dressing and the sac will eventually epithelialise over. It is important to treat hydrocephalus at the same time as the closure of the back lesion, as pressure in the system rises and the back incision may leak CSF and fail to heal (see below).

HYDROCEPHALUS

The hydrocephalus associated with spina bifida is caused by obstruction to the normal pathways of flow of CSF in the brain, usually at the aqueduct, although it can occur at any point in the CSF circulation (see Figure 20.2).

The CSF is produced by the choroid plexuses in the ventricles and normally circulates through the ventricular system and around the surface of the brain, where it is absorbed by the arachnoid granulations into the saggital sinus. CSF also circulates around the spinal cord and down the central canal (Figure 20.2). If circulation of CSF is blocked, the fluid cannot be absorbed and pressure builds up.

Hydrocephalus develops in about 80% of children with spina bifida but is less likely to occur in those with lower spinal lesions (McCarthy & Land, 1992). Hydrocephalus often develops after birth when the lesion on the back is closed (see above). This is caused by the rise in pressure caused by closure of the fluid-filled sac, which was previously able to absorb pressure rises. In addition, the Arnold–Chiari malformation may be displaced downwards by rising pressure in the cranium, obstructing the outflow of the foramen magnum and the posterior cisterns.

In the infant, pressure rises are more easily absorbed because the cranium is more flexible, the bones of the skull can be stretched and the head size increases rapidly. In the older child the skull becomes more rigid and the pressure is transmitted to the brain. The ventricular system dilates in three dimensions, stretching the brain and disrupting the architecture. The lateral ventricles themselves can increase the obstruction at the aqueduct by curling round and pressing directly on it.

There was no effective treatment for hydrocephalus until 1956 when John Holter, an engineer who had a son with hydrocephalus, working with Eugene Spitz, a neurosurgeon, perfected a valve and shunt system. This system was designed to provide a bypass for CSF from the cerebral ventricles to the right atrium of the heart, the ventriculoatrial (VA) shunt. Since that time many other types of shunts have been developed with the same principle of providing a bypass for the excess CSF. The most common route now used is from the cerebral ventricle to the peritoneum, a ventriculoperitoneal (VP) shunt, but shunts can also be placed into the lumbar theca, the pleura, or even into a gastric pouch.

In addition to bypasses for CSF, efforts have been made to place a tube into the aqueduct, using neuroendoscopy, or to reduce production of CSF by cauterising the choroid plexus. The use of neuroendoscopy to make a window in the 3rd ventricle to bypass the aqueduct, 3rd ventriculostomy, has been successful in avoiding shunts in some children. This technique can also be used to make windows in cyst walls, or between the ventricles through the septum pellucidum, which is helpful if there is an uneven CSF flow between the two lateral ventricles. This is an exciting way to avoid long-term shunts but is effective only if the ventricular system is very dilated at the time of neuroendoscopy.

MECHANISMS OF ASSOCIATED NEUROLOGICAL PROBLEMS

If hydrocephalus is treated effectively from birth, neurological problems are likely to be reduced. However, some problems are undoubtedly caused by structural neurological abnormalities occurring during brain development and can be identified with magnetic resonance (MR) imaging. The effects of disruption of the immature brain can be inferred from the commonly encountered learning problems and difficulties of attention seen in children with hydrocephalus.

VISION
Pressure on the optic nerve can cause optic atrophy, which reduces visual acuity and can cause blindness. The optic pathways can be disrupted and the visual cortex may be damaged by huge dilation of ventricles, causing visual field defects or more subtle visual association difficulties. Eye movements can be affected by pressure on the oculomotor nerves, especially the 6th nerve, which has a long intracranial route, producing a convergent squint. Upward gaze can also be affected, causing the 'setting sun' appearance.

MUSCLE POWER AND SENSATION
The spinal lesion can affect innervation of the skin, muscles, bladder and bowel in many ways. Since MR scanning became widely available it has become clear that spinal cord abnormalities are very common. The cord may be divided by a bony spur or surrounded by fatty tissue. There may be a cystic swelling of the central canal, a syrinx, which

occurs most commonly in the cervical or lumbar regions. The cord may be adherent to the dural sac or held by the abnormally sited tissue so that it is tethered and this can cause a gradual deterioration in the neurological signs as the child grows, producing loss of muscle power, or skin sensation, or changes in bladder and bowel control.

SPINAL LEVEL OF THE LESION IN SPINA BIFIDA

The spinal level of neurological damage determines the functional abnormality, e.g. which muscles are affected and whether the bladder or bowel function is involved, although it is rare to get the precise cut-off level seen in spinal injury (Figure 20.3).

NEUROLOGICAL BASIS OF ORTHOPAEDIC PROBLEMS

The spinal cord function may be impaired at a certain level or, more commonly, there may be interruption of the corticospinal tracts with isolated reflex activity present. A spastic paraplegia may occur, with some preservation of voluntary movements and sensation. Some children have a hemi-myelomeningocele, with one leg affected and usually some bladder and bowel involvement.

Occult spinal dysraphism occurs when there is disordered closure of the neural tube or its coverings but the lesion is covered by skin. There may be external clues such as a fatty swelling or hairy tuft or haemangioma, a dermoid or dermal sinus. There is usually no neurological abnormality at birth but the lesion should be fully investigated with MR imaging as neurological complications develop with growth.

Low Lesions–Sacral (10% of Cases) or Lumbosacral (20%)

With low lesions, there may appear to be very good neurological function at birth and the legs may look normal. It is important to examine the hips for instability and look at movement of the feet. The weakness of plantar flexion, small muscles of the feet and hip extension may not be immediately obvious. Sensory testing is also difficult but should be attempted in the neonatal period in order to get an idea of the level of lesion. Testing is performed using a firm pin prick from the toes upwards until a pain reaction is elicited. This indicates the spinal level of involvement.

Talipes equinovarus deformities of the feet may be present at birth and it is important to initiate strapping or splinting to maintain a good position. The knees may be either flexed or hyperextended and there may be instability of the hips or frank dislocation, which requires immediate treatment (conservative management) in this group of children who have a good prognosis for walking independently.

Lumbar Lesions (20%)

In higher lesions muscle activity may be limited to hip flexion and adduction with some knee extension. The hips may be dislocated at birth but surgery in these circumstances is not indicated (Fixsen, 1992).

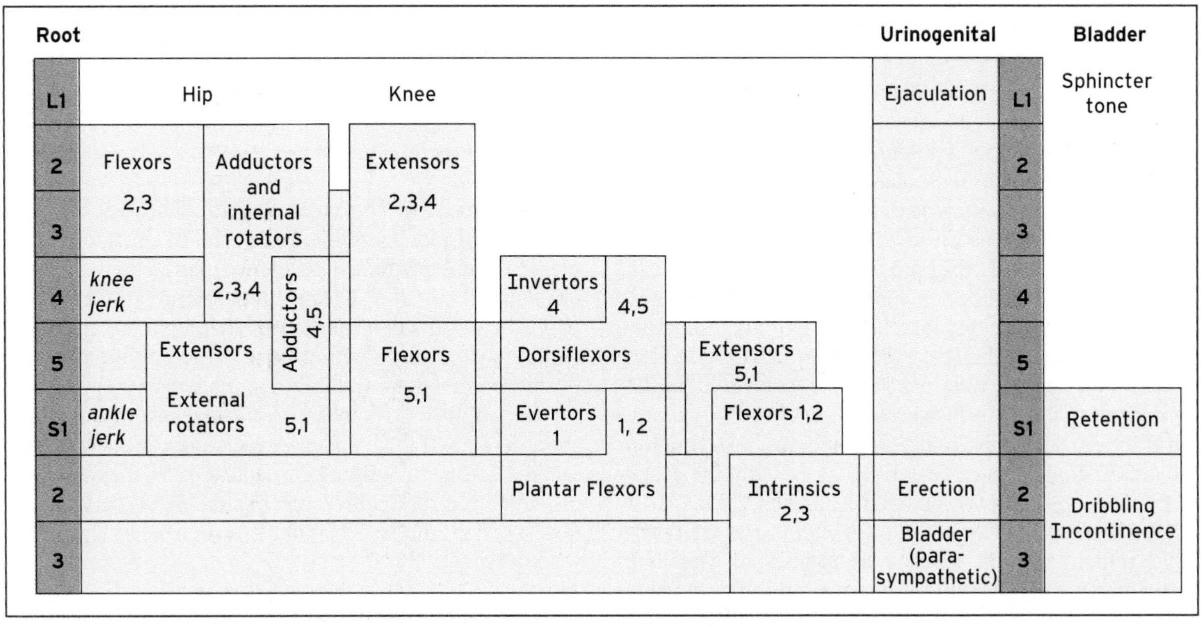

Root	Hip			Knee						Urinogenital	Root	Bladder
L1	Hip			Knee						Ejaculation	L1	Sphincter tone
2	Flexors 2,3	Adductors and internal rotators 2,3,4		Extensors 2,3,4							2	
3											3	
4	knee jerk		Abductors 4,5		Invertors 4	4,5					4	
5	Extensors	External rotators 5,1		Flexors 5,1	Dorsiflexors		Extensors 5,1				5	
S1	ankle jerk				Evertors 1	1,2	Flexors 1,2				S1	Retention
2				Plantar Flexors			Intrinsics 2,3		Erection		2	Dribbling Incontinence
3									Bladder (para-sympathetic)		3	

Figure 20.3 Segmental nerve supply of the lumbar (L1-5) and sacral (S1-3) nerve roots. Reading across from the nerve roots listed on the left of the diagram, the associated muscles of the lower limbs, and bladder, bowel and sexual function can be seen.

High Lesions—Thoracolumbar (50%)

If the lesion is above L1 there is usually no useful muscle activity in the legs. Isolated reflex activity may be present, causing flexion contractures and flexor spasms that are difficult to manage and interfere with postural management and the use of orthoses.

SPINAL DEFORMITY

Spinal curvature may be congenital or may occur as the child develops; the principles of management are similar for both.

Congenital Curve

Spinal deformity may be present at birth, particularly in children with high lesions. There may be a kyphosis with a prominent forward curve. This is usually caused by the underlying vertebral, and sometimes rib, fusion abnormalities.

Paralytic Curves

Paralytic curves are often associated with syringomyelia; they are related to muscle imbalance and appear later than other curves. About 75% of patients with myelomeningocele will develop a spinal curve; the majority are paralytic or mixed, with less than one third being entirely congenital. The incidence of scoliosis is related to the level of the lesion. All patients with a defect at T12 or above have a scoliosis, with the incidence reducing steadily to around 25% at L5 (Morley, 1992).

Management of Spinal Deformity

During growth it is important to hold the spine as straight as possible, using a thoracolumbar spinal orthosis (TLSO). The anaesthetic skin can make bracing difficult, especially in the presence of kyphosis.

Conservative management of spinal deformity is, wherever possible, the best treatment. For this to be effective, the curve must be detected early and referred for specialist management. Bracing is the most commonly used treatment for curves which are flexible and less than 40^0, and for children with remaining growth potential (Morley, 1992).

Where surgery is indicated it is usual to carry out an MR scan of the spinal cord pre-operatively to exclude any underlying abnormalities, including tethering of the cord. Assessment of respiratory function is important, especially in curves involving the chest which may cause reduction of ventilatory capacity. Spinal fusion is carried out at the optimum time, usually between 10 and 13 years, carrying out anterior release, distracting the spine with a Harrington rod and fusing the spine posteriorly by excising the posterior joints and laying on bone grafts (Morley 1992).

Post-operative physiotherapy is vital to ensure that a child returns to full function as quickly as possible. Immediately post-operatively no form of spinal brace is worn, but when the child resumes sitting a removable polypropylene brace must be worn at all times for about 6 months to provide stability. When the child is sitting, care must be taken to prevent traction of the spine during lifting and transferring. Support must be given under the bottom during these procedures either by the lifter or by the use of transfer boards. There is a risk of pressure sores developing on anaesthetic skin and the child must be positioned and lifted to relieve pressure regularly (see below).

The child can usually begin sitting 4 days to 1 week after surgery. While the child is in hospital a programme of exercises needs to be implemented to maintain muscle length and joint range in the lower limbs and to maintain the strength of arm and trunk muscles. Positioning of the ankles and knees to prevent muscle contractures is necessary, with passive movements to prevent decrease in joint ranges (see 'Physical Management').

NEUROPATHIC BLADDER

Bladder function may also be affected by the spinal lesion depending on its anatomical site. If the sphincter is unable to relax during the normal sequence of micturition, there may be incomplete emptying of the bladder. This is often associated with high-pressure contractions of the bladder muscle, the detrusor, which can lead to back pressure on the kidneys, detrusor sphincter dyssynergia (DSD). The combination of high pressure and infection can cause kidney damage, which may occur silently, eventually leading to renal failure.

Bladder activity can be monitored with urodynamic studies (UDS), which can be repeated at intervals. Renal function can also be monitored using different types of scan, e.g. dimercaptosuccinic acid (DMSA) nuclear scan, radionucleotide diethylenetriamine penta-acid (DTPA) scan or glomerular filtration rate (GFR) scanning.

In general there are three types of bladder behaviour: contractile, intermediate, and acontractile. The contractile problem of DSD, which causes obstruction to outflow at the level of the distal sphincter, is recognised as the commonest cause of impaired renal function in children with congenital spinal cord problems. The most vulnerable times for renal function are in the first 5 years of life and the late teens (Borzyskowski, 1992).

Management of the Neuropathic Bladder

The aims of management are to achieve continence and preserve renal function. Continence management depends on bladder function. Clean intermittent catheterisation (CIC) is an effective method of management for some children, particularly with the use of medication to reduce bladder contractions and increase sphincter tone. Children can be taught to catheterise themselves from the age of about 6 years. If the bladder is small and contracts continuously, CIC is not helpful. If medication is not successful in reducing contractions (see Chapter 28), surgery may be necessary to increase bladder size or correct sphincter weakness.

NEUROPATHIC BOWEL

Management of bowel incontinence can be a major problem, particularly for children with low spinal lesions who have poor anal sphincter tone and are active on their feet. The importance of early toiletting to develop a pattern of bowel emptying, even if it is through an incompetent sphincter, cannot be over-emphasised. Other basic areas such as appropriate diet, high fluid intake and the use of laxatives to aid the programme need to be addressed.

The anocutaneous reflex, which has been used in planning bowel movement, is seen in 40% of children with spina bifida regardless of the level of the spinal lesion (Agnarsson et al., 1993). Biofeedback has been used in the treatment of faecal incontinence in myelomeningocele (Whitehead et al., 1986), and relies on the presence of some rectal sensation and a capacity to squeeze the external anal sphincter. Motivation and intelligence are also important for patient selection.

PHYSICAL MANAGEMENT

The physical management of a child with an NTD, as with any disability, requires that the parents and therapists work in partnership to help the child achieve his or her full potential. Ultimately the parents' day-to-day care will have the greatest impact on the child's development and it is therefore vital that they are presented with a positive approach that puts value on their child's life and their ability to influence it. Professionals can give negative attitudes to disability that can be highly influential in shaping parental attitudes (French, 1994). The physiotherapist needs to develop a lasting relationship with the child and family, and recognise the valuable role the parents play in this, by working with them to develop management programmes that can become part of their lifestyle.

The overall objective of physiotherapy in a child with a neural tube lesion is to promote normal development within the limits of the neurological constraints and achieve as much independence as possible.

The main aims of physiotherapy at all stages of an individual's life will include:
- Development of physical skills leading to independence.
- The achievement of independent mobility, either walking or in a wheelchair.
- Prevention of the development of deformity.

Management at different stages from birth to adulthood will now be considered.

NEONATAL PHYSIOTHERAPY

An initial assessment should be made to determine the likely severity of the child's disability. Assessment of the baby's sensation and movement can be the responsibilty of either the paediatrician or the physiotherapist. This assessment will give a fairly accurate picture of the child's future physical ability.

The assessment needs to be done quickly and efficiently, as the child will be in an incubator and unable to tolerate excessive handling. The physiotherapist should first record the baby's resting posture, any active movements and any abnormalities or deformities. Reflexes and muscle groups, rather than individual muscles, are then tested. A definite movement of the tendon or joint must be seen as an indication of the muscle's activity. The examiner should work from the toes upwards, as once normal activity is seen the areas above this should be normal.

The test of sensation needs to be of protopathic (deep) feeling, as testing epicritic feeling (light touch) is not conclusive at this stage. Movements may be elicited due to uncontrolled reflex activity and a reaction to pain is a much more definite sign of sensation. This testing is best done using a firm pin prick.

Once the assessment is completed, a programme of passive movements and stretching exercises can be implemented to maintain and improve muscle length and joint range.

The most common deformities in the neonate with spina bifida are talipes equinovarus (TEV) and congenital dislocation of the hip. The management of TEV follows the same protocol as for idiopathic TEV and varies according to the severity of the deformity and between orthopaedic consultants (Rennie, 1991). The most frequently adopted treatments are strapping with zinc oxide tape, the application of a corrective splint, and serial plastering. Great care must be taken during these techniques as there may be impaired skin sensation and circulation that can lead to the development of pressure sores (see below).

The management of the baby with a congenital dislocation of the hips is conservative unless the lesion is low and the child will be an active independent walker (Fixsen, 1992). The use of abduction splints is thought (from clinical observation) to lead to contractures of the abductors, causing later difficulties, and is not recommended.

During the neonatal period, early positive involvement by parents in their baby's care can aid acceptance of the disability. The main priorities will be the daily programme of stretching exercises and passive movements (see Chapters 24 & 25) and care of the skin.

PRE-SCHOOL PHYSIOTHERAPY

The physiotherapist will often provide an ongoing link between home and hospital. Following the child's discharge from hospital the parents will need regular support as the realities of the child's disability become evident. Visiting the family at home will reduce the unnecessary travelling and allow the child to be treated in a familiar environment. It also enables the physiotherapist to make a clearer assessment of the child's needs in the context of the family.

The physiotherapy programme started in hospital will need to continue and, as the child begins to develop, be updated. Between the ages of 6 and 12 months it is useful to update the muscle chart so that preparations can be made to provide the necessary orthotic equipment.

Passive movements to all lower limb joints should be done at each nappy change to maintain joint range and stimulate the circulation. Once the child begins active arm and upper body movements these should be encouraged and strengthened. Children with spina bifida are often reliant on their arms for ambulation with sticks or crutches so they need to be strong. The child should be positioned as any normal infant in prone, supine and sitting positions to promote the normal developmental milestones of rolling and sitting (see Chapter 18) and maintain muscle length. The physiotherapist should educate parents in strategies to help their child develop and this is more successful through play and stimulation rather than rigid exercise programmes.

Children with high lesions may find developing sitting balance difficult and may require help with positioning so that they can free their hands for play. Trunk support or a wider sitting base may aid balance.

The normal child begins to explore the environment towards the end of the first year and it is important that the child with spina bifida is offered this opportunity even if he or she cannot do it independently. Various items of equipment, such as prone trolleys and small carts, enable the child to propel himself or herself.

Children with spina bifida and hydrocephalus often experience difficulties with perception (Dunning, 1994) including spatial difficulties, impaired hand function, and poor lateralisation and figure–ground discrimination (the ability to identify details from a background and ignore irrelevant information). They may also have poor visual tracking skills so that they cannot track horizontally across the midline and converge and diverge rapidly. The combination of motor and perceptual deficits may result in the child having difficulty with walking as these skills are all needed to manoeuvre in relation to a stable and moving environment. An early opportunity to move about in the environment and experiment with movement may help to reduce these difficulties in later life.

A thorough occupational and physiotherapy assessment should be made to assess the level of the child's perceptual and motor skills, so that the necessary strategies can be implemented to overcome any deficits. Such tests are difficult to perform in detail in the pre-school child but activities involving spatial awareness, e.g. moving over and under objects without touching them, judging speed of moving objects and general ability to move around in the environment, should be observed and any difficulties noted. Occupational therapists use a range of tests from the age of 4 years.

The child is usually ready to begin standing between the ages of 18 months and 2 years. An assessment of the degree of support needed can be made and the type of orthoses required discussed with parents. There are many benefits to standing even if functional walking is not achieved. Mazur et al. (1989) suggested that early mobility and the upright posture are valuable in promoting independence and mobility, decreasing the occurrence of pressure sores, reducing obesity and contractures, and beneficial to the child's psychosocial wellbeing.

Children with a more severe disability who cannot walk will use a wheelchair and will be at high risk of developing postural deformities, so it is important that an assessment of their posture is made. The assessment should consider the child's needs in lying, sitting and standing. For a child who is sitting most of the day there is a risk of hip flexion deformities developing alongside windswept hips and scoliosis. The child should be controlled in a variety of symmetrical postures during the day and night to reduce the risk of developing deformity (see below), and sitting should be limited.

Before the child starts school it is important that a thorough assessment of his or her physical needs is made and that the chosen school has facilities and staff to meet them. Areas that need consideration are: the environment; access to and within the school, including stairs, ramps, doorways, toilet facilities and educational support. Children with hydrocephalus have perceptual difficulties that involve figure–ground discrimination, spatial awareness, motor organisational skills, poor lateralisation of skills, reasoning ability, and number work. These factors may necessitate different learning strategies and the teacher needs to be made aware of these problems.

The choice of mainstream or special school lies with the parents but professionals must ensure that parents are informed of the available options and consider the long-term implications of their decision.

SCHOOL-AGED CHILD

Once the child is in school, the physiotherapist will need to provide ongoing support to the parents and teaching staff. Physiotherapists in many instances provide the link between the medical, home and school environments.

All staff working with children with hydrocephalus must be made aware of the signs that indicate shunt problems; these may include headache, vomiting, weakness or loss of dexterity, decreased levels of consciousness, irritability, slowing of performance, visual problems and worsening of any squint.

During the school years children develop their independence and begin to branch out from their families. This is a worrying time for parents and they need support in allowing their children opportunities to do this within safe boundaries. Teaching staff also need to recognise that a child with spina bifida experiences the same feelings and expectations as other children and should not allow the disability to interfere with the child's development. A child's attitude to his or her disability is likely to reflect the attitude of the adults encountered. If adults perceive the child as a difficulty to be endured, the child's self-esteem will plummet. Imagination is often needed to enable the child to participate in all activities, but solutions can usually be found.

The school environment is much larger than home and the choice of walking or using a wheelchair for different activities may need to be made. Many children find that a wheelchair provides a speed and freedom they do not have when walking. For physical education and games, a wheelchair can be a real asset, as the child's hands are free. Physiotherapists or occupational therapists are responsible for teaching basic wheelchair skills.

During the school years, as a child is expected to take on more daily living and educational tasks, any difficulties with learning will become evident. Dressing and putting on orthoses, intermittent catheterisation, learning the way to and around the school, as well as school work, may prove arduous for children with perceptual, concentration or organisational difficulties. Tasks need to be broken down into manageable units and the use of visual cues introduced. Class room assistants are invaluable in implementing such programmes. The physiotherapist needs to visit the school and/or home regularly to update these programmes.

A child's independence rests to a large extent on mobility—both moving around and transferring. Children need to develop strength and stamina in their arm muscles whether they wish to walk or use a wheelchair as their main form of mobility. To maintain this strength, children should be encouraged to do a regular programme of strengthening exercises, such as push-ups in prone or sitting positions, alongside an active sporting programme, which could include activities such as swimming, cycling with a hand-propelled or low-geared tricycle, and wheelchair basketball. Not only do these activities strengthen muscles, they also increase the circulation and help with weight control, which are both contributory factors in the development of pressure sores.

Children should be taught to transfer safely to and from surfaces at different heights, e.g. from floor to chair, from wheelchair to toilet. It is important that the child is careful not to damage anaesthetic skin during transfers by clearing the surface over which they are moving and not dragging the skin. When a child is not wearing orthoses, he or she needs to make sure the legs are supported during the transfer.

Children who are walking with sticks or crutches need to practice how to fall safely and be able to regain the upright position. They must learn to release their crutches quickly and use their arms to protect themselves. Practice should begin on a soft crash mat and gradually move towards firmer surfaces. Reducing fear of falling is an important confidence booster for entering busy environments.

As the child grows, there is a risk of developing deformity and this must be monitored carefully. The most common deformities seen are hip dislocation and kyphoscoliosis. For children who have high lesions and spend most of their time in a wheelchair, it is essential that they are seated to maintain a symmetrical posture with an even distribution over the weight-bearing surfaces. Although seating cannot correct an existing deformity it can contain postures and decrease the rate of progression (see below).

Muscle contractures of the hip flexors, hamstrings and calf muscles can develop due to spasticity if the child does not continue with a programme of stretching activities (see Chapters 24 & 25). The child needs to stand or lie prone for at least half an hour daily to stretch the hip flexors, to sit in the 'long sitting' position, preferably with orthoses to stretch the hamstrings, and to position the feet in the plantigrade position when sitting or standing.

During the years at primary school, most children with hydrocephalus will undergo a revision of the shunt to lengthen the drainage tube. If a total revision is needed there may be some deterioration in physical skills. Intensive physiotherapy will be needed during these periods to restore the children to their previous levels of function.

ADOLESCENCE

The onset of puberty in children with spina bifida is often early and this can cause problems as they tend to be socially and emotionally immature. Parents and teachers need to be aware of the conflict this creates within children and help them through this confusing period.

By the time children are in their teens, they should be able to take responsibility for much of their day-to-day care. They should also have an understanding of their disability and the implications of leading an independent lifestyle. Time should be spent on educating children in all self-management skills: physical management; catheterisation; application of orthoses; and skin care. They should also know where to seek help.

As children grow they need to take more responsibility for their health and fitness. They should learn to check their skin for signs of pressure, using inspection mirrors, when putting their orthoses on and off, and know the likely danger spots, i.e. toes, heels, behind the knees, buttocks and hips. If they are in wheelchairs for long periods they must do regular lifts, e.g. half-hourly, to relieve the pressure on the buttocks.

During the teenage years, many children with high lesions will need to decide whether to continue walking or opt to become a full-time wheelchair-user. This can be a difficult decision to make and the child should be involved in the discussions.

The growth spurt experienced in adolescence will accelerate the progression of spinal deformities. Orthopaedic surgery of the spine and hips is often undertaken when the growth period is almost over. Pre-operative physiotherapy is important to prepare a child physically for surgery. He or she must be prepared for a change in posture and the need to develop a different sense of balance. Some activities, such as moving the legs for transfers and putting on socks and shoes, may be limited after surgery. New methods of achieving these activities must be found.

ADULTHOOD

During adulthood the role of the physiotherapist becomes less proactive and more supervisory. The young adult of today, if properly educated and cared for during childhood, should be capable of caring for himself or herself, or of seeking care. It is important, however, that therapy services are readily available to adults and, if necessary, treatment or revision of equipment can be provided.

The young adult should be introduced to an adult physiotherapy team before leaving paediatric services so that there is a clear understanding of when and where to seek help. It may be useful for the physiotherapist to undertake an annual review to maintain contact (Chapter 17).

Ambulatory support according to level of paralysis	
Level of paralysis	Equipment required
Above L1	Thoracolumbar spinal othosis (TLSO) with knee-ankle-foot orthoses (KAFOs) hip-guidance orthosis (HGO)
Below L2	TLSO with KAFOs and Lumbar-sacral orthosis (LSO) LSO with KAFOs
Below L3-4	LSO with KAFOs KAFOs alone
Below L5	KAFOs or ankle-foot orthoses (AFOs)
Below S1	AFOs

Table 20.2 Ambulatory support according to level of paralysis.

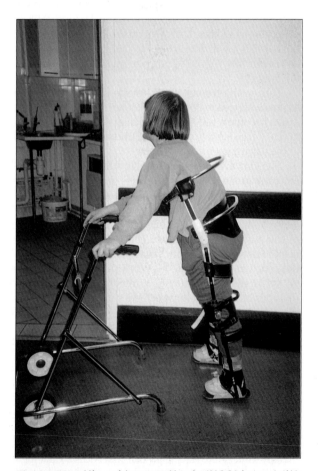

Figure 20.4 Hip guidance orthosis (HGO) in use with a rollator. The HGO is available under various brand names.

Obesity and pressure sores are the main problems encountered in adults and it is important that opportunities to keep fit are offered via sports clubs for their active participation.

ORTHOSES

Orthoses that enable the child to achieve independent walking need to become an integral part of the child's life and should be introduced to the child and family in a positive, enthusiastic manner. The child should be encouraged, but not forced, to wear them and a gradual increase in their use advised. Edwards & Charlton (1996) reviewed orthotic devices used in adult neurological patients. Table 20.2 outlines the level of orthotic support required for different levels of lesion.

Children who require support above the pelvis frequently opt to use a wheelchair as an adult and it is important to be realistic in terms of walking for these children. The support required for a high lesion will include thoracic, lumbar, sacral and lower limb orthoses. The child usually begins walking with a swivel movement, transferring weight from leg to leg, but progresses to a swing-through gait as strength and balance improve. Initially a rollator is used for support but the aim is to move to quadruped sticks and eventually to crutches. The rate of progress will depend on the child's motivation to walk, parental input and physical limitations. The hip guidance orthosis (HGO) was developed for children with high lesions who experience difficulty with walking (Rose *et al.*, 1989). It enables the child to walk at a reasonable speed with a low energy output. The brace consists of a rigid body and leg brace with a fixed hip abduction of 5^0 that allows hip articulation during walking of between 5^0 and 10^0 on a shoe rocker (Figure 20.4).

Swivel walking plates may also aid the development of walking by enabling the child to move in an upright position before walking is possible.

The provision of orthoses to a child adds another very important dimension to the parental care already in place. It is important that parents understand how to apply the orthoses correctly and the need to make regular checks on the child's skin. Anaesthetic skin can easily develop pressure sores and care must be taken to prevent this.

The following guidelines should be implemented:
- A daily check of all anaesthetic skin areas.
- Smooth clothing must be worn under orthoses and cover the whole area of skin contact; vest and socks should fit well and be worn with seams out.
- Toes need to be uncurled when putting shoes on by running a finger underneath them.
- Regular checks on the fit of orthoses and boots should be made.

A more definitive method is needed to assess the energy consumption of children with spina bifida who are walking, in order to assess their prognosis for long-term ambulation and as an indicator as to when ambulation should cease.

Reliable predictive factors could reduce unnecessary surgery for children who will not be ambulant as adults. The Physiological Cost Index (Butler *et al.*, 1986) is a simple method that can be used to measure energy cost.

PRESSURE CARE, POSTURE AND SEATING

The main factors in the development of tissue trauma are:
- Excessive force, causing tissue deformation and restriction of the blood supply.
- Shear forces from friction of retaining a position or changing position.
- Temperature—warm tissues have a better blood supply and therefore are at less risk of developing pressure sores.
- Humidity—wet skin is more vulnerable to damage.

Children with spina bifida are at great risk of developing pressure sores, as most of the above factors are applicable, and where there is anaesthetic skin they are unaware of them. From birth the parents, and later the individual, must be vigilant in reducing these factors. Daily inspection is vital to spot areas that are developing redness. If reddened areas do not subside within 20 minutes of removing the pressure, then there is a real risk of sores developing and the pressure should not be reapplied.

Excessive force can arise from: uneven distribution of weight in sitting; failure to relieve pressure; poorly fitting orthoses; and creased clothing. Relieving pressure during long periods of sitting needs to become a habit alongside frequent orthotic checks.

Shear forces can be created when the person's sitting position does not maintain him or her in a stable posture and there is a tendency to slide down the chair or bed. Postural control systems that distribute pressure evenly and provide sufficient support are needed to prevent this (Fearn *et al.*, 1992). Seating systems for enhancing good posture in wheelchairs are discussed in Chapters 8 & 25 and have been reviewed by Pope (1996). Lightweight, high-performance wheelchairs are now available that are more functional and aesthetically pleasing than older models. Transfers by the child or carer can cause friction if the surface across which he or she is moving is not adequately cleared.

Temperature is difficult to assess where there is no sensation and is likely to fall in non-moving muscles and joints. The child should always be kept warm and learn to feel the skin regularly to check its temperature. Massage can be beneficial in warming the tissues and increasing blood flow. Sheepskin-lined boots can be worn in the winter.

Wet skin can be a danger area in children and adults who are incontinent. This, combined with excessive pressure or shearing forces, can be disastrous for anaesthetic skin. Skin hygiene in susceptible areas must be meticulous and, for later independence, wash-and-dry toilets are recommended.

Conservative management of pressure sores is achieved by relieving pressure on the affected area. For buttocks, contoured cushions and/or use of a self-propelled trolley is indicated. For legs, plaster of Paris or Baycast splinting, changed weekly, can be effective. Minor or plastic surgery is indicated for sores that do not respond to conservative management. Measures must be taken following healing to prevent pressure redeveloping in the same area.

CASE HISTORY

JF was born in April 1989 with a myelomeningocele in the sacral region, L5/S1. The myelomeningocele was closed at 2 days and a shunt to control hydrocephalus inserted at 4 days.

An assessment of her muscle power at 10 days indicated that she would be an active walker with the help of orthoses. To maintain muscle length and joint range, a daily regimen of passive movements to the lower limbs was implemented.

Physiotherapy assessment at 2 months showed an infant with general low muscle tone and poor prone extension. There was no fixed calcaneus deformity; active dorsiflexion was present but no plantarflexion. Stretching of the ankles was recommended at each nappy change. Parents were advised to place JF in the prone position once a day to stretch hip flexors and to encourage active movement with stimulating play activities.

Equinus deformities were seen to be developing at 8 months and night splints to control ankle inversion were fitted. Parents were taught to check her skin regularly for marked areas.

At 12 months JF could roll, sit unaided and take weight in standing. She was attending a specialist nursery once a week and developing into a happy and sociable little girl.

At 17 months she was beginning to pull to standing and at 21 months AFOs were prescribed but she disliked them and preferred walks without them, exhibiting an asymmetrical gait with hip hitch and inverted feet. At 22 months KAFOs were prescribed and gait education begun. Although able to walk without a rollator, she was encouraged to use it to develop a more symmetrical gait pattern.

At 2 years 8 months, JF suffered major shunt problems with infection and disconnection that lasted 4 months and included a bout of peritonitis. This was a very stressful period for her parents and left JF very weak. An intensive period of physiotherapy followed to regain lost muscle strength and mobility. Her left foot had developed an equinus deformity due to lack of splinting while she was ill, so splinting and frequent passive movements were encouraged.

At 4 years 3 months, JF was able to walk independently with KAFOs and a rollator but needed to hip hitch to gain swing through and later implications for her spine were noted. A Physiological Cost Index (PCI) of 1.92 (normal 0.4) indicated that a great deal of effort was required to walk at this stage.

During this year preparations for JF to enter a mainstream school were made and she was awarded a statement of educational needs with ancillary help for 15 hours a week. This time was for educational support for specific learning difficulties related to hydrocephalus and physical support for moving around the school and toiletting. At 5 years, JF began mainstream first school where staff were very concerned about accepting JF, and the specialist health visitor and physiotherapist spent a great deal of time liaising to support her entry into school.

Poor bladder function was successfully controlled with intermittent catheterisation and JF was taught to perform the technique herself. This was a combined gradual approach, led by the specialist health visitor, with the parents and JF's non-teaching assistant.

JF had learnt to use quadruped sticks by the age of 6 years. She was managing well in school, walking independently and beginning to introduce crutches. She could walk independently but the asymmetry of her gait was reduced with sticks. She used a self-propelled wheelchair for long distances and games, rode a low-geared tricycle and swam weekly. These activities contributed to the promotion of specific muscle strength, general fitness and weight control.

At 6 years 6 months, problems with her shunt recurred. This was evident due to a loss of dexterity and general fatigue. She had a shunt revision, which was unsuccessful, followed by 2 weeks exteriorisation of the shunt due to infection. Another very stressful period with a long hospitalisation occurred. Following this there was a considerable loss of balance and strength. JF returned to using a rollator for several weeks and increased her wheelchair use. Physiotherapeutic intervention was aimed at maintaining independent mobility whilst rebuilding muscle strength and fitness to previous levels.

REFERENCES

Agnarsson U, Warde C, McCarthy G, *et al.* Anorectal function of children with neurological problems. I. Spina bifida. *Dev Med Child Neurol* 1993, **35**:893-902.

Butler P, Engelbrecht M, Major RE, *et al.* Physiological cost index of walking for normal children and its use as an indicator of physical handicap. *Dev Med Child Neurol* 1986, **26**:607-612.

Borzyskowski M, Nurse D. The neuropathic bladder. In: McCarthy GT, ed. *Physical disability in childhood.* Edinburgh: Churchill Livingstone; 1992:223-240.

Charney EB. Parental attitudes toward management of newborns with myelomeningocele. *Dev Med Child Neurol* 1990, **35**:14-19.

Cuckle HS, Wald NJ, Cuckle PM. Prenatal screening and diagnosis of neural tube defects in England and Wales in 1985. *Prenat Diag* 1989, **9**:393-400.

Dunning D. *Children with spina bifida and/or hydrocephalus at school.* Peterborough: Association for Spina Bifida and Hydrocephalus (ASBAH); 1994.

Edwards S, Charlton P. Splinting and the use of orthoses in the management of patients with neurological disorders. In: Edwards S, ed. *Neurological physiotherapy: a problem solving approach.* London: Churchill Livingstone; 1996:161-188.

Expert Advisory Group. *Report on folic acid and the prevention of neural tube defects.* London: Department of Health; 1992.

Fearn TA, Green EM, Jones M, *et al.* Postural Management. In: McCarthy GT, ed. *Physical disability in childhood.* Edinburgh: Churchill Livingstone; 1992:401-450.

Fixsen J. Orthopaedic management. In: McCarthy GT, ed. *Physical disability in childhood.* Edinburgh: Churchill Livingstone; 1992:198-201.

French S. Attitudes of health professionals towards disabled people. *Physiotherapy* 1994, **80**:687-693.

Levene MI. The spectrum of neural tube defects. In: Levene MI, Bennett MJ, Punt J, eds. *Fetal and neonatal neurology and neurosurgery.* Edinburgh: Churchill Livingstone; 1988:267.

Mazur JM, Shurtleff D, Menelaus M, Colliver JJ. Orthopaedic management of high level spina bifida. *J Bone Joint Surg* 1989, **71**A: 5661.

McCarthy GT. *Physical disability in childhood.* Edinburgh: Churchill Livingstone; 1992.

McCarthy GT, Cartwright R, Jones M *et al.* Spina bifida. In: McCarthy GT, ed. *Physical Disability in Childhood.* Edinburgh: Churchill Livingstone; 1992:189-212.

McCarthy GT, Land R. Hydrocephalus. In: McCarthy GT, ed. *Physical Disability in Childhood.* Edinburgh: Churchill Livingstone; 1992:213-221.

Morley TM. Spinal deformity in the physically handicapped child. In: McCarthy GT, ed. *Physical disability in childhood.* Edinburgh: Churchill Livingstone; 1992:356-365.

Office of Population Censuses and Surveys. *Congenital malformation statistics notifications.* London: HMSO; 1995.

Pope PM. Postural management and special seating. In: Edwards S, ed. *Neurological physiotherapy: a problem solving approach.* London: Churchill Livingstone; 1996:135-160.

Rennie P. Talipes equino-varus management strategy. *Assoc Paediatr Chartered Physiotherap News* 1991, **Nov**:37.

Rose J, Gamble JG, Lee J, Lee R, *et al.* Energy Expenditure Index: a method to quantitate and compare walking energy expenditure for children and adolescents. *J Paed Orthop* 1981, **11**:571-578.

Wald NJ, Bower C. Folic acid and the prevention of neural tube defects. *Br Med J* 1995, **310**:1019-1020.

Whitehead WE, Parker L, Basmajian L, *et al.* Treatment of faecal incontinence in children with spina bifida: comparison of biofeedback and behaviour modification. *Arch Phys Med Rehab* 1986, **67**:218-224.

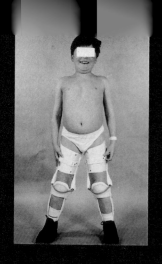

21

N Thompson, T Fahal &
RHT Edwards

MUSCLE DISORDERS
IN CHILDHOOD

CHAPTER OUTLINE

- **The muscular dystrophies**
- **The spinal muscular atrophies**

- **Physical management of neuromuscular disorders**
- **'Social' and psychological issues in neuromuscular disorders**

INTRODUCTION

This chapter deals with the muscular dystrophies of childhood onset as well as the spinal muscular atrophies. Muscle disorders of adult onset were described in Chapter 16. Details of investigations and general management issues are discussed under the section on Duchenne muscular dystrophy (DMD) but most of these also apply to the other disorders. The physical management section applies to all the conditions but prognosis must be taken into account. For a more comprehensive discussion of differential diagnosis and prognosis, clinical features and general management, the reader is referred to Walton *et al.* (1994) and Dubowitz (1995).

THE MUSCULAR DYSTROPHIES

The muscular dystrophies are a group of genetically determined disorders associated with a progressive degeneration of skeletal muscle, without involvement of the central or peripheral nervous system (Emery, 1987). They can be subdivided into various types on the basis of the clinical distribution and severity of muscle weakness, and also the pattern of inheritance (see Tables 16.1 and 16.2).

The Xp21.2 myopathies or dystrophinopathies are the progressive disorders of muscle that include DMD and Becker muscular dystrophy and involve a defect of the protein dystrophin. They are characterised by X-linked

inheritance so that only males are affected and the mothers are carriers. There is a normal appearance at birth (though the level of plasma, creatine kinase [CK] is very high), and an early hypertrophy of muscle, but also weakness, followed by progressive wasting and disability.

DUCHENNE MUSCULAR DYSTROPHY
DMD was first described in the 1860s by Guillaume Duchenne. It is rapidly progressive and is the most severe of all the muscular dystrophies; it is inherited in an X-linked recessive fashion (see Table 16.2). It occurs in 18–30 per 100,000 males at birth with a prevalence in the population of 1.9–4.8 per 100,000 (Emery, 1991).

Clinical and Diagnostic Features
The first clinical manifestations of DMD appear when the child shows delayed motor milestones at 3–5 years. The child is late in sitting, standing and walking and when he does begin to walk, he often falls. If there is no family history the diagnosis is often not suspected. By the age of 5 there is obvious muscle weakness; the child is unable to run or jump. Physical examination reveals enlarged calf muscles due to compensatory hypertrophy but this will develop later into pseudohypertrophy since the muscle is replaced by fat and connective tissue.

Hip and knee extensor weakness results in difficulty getting up from the floor. Initially, in order to rise from the floor, the child must give some assistance to hip and knee extension by pushing off from the thigh with the hand or forearm. With increasing weakness, the child climbs up his legs using both arms, and this is the classic Gowers' manoeuvre which is associated with, though not confined to, DMD. As muscles become weaker the corresponding tendon reflexes become depressed and are eventually lost, but there is no sensory loss.

An abnormal 'waddling' gait is a well recognised presenting symptom (Emery, 1987). Owing to early weakness of the hip abductors, the child is unable to maintain a level pelvis when lifting one leg off the ground. He therefore inclines towards the other leg to bring the centre of gravity of the body over that leg, and as he moves forward this action is continually repeated and accounts for the Trendelenburg sign. This is accompanied by widening of the base of support for increased stability, which contributes to the evolution of hip abduction contractures (iliotibial band tightness).

By 7–8 years of age, contractures of heel cords and iliotibial bands lead to toe walking. Between 8 and 9 years, walking usually requires the use of braces (Figure 21.1) and by the age of 12 years, 95% of patients require wheelchairs (Emery, 1987). Prolonged sitting leads to further flexion contractures of the elbows, hips and knees.

In the early ambulatory phase of DMD, an equinus foot posture is precipitated by relative weakness of the ankle dorsiflexors compared with the better preserved plantar-flexors. Gait analysis has shown that a dynamic equinus is a necessary biomechanical adaptation to maintain knee stability in the presence of gross quadriceps muscle weakness. Forceful action of the ankle plantarflexors provides a torque which opposes knee flexion (Khodadadeh *et al.*, 1986). Thus, contracture of the Achilles tendon, which eventually accompanies disease progression, is secondary to dynamic equinus.

Muscle involvement is bilateral and symmetrical and the proximal muscles are more affected than the distal groups. In the ambulatory stage, the pelvic girdle is slightly more affected than the shoulder girdle. There is more severe weakness in the extensor groups than in the flexors although this differential muscle involvement becomes less clear as the disease progresses, so that ultimately such patterns of weakness are no longer obvious. Finally, contractures become fixed and a progressive scoliosis develops. Scoliosis exacerbates existing respiratory muscle weakness, and in severe cases may render the child bed-bound. Scoliosis occurs in 50–80% of patients and causes additional respiratory problems (Kurz *et al.*, 1983).

Muscle imbalance (caused by the specific pattern of developing weakness) and postural malalignment (resulting from compensatory adjustments to maintain standing equilibrium) are factors precipitating the eventual development of contractures about weight-bearing joints. These are relatively mild while the child remains ambulant but progress rapidly once there is dependence on a wheelchair. These postures combine lumbar lordosis, hip flexion and abduction, and ankle equinus.

The first alteration of body alignment in DMD is a lumbar lordosis due to early weakness of the hip extensors, so that active stabilisation of the hip joint is compromised. In order to maintain the line of force behind the hip joint and prevent collapse into hip flexion, there is an initial posterior alignment of the upper trunk resulting in a compensatory lumbar lordosis. As weakness progresses this is accompanied by an exaggerated anterior tilt of the pelvis which predisposes to contractures of the hip flexors.

It is important to realise that DMD is a multisystem disease and not only a problem of skeletal muscle.

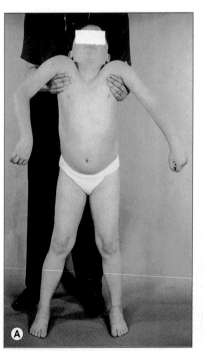
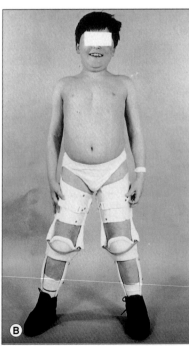

Figure 21.1 Boy with Duchenne muscular dystrophy. (A) At the point of loss of independent walking. (B) Following percutaneous Achilles tenotomies and rehabilitation in lightweight ischial weight-bearing knee-ankle-foot orthoses (KAFOs).

Gastrointestinal problems can be evident clinically through oropharyngeal, oesophageal and gastric dysfunction (Jaffe *et al.*, 1990) and constipation and halitosis are common. About 59% of patients have lower than normal intelligence (IQ 70–85; Billard *et al.*, 1992). Others have normal or above-normal intelligence. The mental retardation does not increase with age. Cardiomyopathy occurs in adolescence and the majority of boys die before their twentieth birthday from respiratory or cardiac failure.

Thus, DMD is an incurable and ultimately fatal disease characterised by muscle weakness, contracture, deformity and progressive disability. However, 'incurable' is not synonymous with 'untreatable'. A variety of therapeutic and surgical measures are available that can help to minimise deformity, prolong independent ambulation and maximise functional capabilities. There is also evidence that improved management strategies are resulting in increased survival rates (Galasko *et al.*, 1992). The principles of successful management are based on an understanding of the natural evolution of patterns of weakness, contracture and deformity, so that intervention can be staged appropriately.

Pathology

Muscle weakness in DMD primarily arises due to the gradual loss of functional muscle fibres, which are replaced by fat and connective tissue; this is evident on muscle biopsy (Figure 21.2). The clinical manifestation of this proliferation of fat and connective tissue is pseudohypertrophy of certain muscle groups, particularly the calf.

Defective production of dystrophin, a protein encoded by the DMD gene, is the primary biochemical defect (Hoffman *et al.*, 1988). It is thought that dystrophin forms a skeleton lattice in the muscle cell membrane and provides integrity to the membrane, particularly during the stress associated with repeated cycles of contraction and relaxation. Absence of dystrophin production may explain a reduction in permeability of the muscle cell membrane, so allowing excessive quantities of calcium to accumulate within the muscle fibre leading to myofibrillar overcontracture, breakdown of myofibrils and various metabolic disturbances that culminate in the death of the muscle fibre (Dubowitz, 1985). Although the precise function of this cytoskeletal protein is not understood, its absence is associated with a generally bad prognosis, whereas in Becker muscular dystrophy, in which there is a capability to produce, albeit abnormal, dystrophin, the prognosis is less severe.

Questions have been raised as to whether the absence of dystrophin is merely an early trigger in the pathogenesis of the dystrophy, with subsequent secondary mechanisms being more important (Dubowitz, 1989). Edwards *et al.* (1984) theorised that the pathogenesis may be related to the largely postural antigravity role of the proximal muscles, rendering them more susceptible to damaging eccentric contractions.

Confirmation of Diagnosis

The tests mentioned in this section are discussed in Chapter 3 and the features relevant to DMD are outlined here and discussed further by Walton *et al.* (1994) and Mastaglia & Laing (1996).

Biochemical Blood Tests
Serum levels of CK (normal range 33–194 IU) are often slightly raised in healthy newborn infants to 200–300 IU; they then drop and remain constant until an

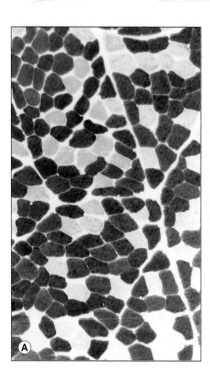
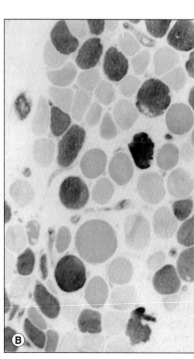

Figure 21.2 Transverse sections through quadriceps muscle biopsies. The sections are stained for myosin ATPase at pH9.6.
(A) From a normal boy aged 5 years, showing a predominance of the dark, type II fibres amongst which are randomly scattered the paler type I fibres. All fibres are of similar size and shape. (B) From a boy, aged 6, with DMD. When compared with the normal muscle, there are more pale, type I fibres, the fibres show more variation in size and shape, with a tendency to hypertrophy, and are separated by bands of fibrous tissue (not stained by this method).
(Courtesy of Dr TR Helliwell, Reader in Pathology, University of Liverpool.)

occasional second slight elevation during the adolescent growth spurt (Gilboa & Swanson, 1976). In early DMD the enzyme is raised up to 50 times greater than normal but the levels drop around the time the boys become confined to wheelchairs, presumably due to the decrease in functioning muscle tissue and reduction of physical activity (Walton *et al.*, 1994). Serum aldolase is raised to 10–20 times the normal range.

Electromyography (EMG)
Changes on EMG are diagnostic of myopathy but not specifically of DMD, and EMG investigations are important to distinguish between a myogenic and a neurogenic disorder. At an early stage the action potentials are reduced in duration and amplitude, with polyphasic potentials more frequent than normal (Walton *et al.*, 1994). Later, with the loss of motor units, there is very little activity.

Percutaneous Needle Biopsy of Muscle
This technique was first advocated by Duchenne in the nineteenth century but was employed as a reliable clinical investigation only more recently (Edwards *et al.*, 1983). Open biopsy under general anaesthesia is no longer necessary, though some clinicians still prefer to do it despite the risks of unsightly scars and, rarely, anaesthetic accidents. Histology shows variation of fibre size, prominent rounded fibres that stain densely with eosin, necrosis with phagocytosis, and eventual fatty replacement. Histochemical staining shows a relative loss of type II fibres (Dubowitz, 1985) and there is no grouping of fibre types (Figure 21.2).

DNA (dioxyribonuclei acid) probes
These tests have been used to identify the abnormal gene location at Xp21 (Mastaglia & Laing, 1996) and are particularly helpful in conjunction with the serum CK test in providing 95% accuracy of female carrier detection (Harper, 1986). They are also used for prenatal diagnosis from amniotic fluid cells at 16 weeks' gestation or chorion biopsy at 10 weeks' gestation.

Dystrophin
Dystrophin measurement from muscle biopsies is useful in confirming the diagnosis. This protein is absent in DMD and truncated in Becker muscular dystrophy (Hoffman *et al*, 1988). The severity of the disease and its rate of progression may vary inversely with the dystrophin level in the muscle.

General Management of DMD
The disease is not curable but much can be done to improve the boy's quality of life. The key milestones in the disease progress that require sensitive management, particularly of the parents, are: (1) suspicion of abnormality; (2) diagnosis; (3) loss of ambulation; (4) consideration of spinal surgery; (5) leaving school and transition from paediatric to adult services; (6) final illness; and (7) bereavement. Management requires a multidisciplinary approach with liaison between the medical care team, and school and parents.

A family may suspect that a child is later in walking than other siblings or friends. The stages of normal childhood motor development, outlined in Chapter 18, are delayed. On average, 50% of patients with DMD fail to start walking until after 18 months (Gardner-Medwin, 1982). Later the child is seen to lag behind, tire easily or fall over whilst playing, such that comparison with other children creates anxiety that there may be something wrong.

Confirmation of the parents' suspicion by a specialist may leave them numb and frightened, with confused emotions of denial, rejection and often the reactions through which the recently bereaved pass. For the parents of a child with DMD or other severe neuromuscular disease, as for the bereaved, it is important to work through these emotions by articulating fears, resentments and worries to a sympathetic person who can explain in an honest but positive way what lies ahead, whilst suggesting means by which the family may achieve a coping strategy.

It is important to ensure that they realise that what may happen in the future, and that the time scale over which deterioration can occur, will depend on how the present problems are dealt with. Patients should be monitored regularly in the clinic throughout life, and changes with each stage anticipated to ease the effects of deterioration on the patient and family.

Management of Disability
The principal approach is that of mechanical correction of the impairment in muscle function, with a view to preserving posture and functions of everyday life. As the muscle weakness progresses, risks of falling, loss of ambulation, contractures and scoliosis require attention. Contributory factors such as lower limb fractures, obesity, convenience and emotional problems may cause premature loss of walking.

Factors accelerating loss of ambulation should be prevented or managed promptly, e.g. lower limb fractures should be treated by a technique that allows continued weight bearing (e.g. internal fixation). Obesity should be prevented and a high-protein, low-fat carbohydrate diet prescribed; weight should be maintained and can be monitored according to percentile charts which have been specifically designed for DMD (Griffiths & Edwards, 1988). Scoliosis is a common and important problem in these patients and surgical correction of scoliosis and stabilisation of the spine have proved successful, improving the quality of life significantly for both patient and carer (Mehdian *et al.*, 1989).

Management of Handicap
The management of handicap addresses psychosocial issues, mobility and education. Promotion of mobility could be achieved by weight control, active and passive exercises, correction of contractures and the use of orthoses (see below). Later on in the disease, tackling the issue of loss of independence can involve provision of adaptation

to accommodation and helpers; most importantly, there must be confidence in the local medical and social support provided.

Respiratory Problems

As the disease progresses, respiratory problems become important and these account for >90% of deaths (Vignos, 1976). Patients with neuromuscular disease characteristically develop a restrictive defect, with a reduction in total lung capacity. This fall in lung capacity is the result of a combination of factors: general immobility; impaired ventilatory musculature; chest wall stiffness (resulting from a combination of kyphoscoliosis and fibrosis of dystrophic chest muscles); pulmonary microatelectasis; aspiration; and impaired clearing of secretions because of reduced ability to cough (Smith et al., 1991a). The earliest detectable abnormality easily recognised by clinical tests is a reduction in static mouth pressures: maximum expiratory pressure is reduced to a greater extent than maximum inspiratory pressure (Griggs et al., 1981).

Other factors contributing to respiratory difficulties include ineffective cough because of impaired glottic function as well as respiratory muscle weakness, impaired CNS ventilatory drive, and upper airway obstruction during sleep. Sleep-related respiratory abnormalities have recently been shown to play a major role in ventilatory failure; nocturnal hypoxaemia develops and contributes to cardiac failure (cor pulmonale) and hypercapnia. Nocturnal hypoxaemia first occurs during REM (rapid eye movement) sleep and may be present when other signs of hypoxaemia, such as daytime hypoxaemia, carbon dioxide retention and associated symptoms, are lacking. DMD and other myopathies have been shown to involve sleep-related hypoxaemia well in advance of other signs of ventilatory failure (Carroll et al., 1991). Since treatment of this process with nocturnal respiratory support is now practical (Heckmatt et al., 1990) and since studies to detect hypoxaemia can be obtained easily and with no morbidity (Carroll et al., 1991), patients with neuromuscular disease must be followed prospectively for the possibility of impending ventilatory difficulties.

Cardiac Problems

Symptomatic cardiac complications are less evident than might be expected in patients with DMD, presumably because of their sedentary lifestyle despite the evidence that cardiac muscle is involved (Hunsaker et al., 1982). Cardiac abnormalities can be detected early in life and increase with age, until present in all patients by the age of 18 years (Nigro et al., 1990).

The Final Illness

Counselling, patient support groups and voluntary work by parents on behalf of others are all important psychological means of dealing with distressed families in their bereavement. The Muscular Dystrophy Group Family Care Officers (see 'Associations and Support Groups') provide important support for families at this sad and difficult time. It is important that there are well structured links with the General Practitioner and social services.

BECKER MUSCULAR DYSTROPHY

Becker muscular dystrophy (Becker MD) is a less severe form of X-linked recessive muscular dystrophy (see Table 16.2), with a prevalence of 1.7–5.5 per 100,000 male live births (Emery, 1991).

Clinical and Diagnostic Features

The distribution of weakness and contractures is similar to that in DMD but the disease is more benign and the time course is slow. The rate of progression can be variable, with some patients becoming chairbound in their twenties while others continue to ambulate into their forties and fifties. It may be possible to prolong standing and/or walking with standing frames or lightweight calipers.

Muscle cramps and calf hypertrophy are early and constant features. Most boys are slow in school sports, with the condition not recognised before the age of 5 years. Walking continues beyond the age of 15 and sometimes into the fourth decade. Cardiomyopathy occurs in about 50% of patients (Steare et al., 1992). Contractures and scoliosis are uncommon and usually late. Death is rare before 21 years and may occur in the forties or later. As patients reach the age when they can father children, the genetic implications are important; whilst none of their sons will be affected, the daughters of people with Becker MD will all be carriers. Laboratory confirmation, EMG and muscle biopsy features are essentially the same as for DMD.

General Management

The principles of management of Becker MD are similar to those for DMD. Attention to the consequences of immobility is required: oedema, obesity, constipation and gastrointestinal problems, bone loss and pressure sores, which are all preventable and mostly treatable (see below). Attention to, and prompt treatment of, respiratory infection can prevent acute respiratory failure, and chronic ventilatory failure can be managed by nasal nocturnal ventilation.

EMERY-DREIFUSS MUSCULAR DYSTROPHY

This is a rare but clinically distinct X-linked recessive MD, in which the defective gene is located at Xq28 and the defective protein is emerin (Mastaglia & Laing, 1996).

Clinical and Diagnostic Features

Emery–Dreifuss MD is characterised by a very slowly progressive weakness that begins in early childhood and is associated with prominent and early contractures of the elbow joints and Achilles tendon, rigidity of the spine, and cardiomyopathy and conduction defects that may lead to sudden death (Bialer et al., 1991). The affected boys are of normal intellect. There is weakness of the muscles of the legs, which is slowly progressive. Most patients survive into their middle life.

General Management

Provided the diagnosis is made sufficiently early, the insertion of a cardiac pacemaker may be life-saving. Management of contractures involves stretching exercises as discussed below.

The associated weakness is usually mild. However, due to rigidity of the spine throughout its length, the patient is unable to compensate for any hip extensor weakness with a lumbar lordosis, as is commonly seen in many of the other neuromuscular diseases. Instead, the patient maintains the centre of mass with increasing equinus at the ankles, leading to secondary contracture of the Achilles tendon. If these contractures become severe, they may in themselves jeopardise mobility and require percutaneous surgical correction. Management should be aimed at controlling the progression of deformity by appropriate strengthening, passive stretching and splinting techniques (see Chapters 24 & 25).

CONGENITAL MUSCULAR DYSTROPHIES

Congenital MDs are two main groups of myopathies inherited in an autosomal recessive fashion; they present at birth with muscle weakness and affecting both sexes. The two groups are: classic (occidental) congenital MD, with no apparent CNS involvement; and the Japanese form, Fukuyama-type, which has significant CNS involvement. Different genetic abnormalities are involved in the two types (Mastaglia & Laing, 1996; Table 16.2). This section describes the more common, classic type.

Clinical and Diagnostic Features

Reduced fetal movements during pregnancy suggest that signs are already present before birth. Features in early infancy consist of muscle weakness and generalised hypotonia, 'floppiness', poor suck and respiratory difficulty (Kobayashi *et al.*, 1996). In childhood, motor milestones are delayed, with severe and early contractures and often joint deformities (arthrogryposis). Weakness is greater in the pelvic girdle and upper leg muscles than in the shoulder girdle and upper arm muscles. On the whole, this condition is relatively slowly progressive and functional ability can improve over time. Contractures at birth are common and may restrict function to a greater degree than weakness if not controlled. It is particularly important to be vigilant for the insidious development of contractures and to treat them promptly.

Other features of the disease are hip dislocation, pes cavus and kyphoscoliosis. The motor development is slow, leading to late sitting, standing and walking. Intelligence is normal. Serum CK activity is usually very high in the early stages. The EMG shows short-duration, small-amplitude and polyphasic motor potentials. There may be variable respiratory difficulties due to associated diaphragmatic involvement, at both presentation and later in adolescence.

General Management

Attention to feeding and breathing is important in the neonatal period. Later on, useful mobility should be maintained for as long as possible. Regular exercise should be encouraged and obesity avoided. Regular gentle stretching is required to avoid or control contractures (see below). Nocturnal hypoventilation may develop in the second decade and responds to nocturnal nasal ventilation.

THE SPINAL MUSCULAR ATROPHIES

The spinal muscular atrophies (SMAs) are a group of neurogenic disorders in which there is degeneration of the anterior horn cells of the spinal cord, resulting in muscle weakness. They are the most common neuromuscular disease in childhood after DMD and affect both sexes. The mode of inheritance is mainly autosomal recessive but can vary, with dominant or X-linked traits (Emery, 1971). The genetic defects lies on the long arm of chromosome 5 (Brzustowicz *et al.*, 1990). Weakness is symmetrical, is greater proximally than distally, and the pelvic girdle is usually slightly more affected than the shoulder girdle. Weakness is generally non-progressive, although as a result of increasing height and weight there may be some loss of functional activities over time. There is no facial weakness and intellectual development is normal. Classification of SMAs is most usefully based on clinical severity (Dubowitz, 1995):

Severe: Unable to sit unsupported.

Intermediate: Able to sit unsupported; unable to stand or walk unaided.

Mild: Able to stand and walk.

The clinical and diagnostic characteristics, as well as general management, are now discussed for each type of SMA.

SEVERE SMA (TYPE 1 OR WERDNIG-HOFFMAN DISEASE)

This is a progressive infantile type of SMA that is inherited in an autosomal recessive manner. Children with severe SMA present neonatally as 'floppy' babies with progressive, severe, generalised weakness in the first few months of life. There is marked respiratory involvement and as a result they rarely survive beyond 2 years of age. Treatment will be mainly supportive.

The infant is unable to move out of a lying position and the upper limbs adopt an internally rotated 'jug-handle' position and the lower limbs a flexed and abducted 'frog position'. Limb contractures may develop related to these positions and, if untreated, activities such as dressing and lifting will become uncomfortable. Regular passive stretching techniques can become part of the daily routine at bathtimes and nappy changes. Moulding of the ribs can occur if the infant is always positioned on one particular side. This will further compromise respiratory capacity, and so alternation of sleeping positions is recommended.

The child will not achieve a sitting position unaided and is best supported in a slightly reclined, rather than upright, sitting position so that the diaphragm is not restricted and the head is supported. A supportive spinal jacket with a diaphragmatic aperture may be useful in helping to maintain a sitting position. The child is unlikely to have any antigravity strength and toys need to be small and lightweight.

The intercostal muscles are severely affected and breathing is almost entirely diaphragmatic, giving a characteristic bell-shaped chest. Cough is weak and bulbar weakness may give rise to sucking and swallowing difficulties. The child will be prone to recurrent respiratory infections that should be treated promptly with antibiotics and chest physiotherapy.

INTERMEDIATE SMA (TYPE 2)

Weakness develops usually between 6 and 12 months and the child presents with inability to stand or walk. Long-term prognosis is dependent on respiratory function, and rapidly progressive scoliosis is a common complication associated with this group. Early spinal bracing will help to control the rate of progression, but spinal fusion may be necessary. Limb joints are often hyperextendable, particularly at the elbow and hands, but are prone to contractures related to positioning.

A major aim of management would be to promote standing and/or walking and the ability to achieve this will be dependent on residual muscle strength, particularly in the trunk and pelvic girdle, which should be carefully assessed. Some children show functional improvement and, with appropriate training, progression from standing in a frame to walking with calipers is possible. Since muscle weakness is not generally progressive, the ability to walk using ischial weight-bearing knee–ankle–foot orthoses (KAFOs) may be maintained over many years, helping to control both joint contractures and scoliosis. It should be noted that spinal bracing and spinal fusion are not normally compatible with continued mobility in calipers, since they limit compensatory trunk side flexion which aids weight transference when the hip abductors are weak.

MILD SMA (TYPE 3 OR KUGELBURG-WELANDER DISEASE)

Mild SMA may be inherited in an autosomal dominant or recessive manner. The ability to walk is achieved at the normal age or slightly late and the child often presents with difficulty hopping, running and jumping. Proximal weakness, which is slightly more marked in the lower limbs, may give rise to a Gowers'-type manoeuvre when getting up off the floor. Strengthening programmes should be targetted to functional difficulties. Joint contractures and progressive scoliosis are rare in this group (Carter *et al.*, 1995). Weakness is generally relatively static, but rapid periods of growth may result in loss of ambulation, and rehabilitation can be achieved in lightweight calipers.

PHYSICAL MANAGEMENT OF NEUROMUSCULAR DISORDERS

This section highlights the areas of management which are specific to muscle disorders, both in adulthood and childhood. Details of treatment concepts and techniques are found in Chapters 22 & 24, respectively. A problem-solving approach is preferable and a model of this is described in Chapter 7 in relation to stroke. Treatment planning should involve the multidisciplinary team (MDT), the patient, parents and preferably a carer at school.

ASSESSMENT

Thorough, standardised and regular assessment of children is essential because they change rapidly. Assessment is important both for guiding clinical management and for evaluating therapeutic outcome for research purposes. Aspects of assessment pertinent to muscle disorders are measurement of muscle strength, performance and lung function, and principles of assessment are discussed in Chapter 4.

Measurement of Muscle Strength

Strength assessments provide information for the planning and monitoring of intervention as well as diagnostic information.

Manual Muscle Testing

Manual muscle testing is the most widely used means of assessing muscle strength in clinical practice and has been recommended as an outcome measure for therapeutic trials in neuromuscular disease (Brooke *et al.*, 1981). The Medical Research Council scale of grading muscle strength is probably the most widely known grading system and is based on an ordinal scale of 0 to 5 (see Chapter 4).

Whilst no special equipment is needed, and manual muscle testing is a rapid method of determining the distribution and severity of weakness over a large number of muscle groups, the major criticism of this method is the subjectivity in grading strengths. There are no standardised joint positions at which testing should be performed and the point at which counterforce is administered is also self-selected. The proportion of maximum strength required to overcome gravity is markedly different between muscle groups (Wiles *et al.*, 1990), and a loss of strength in excess of 50% may develop before weakness can be detected by manual muscle testing (Fisher *et al.*, 1990).

Dynamometry

Force can be measured directly with dynamometers; these quantitative measurements of muscle force are superior to manual muscle testing and provide the most direct method of assessing a particular muscle group. The design of the dynamometer has been gradually refined to produce a simple hand-held electrodynamometer which can measure maximal isometric strength of many different muscle groups as both a research and clinical tool (Hyde *et al.*, 1983).

Myometry readings are highly reproducible, provided standardised techniques are used and the same observer performs the measurement on each occasion (Bohannon, 1986; Lennon & Ashburn, 1993). Serial measurements of a single patient will be the most useful means of evaluating the distribution and rate of change of muscle weakness, whilst the degree of weakness can be established by comparison with published normal values of muscle strength (Wiles *et al.*, 1990). Muscle strength is a valid measure in that force is related to functional performance (Bohannon, 1989).

Hand-held dynamometers are useful only when muscles are weak, since their use is restricted by the strength of the operator to oppose the patient's efforts. Strain gauges attached to rigs, and also commercially available isometric and isokinetic machines, are available (see Chapter 4).

Measurement of Joint Range

The development of joint contractures should be monitored carefully and joint ROM can be measured using a goniometer. However, caution must be taken with this method as it shows variable inter-rater reliability and measurements should be made by the same assessor where possible (Pandya *et al.*, 1985).

Measurement of Functional Performance

The quantitation of muscle strength has proved to be of value in the assessment and management of many muscle diseases, but it can be seen that this is a measure of impairment and is incomplete without concomitant measures of disability and ultimately the handicap to the patient. Measures of functional performance range from simple tests, such as the ability to rise from the floor (Rideau, 1984), to more detailed measures of motor ability and gait (Sutherland *et al.*, 1981; Khodadadeh *et al.*, 1986). These measurements are susceptible to the effects of impairments other than strength, but it is important in terms of patient management to determine whether a change in disability can properly be attributed to a change in the strength of the muscles measured.

There may be disparities between strength and disability in muscle for a variety of reasons. These include: a failure to assess the relevant muscle groups that cause disability; a failure to note progressing severe weakness in an important group, perhaps because of the averaging of many groups; or the intrusion of other relevant factors, such as the development of compensatory biomechanical manoeuvres or a gain in weight or height. It is of paramount importance that the measure of physical performance is both valid and reliable and these factors need to be recognised.

Motor Ability Tests

Whilst the Vignos scale was associated with the assessment of functional ability, particularly in DMD, it was originally designed as a functional classification and its sensitivity as an objective measure of function is doubtful. The Hammersmith motor ability score (Table

Hammersmith score of motor ability	
Motor ability	**Score: 2, 1 or 0**
Lifts head	
Supine to prone over right	
Supine to prone over left	
Prone to supine over right	
Prone to supine over left	
Gets to sitting	
Sitting	
Gets to standing	
Standing	
Standing on heels	
Standing on toes	
Stands on right leg	
Stands on left leg	
Hops on right leg	
Hops on left leg	
Gets off chair	
Climbing step, right leg	
Descending step, right leg	
Climbing step, left leg	
Descending step, left leg	
Total score out of 40	

Table 21.1 Hammersmith score of motor ability. Scoring: 2 for every completed movement; 1 for help and/or reinforcement; 0 if unable to achieve the movement. All movements are attempted and scored. (Redrawn from Scott *et al.*, 1982, with permission from John Wiley & Sons Inc.)

21.1) is a measure of disability that was developed and validated to measure functional ability in progressive neuromuscular conditions and has been shown to correlate closely with changes in muscle strength (Thompson *et al.*, 1996). Its 20 motor activities are biased towards activities involving the lower limbs, making it a more suitable assessment for ambulant patients. The patient sequentially performs a succession of movements that are scored on a 3-point scale, and the motor ability score is a numerical value obtained out of a possible maximum of 40 points. The method of scoring had high inter-rater reliability (Smith *et al.*, 1991b).

Timed Tests

Timed performance tests are commonly recommended as supplementary measures of physical performance (Brooke *et al.*, 1981). The most common tests, chosen to reflect progressive weakness in children with DMD, are walking speed over a set distance and the time taken to get up from the floor, i.e. using Gowers' manoeuvre. In the latter, supine lying is a more reproducible starting position than is sitting.

Lung Function

Spirometry forms part of the regular assessment to monitor changes in lung function. Inspiratory and expiratory mouth pressures can also be measured to assess the strength of the respiratory muscles. Details of lung function tests can be found elsewhere, e.g. in the chest, heart and vascular disorders book in this series (Place & Connellan, 1998), and in Griggs *et al.* (1981) and Hough (1991).

TREATMENT PRINCIPLES

The benefits of an active approach to the physical management of neuromuscular disease are increasingly recognised. These include not only minimising complications in order to maximise abilities but also maintaining the patient in the best possible physical condition so that he or she could benefit from new treatments. Exciting developments in molecular genetics make the latter suggestion a possibility.

The main principles of treatment are:
- To maintain muscle strength and retard contracture progression to maximise function.
- To promote or prolong ambulation with appropriate orthoses.
- To delay or control the development of scoliosis.
- To treat promptly any respiratory complications.

Treatment concepts (see Chapter 22) and details of techniques (see Chapter 24) are not discussed here but the principles relevant to patients with muscle disorders are outlined.

Maintenance of Muscle Strength

The results of resistance exercise programmes in progressive MDs have shown limited increases in strength, with no negative effect on muscle function (e.g. Milner-Brown & Miller, 1988). Greatest effects occur in patients with mild to moderate weakness and in the more slowly progressive myopathies, whilst patients with severely weak muscles do not generally benefit from strengthening programmes. It appears in normal subjects that a prerequisite for successful strength training is a high content of type II fibres (Jones *et al.*, 1989). The relative deficiency of type II fibres in DMD (Dubowitz, 1985) may contribute to the poor force-generating capacity of dystrophic muscle and could also be a limiting factor in the eventual benefit of a strengthening programme.

Eccentric muscle training is increasingly being used in the training of athletes to facilitate the development of muscle power, i.e. the rate of force generation. Eccentric exercise can cause appreciable morphological damage to muscle fibres (Newham *et al.*, 1986) and damage of this nature is commonly seen in the muscles of patients with myopathic diseases. Whilst normal muscle recovers from this damage, eccentric exercise would seem best avoided in muscle disease, in favour of more traditional concentric protocols.

Edwards *et al.* (1987) documented important differences in the rate of progression of various muscle groups and highlighted a particularly rapid loss of force in the hip and knee extensors. Insufficiency of these muscle groups has been shown to be the key deficit in functional decline and gait deterioration in DMD (Sutherland *et al.*, 1981). Whilst maximising muscle strength to achieve optimal or improved functional ability is a primary objective of treatment, the effect of specific muscle strengthening programmes on function in neuromuscular disorders awaits objective evaluation. To devise a strengthening programme, the required functional gain should be considered, and appropriate muscle groups targetted.

It is well accepted that in normal individuals physical exercise increases muscle strength, whilst inactivity causes deconditioning, and there is also widespread observation amongst clinicians that severe restriction of activity causes rapid weakening of muscle in dystrophic conditions and should be avoided. It is therefore important that the duration of enforced immobilisation during any acute illness, and after surgery, should be kept to a minimum so that the patient's return to mobility is not compromised by muscle atrophy.

Weakness occurs when a muscle is held in a shortened position due to joint deformity, and also when it is contracting over a reduced range (Gossman *et al.*, 1982). The establishment of compensatory postures long before the development of fixed contracture means that the muscle is biomechanically disadvantaged earlier than is obvious, since it is continually contracting over a shortened range. This could be a major factor in further progression of the disease as optimal function of the muscle is prevented. Joint positioning during strengthening may therefore be important but research in these patients is required.

Electrical stimulation of normal muscle can improve strength and fatiguability but evidence that the technique is safe, as well as beneficial, in muscle disorders has yet to be produced (see Chapter 24).

Of the many drugs tested in the treatment of DMD, prednisolone was shown to have a beneficial effect on muscle force but the side effects associated with steroid therapy were unacceptable. Research continues to seek a balance between beneficial and side effects using intermittent, low-dose protocols (Sansome *et al.*, 1994).

Gene therapy using myoblast transfer, in which the gene for dystrophin is inserted into the muscle, is a possible method for preventing loss of muscle tissue but is only at the experimental stage (Partridge *et al.*, 1989). The technique has been successful in animal models but clinical trials in humans have so far been negative.

Retarding Contracture Progression

The management of contractures is one of the major contributions of physiotherapy in neuromuscular disease. The aim is not only to retard the progression of contracture but, more importantly, to promote or prolong independent ambulation and functional ability. Impairment of mobility caused by contractures compromises the strength of the muscles working across the involved joint or joints. The force-generating ability of a muscle is influenced by the length at which it contracts (Jones & Round, 1990) and thus the strength of a muscle held in a shortened position is reduced. In the presence of profound weakness, the maintenance of full joint range of motion is essential for optimal muscle function.

A sustained programme of splinting and passive stretching in the early stages of DMD can retard the development of lower limb contractures. Various types of splints may be used to maintain the joints in position and ankle–foot–orthosis (AFO) night splints are recommended.

Scott *et al.* (1981) carried out a prospective study on 59 boys (aged 4–12 years) to evaluate the effect of below-knee night splints and daily passive stretching of lower limb contractures. The development of contractures of the Achilles tendon was delayed, compared with a control group. A direct relationship was demonstrated between the development of lower limb contractures and loss of ambulation, and the study concluded that independent ambulation could be prolonged for as much as 2 years using passive stretching and night splints. The combination of stretching and splints was found to be more effective than stretching alone. Harris & Cherry (1974) examined the effect on 100 boys with DMD of a physiotherapy programme which emphasised daily passive stretching of weight-bearing joints. Stair-climbing ability and independent walking were prolonged by 2 years. These studies are in agreement concerning the importance and effectiveness of management aimed at minimising lower limb contractures.

Whilst independently ambulant, the provision of AFOs for control of Achilles tendon contracture should be confined to night use only. Gait analysis has shown that an equinus position of the foot is used as a compensatory manoeuvre to increase knee stability during the stance phase. Khodadadeh *et al.* (1986) observed that boys with DMD necessarily adopt a dynamic equinus during gait in order to maintain a knee-extending moment in the presence of gross quadriceps weakness. AFOs intended to correct the foot position by reducing the equinus during walking will have biomechanical effects which will destabilise the knee. If there is significant quadriceps weakness the knee will buckle. Thus AFOs used in this way reduce the available compensatory manoeuvres and can result in premature loss of ambulation.

Promoting or Prolonging Ambulation

Following the cessation of independent walking, the duration of useful ambulation in children can be prolonged with an immediate programme of percutaneous Achilles tenotomy and rehabilitation in lightweight ischial weight-bearing KAFOs and intensive physiotherapy. The gains in additional walking time have varied in different centres but on average an extra 2 years of walking can be achieved and sometimes up to 4 years (Heckmatt *et al.*, 1985). This approach is now generally accepted as a means of maintaining mobility after independent walking ceases and has been shown to impede the development of both lower limb contractures and scoliosis (Vignos, 1988).

The accurate timing of intervention and prompt provision of orthoses are crucial to the success of prolonging ambulation. The optimal time for the provision of the orthoses is when the child has lost useful walking but is still able to stand or walk a few steps. There is no advantage in providing orthoses earlier than this. Two of the important factors used to predict successful outcome are the absence of severe hip and knee contractures, and the percentage of residual muscle strength (Hyde *et al.*, 1982). Swivel walkers may be appropriate to allow walking over short distances at home or school. Once the child has been wheelchair-bound for even a short time, fixed lower limb deformities and muscle weakness rapidly progress, and therefore any delay in undertaking this programme may compromise a successful outcome.

Maintenance of Activities

A positive management strategy is to introduce a variety of aids to sustain a broad range of normal activities for as long as possible, as outlined above. In children, calipers are initially used to prevent contractures and sustain upright standing posture as well as for walking (see Figure 21.1). Later, a standing frame allows the patients to stand for several hours a day with a view to delaying spinal curvature and contractures of hips, knees and ankles. Lastly, a wheelchair can be introduced as a means to improve mobility and independence. Adults should be encouraged to perform exercise to reduce contractures and thus be able to enjoy physical leisure activities.

Management of Scoliosis

Scoliosis is a serious complication of DMD and intermediate SMA. Whilst scoliosis is also associated with other neuromuscular disorders, it is rapidly progressive in these two conditions unless treated.

In DMD, scoliosis may become clinically apparent as ambulation becomes increasingly limited. The period of most rapid deterioration is once the child has become dependent on a wheelchair and corresponds most closely with the adolescent growth spurt between the ages of 12 and 15 years (McDonald *et al.*, 1995). Progressive scoliosis is also a threat in the adolescent years of patients with SMA, but due to the profound weakness that is present from early infancy it may become a problem at a much earlier age.

The curve often develops in a paralytic long C pattern in the thoracolumbar areas and is associated with increasing pelvic obliquity. It further compromises respiratory capacity, which is already restricted by involvement of the respiratory muscles. Kurz et al. (1983) reported that for each 10^0 of thoracic scoliosis, the FVC is decreased by approximately 4%, in addition to the 4% loss per year due to progressive muscle weakness in DMD. An increasing scoliosis also leads to difficulty in sitting and maintaining head control, and can cause discomfort and pressure areas. Patients will often need to use their elbows for support in maintaining an upright position, so preventing them from using the arms for other functions. Untreated, the scoliosis may cause patients to become bedridden.

One of the major benefits of treatment aimed at maintaining an upright posture is that it will help to delay the progression of scoliosis significantly. Once the patient is dependent on a wheelchair, the main means of managing scoliosis are conservative, using a spinal orthoses, or surgical spinal stabilisation (see below).

The spine should be monitored carefully where scoliosis is a likely complication of the disease, in conjunction with the respiratory capacity using simple spirometry (see above). Once a curve is clinically apparent, any progression is most accurately measured from radiographs using Cobb's angle. Prompt provision of a spinal orthosis is advisable, to be worn during the day whilst the patient is upright. The orthosis should be corrective rather than supportive; ideally, radiographs should be taken during the fitting process to evaluate the degree of correction achieved. It is recognised that spinal bracing is not the definitive treatment in curves that are known to be rapidly progressive, but it is important in slowing the rate of progression of the curvature (Seeger et al., 1984) and can be used effectively for skeletally immature patients in whom spinal fusion is not yet indicated.

Close monitoring continues whilst the patient is wearing a spinal orthosis, so that surgery can be offered before cardiopulmonary function deteriorates to a point where anaesthesia presents an unacceptably high risk. Spinal bracing in a patient with established severe scoliosis may cause appreciable respiratory impairment when there is respiratory muscle invovlement, and is less likely to be tolerated than early prophylactic bracing (Noble-Jamieson et al., 1986).

The Luque technique of segmental spinal instrumentation (Luque, 1982) has been a major advance in the limitation of scoliosis in neuromuscular disease, and is increasingly recommended as the treatment of choice. Early intervention has been shown to be beneficial in achieving maximum curve correction and minimising respiratory complications. It is recommended that surgery should be offered when the patient still has adequate respiratory and cardiac function to allow him or her to undergo the procedure safely. In DMD, vital capacity increases with age and growth in the early years, then reaches a plateau, and then declines in the early teens, so there is a window of opportunity when surgery can be performed safely. The necessary vital capacity is associated with a relatively mild degree of spinal curvature so that surgery is often proposed soon after the child has ceased to walk (Rideau, 1984; Galasko et al., 1992).

Luque instrumentation permits early postoperative mobilisation in a wheelchair and postoperative casts or orthoses are not normally required. In the immediate postoperative period, respiratory therapy to aid removal of secretions will be necessary in patients who are unable to achieve this unaided. It is possible for a lumbar lordosis and dorsal kyphosis to be moulded into the rods (Galasko et al., 1992), which helps facilitate head control in sitting when weakness of the neck and trunk musculature is likely to be advanced. However, seating requirements will need to be reassessed postoperatively. For example, due to significant upper limb weakness the child is likely to utilise upper trunk flexion to help get his mouth down to his hands for feeding purposes. Following surgery the height of wheelchair arm supports or table height will need to substitute for a fused spine.

Management of Respiratory Complications

Chest infections are a serious complication to vulnerable patients with respiratory muscle weakness and a poor cough. Longstanding weakness may lead to more serious secondary problems, including widespread microatelectasis with reduced lung compliance, a ventilation perfusion imbalance, and nocturnal hypoxaemia (Smith et al., 1991a).

Chest infections should be promptly treated with physiotherapy, postural drainage, antibiotics and, when appropriate, assisted ventilation. Spinal orthoses that control scoliosis may reduce respiratory capacity and should be temporarily removed if causing distress or interfering with treatment. The aim of treatment is to help clear the lungs of secretions effectively in the shortest possible time without causing fatigue. Thoracic expansion exercises will allow increased airflow through small airways and the loosening of secretions, while forced expiration techniques, the use of intermittent positive pressure breathing (IPPB) and assisted coughing will aid removal of secretions (Webber, 1988). Diaphragmatic weakness may limit the use of supine or tipped positions for postural drainage. Parents of children prone to recurrent chest infections can become competent at administering chest physiotherapy but will require support that is readily accessible if children become distressed.

There has been no observed benefit of inspiratory muscle training on a declining respiratory function (Martin et al., 1986; Rodillo et al., 1989) and it may in fact be detrimental where there is severe weakness. However, the potential benefit of prophylactic training before symptoms arise awaits assessment.

Respiratory failure may be precipitated by chest infection or it may occur as a result of increasing nocturnal hypoventilation and hypoxia. The onset is often insidious but symptoms include morning drowsiness, headache or confusion and night-time restlessness, and can be confirmed by sleep study. Symptoms can be dramatically improved by night-time ventilation (Heckmatt et al., 1990). Long-term ventilation of patients in the advanced stages of DMD remains a controversial aspect of treatment, with ethical implications (Miller et al., 1988).

'SOCIAL' AND PSYCHOLOGICAL ISSUES IN NEUROMUSCULAR DISORDERS

A complexity of factors influence management at different stages of the patient's life. For lifelong disorders, these influences pose similar problems as in other disabling conditions, as discussed, for example, in Chapter 19 in relation to cerebral palsy. The need for more training and support for professionals managing these patients was highlighted in a survey by Heap et al. (1996).

PRESCHOOL YEARS

The time of diagnosis will be traumatic for the parents and sensitive support will be needed. If not already known to the family, the genetic implications will need to be discussed and family members offered genetic counselling. A realistic picture of the future should be given, with appropriate information to prepare for each stage as it comes. Precise details of the end stages would not be appropriate, for obvious psychological reasons; also, they may not apply 20 years ahead as medical advances may have occurred by that time.

THE SCHOOL YEARS

Optimal management can be achieved only if there is good communication between the medical team, parents and carers at school. Facilities at school and integration with able-bodied children are important. Physical management programmes should involve realistic goals and take into account other aspects of life which may demand the child's time, particularly, for example, at exam times. The timing of surgery should also consider such issues and not just the medical considerations.

Preparation for leaving school should include organisation for continuation of support services as well as careers advice.

TRANSITION FROM CHILDHOOD TO ADULTHOOD

There is a lack of provision of services for the young disabled adult. On leaving school, the support system often ceases and, apart from occasional visits to the hospital consultant, physiotherapy and other services are not always offered. Patients whose disorder begins in adulthood may never be offered any services or treatment, or even referred to a specialist, despite having a significant disability.

There is a need for centres that provide specialist advice and treatment from therapists and offer an environment for social interaction and training for vocational and leisure activities. This would enable children to continue with their physical management programmes as adults, taking responsibility for their own treatment but receiving help for monitoring and modification of treatment. Those with disorders of adult onset could be educated in physical management strategies by therapists and other patients, and learn how to maximise their abilities and remain functional for as long as possible. Other areas, such as weight control and sexual counselling, could also be dealt with or referral made where appropriate.

Patients with neuromuscular disorders, particularly adults, often feel isolated in the community and some do not lead as full a life as they have the potential for because of lack of support and education about their condition. Some give up employment or even going out of the house. Specialist centres could provide an important function and fill a major gap in care and support.

In the terminal stage of illness, support from the care team, particularly the general practitioner, is essential and bereavement counselling may be required. The Muscular Dystrophy Group Family Care Officers (see 'Association and Support Groups') play a very important role at all stages, particularly during the final illness in guiding and supporting families.

Acknowlegements
The support of the Muscular Dystrophy Group of Great Britain and Northern Ireland is gratefully acknowledged.

REFERENCES

Bailer MG, McDaniel NL, Kelly TE. Progression of cardiac disease in Emery-Dreifuss muscular dystrophy. *Clin Cardiol* 1991, **14**:411-416.

Billard C, Gillet P, Signovet JL. Cognitive functions in Duchenne muscular dystrophy: a reappraisal and comparison with spinal muscular atrophy. *Neuromusc Dis* 1992, **2**:371-378.

Bohannon RW. Test-retest reliability of hand-held dynamometry during a single session of strength assessment. *Phys Ther* 1986, **66**:206-209.

Bohannon RW. Correlation of lower limb strengths and other variables with standing performance in stroke patients. *Physiother Canada* 1989, **41**:198-202.

Brooke MH, Griggs MD, Mendell JR, et al. Clinical trial in Duchenne dystrophy. 1. The design of the protocol. *Muscle Nerve* 1981, **4**:186-197.

Brzustowicz LM, Lehner T, Castilla LH, et al. Genetic mapping of chronic childhood-onset spinal muscular atrophy. *Nature*, 1990, **344**:540[Letter].

Carroll N, Bain RJI, Smith PEM, et al. Domiciliary investigation of sleep-related hypoxaemia in Duchenne muscular dystrophy. *Eur Resp J* 1991, **4**:434-440.

Carter GT, Abresch RT, Fowler WM, et al. Profiles of neuromuscular disease: Spinal muscular atrophy. *Am J Phys Med Rehab* 1995, **74**:150-159.

Dubowitz V. Muscle biopsy: *A practical approach, 2nd edition.* London: Ballière Tindall; 1985.

Dubowitz V. The Duchenne Dystrophy story: From phenotype to gene and potential treatment. *J Child Neurol* 1989, **4**:240-249.

Dubowitz V. *Muscle disorders in childhood, 2nd edition.* London: WB Saunders; 1995.

Edwards RHT, Chapman SJ, Newham DJ, et al. Practical analysis of variability of muscle function measurements in Duchenne Muscular Dystrophy. *Muscle Nerve* 1987, **10**:6-14.

Edwards RHT, Newham DJ, Jones DA, *et al*. Role of mechanical damage in pathogenesis of proximal myopathy in man. *Lancet* 1984, March 10:548-552.

Edwards RHT, Round JM, Jones DA. Needle biopsy of skeletal muscle: a review of 10 years' experience. *Muscle Nerve* 1983, **6**:676-683.

Emery AEH. The nosology of the spinal muscular atrophies. *J Med Genet* 1971, **8**:481-495.

Emery AEH. *Duchenne muscular dystrophy*. Oxford: Oxford University Press; 1987. (Oxford monographs on medical genetics, No. 15).

Emery AEH. Population frequencies of inherited neuromuscular diseases- a world survey. *Neuromusc Dis* 1991, **1**:19-29.

Fisher NM, Pendergast DR, Calkins EC. Maximal isometric torque of knee extension as a function of muscle length in subjects of advancing age. *Arch Phys Med Rehab* 1990, **71**:729-734.

Galasko CSB, Delaney C, Morris P. Spinal stabilisation in Duchenne Muscular Dystrophy. *J Bone Joint Surg* 1992, **74B**:210-214.

Gardner-Medwin D. The natural history of Duchenne muscular dystrophy. In: Wise GB, Blaw ME, Procopis PG, eds. *Topics in child neurology, vol. 2*. New York: SP Medical & Scientific Books; 1982.

Gilboa N, Swanson JR. Serum creatine phosphokinase in normal newborns. *Arch Dis Child* 1976, **51**:283.

Gossman MR, Sahrmann SA, Rose SJ. Review of length associated changes in muscle. *Phys Ther* 1982, **62**:1799-1808.

Griffiths RD, Edwards RHT. A new chart for weight control in Duchenne muscular dystrophy. *Arch Dis Child* 1988, **63**:1256-1258.

Griggs RC, Donohoe KM, Utell MJ, *et al*. Evaluation of pulmonary function in neuromuscular disease. *Arch Neurol* 1981, **38**:9-12.

Harper PS. Isolating the gene for Duchenne muscular dystrophy. *Br Med J* 1986, **293**:773-774.

Harris SE, Cherry DB. Childhood progressive muscular dystrophy and the role of physical therapy. *Phys Ther* 1974, **54**:4-12.

Heap RM, Mander M, Bond J, *et al*. Management of Duchenne muscular dystrophy in the community: views of physiotherapists, GP's and school teachers. *Physiotherapy* 1996, **82**:258-263.

Heckmatt JZ, Dubowitz V, Hyde SA, *et al*. Prolongation of walking in Duchenne muscular dystrophy with lightweigth orthoses: review of 57 cases. *Dev Med Child Neurol* 1985, **27**:149-154.

Heckmatt JZ, Loh L, Dubowitz V. Clinical practice. Night-time nasal ventilation in neuromuscular disease. *Lancet* 1990, **335**:579-582.

Hoffman EP, Fischbeck KH, Brown RH. Characterisation of dystrophin in muscle-biopsy specimens from patients with Duchenne's or Becker's muscular dystrophy. *N Engl J Med* 1988, **318**:1363-1368.

Hunsaker RH, Fulkerson PK, Barry FJ, *et al*. Cardiac function in Duchenne's muscular dystrophy. Results of 10-year follow up study and noninvasive tests. *Am J Med* 1982, **73**:235-238.

Hyde SA, Scott OM, Goddard CM, *et al*. Prolongation of ambulation in Duchenne muscular dystrophy. *Physiotherapy* 1982, **68**:105-108.

Hyde SA, Scott OM, Goddard CM. The myometer: the development of a clinical tool. *Physiotherapy* 1983, **69**:424-427.

Jaffe KM, McDonald CM, Ingman E, *et al*. Symptoms of upper gastrointestinal dysfunction in Duchenne muscular dystrophy: case-control study. *Arch Phys Med Rehab* 1990, **71**:742-744.

Jones DA, Round JM. *Skeletal muscle in health and disease*. Manchester: Manchester University Press; 1990.

Jones DA, Rutherford OM, Parker DF. Physiological changes in skeletal muscle as a result of strength training. *Q J Exp Physiol* 1989, **74**:233-256.

Khodadadeh S, McClelland MR, Patrick JH, *et al*. Knee moments in Duchenne muscular dystrophy. *Lancet* 1986, September **6**:544-555.

Kobayashi O, Hayashi Y, Arahata K, *et al*. Congenital muscular dystrophy. *Neurology* 1996, **46**:815-818.

Kurz LT, Mubarek SJ, Schultz P. Correlation of scoliosis and pulmonary function in Duchenne muscular dystrophy. *J Paed Orthop* 1983, **3**:347-353.

Lennon SM, Ashburn A. Use of myometry in the assessment of neuropathic weakness: testing for reliability in clinical practice. *Clin Rehab* 1993, **7**:125-133.

Luque ER. Segmental spinal instrumentation for correction of scoliosis. *Clin Orthop* 1982, **163**:192-198.

Mastaglia FL, Laing NG. Investigation of muscle disease. *J Neurol Neurosurg Psych* 1996, **60**:256-274.

McDonald CM, Abresch RT, Carter GT, *et al*. Profiles of neuromuscular disease. Duchenne muscular dystrophy. *Am J Phys Med Rehab* 1995, **74**:70-92.

Mehdian H, Shimizu N, Draycott V, *et al*. Spinal stabilisation for scoliosis in Duchenne muscular dystrophy. Experience with various sublaminar instrumentation systems. *Neor Orthop* 1989, **7**:74-82.

Miller JP, Colbert AP, Schock AC. Ventilator use in progressive neuromuscular disease: impact on patients and their families. *Dev Med Child Neurol* 1988, **30**: 200-207.

Miller-Brown HS, Miller RG. Muscle strengthening through high-resistance weight training in patients with neuromuscular disorders. *Arch Phys Med Rehab* 1988, **69**:14-19.

Newham DJ, Jones DA, Edwards RHT. Plasma creatinine kinase changes after eccentric and concentric contractions. *Muscle Nerve* 1986, **9**:59-63.

Nigro G, Comi LI, Politano L, *et al*. The incidence and evaluation of cardiomyopathy in Duchenne muscular dystrophy. *Int J Cardiol* 1990, **26**:271-277.

Noble-Jamieson CM, Heckmatt JZ, Dubowitz V, *et al*. Effects of posture and spinal bracing on respiratory function in neuromuscular disease. *Arch Dis Child* 1986, **61**:178-181.

Pandya S, Florence JM, King WM, *et al*. Reliability of goniometric measurements in patients with Duchenne muscular dystrophy. *Phys Ther* 1985, **65**:1339-1342.

Partridge TA, Morgan JE, Coulton GR, *et al*. Conversion of mdx myofibres from dystrophin-negative to positive by injection of normal myoblasts. *Nature* 1989, **337**:176-179.

Place M, Connellan SJ. Chest assessment and use of lung function tests. In: Smith M, ed. *Chest, heart and vascular disorders*. London: Mosby. (In preparation).

Rideau Y. Treatment of orthopaedic deformity during the ambulatory stage of Duchenne Muscular Dystrophy. In: Serratrice G, Cros D, Desnuelle C, *et al*., eds. *Neuromuscular diseases*. New York: Raven Press; 1984:557-564.

Rodillo E, Noble-Jamieson CM, Aber V, *et al*. Respiratory muscle training in Duchenne muscular dystrophy. *Arch Dis Child* 1989, **64**:736-738.

Sansome A, Royston P, Dubowitz V. Steroids in Duchenne muscular dystrophy: a pilot study of a new low-dosage schedule. *Neuromusc Disord* 1994, **3**:567-569.

Scott OM, Hyde SA, Goddard C, *et al*. Prevention of deformity in Duchenne muscular dystrophy. *Physiotherapy* 1981, **67**:177-180.

Scott OM, Hyde SA, Goddard C, *et al*. Quantitation of muscle function in children: a prospective study in Duchenne Muscular Dystrophy. *Muscle Nerve* 1982, **5**:291-301.

Seeger BR, Sutherland A, Clark MS. Management of scoliosis in Duchenne muscular dystrophy. *Arch Phys Med Rehab* 1990, **65**:83-86.

Smith PEM, Edwards RHT, Calverley PMA. Mechanisms of sleep-disordered breathing in chronic neuromuscular disease: implications for management. *Q J Med* 1991a, **296**:961-973.

Smith RA, Newcombe RG, Sibert JR, *et al*. Assessment of locomotor function in young boys with Duchenne muscular dystrophy. *Muscle Nerve* 1991b, **14**:462-469.

Steare SE, Benatar A, Dubowitz V. Subclinical cardiomyopathy in Becker muscular dystrophy. *Br Heart J* 1992, **68**:304-308.

Sutherland DH, Olshen R, Cooper L, *et al*. The pathomechanics of gait in Duchenne muscular dystrophy. *Dev Med Child Neurol* 1981, **23**:3-22.

Thompson N, Choudhary P, Hughes RAC, *et al*. A novel trial design to study the effects of intravenous immunoglobulin in chronic inflammatory demyelinating polyradiculoneuropathy. *J Neurol* 1996, **243**:280-285.

Vignos PJ. Respiratory function and pulmonary infection in Duchenne muscular dystrophy. In: Robin GC, Falewski de Leon G, eds. *Muscular dystrophy*. Basel: Karger; 1976:123-130.

Vignos PJ Jr. Management of musculo-skeletal complications in neuromuscular disease: limb contractures and the role of stretching, braces and surgery. *Phys Med Rehab* 1988, **2**:509-535.

Walton JN, Karpati G, Hilton-Jones D. *Disorders of voluntary muscle, 6th edition*. Edinburgh: Churchill Livingstone; 1994.

Webber BA. *The Brompton Hospital guide to chest physiotherapy*. Oxford: Blackwell Scientific Publications; 1988.

Wiles CM, Karni Y, Nicklin J. Laboratory testing of muscle function in the management of neuromuscular disease. *J Neurol Neurosurg Psych* 1990, **53**:384-387.

SECTION 4

TREATMENT APPROACHES TO NEUROLOGICAL REHABILITATION

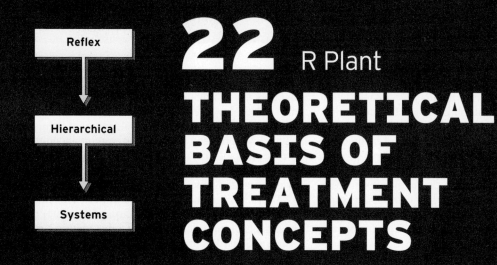

22 R Plant

THEORETICAL BASIS OF TREATMENT CONCEPTS

CHAPTER OUTLINE

- Issues of motor control
- Classic treatment approaches

INTRODUCTION

The challenge for physiotherapists involved in the rehabilitation of individuals with neurological impairments is to develop a model of practice in which treatment methods selected are grounded in a clear understanding of the scientific, physiotherapeutic and practical knowledge base. The development of such a model of practice requires the examination not only of the treatment approaches themselves but also of the theories of motor control to which they relate. This is by no means a straightforward or simple task. However, it is the intention of this chapter to illustrate how some of the basic concepts underlying motor control have evolved and to consider how such concepts relate to developed and developing treatment approaches and techniques.

A brief overview of the major treatment concepts will be given and the scientific evidence on which they are based will be discussed. There are many excellent sources of information available documenting the application of specific treatment approaches and detailing the background neurophysiological and behavioural concepts. This chapter will not repeat such detailed information but rather provide the reader with reference to the appropriate sources in this book and other texts. It is hoped that this chapter will provide the basis for physiotherapists to be able to recognise and understand the theoretical foundations of treatment approaches and to be able to select and apply new theoretical developments to advance their practice (Charlton, 1994).

BACKGROUND

Although there remains debate with respect to terminology and categorisation (Scrutton, 1984; Bower, 1993; Ashburn, 1995), physiotherapy practice in neurology can be considered to fall into three broadly distinct areas:

1. **Neurodevelopmental (or neurophysiological)**
   e.g. Knott & Voss (1968); Bobath (1969, 1990); Bobath & Bobath (1975); Johnstone (1987a, b); 'Rood' (Goff, 1986); 'Brunnstrom' (Sawner & LaVigne, 1992).

2. **Motor learning and relearning**
   e.g. Cotton & Kinsman (1983); Carr & Shepard (1987); Shumway-Cook & Woollacott (1995).

3. **Eclectic**
   In this approach, the physiotherapist selects aspects from different treatment approaches that seem appropriate for the individual patient, e.g. Levitt (1982). This category is included to reflect the real world of physiotherapy practice, which does not always fit neatly within one particular treatment paradigm or the treatment of one isolated condition.

Historically, treatment approaches have largely been developed on a disease- or condition-specific basis, with stroke and cerebral palsy clearly having the highest concentration of specific methodologies (Bower, 1993;

Ashburn, 1995). Treatments for other neurological conditions, such as Parkinson's disease and multiple sclerosis, have tended to utilise and adapt approaches and techniques from a variety of sources rather than to develop condition-specific methodologies (Turnbull, 1992).

Difficulties in defining specific treatment methodologies, the lack of appropriate outcome measures and the multiplicity of variables involved in the treatment process have meant that meaningful evaluation of the effectiveness of overall treatment regimens, or their component parts, has been problematical. Studies have largely produced equivocal results (Partridge *et al.*, 1993). This is not surprising given the multivariate nature of appropriate outcome measures. However, there is a clear need for more thorough and appropriately designed evaluations to be undertaken.

Whilst research into the effectiveness of treatment approaches and techniques is clearly an important aspect of the validation of clinical practice, central to its success is the need for a fundamental shift in the way that physiotherapists perceive and contextualise the treatment modalities they undertake and prescribe. It is no longer acceptable, from the perspectives of audit and service, to undertake treatment without being able to demonstrate patient satisfaction and cost effectiveness. Neither is it valid in research terms to employ treatment methods simply because historically they have always been used in a particular way. Neither, therefore, should practising physiotherapists expect themselves, or their clients, to be satisfied with received wisdom with respect to the underlying theoretical basis of their treatment approaches. Physiotherapy practice in neurology is complex, fluid and esoteric in nature. In order to practise effectively within a multidisciplinary environment, physiotherapists need to make explicit the knowledge-based framework (Higgs & Titchen, 1995) that underpins and develops their clinical practice.

ISSUES OF MOTOR CONTROL

Before considering the detail of the classic treatment approaches used in neurological physiotherapy, it is important to gain an understanding of the scientific frameworks on which they are based. This section will therefore consider the development of theories of motor control upon which therapeutic methodologies are broadly based. A framework will be proposed with which to aid the practising physiotherapist in making reasoned and evidence-based clinical decisions in the selection and development of treatment methodologies and techniques. Details of relevant neuroanatomy, neurophysiology, normal motor control and recovery mechanisms can be found elsewhere in this book and in other key publications (e.g. Kandel *et al.*, 1991; Kidd *et al.*, 1992; Cohen, 1993; Rothwell, 1994).

Historically, many of the approaches used in neurological physiotherapy were developed on a largely empirical basis, when existing methods were found to be inappropriate in the treatment of current problems (Gordon, 1987; Ada & Canning, 1990). This is not to say that they made little use of existing scientific knowledge but rather to infer that clinical observations and responses were central to the development of theory and practice. This in itself is not an uncommon phenomenon in other disciplines, such as medicine and psychology, where advances in knowledge are often based on the observation and reporting of single cases.

There have been significant advances over the past decade in the development of meaningful and appropriate models of motor control from a therapeutic perspective (e.g. Schenkman & Butler, 1989; Carr & Shepherd, 1990; Connolly & Montgomery, 1991; Mathiowetz & Haugen, 1994). However, consideration of models of motor control has tended to be made with respect to classic treatment approaches (e.g. those of Bobath or Carr & Shepherd) rather than individual treatment techniques (e.g. functional electrical stimulation, vibration and sensory cueing). The eclectic use of treatment techniques is increasing, as is the adaptation of the classic approaches for use in other conditions. These developments reflect the increasing scope of professional practice and require the physiotherapist to be able to apply theoretical concepts of motor control across treatment approaches, techniques and conditions. The rest of this section will consider treatment approaches and techniques as part of the same continuum.

FRAMEWORK

A useful framework for considering the relationship between motor control and treatment approaches has been proposed by Mathiowetz & Haugen (1994). They consider the three overarching models of motor control to be reflex, hierarchical and systems (see Figure 22.1).

To varying degrees these models can be considered to have components taken from neurophysiology, biomechanics and behavioural psychology. Each model contributes to traditional and contemporary theories of motor development and learning. Together, the models and theories lead to the development and application of specific central nervous system (CNS) treatment approaches. These approaches were defined by Mathiowetz & Haugen (1994) as: muscle re-education; neurodevelopmental; motor relearning programme; and contemporary task-oriented.

Using a framework such as this it should be possible for physiotherapists to select the most appropriate treatment approach and technique based on a clear understanding of its theoretical basis. For example, following injury to the spinal cord it may be entirely appropriate to adopt a reflex model of motor control, utilising a muscle-strengthening technique, such as functional electrical stimulation, to re-educate the weakened muscle. However, the adoption of a systems model of motor control, utilising a task-oriented approach, which incorporates cognitive and perceptual techniques, would be appropriate in re-educating the activity parameters of the whole muscle group.

No delineation of theoretical models or concepts would appear to be totally satisfactory; they are constantly changing and developing, as is their relationship to treatment (Shumway-Cook & Woollacott, 1995). This reflects the complexity, scope and changing nature of physiotherapy practice. Futhermore, overlap exists between the stated and applied basis of different treatment approaches and techniques. The following outline is not intended to be considered as complete, fixed or immovable, but rather to be seen as a tool by which treatments can be understood, evaluated, explored and developed.

Models of motor control, together with theories of motor development and learning, will be considered under the headings of reflex, hierarchical and systems. The second section of this chapter will consider treatment approaches used in CNS dysfunction.

Each model of motor control will be considered with respect to:
- The basic premises of the model.
- The theoretical implications of the model.
- The implications of the model for physiotherapy practice.
- The limitations of the model.

REFLEX MODEL

Reflex components of motor behaviour have been well documented and explored since the observations of Sherrington (1906). The classic component is that of the reflex arc, the key element of which is the concept of stimulus → response. The simplest reflex pathway could be considered to consist of: stimulus of a receptor organ (e.g. stretch of the muscle spindle); transmission along an afferent nerve to a central neurone (e.g. an α-motoneurone); transmission along an efferent nerve; followed by a response in an effector organ (e.g. contraction of muscle fibres). Reflex control of movement has been shown to: involve spinal, supraspinal and long-loop pathways (Matthews, 1991); be modified by various inhibitory mechanisms (Hultborn et al., 1971; Day et al., 1984; Iles & Roberts, 1986); operate differentially during different movement tasks (Tanaka, 1980; Dietz et al., 1990; Plant & Miller, 1993); and to be affected in various neurological conditions (Yanagisawa et al., 1976; Lee et al., 1983).

A reflex model of motor control can be considered to operate largely as a closed-loop system (Adams, 1971). The basic premise of a closed-loop system is that feedback, error detection and correction are all part of a self-regulating system (Mulder, 1993). Thus, when an individual performs a movement the following processess occur: (1) the movement is initiated from a stored memory trace (which selects and starts movement); (2) sensory feedback then allows comparison to be made with a perceptual trace (stored movement traces based on previous movements); and (3) adjustments are then made to match the traces with the intended movement (Adams, 1971). The notion of a closed-loop system brings together previous understanding of sensorimotor reflex behaviour. In simplistic terms, once movement has been initiated then it is the role of reflex feedback, from a number of different sources, that determines the ability and precision with which the movement is made.

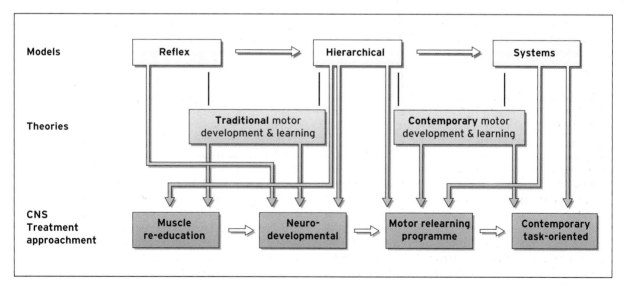

Figure 22.1 The historical relationship between the development of models, theories and treatment approaches used in the treatment of neurological dysfunction. The upper part shows models of motor behaviour and the arrows indicate the major shifts in understanding. The middle part of the figure indicates the influence of the models on traditional and contemporary theories of motor development and learning. The lower part shows the evolution of CNS treatment approaches over time. The downward arrows indicate the models and theories that have influenced the approaches. (Redrawn from Mathiowetz & Haugen, 1994, with permission.)

The basic premises of the reflex model are:
- A closed-loop system.
- Sensory feedback is key to movement ability.
- Perceptual traces are stored centrally as a type of motor programme.

The theoretical implications of the reflex model are:
- Memory traces exist in all individuals who were undamaged before the illness.
- Perceptual traces can be altered.
- Incorrect sensorimotor feedback will lead to altered performance.

The implications for physiotherapy practice are:
- Individuals with perinatal damage need to develop normal memory traces; if they do not, normal movement will never occur.
- Individuals with developed memory traces at the onset of morbidity already have stored the concept of normal movement; this raises the question as to the benefit of developmental sequencing in treatment.
- Sensorimotor feedback can be used to alter the perceptual memory trace, which has become distorted following injury.
- Uncorrected movement patterns and behaviours will reinforce the abnormal perceptual trace; this suggests that such measures as splinting, positioning, assistive aids and appliances, may be of use.

The limitations of the reflex model are:
- Human movement can take place without sensory input.
- Cognitive override is not considered.
- Normal movement control does not necessarily appear once reflexes have been normalised.

HIERARCHICAL MODEL

The hierarchical model, as the name implies, considers that the nervous system is organised and controlled in such a way that higher centres control and influence lower centres on a strictly hierarchical basis. This model can be considered to operate largely according to the concept of an open-loop system (Jackson & Taylor, 1932). The key to the open-loop system is that motor programmes are stored centrally within multiple motor areas in the brain. Thus, the performance of a motor activity is initiated, co-ordinated and controlled by central mechanisms that act on a hierarchical basis. For example, in performing a reaching and retrieving movement: (1) the component parts of the stored movement programme in the brain are activated; (2) these in turn exert either a facilitatory or inhibitory influence on spinal neurones and interneurones via corticospinal pathways; and (3) neuromuscular activity is finally initiated to complete the task.

Latterly the hierarchical model has been modified to incorporate the concept of programmes stored not only in the brain but in other parts of the CNS. For example, the existence of pattern generators located in both the brain

and the spinal cord has been proposed from work on animal models (Grillner, 1975, 1976; Halbertsma et al., 1976). Studies using positron emission tomography (PET) scans in normal human subjects and in individuals with Parkinson's disease have indicated that a particular set of neuronal links are made (at discrete onset times) between diverse parts of the brain (Hallet, 1994). This neuronal pattern of activity appears to be task-specific and, furthermore, activity has been demonstrated before, during and after movement (Evarts & Tanji, 1976; Brooks, 1994). The key premise of the open-loop system is that, once it has been learnt, movement can be performed without the need for peripheral feedback.

The basic premises of the hierarchical model are:
- An open-loop system.
- Motor programmes are mainly stored centrally, with some stored at a spinal level.
- Learnt movements are executed by pattern generators.

The theoretical implications of the hierarchical model are:
- Movements are executed according to programme sets or patterns.
- Programmes exist for all movement patterns.
- Peripheral input does not affect the central set.
- If central control centres are damaged then lower level reflex behaviour becomes dominant.

The implications for physiotherapy practice are:
- If programme sets are stored centrally, then the key to therapy is the access of these basic programmes; this could be achieved by enabling the individual to skip the part of the programme that is damaged.
- Normalisation of released reflexes may compensate for loss of central control.
- Task-oriented techniques and approaches will be effective, as these are likely to reflect the programmes stored.

The limitations of the hierarchical model are:
- The lack of an ongoing role for sensory input in motor control.
- The presupposition that every possible movement combination is stored centrally.

SYSTEMS MODEL

As already indicated, the classification of motor control into three distinct models is somewhat artificial as the boundaries between each tend to overlap. This is nowhere more evident than in consideration of the systems model, which has evolved historically from the reflex and hierarchical models of motor control. In its development it has also encompassed the perspectives of other disciplines such as biomechanics and behavioural psychology. The systems model is the model of choice underpinning current developments in the understanding of motor control. It has given rise to a number of theories of motor development and learning, such as motor relearning (Carr & Shepherd, 1987; Gordon, 1987), problem solving (Schenkman &

Butler, 1989) and, more latterly, the task-oriented approach (Horak, 1992; Mathiowetz, 1994; Shumway-Cook & Woollacott, 1995), dynamic pattern theory (Scholz, 1990) and parallel processing (for review see Shumway-Cook & Woollacott, 1995).

As indicated, a systems model takes its basis from a wider perspective than pure neurophysiology as it also incorporates biomechanics and learning behaviour. It was usefully described by Crutchfield & Barnes (1993) as a heterarchical model, in so far as it considers the context, the environment and cognition as key factors in the performance and relearning of motor tasks (Newell, 1991).

Schema Theory

In understanding the development of the systems model it is useful to consider the schema theory proposed by Schmidt (1975), which combined some of the aspects of the open- and closed-loop systems described previously. In essence the schema model considers that there is a generalised motor programme stored within the CNS that is class- or task-specific (Schmidt, 1988). Therefore, when a motor activity is to be undertaken: (1) a basic template already exists; (2) the template is then modified according to the required parameters (such as force, time and direction); and (3) the movement is then performed.

Mulder (1993) identified four kinds of information stored on the basis of a movement performed, according to the Schmidt schema theory:

1. The response specifications (parameters such as force, direction and time).
2. The initial conditions (position of the body).
3. The sensory consequences (all response-produced information).
4. The result (the environmental effect).

The relationship between the above elements is then stored for future use, either as a generalised motor programme to initiate movement (recall schema), or as a method of detecting error (recognition schema). This model can then be considered to combine elements of both reflex (closed-loop) and hierarchical (open-loop) models.

The basic premises of the schema model are:
- Generalised motor programmes.
- Feed-forward mechanisms based on the parameters of the intended movement.
- Feedback and alteration of the programme based on the experience of movement.

The theoretical implications of the schema model are:
- Movement programmes are stored as generalised sets.
- Experience and motor learning adjust and adapt the sets.
- Sensory feedback and environment are central to schema formation.

The implications for physiotherapy practice are:
- Movement patterns and parameters can be altered through peripheral and environmental manipulation.

- Generalised tasks rather then specific actions are more important as they form the basis of future action.
- Practice of movement patterns allows the development of meaningful and useful sets.

The limitations of the schema model are:
- The processing parameters are unclear.
- How schema are initially formed is unclear.
- The theory remains general, i.e. specifics such as neuronal connections are not described.

Systems Theory

The systems model continues to undergo development from a number of different disciplines and it is therefore, as yet, impossible to provide a definitive version of the model. What follows is an attempt to describe broadly the current issues. For the purposes of simplicity these will be considered in terms of input, processing and output. This is not to imply, however, that in the systems model, these occur in a linear sequence.

Input

The roles of sensory and kinaesthetic input remain important in the systems model. Skin, joint and muscle receptors discharge during active or passive movement. These receptors discharge differentially under active and passive conditions and during different phases of movement (Hulliger, 1979; Burke et al., 1988). In contrast to open-loop theories such as the servohypothesis (Merton, 1953), it is held that all types of receptors provide proprioceptive information about movement. Furthermore, such feedback is critical when learning a new skill (Gandevia & Burke, 1994) and therefore perhaps also in skill reacquisition. It is clear that the mechanisms controlling reflexes and perception may be set differently during the same movement and may also differ during isometric and isotonic activity. The reflex contribution to human movement has been considered elsewhere in this book (see Chapter 2) and it has been demonstrated that afferent feedback influences both spinal and supraspinal loops (Matthews, 1991), changing the gain of the system appropriate to the demands of a task. There is also evidence of feedforward mechanisms in which cortical activity can be demonstrated to take place before perceptual recognition is made of the desire to move in response to an external stimulus.

In essence the CNS has access to a variety of peripheral information from skin, muscle and joint receptors in addition to centrally generated signals of timing, grading and destination of motor output (which can be amended through conscious control). Movement can take place without peripheral feedback, which can even become redundant in 'practised' motor skills. However, a full movement repertoire cannot be achieved without peripheral feedback to adjust, update and amend spinal and supraspinal control mechanisms. The implications for therapeutic intervention are that when feedback is removed reliance is placed on central commands. These commands may be sufficient to perform simple learnt movements but feedback is essential when movements involve precise contractions, when disturbances occur, or during the learning process (Gandevia & Burke, 1994).

Processing

As indicated above, systems theory considers that processing takes place in parallel rather than in series. However, the concept of a generalised programme from which a number of similar movements are controlled (rather than there being individual and distinct programmes for every type of movement) indicates that it is at least in part a serial process. Stowell (1995) suggested that 'the biological nervous system is a neural network not a nineteenth century telegraph machine'. This is a useful analogy if one considers the processing method as rather like a telephone system. If it is comprised of private lines, i.e. discrete units controlling particular movements, then when a line is cut no recovery is possible. If, however, the system is organised on a temporal and spatial basis, i.e. flexible combinations of units, then recovery and adaption of the system are possible as other lines can be used to achieve the same functional outcome.

Mulder (1993) offered a helpful reworking of Schmidt's original schema model which centres on the processing of information. The components of the information processing model which are considered key to motor control are shown in Table 22.1.

Feedback and feedforward are central to the information processing model. Feedback loops update programming rules. Feedforward tunes the system before the arrival of commands, which is particularly important in environmentally unstable situations. In the selection of treatment approaches and techniques, the information processing model indicates that it is not possible to separate cognitive and motor processes (which are both related to the environment). Furthermore, motor control is not based on muscle-specific programmes but on abstract rules. Treatment therefore involves not simply re-education of movement but also the re-education of the information processing system that sets the movement rules. Mulder (1993) stated that there are three key factors in the re-education or development of movement rules:

1. Variability of practice—treatment and practice must take place in different environmental contexts to develop flexible rules.
2. Identical elements—there must be maximum overlap between re-education occurring in the therapeutic situation and in daily life for transfer to occur.
3. Consistent use of feedback—the acquisition of the knowledge of results (at a cognitive and automatic level) is key in developing movement rules; negative and positive results are equally important in this process.

Output

From a biomechanical perspective the question has been addressed as to how neural commands are represented and controlled in the activation of muscle. The eqilibrium-point hypothesis (Bizzi et al., 1984) suggests that centrally planned motor intentions are expressed and transmitted according to a virtual trajectory. This approach obviates the need for complex calculations and commands as the length–tension relationship between

Table 22.1 Components of the information processing model.

Mulder 1993

Components of the information processing model	
Intention	Must be functionally specific
Activation	Basic level of neurophysical and neuropsychological activation required for motor behaviour to occur
Sensory input selection and appropriate stimulus recognition	The ability to select and recognise the sensory stimulus through memory mechanisms and functional significance
Response selection	An abstract representation of the task rather than muscle-specific records or engrams
Programming	Takes place in the interface between cognition and action; consists of two subprocesses – planning and parametric specification

agonist and antagonist muscles will ensure that the final limb position is one of equilibrium. It would seem from the evidence that slow simple movements around a single joint can be expressed in terms of such a virtual trajectory and that such a hypothesis would allow for a variety of different movements with the trajectory as its basis. So, for example, in reaching towards an object, central commands would 'switch on' the virtual trajectory and a virtual position (or equilibrium) would be reached from which the actual position could then be achieved.

The dual-strategy hypothesis (Gottlieb *et al.*, 1989) proposes that there are two different sets of rules that control and regulate movement (Corcos, 1991): one that controls speed-insensitive movements, and one that controls speed-sensitive movements. Speed-sensitive movements are controlled by increasing the intensity of activation of the motoneurone pool. Speed-insensitive movements involve changes in duration of activation of motoneurones.

Such observations have been made largely, though not exclusively, over single joints with one degree of freedom. Degrees of freedom refers to the number of joint complexes involved in the performance of a task (Berstein, 1967). Functional activities clearly involve more than one degree of freedom. Although an understanding of muscle kinematics is important for physiotherapy, for it to be relevant to individuals with neuro- logical deficit it needs to be applicable to functional situations and activities.

CURRENT POSITION

Current debates and issues in motor control (for review see Cordo & Harnad, 1994) would seem to suggest broad agreement on the following:

- Motor control cannot be explained by the storage of hard-wired information for each movement.
- Movement patterns are stored as abstract rather than literal interpretations.
- Both parallel and serial processing occurs within the CNS.
- Movement control is non-linear.
- Kinaesthetic feedback is central to the performance of normal movement.
- Under normal conditions feedback may become redundant.
- Spinal pattern generators are task-dependent.

The overall implications of current understanding of the systems model for physiotherapy practice are:

- Practice and repetition are prerequisites for all motor skill acquisition—especially practice of deficient strategies.
- Functional tasks should be practised in their entirety.
- Learning and relearning of motor sets or patterns/activities needs to take place in different environmental contexts for transfer to occur.
- Cognition and motivation positively influence motor behaviour.

- The human motor system has some components that act in series but the majority act in parallel; therefore treatment modalities need to combine both hierarchical and heterarchical methods in order to be effective in the natural environment.
- Strength training of weak muscles has a role in improving movement ability across all neurological conditions.
- Identification of primary problems is key—are they associated with input, processing or output, or a combination of all three?

SUMMARY OF MOTOR CONTROL MODELS

In essence, current thinking appears to be reluctant to dismiss in toto any of the traditional models of motor control. It appears to recognise a place for predetermined (genetic) motor patterns upon which experience and learning determine abstract motor sets (through synaptic weight or gain). However, there remains a distinct gap between neurophysiological evidence gained from electrophysiological studies (in both animal and human models) of, for example, spinal reflex and cortical behaviour and the mainly theoretical models of how the CNS organises and controls movement. Clearly, evidence of types of normal and altered reflex behaviour are important to practice, as is an understanding of muscle physiology, biomechanics and neuromuscular plasticity. However, rehabilitation at the functional level requires hard evidence of overall control mechanisms because it is the reordering of such mechanisms that constitutes the scientific outcomes of treatment. For example, intrathecal baclofen and phenol nerve blocks are used in the pharmacological treatment of spasticity and their effect on peripheral mechanisms has been demonstrated (Barnes *et al.*, 1993). Functional improvement is to some extent a byproduct of the technique. In contrast, the aim of therapy in neurological conditions is the re-education of function; reduction of spasticity may be seen as part of this process, but the end point is the effect on functional motor control.

At present there are a number of models that can be used to explain motor control. There is increasing evidence of specific peripheral, spinal, supraspinal and environmental mechanisms that may contribute to this control. It is in the gap between the theoretical and scientific evidence that physiotherapy attempts to practice. Table 22.2 gives a summary of the theoretical basis of each model and the relationship to physiotherapy treatment approaches and techniques.

CLASSIC TREATMENT APPROACHES

This section will overview the classic treatment concepts used in neurological physiotherapy. It will not give detailed guidelines of how to undertake the specific approaches but will consider their theoretical background and key features. References to texts detailing application are cited throughout. The treatment approaches discussed, in no particular order, are:

The scientific concepts associated with the three classic models of motor control		
Motor control model	**Theoretical basis**	**Physiotherapy approaches**
Reflex	Closed loop	Muscle re-education, e.g. functional electrical stimulation, PNF
Hierarchical	Open loop	Neurodevelopmental, e.g. Bobath, Johnstone, Rood, Brunnström
Systems	Multisystem Schema theory Information processing Parallel processing	Motor learning and relearning, e.g. Carr & Shepherd, Conductive Education, task-orientated *
* Shumway-Cook & Woollacott, 1995; Mathiowetz & Haugen, 1994		

Table 22.2 The scientific concepts associated with the three classic models of motor control. Examples of the physiotherapy approaches based on each model are given. (Abbreviation: PNF, proprioceptive neuromuscular facilitation.)

1. Bobath.
2. Johnstone.
3. Proprioceptive neuromuscular facilitation.
4. Brunnström.
5. Rood.
6. Conductive education.
7. Motor relearning (Carr & Shepherd).

A less widely used method, the Hare approach, which is used in the treatment of brain injury and cerebral palsy, is considered in Chapters 8 & 19.

Table 22.3, at the end of this section, outlines some of the major features of the classic approaches and should provide a useful framework for physiotherapists to examine and select appropriate methods from a sound theoretical basis.

BOBATH

The Bobath approach to the treatment of neurological deficit developed specifically from observations of abnormal postural tone in children with cerebral palsy (Bobath & Bobath, 1975). These observations led to the formation of an approach which was considered to be neurodevelopmental in nature. The theory proposed suggested that in order for accurate diagnosis and treatment to be undertaken, comparison needed to be made with normal developmental milestones. The key feature within this paradigm is the notion that development follows a sequential and hierarchical sequence. Accordingly, treatment of children with cerebral palsy or motor delay was advocated on the basis of reducing abnormal tone and

posture, thus preparing and enabling the child to reach the normal developmental reactions expected on the basis of age and stage of development. Specific guidelines on the actual method of treatment are not well published (Bower, 1993) and it has been largely the preserve of individual therapists to implement the theory in practice.

Subsequent extension of this approach into the treatment of adult hemiplegia was originally based on neurodevelopmental theory. However, although some conceptual similarities remain, the current paradigm is more clearly based on neurophysiological principles, in particular reflex inhibition. Central to the Bobath approach is the normalisation of tone in the affected limb or limbs, through inhibiting techniques and postures and the facilitation of correct movement through handling by the physiotherapist (Ashburn, 1995). In contrast to cerebral palsy, treatment of the individual who has had a stroke is documented in some detail (Bobath, 1990). However, the specifics still largely remain the domain of the individual therapist. Furthermore, as in common with other techniques, the neurophysiological basis has been poorly explained and sometimes misunderstood.

The approach follows a broadly hierarchical treatment regimen, dependent on the stage of recovery (i.e. flaccid, spastic and relative). Subsumed within each of these stages are patterns of activities that are intended to prepare patients for subsequent volitional control. For example, sitting to standing is achieved through preparation in supine and side lying and in these positions the aim is to facilitate control of the leg, arm and trunk using various techniques. In theory the individual is not allowed to progress until normal postural activity can be demonstrated and maintained for that activity. Volitional movement is permitted only on the basis of normal automatic postural control. Successful accomplishment is determined by the therapist, who is also, by and large, key to its success, through the use of skillful handling of 'key points'. These key points tend to be located at proximal points at the junction of the appendicular and axial skeleton. The theory is that through judicious handling, normal afferent input and postural tone will be facilitated, resulting in the experience of normal patterns of movement.

JOHNSTONE

The Johnstone approach (Johnstone 1987a, b) was developed specifically for the treatment of stroke and is based on similar principles to that of the Bobath approach. Control of abnormal reflex activity is central, and particular attention is paid to the normalisation of postural reflexes. Central to this approach is the concept of developmental sequences of movement control and proximal to distal limb control. The control of abnormal muscle tone, defined by Johnstone as spasticity, is seen as a precursor to successful rehabilitation.

This approach stresses the importance of sensory stimulation in the achievement of normal functioning. This is accomplished through the use of such techniques as pressure splints and rhythmic stabilisations. Techniques are selected for use on the premise that they lead to a final functional outcome, such as independent walking. The treatment sequence is hierarchical, with the individual not being allowed to progress to the whole until each component part has been achieved. The therapist remains key to this approach with respect to determining progression and in the control of limb movement through passive, assisted and active–assisted stages. However, the individual is active in achieving and maintaining the positions required. Inhibition of spasticity is paramount from day 1. The use of pressure splints and weight-bearing through the affected limbs in corrective patterns are considered essential to control abnormal postural reflex mechanisms. In general the Johnstone approach places more emphasis on the upper limb than any other approach.

PROPRIOCEPTIVE NEUROMUSCULAR FACILITATION

The techniques of proprioceptive neuromuscular facilitation (PNF) were developed by Knott & Voss from the observations of Kabat (Knott & Voss, 1968). Kabat observed that movement patterns in the normal population take place in spiral or diagonal sequences and are always purposeful in direction. The original premise of the approach was neurodevelopmental in nature, using patterns of movement that were based on observations of primitive patterns and related to postural reflex mechanisms. Key to the approach was the application of maximal resistance throughout the range of movement, stretch applied to muscle groups, synergistic action over more than one joint, and reinforcement through repeated contractions, rhythmic stabilisations and slow reversals. PNF was originally used in the treatment of poliomyelitis and has been used in other areas of musculoskeletal rehabilitation

The principles underlying practice tend to be esoteric in nature, although there are very clear guidelines of how to perform the individual facilitation techniques (see Chapter 24). These fall into two broad areas: those initiated by the therapist, and those requiring the co-operation and effort of the individual undergoing treatment. There are clear specifications for stimulating muscle activity through manual handling and through verbal (and visual) commands and communication. Although not stated explicitly, PNF recognises a role for cueing, reinforcement and effort in the rehabilitation process. Knott & Voss, whilst retaining the original techniques, expanded the context of their usage, with particular respect to developmental sequences, which are considered neccessary pre- requisites for recovery to occur. These sequences and activities are broadly hierarchical in order, the individual having to demonstrate the ability to maintain one position before progressing to the next. However, the timing of such progression may be fairly swift and can occur within one treatment session.

BRUNNSTRÖM

Brunnström (Sawner & LaVigne, 1992) developed a technique for maximising recovery following stroke, based on observations of a large number of individuals. The primary observations were that movement recovery tended to be stereotypical in nature and was expressed through altered synergistic control of the affected limb. Basic limb synergies (as in reflex responses) are considered to recover first, with the dominant muscle groups (e.g. elbow flexors, knee extensors) controlling the pattern of responses. As recovery progresses, independent voluntary movements begin to become possible outside of the dominance of basic patterns and synergies. Movement within basic limb synergies is considered easier to achieve than non-synergistic movements, and the key to successful progression from one to the other appears to be the presence, or otherwise, of spasticity. The parallel is drawn in this approach between recovery from stroke and normal development, i.e. reflex → voluntary; gross → fine movement; and proximal → distal control.

From this premise, reflex activity is used as the basis for voluntary movement and treatment is dependent on the stage of recovery reached. The Brunnström approach recognises the need for goals set to be seen as achievable by the individual and describes the technique not as treatment but as training procedures. Little use is made in these procedures of supine lying positions, the individual being encouraged to undertake activities in the sitting position as soon as possible. Based on observations of recovery following stroke, this approach makes use of associated reactions, tonic reflexes and the development of basic synergies to facilitate movement. However, the use of such characteristics is considered to be of a temporary nature which, together with sensory stimulation, verbal and manual support, needs to be withdrawn in order for voluntary control to develop. Stretching of muscles, the use of traction, rhythmic repetitions, verbal commands and cutaneous stimulation (such as stroking and brushing) are all features of this approach. Facilitation of the recovery process is seen to take place in developmental stages. However, these stages have only to be achieved and not perfected before attempts at the next stage may begin.

ROOD

The Rood approach to treatment (Goff, 1986) developed from the concept that different types of skeletal muscle have different properties and functions in achieving motor output. This approach considers that differences between motor unit type and muscle property determines the type of stimulus required either to facilitate or inhibit muscle activity. The approach was not developed specifically for use in neurological conditions.

In essence, treatment is based on neurodevelopmental reasoning, selecting appropriate positions from total body patterns exhibited during childhood development. From this baseline a variety of afferent stimuli are utilised to achieve (1) proximal control and (2) distal, selective movement. Stimuli may be: cutaneous (fast brushing, slow stroking, cold); stretch (slow stretch, quick stretch); volitional (non-resisted, repeated, small range); compression and pressure; bone tapping; and positional (see Chapter 24). Movement patterns and stimuli are used in different combinations dependent on the presenting syndrome under the broad headings of hypokinesia, bradykinesia and spasticity. The specificities of treatment are not prescribed as such and are determined by assessment of the individual. Central to the approach, however, is the theory of cephalocaudal development of postural control and ontogenesis of movement function.

CONDUCTIVE EDUCATION

The conductive education approach was developed by Peto in Budapest, Hungary, to deal with the educational handicaps of children with severe motor disability (Cotton & Kinsman, 1983; Kinsman et al., 1988). This approach is grounded in practice and the theoretical basis (although difficult to define) appears to have major links with Eastern European psychology (Cottam & Sutton, 1986). The aim of the approach is to facilitate the ability of the individual to function in society without the use of aids or assistive devices. It does not seek to ameliorate the underlying medical condition but rather to promote what is termed 'orthofunction'. In essence, the approach is not condition-specific, its principles being used with individuals with Parkinson's disease, multiple sclerosis, paraplegia and spina bifida. However, it is most commonly used by western physiotherapists in the treatment of cerebral palsy and adult hemiplegia.

The key principles are that the individual is viewed as a whole person, that education is facilitated by a conductor and that work takes place in groups. Functional activities are broken down into their component parts and, through the use of repetition and reinforcement, tasks are learnt and achieved by the individual. The term 'rhythmic intention' is used to describe how individuals are instructed to use language to organise, plan and carry out movements. A hierarchy of tasks exists; once the movements become automatic the next task in the sequence can be begun. The control and power base in this approach lies with the individual, who takes responsibility for his or her own treatment and progression through his or her own efforts and initiative. The therapist or conductor acts in a facilitatory role, providing the optimum environment and tools with which the individual can practice and develop skills. The approach is structured and controlled throughout the whole of the day.

MOTOR RELEARNING (CARR & SHEPHERD)

Carr & Shepherd (1980, 1987) originally developed a theoretical model, that of motor learning, for use in the rehabilitation of individuals following stroke. The underlying assumptions are clearly stated and have been modified in the light of new knowledge. The theoretical model led to the development of a motor relearning programme comprising seven sections: upper limb function; orofacial function; motor tasks whilst sitting; motor tasks whilst standing; standing up; sitting down; and walking. Subsumed in each of these sections are four steps: (1) task analysis; (2) practice of missing components; (3) practice of the task; and (4) transference of training. There is no requirement to be successful in one section before progressing to another section.

Carr & Shepherd (1990) stated that physiotherapy has a unique contribution to make to the rehabilitation process, and in particular motor control, based on an understanding of the kinematics and kinetics of normal movement, motor control processes and motor learning. The theoretical assumptions are four-fold: (1) performance of motor tasks requires learning and accordingly the process of teaching and learning has to be understood; (2) motor control is both anticipatory and ongoing, and postural control and specific limb activities are interrelated; (3) practice of specific motor tasks leads to ability to perform the task, which should be practised in the appropriate environment; and (4) sensory input modulates the performance of motor tasks.

The individual follows a programme based on a model of normal motor learning, which involves: the elimination of unnecessary muscle activity; feedback; practice; and the interrelationship between posture and movement. Thus, the individual is engaged in a process of motor relearning. The approach comprises techniques found in other treatment approaches, such as verbal commands, approximation and cutaneous stimulation. However, the therapist is instructed to apply techniques only on the basis of assessment and theoretical applicability. This approach is designed to discourage compensatory behaviour and facilitate learning through the active involvement of the individual. Motor tasks are practised in their entirety, explanation and demonstration are used as key techniques, and activities are progressed as soon as the individual has demonstrated some control. The individual is encouraged to use his or her own observations and experiences as part of the relearning process. The reduction of spasticity is not seen as central in this approach.

Table 22.3 outlines the major treatment approaches and gives an indication of reasoning and practice with respect to various central parameters. Evidence has been taken from the literature rather than individual practice and it is recognised that some aspects are open to debate and potential modification. It should be read as a framework for understanding and enquiry rather than a definitive account. Some indication has been given as to the conditions for which the approach was developed and/or is commonly used. This is not to infer that these are the only conditions to which they can be applied. It is suggested that the reader uses this framework, together with other information in this chapter and the wider literature, to make connections between these approaches and other pathologies which use a more eclectic combination of techniques.

CONCLUSION

The theoretical concepts underpinning treatment approaches and techniques used in neurological physiotherapy have clear historical antecedents. Current evidence and knowledge from the behavioural and neurosciences suggests that there is no single model that adequately explains motor behaviour. As investigative techniques and modelling methods are developed, the knowledge base will increase and perhaps, at some time in the future, a definitive model will emerge. In the meantime physiotherapists should ensure that they use approaches and techniques, in combination, based on a clear understanding of their effect and outcome. The challenge to physiotherapists is to be selective and innovative and not to be driven by prescription or dogma. Not only do physiotherapists need to be able to explain clearly what they do but they also need to contribute to the debate by developing and expanding their frame of reference.

A. The classic physiotherapy approaches used in the treatment of neurological dysfunction and their relationship with parameters	
Treatment approach	**Bobath**
Conditions	Stroke; cerebral palsy
Basis of approach	Neurophysiological in adults. Neuro-develpmental in children
Recovery theory	Hierarchical sequence (flaccid, spastic and relative), based on developmental milestones, reflexes and patterns. Proximal control > distal function
Key features/techniques	Inhibition of abnormal reflexes and movements Facilitation of normal patterns through handling of key points
View of tone	Inhibition of abnormal tone central
Control of reflexes	Primitive and associated reactions inhibited Postural reflexes facilitated. Balance reactions facilitated
Task specific (ADL)	Pattern-centred rather than goal or task specific. Need for transferable skills recognised
Cognitve features	None
Volition	Therapist controlled volition permitted only on background of postural activity

Table 22.3 Classic physiotherapy approaches used in the treatment of neurological dysfunction. Seven approaches are outlined in sections A-E, and are not in any particular order.

B. The classic physiotherapy approaches used in the treatment of neurological dysfunction and their relationship with parameters

Treatment approach	**Johnstone**
Conditions	Stroke
Basis of approach	Neurophysiological
Recovery theory	Hierarchical sequence (passive, assisted and active assisted). Control of postural reflexes key
Key features/techniques	Air splints, positioning, rhythmic stabalisations in corrective pattern
View of tone	Inhibition of 'spasticity' central
Control of reflexes	a.a. from proximal to distal
Task specific (ADL)	Pattern-centred
Cognitve features	None
Volition	Individual active in achieving and maintaining correct positions

C. The classic physiotherapy approaches used in the treatment of neurological dysfunction and their relationship with parameters

Treatment approach	**Proprioceptive neuromuscular facilitation**
Conditions	Poliomyelitis; not condition-specific
Basis of approach	Neurophysiological/neurodevelopmental
Recovery theory	Hierarchical in developmental sequence
Key features/techniques	Mass patterns of spiral/diagonal movements and proprioceptive input. Use of stretch, repetition, stabalisations, reversals and verbal commands
View of tone	Not specifically mentioned
Control of reflexes	Control of abnormal postural reflexes through mass patterns of movement
Task specific (ADL)	Mass pattern-specific
Cognitve features	Some, e.g. use of verbal stimuli. Evidence of underlying notion of motor learning
Volition	Manual handling by therapist but co-operation of individual required

D. The classic physiotherapy approaches used in the treatment of neurological dysfunction and their relationship with parameters

Treatment approach	Brunnström
Conditions	Stroke
Basis of approach	Developmental based on observations of recovery from stroke
Recovery theory	Stereotypical recovery based on synergistic control. Hierarchy reflects normal development: reflex > voluntary; gross > fine movement; proximal > distal control
Key features/techniques	Facilitation of synergistic and then non-synergistic movement using reflex activity and sensory stimulation
View of tone	Spasticity key to progression from synergistic to non-synergistic movement. However, no attempt to normalise tone
Control of reflexes	Associated reactions, tonic reflexes and basic synergies used to facilitate movement – withdrawn as voluntary control develops
Task specific (ADL)	Recovery rather than ADL specific
Cognitve features	Need for goal to be seen as achievable by individual recognised. Techniques described as training procedures rather than treatment
Volition	Volition progresses with stage of recovery

E. The classic physiotherapy approaches used in the treatment of neurological dysfunction and their relationship with parameters

Treatment approach	Rood
Conditions	Not condition-specific
Basis of approach	Neurophysiological/neurodevelopmental
Recovery theory	Hierarchical: cephalocaudal development of postural control; ontogenetic development of movement functions. Muscle properties defined and plastic changes facilitated
Key features/techniques	Body positions selected from developmental sequence. Afferent stimuli, cutaneous, stretch, volitional and pressure, used in combination dependent on presenting syndrome (hypokinesia, bradykinesia, spasticity)
View of tone	Level of tone defines broad headings for treatment
Control of reflexes	Postural reflex control stimulated at an autonomic level
Task specific (ADL)	Movement patterns and stimuli used to facilitate control of developmental tasks rather than ADL
Cognitve features	Links between somatosensory, autonomic and psychological functioning made
Volition	Non resisted, repeated and small range movements used dependent on stage of recovery

F. The classic physiotherapy approaches used in the treatment of neurological dysfunction and their relationship with parameters

Treatment approach	Conductive education
Conditions	Motor disability in children and adults
Basis of approach	Educational psychology
Recovery theory	Facilitation of functioning in society, without use of aids and assistive devices
Key features/techniques	24-hour, planned, group activities co-ordinated by a conductor. Facilitations include: rhythmic intention, motivation, continuity, self and manual facilitation
View of tone	None
Control of reflexes	None
Task specific (ADL)	Hierarchy of functional specific tasks broken down into component parts
Cognitve features	Individual progresses through own efforts and initiative. Feedback, motivation and conscious control of movement and language central
Volition	Key strategies to overcome failure through self control of physical ability

G. The classic physiotherapy approaches used in the treatment of neurological dysfunction and their relationship with parameters

Treatment approach	Carr & Shepherd
Condtions	Stroke and other brain disorders
Basis of approach	Motor learning-based on theories of motor control, kinematics and kinetics of normal movement
Recovery theory	Motor relearning programme comprises seven sections and four steps. Non-hierarchical
Key features/techniques	Motor tasks practised in entirety. Teaching and learning and manual guidance techniques used
View of tone	Spasticity not seen as a major problem
Control of reflexes	Specifically none – although compensatory behaviour is discouraged
Task specific (ADL)	Key-functional tasks practised in appropriate environment
Cognitve features	Learning, understanding, motivation, practice, progression and relevance central
Volition	Key

REFERENCES

Ada L, Canning C. *Key issues in neurological physiotherapy*. London: Butterworth Heinemann; 1990.

Adams JA. A closed loop theory of motor learning. *J Motor Behav* 1971, 3:111-150.

Ashburn A. A review of current physiotherapy in the management of stroke. In: Harrison M, ed. *Physiotherapy in stroke management*. Edinburgh: Churchill Livingstone; 1995.

Barnes MP, McLellan DL, Sutton RA. Spasticity. In: Greenwood R, Barnes MP, McMillan, TM, *et al.*, eds. *Neurological rehabilitation*. Edinburgh: Churchill Livingstone; 1993:161-172.

Berstein N. *The co-ordination and regulation of movements*. London: Pergamon Press; 1967.

Bizzi E, Accornerno N, Chapple W, Hogan N. Posture control trajectory during arm movement. *J Neurosci* 1984, 4:2738-2744.

Bobath B. The treatment of neuromuscular disorders by improving patterns of co-ordination. *Physiotherapy* 1969, 55:18-22.

Bobath B. *Adult hemiplegia: evaluation and treatment, 3rd edition*. Oxford: Butterworth Heinemann; 1990.

Bobath B, Bobath K. *Motor development in the different types of cerebral palsy*. London: Heinemann; 1975.

Bower E. Physiotherapy for cerebral palsy: a historical review. In: Ward C, ed. *Baillière's clinical neurology: rehabilitation of motor disorders*. London: Baillière Tindall; 1993:29-55.

Brooks DJ. Functional imaging studies of movement. *Movement Disorders*, 1994, 9(suppl. 1):11.

Burke D, Gandevia SC, McKeon B. Responses to passive movement of receptors in joint, skin and muscle of the hand. *J Physiol* 1988, 432:445-458.

Carr J, Shepherd R. *Physiotherapy in disorders of the brain*. London: Heinemann; 1980.

Carr J, Shepherd R. *A motor relearning programme for stroke, 2nd edition*. Oxford: Butterworth Heinemann; 1987.

Carr J, Shepherd R. A motor learning model for the rehabilitation of the movement disabled. In: Ada L, Canning C, eds. *Key issues in neurological physiotherapy*. London: Butterworth Heinemann; 1990:1-24.

Charlton JL. Motor control issues and clinical applications. *Physiother Theory Prac* 1994, 10:185-190.

Cohen H. *Neuroscience for rehabilitation*. Philadelphia: Lippincott; 1993.

Connolly B, Montgomery P. *Motor control and physical therapy: theoretical framework and practical applications*. Tennessee : Chatanooga ; 1991.

Corcos DM. Strategies underlying the control of disorded movement. *Phys Ther* 1991, 71:25-38.

Cordo P, Harnad S, eds. *Movement control*. Cambridge: Cambridge University Press; 1994.

Cottam PJ, Sutton A, eds. *Conductive education: a system for overcoming motor disorder*. London: Croom Helm; 1986.

Cotton E, Kinsman R. *Conductive education for adult hemiplegia*. Edinburgh: Churchill Livingstone; 1983.

Crutchfield CA, Barnes MR. *Motor control and motor learning in rehabilitation*. Atlanta: Stokesville; 1993.

Day BL, Marsden CD, Obeso JA, Rothwell JC. Reciprocal inhibition between the muscles of the human forearm. *J Physiol* 1984, 349:519-534.

Dietz V, Faist M, Pierrot-Deseillgny E. Amplitude modulation of the quadriceps H-reflex during the early stance phase of gait. *Exp Brain Res* 1990, 79:221-224.

Evarts EJ, Tanji J. Reflex and intended responses and motor cortex pyramidal tract neurones of monkeys. *J Neurophysiol* 1976, 39:1069-1080.

Gandevia SC, Burke D. Does the nervous system depend on kinesthetic information to control natural limb movements? In: Cordo P, Hanard S, eds. *Movement control*. Cambridge: Cambridge University Press; 1994.

Goff B. A neurophysiological approach. In: Banks MA, ed. *International perspectives in physical therapy: stroke*. Edinburgh: Churchill Livingstone; 1986.

Gordon J. Assumptions underlying physical therapy intervention: theoretical and historical perspectives. In: Carr JH, Sheperd, RB, Gordon J, *et al.*, eds. *Movement science: foundations for physical therapy in rehabilitation*. London: Heinemann; 1987.

Gottlieb GL, Corcos DM, Agarwal GC. Strategies for the control of single mechanical degree of freedom voluntary movements. *Behav Brain Sci* 1989, 12:189-210.

Grillner S. Locomotion in vertebrates: central mechanisms and reflex interactions. *Physiol Rev* 1975, 55:247-307.

Grillner S. Some aspects on the descending control of spinal circuits generating locomotor movements. In: Herman RM, Grillner S, Stein PSG, Stuart DG, eds. *Neural control of locomotion*. New York: Plenum Press; 1976.

Halbertsma J, Miller S, Van der Meche FGA. Basic programmes for the phasing of flexion and extension movement of the limbs during locomotion. In: Herman RM, Grillner S, Stein PSG, Stuart DG, eds. *Neural control of locomotion*. New York: Plenum Press; 1976.

Hallet M. Physiological studies of abnormal movement. *Movement Disorders* 1994, 9(suppl. 1):11.

Higgs J, Titchen AT. The nature, generation and verification of knowledge. *Physiotherapy* 1995, 81:521-530.

Horak F. Assumptions underlying motor control for neurologic rehabilitation. In: Lister MJ, ed. *Contemporary management of motor control problems*. Proceedings of the II step conference. Alexandria, Virginia: American Physical Therapy Association; 1992.

Hulliger M, Nordh E, Thelin AE, Valbo AB. The reponses of afferent fibres from the glabrous skin of the hand during voluntary finger movements in man. *J Physiol* 1979, 291:233-249.

Hultborn H, Jankowska E, Lindstrom S. Recurrent inhibition of interneurones monosynaptically activated from group Ia afferents. *J Physiol* 1971, 215:613-636.

Iles JF, Roberts RC. Presynaptic inhibition of monosynaptic reflexes in the lower limbs of subjects with upper motor neurone disease. *J Neurol Neurosurg Psych* 1986, 49:937-944.

Jackson JH, Taylor J, eds. *Selected writings of John B Hughlings*, I and II. London: Hodder & Stoughton; 1932.

Johnstone M. *Restoration of motor function in the stroke patient, 3rd edition*. Edinburgh: Churchill Livingstone; 1987a.

Johnstone M. *The stroke patient, 3rd edition*. Edinburgh: Churchill Livingstone; 1987b.

Kandel E, Schwartz JH, Jessell TM, eds. *Principles of neuroscience, 3rd edition*. New York: Elsevier; 1991.

Kidd G, Lawes N, Musa I. *Understanding neuromuscular plasticity: a basis for clinical rehabilitation*. London: Edward Arnold; 1992.

Kinsman R, Verity R, Walker J. A conductive education approach for adults with neurological dysfunction. *Physiother* 1988, 74:277-230.

Knott M, Voss DE. *Proprioceptive neuromuscular facilitation, 2nd edition*. Philadelphia: Harper & Row; 1968.

Lee RG, Murphy JT, Tatton WG. Long latency myotatic reflexes in man: mechanisms, functional significance and changes in patients with Parkinson's disease or hemiplegia. In: Desmedt JE, ed. *Advances in neurology*. New York: Raven Press; 1983.

Levitt S. *Treatment of cerebral palsy and motor delay, 2nd edition*. Oxford: Blackwell; 1982.

Mathiowetz V, Haugen JB. Motor behavior research: implications for therapeutic approaches to central nervous system dysfunction. *Am J Occup Ther* 1994, 48:733-745.

Matthews PBC. The human stretch reflex and the motor cortex. *Trends Neurosci* 1991, 14:87-91.

Merton PA. Speculation on the servo control of movement. In: Malcolm JL, Gray JAB, Wolstenholme GEW, eds. *The spinal cord*. Boston: Little Brown; 1953.

Mulder T. Current topics in motor control: implications for rehabilitation. In: Greenwood R, Barnes MP, McMillan TM, *et al.*, eds. *Neurological rehabilitation*. Edinburgh: Churchill Livingstone; 1993:125-134.

Newell KM. Motor skill aquisition. *Ann Rev Psych* 1991, 42:213-237.

Partridge C, Cornall C, Lynch M, Greenwood R. Physical therapies. In: Greenwood R, Barnes MP, McMillan TM, *et al.*, eds. *Neurological rehabilitation*. Edinburgh: Churchill Livingstone; 1993:189-198.

Plant RD, Miller S. Task dependent inhibition in spastic hemiplegia. In: Thilman AF, Burke DJ, Rymer WZ, eds. *Spasticity: mechanisms and management*. Berlin: Springer Verlag; 1993.

Rothwell JR. *Control of human voluntary movement, 2nd edition*. London: Chapman & Hall; 1994.

Sawner KA, LaVigne JM. *Brunnstrom's movement therapy in hemiplegia, 2nd edition*. Philadelphia: Lippincott; 1992.

Schenkman M, Butler RB. A model for multisystem evaluation, interpretation and treatment of individuals with neurologic dysfunction. *Phys Ther* 1989, **69**:538-547.

Schmidt RA. A schema theory of discrete motor learning. *Psych Rev* 1975, **82**:225-260.

Schmidt RA. *Motor control and learning: a behavioral emphasis, 2nd edition*. Champaign, Illinois: Human Kinetics; 1988.

Scholz JP. Dynamic pattern theory: some implications for therapeutics. *Phys Ther* 1990, **70**:827-843.

Scrutton D. Management of the motor disorders of children with cerebral palsy. *Clin Dev Med* 1984, **90**:1-6.

Sherrington C. *The integrative action of the nervous system*. New York: Scribners; 1906.

Shumway-Cook A, Woollacott MH. *Motor control: theory and practical applications*. Baltimore: Williams & Wilkins; 1995.

Stowell H. Networks for pain. *Nature Med* 1995, **1**:976. [letter]

Tanaka R. Inhibitory mechanisms in reciprocal innervation in voluntary movements. In: Desmedt JE, ed. *Progress in clinical neurophysiology*. Basel: Karger; 1980.

Turnbull GI. *Physical therapy management of Parkinson's disease*. New York: Churchill Livingstone; 1992.

Yanagisawa N, Tanaka R, Ito Z. Reciprocal inhibition in spastic hemiplegia in man. *Brain* 1976, **99**:555-574.

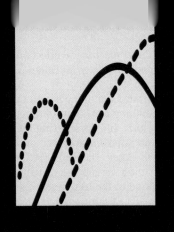

23 E Panturin & M Stokes

MUSCULOSKELETAL TREATMENT CONCEPTS APPLIED TO NEUROLOGY

CHAPTER OUTLINE

INTRODUCTION

Some treatment approaches that were developed in orthopaedic physiotherapy and are now being used in the management of neurological patients are introduced in this chapter. Two techniques not covered here but discussed in Chapter 24 are acupuncture and the gymnastic ball. The two concepts discussed in Sections One and Two of this chapter are adverse neural tension (ANT) and muscle imbalance. They are dealt with separately from the concepts included in Chapter 22 because they are still only emerging in the musculoskeletal field. It is not possible, in this brief review, to give details of the techniques involved, to enable the reader to perform them. The intention is only to introduce the concepts.

Research is still required to provide evidence for the theoretical bases of ANT and muscle imbalance, and to evaluate the effectiveness of the treatment techniques involved. Some aspects of the assessment and treatment techniques designed for the orthopaedic patient will need to be adapted for the neurological patient, and this will also require research to produce appropriate clinical guidelines for different patient groups.

SECTION ONE: ADVERSE NEURAL TENSION–NEURODYNAMICS

The purpose of physiotherapy treatment in general, and of physiotherapy of neurological conditions in particular, is to help the individual to return to full function of as near to normal quality as is achievable (depending, obviously, on the severity of the condition).

There are many causes that may prevent normal function in people, e.g. limited joint movements, muscle weakness, shortening of soft tissues, increased and/or decreased muscle tone, sensation, cognitive and perceptual restrictions. Over recent years, orthopaedically oriented physiotherapists such as Elvey (1986), Maitland (1986) and Butler & Gifford (1989) have all mentioned another cause for restricted function, which is restricted movement of the nervous system, termed adverse mechanical, or neural, tension (AMT or ANT). That is to say, impairment of movement and/or elasticity of the nervous system may cause symptoms from within its own tissues.

Recently, Shacklock (1995a, 1995b) emphasised not only the mechanics of the nervous system, but also the link between the pathomechanics and pathophysiology of the nervous system. Shacklock suggested using the term 'neurodynamics' when discussing interaction between nervous system mechanics and physiology.

Can we presume that the difficulty in the person with hemiplegia or severe head injury to straighten his or her knee on heel strike when walking is always due to a restriction in the knee joint itself? Perhaps it may be caused by increased tone, shortening of the gastrocnemius muscle or hamstrings or, possibly, by an abnormality in the movement of, or physiological changes in, the nervous system. Following this theme, why may a person suffering central nervous system (CNS) damage have difficulty in extending his or her hip in the stance phase? Or, are we aware of all the causes of pain and restriction of movement in the shoulder of the person with hemiplegia or incomplete spinal cord injury? Do we know why the person is unable to stretch out his or her arm to pick up an object or grasp a glass in a normal manner?

In central neurological, as in orthopaedic, conditions one must always look for further causes of restricted function: (1) by examining the ability of movement, or elasticity, of the nervous system; and (2) by understanding the effect of the physiological changes of the nervous system caused as a direct result of the injury itself. According to Butler (1991a) the nervous system should be considered as another organ of the body, where a change occurring in part of the system may cause repercussions in the system as a whole. This is an inevitable phenomenon in a continuous tissue tract, and as the peripheral, central and autonomic nervous systems form such continuous tracts they can be considered as a body organ system.

This relatively new concept of ANT is beginning to be applied to neurological practice; a brief overview of its proposed mechanisms and applications is given here, and the reader is referred to the growing literature on this subject.

MOVEMENT OF NEURAL TISSUE

The nervous system is a continuum and can be likened to the letter H in that it joins together all the parts of the body (Butler, 1991a). We can therefore understand how movement in one part of the body can produce either an enhancing or a restricting effect in other parts of the body.

A study in the monkey showed that the addition of dorsiflexion on straight leg raising may either stretch and/or move the nervous system up as far as the cerebellum (Smith, 1956). The spinal cord is moved, and the meninges stretched as far as the sciatic nerve, by passively flexing the neck (Breig, 1978). Breig & Troup (1979) demonstrated the influence of dorsiflexion on the lumbosacral nerve roots. Referring to the upper limb, movement of the wrist has been shown to produce a direct mechanical effect on the nervous system in the upper arm (e.g. McLellan & Swash, 1976).

In 1980, Maitland demonstrated that the position of the head whilst performing the slump test (slump sitting, neck in flexion, straightening knee and dorsiflexing the foot) altered the amount of dorsiflexion achieved and affected the ability to extend the knee. Davidson (1987) demonstrated that, while extending the hip in side lying with the knee flexed, the position of the head alters the amount of hip extension achieved, i.e. 'slump–prone knee bending' (SPKB).

A direct connection has been shown between movement of the nervous system and the symptoms displayed by patients with orthopaedic problems. One of the first to demonstrate the clinical effect was Maitland (1979) while performing the slump test in sitting. Symptoms in an arm were shown by Elvey (1986) to be provoked and/or altered by movement of the contralateral arm or by a straight leg raise (SLR). Sciatic brachialgia syndrome, in which an SLR caused pain in the leg and shoulder, was described by Breig (1979). Many further examples can be seen in the growing literature on this topic.

TREATMENT IN ORTHOPAEDIC PRACTICE

The concept of ANT treatment of orthopaedic injuries has been developed based on previous observations (Elvey, 1986; Butler & Gifford, 1989; Butler, 1991a). Various techniques for examining and treating movement of the nervous system have been devised, using passive neck flexion (Troup, 1981); SLR prone knee bending (Maitland, 1979; Davidson, 1987); SPKB (Davidson, 1987); and the upper limb tension test (ULTT) 1 (Elvey, 1986; Butler, 1991a). Modification of the ULTT 1 was suggested by Yaxley & Jull (1991); ULTT 2 and 3 were developed by Butler & Gifford (1989) and by Butler (1991a). All these tests, or treatments, emphasise movement of a certain nerve, e.g. ULTT 1 examines the median nerve (see 'Case history').

A relationship has been observed between the appearance of symptoms in the ULTT and those of Colles' fracture (Young & Bell, 1991), tennis elbow (Yaxley & Jull, 1993) and whiplash injury (Quintner, 1989). Positive signs of neural tension have also been observed in asymptomatic sportsmen, e.g. swimmers (Heighway & Monteith, 1991).

Each nerve can be moved according to its anatomical pathway and this fact will lead to further tests and treatments, according to the individual nerves. It has been established that the effect of the examination may be altered according to the position of the person being tested and whether it is performed passively or actively (Butler, 1991a). It should be remembered that physiological changes in the nerve, such as occur in diabetic patients, may also affect the result (Shacklock, 1995b).

PROPOSED EXPLANATION OF THE ANT PHENOMENON

Examples of movement of the nervous system can be observed in peripheral nerves and the spinal cord. Shortening of the ulnar nerve, and elongation of the radial and median nerves, occurs on flexing the elbow. The bed of the median nerve is 20% longer when the elbow and wrist are extended than when they are flexed (Millesi, 1986). The spinal canal is 5–9 cm longer in flexion than in extension of the spine (Breig, 1978; Louis, 1981).

The nervous system possesses an adaptive mechanism of movement and, according to Butler (1991a), this is achieved by:
1. The presence of excess length in the nervous system (Breig, 1978; Millesi, 1986).
2. The nerve moving in relation to the tissue surrounding it (e.g. the posterior interosseous branch of the radial nerve moves within the supinator muscle) or movement within the nerve itself when the fascicles move against the external epineurium and each fascicle moves against its neighbour (Butler, 1991a).

As already stated, the connection between movement of the nervous system and symptoms demonstrated by orthopaedic patients can be explained by the fact that the nervous system may be damaged by physical injury, endangering the neural and connective tissues. The pathology caused may be extra- and/or intraneural. Normally the nerve is situated in contact with various tissues, named by Butler (1989) as mechanical interfaces ,and defined as 'that tissue or material adjacent to the nervous system that can move independently to the system'. The mechanical interfaces may be pathological features, such as haemorrhage, oedema or scar tissue, or plaster casts, and perhaps muscle in spasticity (suggestion of the author EP).

The injury may be to the blood supply of the nerve, to the nerve itself or to the axoplasmic flow. The nervous system consumes 20% of the oxygen in the arterial circulation and this is required for impulse conduction (Dommisse, 1994). An increase of 8% of the normal length of a nerve decreases the blood flow and an increase of 15% in nerve length will cause complete occlusion of the blood supply (Ogata & Naito, 1986). The blood vessels in the spinal cord and of the peripheral nerves possess extra length and anatomical organisation affording both movement and normal blood flow (Breig, 1978).

The axoplasmic flow includes anti- and retrograde movement of substances, and their function and importance are described by Butler (1991b). Changes in the flow are expressed by trophic changes in the target tissue, damage to the neurone and its axon and in the action potential of the nerve. It was found, in rabbits, that axoplasmic flow was affected by very low pressures (Shacklock, 1995a,b), so it may be possible that spasticity could have an effect, though as yet there is no proof. Furthermore, mobilisation of the nervous system may influence axonal transport (Shacklock, 1995a, b).

As the nervous system is a continuum, symptoms may develop in various areas distant from the area of injury (Butler, 1991a). This fact has been discussed in many sources as the 'double crush' phenomenon (appearance of symptoms in a part of the body, or nervous system, distant from the original injury and symptoms), a concept first described by Upton & McComas (1973). The concept was further developed by Butler (1991a) who described the 'multi crush syndrome' and its many causes. The general orthopaedic therapeutic conclusion is that careful and exact movement in one area of the body can influence the symptoms in other areas, and therefore the movement is in itself therapy.

NEURAL TENSION IN NEUROLOGICAL DISORDERS

It appears that the effect of movement of the nervous system on various orthopaedic conditions may also apply to injuries of the CNS, according to Davies (1994), to the author's (EP) clinical experience and to Simionato et al. (1988), who described neural tension signs in Guillain–Barré syndrome.

When examining patients with head injuries, hemiplegia, incomplete spinal cord injuries or cerebral palsy, it can be observed frequently that the range of motion in one part of the body is altered by passive movement of another part distant from the original movement (Davies, 1994).

Clinical experience shows that lifting the head of a person with cerebral palsy increases the range of movement in SLR. With hemiplegic patients, passive SLR may affect the movement of the plegic shoulder, movement of the head affects the range of movement of the shoulder or elbow, and performing a ULTT 1 on the unaffected arm can affect movement and pain of the plegic arm. It has also been observed clinically (by the author EP in as yet unpublished research) that hip flexion in SLR is affected by hip extension in SPKB and vice versa. The slump test technique reduces tension in the involved upper extremity and may cause retraction of the scapula in the patient with hemiparesis (Davies, 1994). Davies also suggests using abduction of the hip in the slump technique in cases of adductor spasticity.

Davies (1994) recommended including the techniques of ANT within holistic treatment, giving an example of the positive effects of treatment in head-injured persons even 10 years after injury. The physiotherapist must, therefore, remember that treatment by movements means not only moving joints or muscles, or inhibiting or facilitating tone, but also moving the nervous system. It is therefore suggested that the physiotherapist include: (1) movement of a part distal to all movements performed during treatment; and (2) movement of the trunk, which enhances movement of the nervous system and affects the sympathetic chain (Breig, 1978; Butler, 1991a; Davies, 1994).

Where does treatment begin? Physiotherapy is symptomatic and, therefore, carefully selected movements of different parts of the body and their effect on the

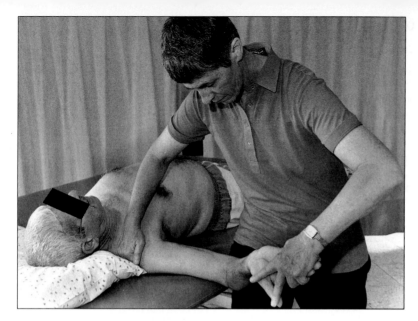

Figure 23.1 Upper limb tension test (ULTT) 1. Abduction of glenohumeral joint to 90-100°, extension of wrist and fingers, supination of forearm, lateral rotation of glenohumeral joint and elbow extension. Restriction of finger, wrist and elbow extension is demonstrated.

functional ability of the patient must be observed. The variety of available movements is very large, and the effect is varied and individual to each patient. For example, while performing ULTT 1 on a plegic arm, a similar movement of the other arm may improve movement of the affected arm in some hemiplegics, whilst in others it may increase pain and restrict movement (Davies, 1994).

When does treatment begin? In order to preserve free mobility of the joints, muscles and nervous system, and knowing that axoplasmic flow is influenced by movement, treatment should start as early as possible (Davies, 1994).

Treatment of the patient with a neurological condition should not be solely passive and local. The integration of ANT into general treatment and active function is desirable. Each improvement in range gained passively needs to be integrated immediately into the patient's active control and function, depending on the degree of damage (Davies, 1994). If no active ability exists, passive techniques contribute greatly to the patient's wellbeing and help to prevent contractures.

CASE HISTORY

HG, an active 64-year-old man with right hemiparesis following CVA, complained of difficulty in grasping objects with his paretic hand or with both hands. He also did not extend his right hip sufficiently when standing or walking. The aim of treatment was to improve his ability to drink from a cup, held in both hands, whilst sitting and standing.

As part of HG's holistic care, some therapeutic components of ANT were included. Treatment possibilities were many, and started with movements of the trunk and scapula. This was followed by performing ULTT 1 in lying (Figure 23.1). The sequence of ULTT 1 is: abduction of the arm to between 90° and 100°, wrist and finger extension,

supination, external rotation of the arm, careful extension of the elbow and, if achievable, lateral flexion of the neck towards the contralateral side (Butler, 1991a). This test produced tension, causing restriction of wrist, fingers and elbow extension, and HG complained of slight pain.

Other movements of the body that might alter these restrictions and pain were then sought. Of the many possibilities, ULTT 1 of the opposite limb was chosen and was found to reduce the restriction and pain in the plegic arm. If symptoms had been increased by this manoeuvre, it would not have been repeated. Attempts were also made to find movements in other limbs (such as SLR) that might alter the restriction and relieve the pain. (If symptoms are worsened by ANT tests of the upper limb, focus should be centred on performing pain- and tension-free controlled movements of the paretic limb, or side flexion of the neck after releasing the affected limb.)

Since the ULTT 1 on the contralateral arm improved symptoms in HG, this was followed by straightening the elbow and wrist of the paretic arm. Passive movements of the wrist were performed whilst the elbow was flexed, as well as passive movements of the elbow whilst the wrist was released from tension. Active movements followed immediately after the passive movements, e.g. straightening the elbow whilst maintaining extension of the wrist.

Another treatment possibility is performing ULTT 3 and this was used on HG. The sequence of this test, according to Butler (1991a) is: extension of wrist and fingers, supination and flexion of the elbow, external rotation of the arm, depression of the shoulder girdle, abduction of the arm and, if attainable, lateral flexion of the neck towards the contralateral side. This should be followed immediately by active movements.

Attention was then paid to the restricted extension of the hip joint. Here, also, many possibilities of treatment were available, all beginning with movements of the

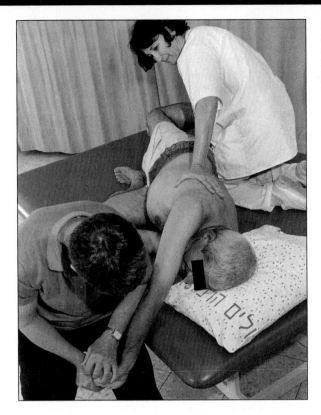

Figure 23.2 Movement of the trunk and affected upper extremity (supination and extension of the wrist and fingers) whilst maintaining 'slump-prone knee bend'. SPKB involves side lying with lower hip and knee fully flexed, upper hip extended and upper knee flexed.

trunk. Extending the affected hip in side lying (SPKB) was chosen for HG, with both knees flexed. The passive movements were again followed immediately by active extension of the hip. Still in side lying, the patient rotated his upper trunk towards the bed, enabling increased hip extension, extended his arm diagonally downwards, while the therapist added supination and extension of the wrist and fingers and performed various assisted active movements (Figure 23.2). Thus, a combination of the two functional aims of the treatment could be attained. The treatment ended with a re-evaluation of the function. The patient was encouraged to perform suitable movements at home.

PRECAUTIONS WITH ANT TREATMENT

1. Some neurological patients will have a history of back pain and symptoms may still be present; the therapist must therefore always perform neurological examinations and treatments with the greatest caution and care (Butler & Gifford, 1989).
2. All movement and treatment progress must be performed slowly as the nervous system is delicate, and in certain areas superficial (Butler & Gifford, 1989).
3. Joints must be in normal alignment during each movement.
4. Attention must be given to the effect of every movement on the body as a whole.
5. Special care should be taken when treating unconscious patients or those without sensation (Davies, 1994).

6. Pain of neural origin can appear some hours after the nerve has been irritated.
7. Clinical experience shows that, despite the resistance to movement that may be felt by the therapist, the patient may not feel any discomfort or limitation; in this instance, the therapist must treat according to the symptoms he or she feels (Butler & Gifford, 1989; Davies, 1994).
8. It has been demonstrated that frequent repetition of SLR in a healthy person can give rise to symptoms such as headache, nausea and 'floating'; a possible explanation may be that SLR moves the sympathetic chain (Breig, 1978).
9. The pathomechanical and pathophysiological aspects of both symptoms and treatment must be considered (Shacklock, 1995a,b).

CONCLUSION

As yet, there is no scientific research or direct proof of the effect of using ANT techniques in neurological treatments. There is also insufficient knowledge available to explain the physiological effect of the treatment. Clinical experience in this field is growing, and research is required to underpin its use and develop it further.

The therapist must remember that treatment of the neurological patient is holistic, and that the use of ANT techniques is only one part of the integral treatment. In the opinion of the author (EP), ANT techniques can be successfully integrated within other treatment concepts outlined in Chapter 22.

SECTION TWO: MUSCLE IMBALANCE IN NEUROLOGICAL CONDITIONS

Muscle imbalance is said to occur when relative changes in muscle length and recruitment patterns take place between synergists and between antagonists. The ratio of muscle strength and flexibility alters, and functional consequences include abnormal movement patterns, pain and instability.

The concept of muscle imbalance is not new but there has been a recent resurgence of interest amongst orthopaedic physiotherapists. This is a welcome addition to orthopaedic practice which was tending to focus on skeletal mobilisation techniques, with little consideration for the role of the musculature in dysfunction and restoration of normal function. Early clinical observations of muscle imbalance were made in patients with polio, in whom it was recognised that functional recovery largely depended on maintaining joints in a neutral position to prevent changes in muscle length (e.g. Kendall & Kendall, 1938).

Theories of muscle imbalance in orthopaedic conditions have been developed over the last two decades by several authors including Janda, Sahrmann, Jull and Richardson (see below for references). Their work is mainly concerned with muscle function in relation to stabilisation of joints of the lumbar spine. Most of the research has focused on the scientific basis of the theoretical concept, which is an important first step. Despite the popularity of educational courses on muscle imbalance and use of the analysis and correction techniques, there is no scientific evidence of their effectiveness. That is not to say that the techniques do not work or should not be used, but research of treatment outcome is urgently needed. There is also a paucity of literature on the subject; most is published in conference proceedings and book chapters which are not easily accessible on literature searches. More research, and publication in scientific and professional journals, would help to rectify this situation.

The present chapter will give a brief introduction to this emerging field by presenting overviews of the theories of muscle imbalance and the techniques for its correction.

THEORETICAL BASIS OF MUSCLE IMBALANCE

Since the basic concept of muscle imbalance relates to changes in muscle length, the theories describe how length changes alter different aspects of muscle function. The three main theories are concerned with weakness due to stretch and position, and altered recruitment. The classification of muscle types is also an important consideration when discussing these theories, since the type of muscle determines its tendency to shorten or lengthen under stress.

FUNCTIONAL CLASSIFICATION OF MUSCLE TYPES

Two classification systems for describing the function of muscles in relation to muscle imbalance were discussed by

Norris (1995a). They both relate to the physiological and biochemical properties of muscles, which are largely determined by the fibre-type composition (see Chapter 1 for details of muscle fibre types). Norris (1995a) described Janda's classification of muscles into postural and phasic types. It is misleading to use this classification since Janda developed a unique meaning for the terms which does not fit in with the more conventional way of describing postural and phasic muscles in relation to their fibre-type characteristics. It may therefore be more appropriate to use Janda's functional description of the tendency of the muscles to tighten or lengthen.

As Richardson (1992) summarised, different relationships between muscle groups are required to maintain balance to support and protect joints. These involve balance between agonists and antagonists, synergists (muscles involved in the same action to move and stabilise a joint), and between muscles supporting and moving adjacent body segments. In the two classifications described below, the tighten/lengthen categorisation relates to agonists and antagonists, whilst the second classification relates to synergists, describing two types (movement and stability synergists).

Tendency to Shorten or Lengthen

The behaviour of muscle types has been characterised in relation to muscle imbalance syndromes by their tendency to shorten or lengthen (Jull & Janda, 1987). Muscles that tend to tighten also tend to be stronger, develop painful trigger points, have a lower recruitment threshold and to be biarticular. Conversely, the muscles that tend to lengthen also tend to be inhibited and weaker in inner range, and to be uniarticular.

Examples of trunk muscles prone to tightening include erector spinae, iliopsoas and quadratus lumborum, while those prone to lengthening include the gluteii. Muscles of the lower limb that tend to tighten are tensor fascia lata, rectus femoris, hamstrings and gastrocnemius. Muscles of the lower limb that lengthen include quadriceps (the three vastii), tibialis anterior and the peronei. In the upper limb, muscles that tighten include the limb flexors, pectoralis major and upper trapezius, and those that lengthen include the limb extensors, serratus anterior and lower trapezius (Jull & Janda, 1987).

Movement and Stability Synergists

This classification of muscles in relation to imbalance takes into account the anatomical, biomechanical, physiological and biochemical properties of the muscles, and the motor control patterns in which they are involved. Richardson (1992) focused on synergistic muscles since they are commonly involved in imbalance syndromes, i.e. where static postures need to be held during work or leisure activities or where dynamic tasks are continually repeated.

The classification is similar to that of the tighten/lengthen categorisation in that stability synergists tend to equate to lengthened muscles and movement synergists to shortened muscles. Problems with terminology arise if the terms postural and phasic muscles are used, as the two systems no longer appear to concur due to Janda's altered meaning of the words. Some differences which occur include tensor fascia lata, hamstrings and gastrocnemius, which are movement synergists in one classification (Richardson, 1992) and postural muscles in the other (Jull & Janda, 1987). Inconsistencies do not occur so much if the tighten/ lengthen terms are used and it may help to bear this in mind when reading any literature by Janda or any reviews which mention this classification (e.g. Norris, 1995a).

There is some experimental evidence to support the stability/movement classification in normally functioning muscles, in that rapid movements which mainly involve type II muscle fibres have been shown to favour muscles in the movement synergist category. Examples include: rapid knee extension involving more rectus femoris activity than vastii activity (Richardson & Bullock, 1986); rapid ankle plantarflexion producing greater activity and a training effect in gastrocnemius rather than soleus (Ng & Richardson, 1990); rapid trunk flexion involving greater activity of rectus abdominis than the oblique abdominal muscles (Thorstensson et al., 1985; Wohlfahrt et al., 1993); and, in cyclists, lengthening and reduced activity of gluteus maximus (Richardson & Sims, 1991).

Stability synergists tend to be uniarticular, deep, have extensive aponeuroses rather than long tendons and have properties of predominantly type I fibres. In muscle imbalance syndromes, Richardson (1992) suggested that the movement synergists take over the stability role, as the stability synergists are activated less than the movement synergists.

Since the stability synergists are thought to be used less in muscle imbalance syndromes, they tend to lengthen and the reduction in their tonic activity and increase in phasic activity causes loss of endurance. The movement synergists become more active and increase their tonic activity to take over the stabilising role of the joint.

The stability/movement classification proposed by Richardson (1992) therefore provides a clear means of describing synergistic muscle types in the normal situation, as well as a basis for explaining the development of muscle imbalance between synergists.

The characteristics of the two functional classification types of muscle involved in imbalance syndromes are summarised in Table 23.1. The terminology problem is recognised in the field of muscle imbalance and the terms multijoint (biarticular) *versus* monoarticular tend to be used (Richardson & Jull, personal communication) but this has not yet reached the literature.

CAUSES OF MUSCLE IMBALANCE

Several factors have been suggested as causes of muscle imbalance, based on clinical observation (reviewed by Norris, 1995a). Habitual poor posture and alignment problems have been suggested as a major cause of muscle imbalance (Sahrmann, 1987). Pain may also cause postures that reduce pain but lead to imbalance and abnormal alignment. Joint pathology can cause reflex inhibition of muscle activity, which tends to inhibit selectively certain muscles associated with a joint (Stokes & Young, 1984) and might therefore lead to imbalance. Muscle imbalance has been suggested as a cause of injury (Grace, 1985). Richardson (1992) proposed that modern lifestyle activities at work and in sport may lead to muscles changing their activation pattern and thus functional role, therefore leading to imbalance. Clearly, any of these causal factors can become involved in a vicious cycle in which it may not be possible to state which came first, i.e. imbalance, altered length or recruitment, or injury.

PHYSIOLOGICAL CONSEQUENCES OF ALTERED MUSCLE LENGTH

The strength and excitability of a muscle alter with changes in length, and three theories explain these functional adaptations which all relate to Sahrmann's 1987 suggestion of 'faulty static [structural length] and/or dynamic [contractile strength or pattern of recruitment]

Classification of muscle types according to their functional characteristics in relation to muscle imbalance syndromes	
Shorten/Tighten	**Lengthen**
Stronger in inner range	Weaker in inner range
Movement synergist	Stability synergist
Increased tonic activity	Reduced tonic activity
Low recruitment threshold	High recruitment threshold
Biarticular/multijoint	Monoarticular

Table 23.1 Classification of muscle types according to their functional characteristics in relation to muscle imbalance syndromes.

properties of muscle that alter the ideal relationship between antagonists and synergist.' Pain and reduced range of movement (ROM) are other consequences of muscle shortening. Gossman et al. (1982) and Norris (1995a) reviewed the literature on length-associated changes in muscle and discussed their clinical implications, some of which are outlined briefly here.

Stretch Weakness Theory
The stretch weakness theory was put forward by the Kendalls and based on their clinical observations (Kendall et al., 1993). It refers to muscles that lengthen when maintained in an elongated position, beyond their normal resting length, and become weak in inner range. This theory is supported by experimental evidence (Williams & Goldspink, 1978; Goldspink & Williams, 1990).

Positional Weakness Theory
The effect of immobilising muscles in lengthened and shortened positions on their anatomical structure and function were demonstrated in animal studies by Williams & Goldspink (1978). The lengthened muscles gained sarcomeres and shortened muscles lost sarcomeres, with normal sarcomere numbers being restored when immobilisation was discontinued.

The effects of these adaptations on physiological function is to cause a shift in the length–tension relationship. In lengthened muscles, the curve is shifted to the right, so that peak tension occurs at a longer length than normal (in the position in which it has been immobilised). Also, because the muscle is longer and has a greater mechanical advantage, its absolute peak tension is greater than that of a muscle of normal length (Figure 23.3). In the shortened muscle, the curve is shifted to the left of normal, giving a lower peak tension.

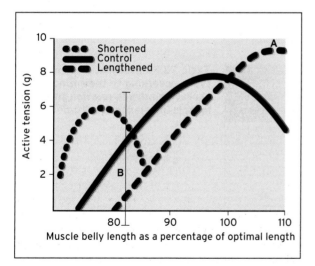

Figure 23.3 Changes in the length-tension curve for muscles immobilised in lengthened and shortened positions. (Redrawn from Norris, 1995a (adapted from Gossman et al., 1982), with permission.)

Lengthened muscles are therefore stronger than normal, and short muscles weaker than normal, when tested at their optimal lengths, which can be achieved under laboratory conditions. The optimal length of a lengthened muscle (Point A in Figure 23.3) can produce a peak tension which is up to 35% greater than that of a muscle of normal length (Williams & Goldspink, 1978). However, muscles are clinically tested in inner range which is approximately just over 80% of the optimal length for a muscle of normal length (Point B in Figure 23.3). At this point of the range, optimal length is not achieved for any length of muscle and favours greatest tension for the shortened muscle. This is because, in inner range, the myofilaments of the lengthened muscle would overlap too much to allow enough cross-bridge formation to produce as much force as the normal length or short muscle, in which more cross-bridges would form.

Under clinical conditions, therefore, lengthened muscles appear weaker than short muscles, as testing is performed in inner or middle range. Isometric manual muscle testing is therefore more appropriate for detecting this positional weakness than methods aimed at measuring total strength, which are less relevant for this type of dysfunction.

Preferential Recruitment Theory
The suggestion that shortened muscles are recruited first in a movement pattern was based on the clinical observations of Sahrmann (1987). It was thought that this biased recruitment led to the short muscle becoming stronger, thus determining alignment. Furthermore, selective recruitment of short muscles would cause reciprocal inhibition of the lengthened antagonistic muscles. This theory lends itself to confirmation by scientific investigation by electromyography (EMG), and such a study showed reduced activation of the lengthened gluteus maximus in cyclists (Richardson & Sims, 1991).

This theory fits in with the stability/movement synergist theory in which Richardson (1992) described altered recruitment of shortened movement synergists which take on a stabilising role. It also concurs with the length theory and it is not possible to say which change comes first.

It has been suggested that muscle imbalance may occur due to a difference existing in the motor control mechanism of muscles that tend to tighten and those that lengthen and become weak (Jull & Janda, 1987). It was further suggested that this concept is supported by the typical patterns of spasticity seen with CNS damage. For example, in hemiplegia, the patterns of shortening are similar to those in musculoskeletal conditions but are more extreme due to the spasticity.

Pain Associated with Tightened Muscles
Painful trigger points, which are areas of hypersensitive tissue, can occur in shortened muscles (Travell & Simons, 1983). There is deep tenderness and increased tone which is palpable.

Changes in Range of Joint Motion

Short muscles will limit the ROM of a joint and lengthened muscles will allow excessive motion. It is clear that neither of these situations is desirable.

ASSESSMENT OF MUSCLE IMBALANCE

Aspects of function which should be included in assessment are postural alignment, muscle length, strength and holding capacity, and movement patterns (Norris, 1995a). Analysis of muscle imbalance deals with the peripheral aspects of motor control.

POSTURAL ALIGNMENT

Examination of posture provides information on the resting position of muscles. Posture in standing is assessed using a plumbline which should pass through certain anatomical landmarks, and deviations from this indicate altered alignment. In relation to orthopaedic conditions of the spine, four abnormal posture types have been identified (Kendall *et al.*, 1993; Norris, 1995a). Assessment of standing posture will not always be possible in the neurological patient but alignment of body segments in sitting and lying can still be examined.

MUSCLE LENGTH

Muscle length tests are performed to determine their relative lengthening or shortening. Examples of length testing of muscles of the lumbar spine and pelvic girdle can be seen in Jull & Janda (1987), Richardson (1992) and Norris (1995a). Muscle length tests are described in detail for all areas of the body by Kendall *et al.*, (1993). Examples around the pelvic girdle, which are described in the references given above, include hip flexor tightness using the Thomas test and hamstring tightness using the SLR.

MUSCLE STRENGTH

As explained above, absolute strength is not relevant to the ability to generate and maintain force in different parts of the functional range of motion. It is therefore more appropriate to determine the force required to move the limbs and trunk rather than that required to move an external resistance applied during strength testing. Graded strength-testing regimens, which involve using parts of the body as the load, have therefore been developed for different muscles groups, e.g. trunk muscle strength using a trunk curl with grades of increasing difficulty, or a leg lowering test to see if posterior pelvic tilt can be maintained throughout the range (Kendall *et al.*, 1993; Jull & Richardson, 1994; Norris, 1995a).

HOLDING CAPACITY

The ability of antigravity muscles (postural muscles in the traditional sense and stability synergists) to maintain low force isometric contractions is vital to their functional requirements. This ability can be tested in the usual muscle testing positions in the middle or inner range, by asking the subject to hold the contraction. It is not the total time of static hold that is of interest, but the length of time the contraction is held without jerky (phasic) movements occurring (Richardson, 1992).

MOVEMENT PATTERNS

Muscle imbalance leads to abnormal movement patterns in which a functional activity may be achieved and be apparently normal but compensatory strategies and 'trick movements' may have been used (Jull & Janda, 1987; Kendall *et al.*, 1993). Analysis of functional movement patterns is necessary to detect these abnormalities so that treatment can be planned for their correction.

CORRECTION OF MUSCLE IMBALANCE

The priority in restoring muscle balance is not to strengthen but to normalise activation patterns (Richardson, 1992) and muscle length (Norris, 1995a). Only when these have been achieved should strengthening be considered. Postural correction and reduction of repetitive work are important but the following more specific techniques can be used.

RETRAINING MUSCLE ACTIVATION

Muscle activation patterns could be altered by increasing tonic input to the stability synergists or by reducing tonic input to the movement synergists. Richardson (1992) explained that the former method was thought to be more effective clinically and described strategies for retraining tonic activity. The first step is to isolate the stability synergist so that the movement synergist is not contracting.

Tonic activity to re-educate slow-twitch muscle fibre function can be achieved by voluntary exercise or electrical stimulation. Richardson (1992) suggested voluntary activity involving low force (20–30% of maximum voluntary contraction), sustained contractions of about 10 seconds each. Presumably rest periods, numbers of repetitions and frequency of exercise have yet to be researched but would also depend on the individual. Low-frequency electrical stimulation can be used to change the muscle fibre properties but care must be taken as this can weaken muscle, and further research is required to establish appropriate frequency patterns (see Chapter 24).

RESTORATION OF MUSCLE LENGTH

Techniques for restoring muscle length were described by Kendall *et al.* (1993). Briefly, shortened muscles can be lengthened using standard manual stretching or proprioceptive neuromuscular facilitation (PNF) techniques (see Chapter 24). Lengthened muscles can be shortened by exercising them using low-load contractions held for about 10 seconds, in the shortened, inner range or by splinting them in this position (Kendall *et al.*, 1993).

Norris (1995a) discussed the problems of muscle imbalance around the lumbar spine and techniques for correcting length changes in specific muscle groups.

RESTORING STABILITY

The functional interaction between synergists is restored by gradually increasing loads and speed (Richardson, 1992). Exercise programmes have been developed to improve the stability of the lumbar spine (Sahrmann, 1983; Jull & Richardson, 1994; Norris, 1995b). The principles of restoring stability fall into four stages which were summarised by Norris (1995b) and involve: re-education of stabilising muscles; exercise progressions for static stabilisation; exercise progressions for dynamic stabilisation; and occupational/activity-specific stabilisation. Jull & Richardson (1994) described the use of feedback devices to aid in the isolation of specific muscles for assessment and retraining purposes.

MUSCLE IMBALANCE IN NEUROLOGICAL CONDITIONS

Little has been published on the application of the muscle imbalance concept to neurology but it is certainly being used clinically in many centres. Sahrmann (1987) gave an example of a muscle imbalance syndrome in hemiplegia, involving the tightness of the iliotibial band (ITB). The posture adopted by the paretic lower limb, of hip abduction and medial rotation with knee extension, favours the shortened ITB.

The use of a cycle ergometer and EMG biofeedback was proposed for correction of muscle imbalance in stroke patients (Brown & DeBacher, 1987). Treatment involved retraining of activation of antagonistic muscle groups of the hemiplegic limb, as well as reciprocal exercise with some symmetry between the two limbs.

Muscle imbalance techniques developed for assessment and treatment of orthopaedic conditions can be applied to patients with neurological conditions but studies are required to demonstrate their effectiveness and produce guidelines for their appropriate use in neurological patients.

SUMMARY

The potential impact of the muscle imbalance concept for improving the effectiveness of physiotherapy appears to be substantial but its future depends on research to establish its place in clinical practice. Collaborative research between physiotherapists, physiologists and biomechanical engineers should prove fruitful in elucidating the theory, producing guidelines for assessment and treatment, and providing evidence of the effectiveness of corrective techniques. Neurological physiotherapists need to take part in research in this area so that application of the concept to neurological patients is applied and evaluated appropriately.

Acknowledgements
The author (MS) wishes to thank Dr Carolyn Richardson (Senior Lecturer) and Gwendolen Jull (Associate Professor) of the Department of Physiotherapy, University of Queensland, for their helpful comments on this section of the chapter. The author's understanding of muscle imbalance was clarified by attending a course by Mark Camerford held at the Royal Hospital for Neuro-disability, Putney, London.

REFERENCES

Section One:

Breig A, Troup JDC. Biomechanical considerations in the SLR test. *Spine* 1979, **4**:242-250.

Butler D. Adverse mechanical tension in the nervous system: a model for assessment and treatment. *Aust J Physiother* 1989, **35**:227-238.

Butler D. *Mobilisation of the nervous system*. Melbourne, Australia: Churchill Livingstone; 1991a.

Butler D. Axoplasmic flow and manipulative physiotherapy. In: *Proceedings of 7th Biennial Conference of Manipulative Physiotherapists Association*. Australia, New South Wales; 1991b:206-213.

Butler D, Gifford L. The concept of adverse mechanical tension in the nervous system, *Physiother* 1989, **75**:622-636 .

Davidson S. Prone knee bend: an investigation into the effect of cervical flexion and extension. In: Dalziell RA,Snowcill JC, eds. *Proceedings of the Manipulative Therapist Association of Australia 5th. Biennial Conference*. Melbourne; 1987:235-246.

Davies PM. *Starting again*. London: Springer Verlag; 1994:121-179.

Dommisse GF. The blood supply of the spinal cord. In: Boyling JD, Palastanga N, eds. *Grieve's modern manual therapy - the vertebral column, 2nd edition*. London: Churchill Livingstone; 1994:3-20.

Elvey RL. Treatment of arm pain associated with abnormal brachial plexus tension. *Aust J Physiother* 1986, **32**:225-230.

Heighway S, Monteith G. Swimmers shoulder: incidence of upper limb neural tension signs in swimmers. *Aust J Physiother* 1991, **37**:52.

Louis R. Vertebroradicular and vertebromedullar dynamics. *Anat Clin* 1981, **3**:1-11.

Maitland GD. Movement of pain sensitive structures in the vertebral canal in a group of physiotherapy students. South Af *J Physiother* 1980, **36**:4-12.

Maitland GD. Negative disc exploration: practical canal signs. *Aust J Physiother* 1979, **25**:129-134.

Maitland GD. *Vertebral manipulation, 5th edition*. London: Butterworths; 1986.

McLellan DL, Swash M. Longitudinal sliding of the median nerve during movements of the upper limb. *J Neuro Neurosurg Psych* 1976, **39**:556-570.

Millesi H. The nerve gap: theory and clinical practice. *Hand Clinics* 1986, **4**:651-663.

Ogata K, Naito M. Blood flow of peripheral nerve effects of dissection, stretching and compression. *J Hand Surg* 1986, **11**(b):10-14.

Quintner TI. A study of upper limb pain and paraesthesia following neck injury in motor vehicle accidents: assessment of the brachial plexus tension test of Elvey. *Br J Rheum* 1989, **28**:528-533.

Shacklock M. Neurodynamics. *Physiother* 1995a, **81**:9-16.

Shacklock M. Clinical application of neurodynamic. In: Shacklock M. *Moving in on pain*. Australia: Butterworth Heineman; 1995b.

Simionato R, Stiller K, Butler D. Neural tension signs in guillain barre syndrome: two case reports. *Aust J Physiother* 1988, **34**:257-259.

Smith CG. Changes in length and posture of the segments of the spinal cord with changes in posture in the monkey. *Radiol* 1956, **66**:259-265.

Troup JDG. Straight leg raising (SLR) and the qualifying tests for increased root tension. *Spine* 1981, **6**:526-527.

Upton ARM, McComas AJ. The double crush in nerve entrapmentsyndromes. *Lancet* 1973, **2**:359-362.

Wohlfahrt DA, Jull GA, Richardson CA. The relationship between the dynamic and static function of the abdominal muscles. *Aust J Physiother* 1993, **39**:9-15.

Yaxley GA, Jull GA. A modified upper limb tension test: an investigation of responses in normal subjects. *Aust J Physiother* 1991, **37**:143-152.

Yaxley GA, Jull G. Adverse tension in the neural system. a preliminary study of tennis elbow. *Aust J Physiother* 1993, **39**:15-22.

Young L, Bell A. The upper limb tension test response in a group of post colles fracture patients. In: *Proceedings of 7th Biennial Conference of Manipulative Therapists Association*. Australia, New South Wales; 1991: 226-231.

Section Two:

Brown DA, DeBacher GA. Bicycle ergometer and electromyographic feedback for treatment of muscle imbalance in patients with spastic hemiparesis. *Phys Ther* 1987, **67**:1715-1719.

Goldspink G, Williams PE. Muscle fibre and connective tissue changes associated with use and disuse. In: Ada L, Canning C, eds. *Key issues in neurological physiotherapy*. Oxford: Butterworth Heinemann; 1990: 197-218.

Gossman MR, Sahrmann SA, Rose SJ. Review of length-associated changes in muscle: experimental evidence and clinical implication. *Phys Ther* 1982, **62**:1799-1808.

Grace TG. Muscle imbalance and extremity injury: a perplexing relationship. *Sport Med* 1985, **2**:77-82.

Jull GA, Janda V. Muscles and motor control in low back pain: assessment and management. In: Twomey L & Taylor JR, eds. *Physical therapy of the low back, 1st edition*. Edinburgh: Churchill Livingstone; 1987:253-278.

Jull GA, Richardson CA. Rehabilitation of active stabilisation of the lumbar spine. In: Twomey L & Taylor JR, eds. *Physical therapy of the low back, 2nd edition*. Edinburgh: Churchill Livingstone; 1994:251-273.

Kendall HO, Kendall FP. Care during the recovery period in paralytic poliomyelitis. *Pub Health Bull* 1938, **242**:1-9.

Kendall FP, Kendall McCreary E & Provance PG. *Muscles, testing and function, 4th edition*. Baltimore: Williams & Wilkins; 1993.

Ng G, Richardson CA. The effects of training triceps surae using progressive speed loading. *Physiother Prac* 1990, **6**:77-84.

Norris CM. Spinal stabilisation: 4. Muscle imbalance and the low back. *Physiother* 1995a, **81**:127-138.

Norris CM. Spinal stabilisation: 5. An exercise programme to enhance lumbar stabilisation. *Physiother* 1995b, **81**: 138-145.

Richardson CA. Muscle imbalance: principles of treatment and assessment. In: *Proceedings of the New Zealand Society for Physiotherapists Challenges Conference*. New Zealand, Christchurch; 1992:127-138.

Richardson CA, Bullock MI. Changes in muscle activity during fast, alternating flexion-extension movements of the knee. *J Rehab Med* 1986, **18**:51-58.

Richardson CA, Sims K. An inner range holding contraction. An objective measure of stabilising function of an antigravity muscle. In: *Proceedings of the World Confederation for Physical Therapy, 11th International Congress*. London; 1991:829-831.

Sahrmann S. A program for correction of muscular imbalance and mechanical imbalance. *Clin Manage* 1983, **3**:23-28 .

Sahrmann S. Muscle imbalances in the orthopaedic and neurological patient.In: *Proceedings of the 10th International Congress of the world Confederation of Physical Therapy*. Australia, Sydney; 1987:836-841.

Stokes M, Young A. The contribution of reflex inhibition to arthrogenous muscle weakness. *Clin Sci* 1984, **67**:1-14.

Thorstensson A, Oddsson L, Carlson HJ. Motor control oc voluntary trunk movements in standing. *Acta Physiol Scand* 1985, **125**:309-321.

Travell JG, Simons DG. *Myofascial pain and dysfunction*. Baltimore: Williams & Wilkins; 1983.

Williams PE, Goldspink G. Changes in sarcomere length and physioloigcal properties in immobilized muscle. *J Anat* 1978, **127**:459-468.

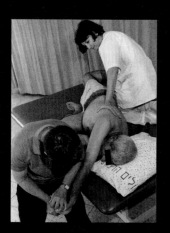

24 J Jackson

SPECIFIC TREATMENT TECHNIQUES

CHAPTER OUTLINE

- **Facilitation**
- **Inhibition**
- **Exercise and movement**

- **Electrical stimulation techniques**
- **Other techniques**

INTRODUCTION

A huge variety of techniques are employed by physiotherapists working in neurological rehabilitation. When examining treatment approaches from different philosophical backgrounds, it is apparent that similar techniques may be utilised within them (see Chapter 22). A technique can be defined as a 'means of achieving one's purpose, especially skillfully' (*Concise Oxford Dictionary*). With this definition in mind it is important to consider to what purpose different techniques are employed and that, in order to be effective, the technique must be appropriate to help meet the treatment goals.

This chapter illustrates the diversity of the techniques used by physiotherapists. It is clear that there is a wealth of research supporting the use of some techniques and a great lack of scientific evidence to justify the use of others. Many techniques rely on anecdotal evidence to support their use. In this chapter a variety of techniques are reviewed and the evidence available to support their use is considered. Some of the work cited is fairly old and that reflects the need for more research in the field of specific treatment techniques.

The chapter is divided into sections; some techniques have mixed effects such that they could be included in more than one section. They will be found in the section which reflects their main usage, with the exception of ice and passive stretching, which will be considered in both the sections on facilitation and inhibition. The section on inhibition mentions techniques used to reduce spasticity

but the specific management of muscle tone is dealt with in Chapter 25. This is not intended as a recipe-type guide to treatments but rather as a brief overview of the different treatments available, their proposed effects and their indications for use. Details of how to apply the techniques can be found in the relevant literature, some of which is cited here. Examples of where the techniques may be applied can be seen in the chapters on specific neurological conditions in this text.

FACILITATION

Many of the techniques used in neurological rehabilitation are applied to facilitate and enhance muscle activity and thus help achieve improved control of movement. Some of those most commonly used are outlined below.

BRUSHING

In the 1950s Rood proposed that fast brushing, using a battery-operated brush, of the skin overlying a muscle could be used to facilitate a muscle contraction. Brushing has been used widely by physiotherapists, applied either using an electrically operated brush or manually using a 'bottle' brush, but there is little indication given about the required rate or duration of the brushing, or pressure to be applied. It would make sense that the skin being brushed and the muscle being facilitated should be supplied by the same spinal segment.

Rood stated that the maximum effect of brushing would be achieved 30 minutes after stimulation and this would suggest that it should be applied prior to other forms of stimulation so that full benefit is obtained. Brushing for 3–5 seconds and again after a further 30 seconds has been recommended (McCormack, 1990).

There is little evidence to support the effectiveness of brushing (Sullivan, 1988), although Garland & Hayes (1987) observed an effect in hemiplegic subjects with foot drop. In subjects who received a combination of brushing preceded by voluntary contraction of the tibialis anterior, a significant change in electromyographic (EMG) activity was seen both immediately and 30 minutes after stimulation. Brushing may be a powerful method of facilitation but it is clearly not well researched in terms of its effects, particularly as much of the work has been done on subjects with no neurological impairments. It is worth noting that several authors urge caution in its use (Farber, 1982; Umphred & McCormack, 1990).

ICE

Ice has two opposing uses in neurological rehabilitation: it can be used to facilitate a response from muscle, or to inhibit unwanted muscle activity. Ice uses a combination of coolness and pain sensations to produce the desired response.

In order to facilitate a motor response, an ice cube is quickly 'swept' over the chosen muscle belly (Umphred & McCormack, 1990). Following each swipe the iced area is 'blotted' with a towel. After three swipes the patient is asked to produce an active muscle contraction. If ice is being used to facilitate lip closure and encourage feeding and sucking, an ice lolly can be placed in the mouth with pressure on the tongue (Farber, 1982).

When using ice as a stimulating technique it is important to remember that it can be a potent stimulus and results can be unpredictable. Putting ice on the face above the level of the lips should be avoided, as it has been reported that undesirable behavioural and autonomic responses may be provoked (Umphred & McCormack, 1990).

TAPPING

Tapping is the use of a light force applied manually over a tendon or muscle belly to facilitate a voluntary contraction. Tapping over a tendon would usually be used to assess reflex activity. A normal response would be a brisk muscle contraction. It is not therefore recommended that tendon tapping be used in a treatment situation, as the response is a crude muscle contraction and will be of little use to help a patient produce a graded, functional movement (Umphred & McCormack, 1990).

Rood recommended 3–5 taps over the belly of the muscle being facilitated (McCormack, 1990). In addition, tapping can be applied to a muscle that has been stretched by the effect of gravity. Once the muscle responds to the stretch produced by gravity the therapist taps the muscle, using the hand, facilitating further activity (Sullivan, 1988). For example, with a patient who is standing, weight-bearing through both legs, if one knee 'gives way' gravity will stretch the quadriceps muscle group. The therapist can then tap the muscle, facilitating a return to full knee extension.

Davies (1985) described the use of sweep tapping to provide an excitatory stimulus to activate the finger extensors in hemiplegia. This is applied by providing support to the affected upper limb with one hand, while the other hand sweeps firmly and briskly over the extensors of the wrist and fingers; the 'sweep' commences just below the elbow and continues over the dorsum of the hand and fingers. In common with other tapping techniques, an active response is requested from the patient following its application.

The use of tapping, like many of the other sensory facilitatory techniques, is supported mainly by anecdotal evidence.

PASSIVE STRETCHING–FAST

Stretching may be applied in different ways to patients with neurological dysfunction to achieve different effects. A quick stretch is applied to facilitate a muscle contraction, and a slow or sustained stretch is given to reduce spasticity or prevent or reduce contractures. It is not within the scope of this chapter to consider the anatomy and physiology of the structures involved, including muscle, tendons and joints, as there are comprehensive texts devoted entirely to such topics (see Chapter 1 for details of the stretch reflex).

A quick stretch is facilitatory and achieves its effect via stimulation of the muscle spindle primary endings. Quick stretching of the agonist muscle will therefore result in reflex facilitation of that muscle. This stretch is normally applied manually by the physiotherapist. Fast stretching is one of the core procedures employed during proprioceptive neuromuscular facilitation (PNF) techniques (see below).

JOINT COMPRESSION (APPROXIMATION)

Receptors in joints are involved with the awareness of joint position and movement. Compression of a joint stimulates these receptors and can produce both inhibitory and facilitatory effects. Joint compression is used either as normal body weight being applied through the longitudinal axis of the bone or as heavy joint compression where the approximation is greater than that produced by body weight (McCormack, 1990).

Bone pounding or jamming is used to inhibit plantarflexion and facilitate co-contraction around the ankle. It can be applied with the patient sitting, by pounding the heel on the floor whilst supporting the knee. Alternatively, with the patient lying prone over a pillow with some degree of flexion at the hips and knees, force can be applied to the heel by the therapist using the ulnar side of a clenched fist.

Other techniques that use joint compression include weight-bearing through a hemiplegic arm to facilitate co-contraction and activation of the muscles around the shoulder joint (Davies, 1985). Weight belts and weighted wrist or ankle cuffs have also been used to increase joint compression. Joint compression can be applied to many joints using a variety of positions or patterns of movement. For example, using four-point kneeling as a starting position, joint compression can be applied to the shoulders and/or hips. Ideally, joint compression should be applied in a functional position but if this is not possible treatment should quickly progress to using the joint in a functional manner. Joint compression is also a procedure used in PNF and is considered in this context below.

Several authors described joint compression, either in terms of normal weight approximation or by other means, but only anecdotal evidence is given to support its use (Farber, 1982; Davies, 1985; McCormack, 1990; Umphred & McCormack, 1990).

VIBRATION

Therapeutic vibration is a directly applied stimulus of high frequency (100–300 Hz) and low amplitude, which stretches the muscle spindle and activates type 1a afferent fibres. Vibration is generally applied directly to the chosen muscle or its tendon. Bishop (1974) identified three motor effects achievable by vibrating a muscle: (1) a sustained contraction of the vibrated muscle (via the tonic vibration reflex); (2) the depression of the motoneurones innervating the antagonistic muscles (reciprocal inhibition or antagonist inhibition); and (3) suppression of the monosynaptic stretch reflexes of the vibrated muscle (during the period of vibration). There appears to be disagreement, however, as to whether vibration has a sustained effect on muscle contractility (Umphred & McCormack, 1990) and thus any long-term benefit.

It would appear that vibration has potential clinical applications via agonist facilitation or antagonist inhibition. Bishop (1974) identified four factors that influenced the strength of the tonic vibration reflex (TVR):
1. The location of the vibrator.
2. The initial length of the muscle.
3. The level of excitability of the CNS.
4. The parameters of the vibratory stimulus.

Application of the vibrator onto the belly of a stretched muscle or over the tendon allows easy facilitation of the TVR. It appears that the tonic neck reflexes and body righting reflexes (see Chapter 1) interact with the TVR; so, treatment in the supine position results in an improved extensor TVR, and that in the prone position results in increased flexor TVR. Finally, increasing the amplitude of the vibration increases the stretch on the muscle but, more significantly, the TVR is greater as the frequency of the vibratory stimulus increases.

Despite the apparent theoretical basis for its use, there are few reports of vibration being used in clinical practice to facilitate muscle contraction.

Another quite different investigation involving vibration was made by Lovgreen et al. (1993) who studied the effects of muscle vibration on the voluntary movements of patients with cerebellar dysmetria. Part of the study was to consider whether vibration could improve movement accuracy and reduce hypermetria. They found that antagonist vibration reduced the amplitude of patients' movements and suggested that vibration had potential for use in both hyper- and hypometria, although the feasibility of its application would require careful thought.

Vibration has the potential to be a potent treatment technique but there are various precautions that must be considered when using it. Key points to remember include: vibration will generate heat at its point of application; and there is potential to cause damage to the skin, particularly at high amplitudes (Farber, 1982). Athetoid-like movements have been reported in patients with cerebellar disease when vibration was applied over muscle and a clear explanation to the patient is always essential.

Umphred & McCormack (1990) recommend that vibrators registering 100–125 Hz be used and noted that most battery-operated hand-held vibrators register only 50–90 Hz. There is a wide range of commercially available vibrators, so the available frequency range should always be checked prior to purchase.

VESTIBULAR STIMULATION

Any static position or movement will have an effect on the vestibular system, so many interventions will result in vestibular stimulation in some way or other. However, specific vestibular stimulation is not widely used in neurological physiotherapy and it is mainly described in relation to a multisensory approach to neurological rehabilitation in paediatrics (see Chapter 19). Advocates of its use are anxious to remind others that vestibular stimulation is a powerful form of stimulation that should be used with care. Umphred & McCormack (1990) stated that the key points to remember are that '... the rate of vestibular stimulation determines the facilitatory or inhibitory effects. A constant, slow rocking tends to be inhibitory whereas a fast spin or linear movement tends to be facilitatory.'

In a study to compare the effect of conventional movement training and trampoline training on balance and gait in chronic hemiplegic patients (Era et al., 1991), the role of the vestibular system in the outcome was not given great consideration. Yet, the effect on the vestibular system while using a trampoline to provide the supporting surface for physiotherapy must be considerable. Zoltan & Ryckman (1990) used vestibular stimulation in the management of head injuries, describing its use as 'essential' for progress. Perhaps the role of vestibular stimulation in neurological physiotherapy should be given more prominence and warrants further investigation.

INHIBITION

When increased tone is proving to be an obstacle to the achievement of normal movement, the physiotherapist may use specific inhibitory techniques (see Chapter 25).

PASSIVE STRETCHING-SLOW

Slow stretch is applied to a muscle or joint such that a stretch reflex is not elicited and the effect is therefore inhibitory in terms of the neural response. The effect of prolonged, slow stretching on muscle is not entirely clear, although it certainly varies depending upon the time for which the stretch is maintained. It appears to have an influence on both the neural components of muscle, via the

Golgi tendon organs and muscle spindles, and the structural components in the long term, via the number and length of sarcomeres (Hale *et al.*, 1995).

Changes in Muscle Length

The presence of increased tone, possibly combined with paresis and/or weakness, can ultimately lead to joint contracture and changes in muscle length. Slow, prolonged stretching is therefore applied to maintain or prevent loss of range of movement (ROM). It has been demonstrated in animal studies that if a muscle is immobilised in a shortened position, sarcomeres will be lost and, conversely, a muscle immobilised in a lengthened position will add on sarcomeres (Goldspink & Williams, 1990). A shortened immobilised muscle will also show an increase in stiffness related to an increase in connective tissue within the muscle (Williams *et al.*, 1988). However, it has been demonstrated in mice that a stretch of 30 minutes daily will prevent the loss of sarcomeres and changes in the connective tissue of an immobilised muscle (Williams, 1990). The time scale relating to changes in the mouse may not be relevant to humans.

Manual Stretching

A prolonged muscle stretch can be applied manually, using the effect of gravity and body weight, or mechanically (by machine or splint). When applied, the stretch should provide sufficient force to 'overcome' the hypertonicity and passively lengthen the muscle. When contractures are already present, it is doubtful whether the use of manual stretching alone will be sufficient to provide a sustained improvement in the range of movement, if any was achieved.

Splinting

Low-force stretching of long duration can be provided by splinting to reduce tone. Different types of splinting and the rationale for use are discussed in Chapter 25, with further details being provided by Edwards & Charlton (1996).

Weight-Bearing

Several studies report the use of weight-bearing to reduce contractures in joints of the lower limb (Richardson, 1991; Bohannon 1993a). These reports illustrate the effectiveness of using a tilt-table to achieve a sustainable position in which a prolonged stretch is applied.

Serial Plastering

Serial plaster casting is another technique used to prevent or reduce contractures, which may be most effective when the contractures result from spasticity. Serial casting methods were described and illustrated by Edwards & Charlton (1996). The use of a soft splint has been shown to be effective in the acute management of elbow hypertonicity (Wallen & Mackay, 1995). This splint has certain advantages over casting in that it is more dynamic in nature, less likely to cause unwanted pressure, and provides neutral warmth (Wallen & O'Flaherty, 1991). However, it is also easily removed and thus a level of compliance is necessary!

When spasticity is present, physiotherapists are often reluctant to use splints or other externally applied devices for stretching as, despite the lack of supporting evidence, it is thought that splinting can lead to an increase in muscle tone. However, it has been demonstrated that inhibitory splinting can reduce contractures without causing detrimental effects to muscle tone (Mills, 1984).

Duration of Stretch to Reduce Spasticity

Although it has been shown that prolonged stretching can reduce spasticity, the time needed is not clear. A recent report addressed this issue and found that the most beneficial duration of stretch applied to reduce spasticity was 10 minutes (Hale *et al.*, 1995). This study used a variety of methods to assess the level of spasticity, including both subjective and objective measures. The results illustrated the difficulties that arise when measuring spasticity (see Chapter 25), and that perhaps the concurrent problems of length-associated changes in muscle required greater consideration.

Duration of Stretch to Prevent Contracture

Tardieu *et al.* (1988) investigated how long it was necessary to stretch the soleus muscle each day to prevent contracture in children with cerebral palsy and concluded that it must be stretched for 6 hours a day.

Much work has been done to evaluate the effect of stretching, mainly on normal subjects. However, it is clear that further work is still required to establish the appropriate stretching techniques and the duration required to produce the desired effect in different situations.

POSITIONING

Positioning is used widely by physiotherapists to prevent the development of contractures and to discourage unwanted reflex activity (Carr & Kenney, 1992; Pope, 1996).

Specific positions are often adopted to achieve a slow maintained stretch on a particular muscle and the thinking behind this has already been explored. Bromley (1985) gave detailed guidelines for the positioning of patients following spinal cord injury and described its importance for: correct alignment of fractures; prevention of contractures; prevention of pressure sores; and inhibiting the onset of severe spasticity.

Indeed, many of the positions advocated by physiotherapists relate to the desire to avoid the development of spastic patterns of movement (Bobath, 1990). Positions are chosen to minimise the influence of the primitive reflexes. The three reflexes, which are normally under cortical control and whose 'release' can be influenced by careful choice and use of positions are: the symmetrical tonic neck reflex; the asymmetrical tonic neck reflex; and the labyrinthine reflex (Carr & Kenney, 1992). These reflexes are outlined in Chapters 1 & 18.

Davies (1985) gave fairly detailed descriptions of desirable positions that should be used following stroke, urging the avoidance of supine lying as in this position the influences of the tonic neck and labyrinthine reflexes are great and this could result in an overall increase in extensor activity throughout the body.

Careful positioning to limit musculoskeletal changes is essential but it appears that there is a lack of consensus about the precise positions necessary to limit the onset of spasticity and unwanted patterns of movement, particularly after stroke (Carr & Kenney, 1992). Certainly, Bobath (1990) identified a need to be more dynamic and advocated the use of reflex-inhibiting patterns of movement, rather than static postures, to inhibit abnormal postural reactions and facilitate automatic and voluntary movements. These concepts are discussed in Chapter 22. Positioning is also discussed in Chapters 7, 8 & 25.

PRESSURE

Pressure is used by physiotherapists both to facilitate and inhibit a response in muscle, more especially in muscle tone. This pressure can be applied in a variety of ways including the use of air-filled splints (Johnstone, 1995), tone-inhibiting casts (Zachazewski *et al.*, 1982) or manually (Umphred & McCormack, 1990). Pressure can be applied directly over a tendon (Leone & Kukulka, 1988) or over the muscle itself (Robichaud *et al.*, 1992). The pressure can be sustained or intermittent, and variable in terms of the degree applied.

Most of the research investigating the effects of a variety of pressure conditions has measured motoneurone excitability, via change in the Hoffman reflex (H reflex). Studies have suggested that the characteristic appearance of the H reflex reflects spinal motor function and therefore it can be used to evaluate the effects of therapeutic interventions that aim to reduce motoneurone excitability (Suzuki *et al.*, 1995). It is important to remember, however, the problems of quantifying that part of muscle tone that occurs as a direct result of reflex activity.

Leone & Kukulka (1988) investigated the effects of Achilles tendon pressure on the H reflex in stroke patients. The assumption was made that any change in motoneurone excitability would be reflected in an associated alteration in tone as, again, no direct measurement of tone was made. Pressure was applied both continuously and intermittently, and under both conditions depression of the H reflex occurred. Intermittent pressure, however, was significantly more effective than continuous. Further investigation revealed that increasing the amount of pressure had no greater effect, and the effect of the pressure was sustained only during its actual application. No carry-over effect was observed but it is suggested that tendon pressure could be used therapeutically; e.g. when a short-term reduction in tone would allow achievement of an improved patient position in bed. Umphred & McCormack (1990) also reported the inhibitory use of tendon pressure applied across the longitudinal axis of a tendon until muscle relaxation was achieved.

The strongest proponent of the use of pressure during treatment was Johnstone (1995), who advocated the use of constant pressure provided by orally inflated splints and intermittent pressure produced by a machine (see Chapter 22).

The uses of the splint are to: reduce the therapist's need for extra hands; provide stability to the limb; divert associated reactions; allow early weight-bearing through the affected limb; and increase sensory input (Johnstone, 1995). It was claimed that when the antigravity muscles of the upper limb are held in a position of sustained stretch using the air splints, tonic and phasic wrist flexor EMG activity is reduced (Johnstone, 1995).

Robichaud *et al.* (1992) supported the use of air-splint pressure to reduce motoneurone excitability of the soleus muscle when circumferential pressure was applied around the lower leg. As in the tendon pressure study, the reduction was not sustained once the pressure had been released. Conversely, an increase in motoneurone excitability following the application of muscle pressure has been reported (Kukulka *et al.*, 1987). This may reflect the different methods employed to apply pressure, which can include tapping and massage (Umphred & McCormack, 1990).

It is clear that the application of pressure has many potential effects, some of which are still not understood. Externally applied pressure over muscle or tendon must also cause a disturbance in the cutaneous mechanoreceptors. Because of the wealth of afferent activity caused by pressure, its application poses many questions yet to be answered.

NEUTRAL WARMTH

When considering exteroceptive input techniques, Umphred & McCormack (1990) identified an additional use for air splints—that of the provision of neutral warmth. Johnstone (1995) also advocated their use to provide sensory stimulation of soft tissues, causing inhibition of the area under which the neutral warmth is applied. Alternative techniques used for achieving neutral warmth are tepid baths, whole body wrapping, and wrapping of isolated body parts. The required range of temperatures that should be utilised for this technique is 35–37^{0}C (Farber, 1982).

There appears to be little research to support the use of this concept of neutral warmth. One study that does exist looked specifically at the effect of a wrapping technique on a passive range of motion in a spastic upper extremity (Twist, 1985). Wrapping (elastic wrap bandages and gloves) was applied to spastic upper limbs for 3 hours, three times a week on alternate days over a period of 2–4 weeks. Results showed statistically significant increases in passive ROM, with subjective reports of reduced pain. Although this study contained several shortcomings (small subject numbers and lack of control) it did indicate an effect.

ICE

Prolonged use of ice reduces afferent and efferent neurotransmission. To be effective in reducing spasticity, the muscle spindles must themselves be cooled. The ice must be applied until there is no longer an excessive reflex response to stretching (Lehmann & deLateur, 1990). It is considered that a reduction of spasticity lasting 1–2 hours can be achieved, such that stretching or active exercises can be applied to greater effect.

The most common form of application of ice to reduce spasticity is local immersion; this is particularly effective for reducing flexor spasticity in the hand. A mixture of tap water and flaked ice is used, in the ratio of one third water to two thirds ice. Davies (1985) advocated that the hand is immersed three times for 3 seconds, with only a few seconds between immersions. The therapist should hold the patient's hand in the ice–water mixture. This procedure can result in a dramatic reduction in spasticity.

General immersion, where the patient sits in a bath of cold water, has been used to reduce spasticity. Patients can tolerate water temperatures of 20–22°C for 10–15 minutes (Lee et al., 1978). Neither local nor general cooling has been found to have any long-term effect on spasticity, so any short-term reduction achieved must be fully exploited.

When using ice it is important to remember that the patient must be receptive to its use. If ice causes the patient distress and anxiety, the inhibitory effect may be blocked (Farber, 1982). A sensory assessment of the patient should be carried out before using ice and the presence of sensory deficits is a contraindication to its use (Umphred & McCormack, 1990).

VIBRATION

Vibration can also be used to produce inhibitory effects. In an effort to support the efficacy of its use to treat patients with disorders of muscle tone, Ageranioti & Hayes (1990) investigated the effects of vibration on hypertonia and hyper-reflexia in the wrist joints of patients with spastic hemiplegia. They found that immediately after vibration, hypertonia and hyper-reflexia were significantly reduced and concluded that in patients with spastic hemiplegia vibration gave short-term symptomatic relief. However, they also acknowledged that despite using a relatively homogeneous group of subjects, there were many different patterns of hyper-reflexia and this could possibly explain previous anecdotal reports where vibration was of no benefit in apparently similar cases.

Vibration has also been used at low frequencies (60–90 Hz) to normalise or reduce sensitivity in the skin (Farber, 1982; Umphred & McCormack, 1990). Hochreiter et al. (1983) found that in the 'normal' hand, vibration increased the tactile threshold, with the effect lasting for at least 10 minutes. There appears to be a lack of clinically applied studies in this area.

Certain precautions need to be considered when applying vibration (Farber, 1982), and these are outlined above in the section on facilitation.

MASSAGE

Massage was a core element of physiotherapy in the UK and has been described as one of the 'roots of our profession' (Murphy, 1993). How widely massage is used or should be used is the subject of much debate that will not be explored here. For an extensive overview of massage, its application and effects, the reader is directed to Hollis (1987).

Massage has two main effects—mechanical and physiological. The inhibitory effects of massage are of particular interest to the physiotherapist working in neurology when the aim is to achieve a reduction in muscle tone or muscle spasm. Slow stroking applied to patients with multiple sclerosis has been found to achieve a significant reduction in the amplitude of the H reflex (a measure of motoneurone excitability). The stroking was of light pressure and applied over the posterior primary rami (Brouwer & Sousa de Andrade, 1995).

Studies on neurologically healthy subjects have found similar results. Goldberg et al. (1992) found that deep massage produced a greater inhibitory response than light massage when applied to the leg. Sullivan et al. (1991) indicated, by their results, a specificity of the effect of massage on the muscle group being massaged. This was contrary to their expectations that the inhibitory effects of massage would extend beyond the muscle being massaged.

It is not clear whether the results of these studies could be transferred to subjects with neurological dysfunction; further studies are essential and must include measures beyond that of H-reflex amplitude as an indication of the efficacy of massage.

EXERCISE AND MOVEMENT

This section includes well established treatments and those that are emerging in neurological rehabilitation. A major area that is not included is gait re-education. This is a vast field and the reader is referred to the chapters in this book on the different neurological conditions as well as to Davies (1985), Payton (1989), Kisner & Colby (1990) and Kerrigan & Sheffler (1995).

HYDROTHERAPY

Emersion in water can enhance the treatment of the neurologically impaired patient and has therapeutic, psychological and social benefits. Hydrotherapy can give an individual with limited independence on dry land an ability to move freely and with confidence. It also allows a recreational activity that can be easily enjoyed by many.

It must be remembered, when hydrotherapy is incorporated into a rehabilitation programme, that the effects of gravity are altered when in water. Many of the problems associated with neurological dysfunction arise from an individual's inability to respond normally to the effect of gravity and, therefore, hydrotherapy is unlikely to be the sole method of treatment. However, water is an environment that permits a freedom of movement seldom achieved elsewhere and its use should be incorporated where possible (Smith, 1990).

Muscle stretching, reducing contractures, re-education of motor patterns, re-education of balance and equilibrium reactions, gait re-training and breathing exercises are all areas covered by Smith (1990), along with details of examples of suitable procedures used in hydrotherapy for neurological rehabilitation. Bad Ragaz techniques, where the buoyancy of the water is used to provide support rather than resistance to the patient, is covered by Davis & Harrison (1988).

As with any technique, careful assessment of the patient before and after treatment will allow the physiotherapist to monitor the effect of hydrotherapy. There are anecdotal reports of increased tone following exercise in hot water but there is little evidence to substantiate this claim. The anxiety experienced by a patient being treated in water should be minimised by the reassurance provided by careful teaching skills (Reid Campion, 1990).

Swimming can form an integral part of hydrotherapy. The Halliwick method of swimming for the disabled (Martin, 1981; Reid Campion, 1990) is suitable for nearly any degree of disability at any age.

For further details of the principles, applications and techniques of hydrotherapy, the reader is directed to Skinner & Thomson (1983), Davis & Harrison (1988) and Reid Campion (1990).

GYMNASTIC BALLS

Gymnastic balls were originally used in orthopaedics but are now used widely by physiotherapists working in neurology. These balls are lightweight, being inflated with air to a high pressure. The ball is used to provide some support to the patient; this could range from a patient lying supine with feet resting on the ball to a patient sitting on the ball with the feet on the ground. When using the gymnastic ball, the principle of 'action–reaction' is followed. The patient is asked to achieve a specific action of the ball that will result in the desired reaction of body movement. With the patient sitting on the ball, feet on the floor, the action required is to roll the ball gently forwards and backwards. The reaction is flexion and extension of the lumbar spine, with associated pelvic tilt.

When using a ball it is important to remember several key points such that its potential is fully exploited. A ball provides an unstable surface; if it is fixed and unable to roll, its effects are significantly altered. The stability of a ball is influenced by the horizontal location of the centre of gravity relative to the base of support. The ball can be used with the patient lying, sitting or standing. Its uses are so extensive that it can be used with patients who have a limited ability to move independently or those who are completely independent. For example, when sitting a patient on a ball, the ball supports the weight of much of the body. Achieving and maintaining a correct sitting position will require continual co-ordinated activity in the muscles of the trunk and limbs to prevent the ball from rolling. This would be more demanding than having the patient sit on a stable surface, yet easier than standing. The patient who is functioning at a higher level can use the ball in a more dynamic manner in which controlled movement of the ball is required.

A comprehensive description of the use of the gymnastic ball can be found in Carriere (1997) and Davies (1990).

Gymnastic balls are available in a variety of different sizes and are now produced by various manufacturers. They should be made of a resilient plastic and inflated to sufficient pressure to withstand adult body weight such that little deformation of the ball occurs. The gymnastic ball is a highly portable, versatile piece of equipment and is available in many neurological physiotherapy departments, yet there is no evidence of its effectiveness and research is required to support its continued use.

PROPRIOCEPTIVE NEUROMUSCULAR FACILITATION (PNF)

PNF was developed as a therapeutic approach over 40 years ago. It is a very labour-intensive method of treatment, in which the physiotherapist facilitates the achievement of specific movement patterns by the patient with particular use of the therapist's hands. The philosophy and conceptual framework of this approach have been discussed in Chapter 22. Some of the basic procedures and techniques which are utilised will be considered here in relation to their use in neurological rehabilitation. For a complete overview of PNF the reader is referred to Voss et al. (1985) and Adler et al. (1993); combined, these texts give an extensive theoretical and practical review of the thoughts of some of the proponents of PNF.

Ten basic procedures for facilitation have been identified by Adler et al. (1993):
1. Resistance.
2. Irradiation and reinforcement.
3. Manual contact.
4. Body position and body mechanics.
5. Verbal commands.
6. Vision.
7. Traction and approximation.
8. Stretch.
9. Timing.
10. Patterns of movement.

The application of manual resistance has been one of the core features of PNF. There has been a shift away from the use of maximal resistance to the use of resistance appropriate to the needs of the patient. How the resistance is applied will reflect the type of muscle contraction being resisted. Concentric and eccentric muscle work should be resisted so the movement is smooth and co-ordinated. Resistance to an isometric contraction should be varied, with a gradual increase and decrease such that no movement occurs. By the correct application of resistance, irradiation or reinforcement will result. An example of this could be the use of resisted hip flexion, adduction and external rotation to facilitate weak dorsiflexion.

These two procedures of resistance and the resulting irradiation and reinforcement are possibly two of the reasons why PNF is no longer used extensively for neurological rehabilitation in the UK. The use of resistance does not fit comfortably with the other neurophysiological approaches, such as the Bobath approach. This, combined with the diagonal and spiral patterns of movement in the three anatomical planes, makes its relevance to normal movement difficult to comprehend. It is interesting to note, however, that Adler et al. (1993) felt that the patterns are not essential for the application of PNF and it is possible to use only the philosophy and appropriate procedures.

The other basic procedures appear to involve the use of techniques widely employed by physiotherapists using other approaches. The use of accurate handling is stressed in PNF; the lumbrical grip is advocated to give the appropriate stimulus to the patient. The therapist's manual contact should give information to the patient, facilitating movement in a specific direction. The position of the therapist relative to the patient allows the therapist to stay in line with the desired motion or force and to use body weight to give resistance. The use of visual feedback is promoted, with the patient following the movement to facilitate a stronger contraction. Traction and approximation may be applied to the trunk or extremities, eliciting a response via stimulation of the joint receptors.

The remaining three procedures—timing, stretch and the use of verbal commands—are extensively used in physiotherapy. Combining these in a variety of ways gives rise to the specific techniques of PNF.

Adler *et al.* (1993) grouped the techniques so that those with similar functions or actions were together. They gave detailed descriptions and examples of the techniques and indications for their use.

Although the core PNF texts previously cited gave examples of its use with neurological dysfunction, PNF is certainly not in common use in neurology gymnasia in the UK. One recent study investigated its effect on the gait of patients with hemiplegia of long and short duration and found its cumulative effects were more beneficial than the immediate effects (Wang, 1994). However, as no control groups were used, the possible inferences from this study are limited. An earlier study by Dickstein *et al.* (1986) compared three exercise therapy approaches including PNF and found that no substantial advantages could be attributed to any of the three therapeutic approaches used.

It has been identified that some of the underlying assumptions of the procedures and techniques used in PNF are now out of date (Morris & Sharpe, 1993) but there still appears to be a vast potential for research involving its use. An attempt has been made to explore the rationale behind the PNF relaxation techniques by studying postcontraction depression of the H reflex (Moore & Kukulka, 1991). The techniques did produce a strong but brief neuromuscular inhibition, but the results of this study, performed on subjects with no neurological dysfunction, cannot be directly applied to patients.

ISOKINETIC EXERCISE
The use of exercise to increase muscle strength in neurological rehabilitation is controversial and many physiotherapists have felt that muscle strength is not an appropriate variable for treatment or measurement. However, recently there have been several studies where muscle strength training has been undertaken in patients with neurological dysfunction (Engardt *et al.*, 1995; MacPhail & Kramer, 1995). Both of these studies employed isokinetic

dynamometers to provide training at predetermined, constant velocities.

Engardt *et al.* (1995) investigated dynamic muscle strength training in stroke patients, monitoring the effects on knee extension torque, EMG activity and motor function. One group was trained using eccentric muscle work, the other using concentric work. From this study it appeared that eccentric knee extensor training was the more desirable mode of training and this is supported by Bohannon (1993b), who also concluded that eccentric exercise appeared to offer more advantages over concentric exercise.

A previous study by Glasser (1986) investigated the effects of isokinetic training on the rate of movement during ambulation in hemiparetic patients and found no difference between a group of subjects who received isokinetic training, in addition to the conventional exercise programme received by the other group. This result may have reflected the inability of the early dynamometers to offer a facility for eccentric muscle work.

In another study, isokinetic strength training was undertaken on adolescents with cerebral palsy who underwent both concentric and eccentric muscle training; significant gains were made in muscle strength and gross motor function (MacPhail & Kramer, 1995). It must be noted that the adolescents in this study were only mildly affected by cerebral palsy but there was no significant change in their spasticity, measured using the modified Ashworth scale and the ankle clonus four-point scale, during or after the training period.

It appears that further studies are warranted in the area of muscle strengthening associated with neurological dysfunction, particularly the use of isokinetic dynamometers which have the potential to be used as a training device and an evaluation tool for both muscle strength and power (Bohannon, 1993b), and spasticity (Firoozbakhsh *et al.*, 1993).

ELECTRICAL STIMULATION TECHNIQUES

The uses of electrical stimulation (ES) include relief of pain, strengthening of muscle and improving endurance, and producing functional movement. Different terms are used for the different applications (see below).

TRANSCUTANEOUS ELECTRICAL NERVE STIMULATION (TENS)
TENS is a term used to describe nerve-stimulating pulses of low intensity, often used to control pain but also used to reduce spasticity.

Pain Relief
The management of pain in neurological rehabilitation would possibly not be identified as a key area for the physiotherapist working in neurology. However, as has been identified clearly, 'The potential for effective pain relief which physiotherapy offers across a wide spectrum of medical care is only slowly becoming generally recognised' (Wells, 1994). Pain management by physiotherapy is an enormous topic

and the reader is directed to an excellent text by Wells *et al.* (1994); this provides a comprehensive overview of pain and its management. Chapter 26 will review the specific management of pain in neurological rehabilitation.

TENS has been used specifically in the management of hemiplegic shoulder pain. High-intensity TENS has been shown to be a valuable technique in the treatment of such shoulder pain, whereas the more traditional low-intensity TENS was not (Leandri *et al.*, 1990). In this study a reduction in pain was achieved and increased passive ROM obtained; both of these effects were sustained to some extent for the month following cessation of treatment.

Details about TENS and its application in pain relief can be found in Low & Reed (1990), which also provides a comprehensive overview of electrotherapy and its principles and practice.

Management of Spasticity using TENS

An alternative use of TENS has been in the treatment of spasticity. Studies investigating its effects on spasticity have had mixed results. Goulet *et al.* (1994) postulated that TENS would have an inhibitory effect on the amplitude of the soleus H reflex. They failed to demonstrate any consistent effects and no significant treatment effects were found following stimulation (at 50 or 99 Hz) on a mixed or sensory nerve. These results could reflect the difficulties of obtaining consistent H reflex amplitudes in normal subjects and in those with neurological dysfunction. Seib *et al.* (1994) used the spasticity measurement scale, in which neurophysiological and biomechanical responses are evaluated, to investigate the effect of cutaneous ES (over the tibialis anterior muscle) on spasticity of the gastrocnemius–soleus–Achilles tendon unit. Using two groups of subjects, one with traumatic brain injuries and the other with spinal cord injuries, a significant reduction in spasticity was found which lasted for 6 hours or more following the stimulation. Based on these results the authors proposed that TENS could be of use for decreasing spasticity prior to other physiotherapeutic interventions such as stretching.

ELECTRICAL STIMULATION (ES) OF MUSCLE

The use of surface ES to produce a muscle contraction via the motor nerves has been used widely in physiotherapy. Muscle ES has five major uses in physiotherapy in general:
1. Strengthening and/or maintaining muscle bulk.
2. Facilitating voluntary muscle contraction.
3. Gaining or maintaining ROM.
4. Reducing spasticity.
5. As an orthotic substitute to produce functional movement.

The latter three uses are those most commonly seen in neurological rehabilitation. All types of ES that produce contraction tend to be termed functional electrical stimulation (FES) but this is inaccurate (see below).

Maintaining ROM is often an important goal in neurological dysfunction. If a patient is unable to maintain range by moving a joint themselves, or having it moved passively, neuromuscular ES may be used to provide assistance or as a

substitute. It can provide a consistent controlled treatment that the patient can apply and use at home (Baker, 1991).

Another study considered the effects of ES on shoulder subluxation, functional recovery of the upper limb and shoulder pain in stroke patients (Faghri *et al.*, 1994). Using radiographs to assess the degree of subluxation, a significant reduction in the amount of displacement was achieved in the experimental group who received ES to supraspinatous and posterior deltoid muscles.

Functional Electrical Stimulation (FES)

FES has been defined as 'the use of artificially generated electrical stimuli to a paralyzed muscle system to produce contractions that result in meaningful movement' (Petrofsky, 1988). The term FES also tends to be used for stimulation of non-paralysed muscle as well as that which does not produce functional movement, but these uses are not strictly FES.

When used as an orthotic substitute, ES can possibly be considered to be truly 'functional'. However, opinions vary as to the efficacy of its use in this area. Petrofsky (1988) identified that FES can be used, often in conjunction with lightweight braces, to provide a method of independent ambulation, but that walking in this way is only part of a comprehensive physical training programme. Melis *et al.* (1995) concluded that the use of ambulatory assistive devices and FES could help patients with spinal cord injuries to regain independent locomotion and improve their quality of life. Much of the literature available about FES of the lower limbs focuses on its use in spinal cord injury. Whalley Hammel (1995) considered the financial implications of FES which, despite two decades of research, still cannot produce a functional level of walking. Another use of FES in this patient group is in the upper limb to improve hand function, but it appears that the fine control required here is as difficult to reproduce as the combination of balance and movement required in walking (Baker, 1991).

The use of FES as part of a rehabilitation programme must be accompanied by an accurate explanation to the patient, including the setting of achievable goals so that the patient's expectations are realistic.

ES for Reducing Spasticity

Establishing the effect of ES on spasticity has been hindered by the difficulties of quantifying spasticity. Vang *et al.* (1995) used a single case study design to investigate the effect of ES on a patient experiencing problems with upper limb function due to spasticity, secondary to cerebral palsy. Using a test of hand function to evaluate the level of spasticity, ES resulted in a measurable reduction in spasticity.

The use of ES to increase the effectiveness of stretching spastic muscles has been reported (O'Daniel & Krapfl, 1989). In this situation, ES was applied to the anterior compartment muscles of the leg while a stretch was applied to the spastic gastrocnemius muscle in a weight-bearing position (using a tilt-table). It is proposed that the reduction of spasticity was achieved by reciprocal inhibition.

Considerations when using ES

It is important to be aware of the safety aspects of using ES and the adverse effects it may have on abnormal neuromuscular systems, as much of the research has so far been conducted on normal muscle. Stokes & Cooper (1989) considered the problems of fatigue when stimulating muscles, the physiological effects of ES and the potential dangers when ES is used indiscriminately for therapeutic stimulation. Indeed, initial studies using stimulation to allow paraplegic and quadriplegic subjects to stand and walk short distances found fatigue limited the distance walked and excessive stress was placed on the cardiorespiratory system and the legs (Petrofsky, 1988). These problems have been partly overcome by the combined use of bracing and FES, and preparation of the muscle for FES by low-frequency conditioning stimulation to improve endurance.

Increased resistance to fatigue in response to conditioning stimulation is achieved by biochemical and physiological adaptations in the muscle (Pette, 1986). Furthermore, the frequency patterns used during conditioning stimulation are important, as a single low frequency can cause muscle weakness but intermittent bursts of high frequency can maintain strength and still improve endurance (Rutherford & Jones, 1988). When ES is used to strengthen muscle, a stimulation pattern similar to the normal motor unit firing pattern has been shown to be more effective than uniform frequency or random frequencies (Oldham *et al.*, 1995). This finding was in patients with rheumatoid arthritis and hand muscle weakness. No such results were found for other muscles, so whilst this approach appears promising, further research is required.

It also appears that further studies are necessary to monitor the effects of ES in specific neuromuscular disorders. Studies such as those which examined the effects of ES on patients with progressive muscular dystrophy (Zupan & Gregoric, 1995) and other neurological disorders (Scott *et al.*, 1986) may allow physiotherapists to make informed decisions about the usefulness of ES as part of a therapeutic programme. Research is also needed to establish appropriate stimulation parameters for the different applications of ES.

OTHER TECHNIQUES

In this section, various unrelated techniques are discussed. Two treatments that were mainly used in orthopaedics before being applied to neurology are acupuncture and adverse neural tension (ANT; see Chapter 23). Another orthopaedic treatment not discussed here is the correction of muscle imbalance (see Chapter 23).

BIOFEEDBACK

Biofeedback has been used widely in physiotherapy, especially in stroke rehabilitation; a detailed description of its use in this area can be found in Barton & Wolf (1993). It has been defined as 'procedures whereby information about an aspect of bodily functioning is fed back by some visual or auditory signal' (Caudrey & Seeger, 1981). Biofeedback therapy seeks to allow subjects to gain conscious control over a voluntary but latent activity (Glanz *et al.*, 1995).

The most commonly used form of biofeedback in neurological rehabilitation is EMG using surface electrodes. Most EMG feedback equipment will provide both auditory and visual feedback to the patient and therapist. For the purposes of providing feedback, changes in the EMG signal can be taken to indicate changes in muscle activity. This does not provide a measure of changes in force, since EMG and force are known to dissociate when muscle fatigues, as shown by the classic experiment of Edwards & Lippold in 1956. EMG biofeedback therefore reflects muscular effort and not force.

Recent reviews of EMG biofeedback therapy assessed its efficacy in rehabilitation following stroke (Glanz *et al.*, 1995) and compared it with conventional physical therapy for upper-extremity function also following stroke (Moreland & Thomson, 1994).

Glanz *et al.* (1995) carried out a retrospective study to determine whether biofeedback could increase the ROM of paretic limb joints after stroke. They reviewed eight published randomised controlled trials and concluded that the efficacy of biofeedback therapy in the rehabilitation of cerebrovascular disease had not been established. A particular problem identified by this meta-analysis was the number of studies with very small sample sizes. A similar conclusion was reached by Moreland & Thomson (1994).

Both these reviews indicated that further research is required to support the use of biofeedback in physiotherapy. The doubts over its efficacy may explain why De Weerdt & Harrsion (1985) found that the use of biofeedback was limited in physiotherapy departments in Great Britain.

Caudrey & Seeger (1981) provided a clear review of biofeedback devices other than EMG which could be used as adjuncts to conventional physiotherapy. These include posture control equipment and the head position trainer, the limb load monitor and devices for improving orofacial control.

Most biofeedback equipment provides immediate, precise feedback to the patient about some aspect of activity. It is important to remember that most physiotherapists utilise verbal feedback when treating patients whether to provide praise, correction or instruction.

ADVERSE NEURAL TENSION

With any form of neurological dysfunction, the normal adaptive lengthening or shortening which occurs within the nervous system may be interrupted. Maintaining and restoring a mobile, extensible nervous system and a knowledge of normal neurodynamics is therefore an essential part of the management of the neurological patient and this topic is discussed in detail in Chapter 23.

ORTHOSES

An orthosis is a device that, when correctly applied to the appropriate external surface of the body, will achieve one

or more of the following (Leonard *et al.*, 1989):
- Relief of pain.
- Immobilisation of musculoskeletal segments.
- Reduced axial loading.
- Prevention or correction of deformity.
- Improved function.

In neurological rehabilitation, orthoses are most frequently used to improve function and occasionally to prevent or correct deformity. Using anatomical and physiological knowledge, functional and biomechanical abnormalities are identified and, as far as is possible, corrected.

A variety of materials and designs can be used in the construction of an orthosis. The word splint suggests an orthotic device designed for temporary use; examples of some splints were considered above in the section on inhibitory stretching. Ideally, most orthoses are designed, made and fitted by an orthotist.

Orthoses tend to be named in relation to the joints they surround. Foot orthoses (FOs) are applied to the foot, either inside or outside the shoe (arch supports, heel lifts). Ankle–foot orthoses (AFOs) encompass the foot and ankle, generally extending to just below the knee. Knee–ankle–foot orthoses (KAFOs) extend from foot to thigh; those extending above the hip are hip–knee–ankle–foot orthoses (HKAFOs) (Edwards & Charlton, 1996). Table 20.2 lists some uses for these orthoses in children with different levels of paralysis.

Orthoses should help the patient meet identified functional objectives; in the case of those applied to the lower limbs, this frequently relates to walking. In order to use orthoses effectively to improve walking, it is essential to consider the normal biomechanics of walking. When using an orthosis, forces are applied to the lower limb as a series of three-point force systems (Leonard *et al.*, 1989). It is essential that these forces are correctly applied so that the desired effect is achieved.

Of particular biomechanical interest is an ability to visualise the ground reaction forces during activities of the lower limb. In a laboratory situation it is possible, using a force plate and video vector generator, to evaluate the effects of an orthosis, using a real-time ground reaction vector. Abnormal moments or turning effects on joints can be noted; energy demand is reduced by minimising the moments that must be resisted during walking, and this can be achieved by altering the forces applied by the orthosis. Butler & Nene (1991) illustrated this clearly in relation to the application of fixed AFOs used in the management of children with cerebral palsy.

Upper limb orthoses used in neurological dysfunction are often used to provide a dynamic force on a joint to reduce contractures (Leonard *et al.*, 1989), a use already outlined above. Perhaps the most common orthotic device used by physiotherapists working in neurology is some form of shoulder support for patients with subluxation following stroke. Various types of shoulder support have been used; one of the most commonly used supports in the UK is based upon a method outlined by Bertha Bobath (Leddy, 1981). A recent study compared four different supports used to correct shoulder subluxation (Zorowitz *et al.*, 1995). There was no evidence to show that the use of supports prevented or reduced long-term subluxation; indeed two of the supports investigated appeared to cause lateral displacement of the humeral head. It is essential that the effects of shoulder supports are carefully evaluated and it may well be that, until evidence is provided to the contrary, there is little justification for their use.

ACUPUNCTURE

Acupuncture was recognised in 1979 by the World Health Organisation (WHO) as a clinical procedure of value that should be taken seriously. Although increasingly used in the musculoskeletal field, acupuncture has not been used extensively by physiotherapists working in neurology. The exception to this is in East Asia where various papers report its use (Johansson, 1993).

In an overview of acupuncture from a medical viewpoint, Gibb (1981) identified its use in chronic pain, analgesia, chronic arthritis, autonomic dysfunction, dysmenorrhoea, insomnia and malignant pain. In a recent paper the question was posed: 'Can acupuncture improve the functional outcome in stroke patients?' (Klingenstierna *et al.*, 1995). In order to answer the question, the authors were undertaking a randomised controlled study in which subjects were assigned to one of three groups. All subjects were receiving conventional physiotherapy (details not given). Subjects in two of the groups were also to receive acupuncture, either with deep needles plus ES on the affected side or with superficially situated needles. The results of this Swedish study were not available at the time of writing.

STRING WRAPPING

Flowers (1988) advocated the use of string wrapping, also referred to as compressive centripetal wrapping, to help control oedema. This is an easily applied method for reducing oedema, particularly in the swollen paralysed hand. Each digit, the thumb and hand are wrapped, from distal to proximal, using string of 1–2 mm diameter. A loop is made as the wrapping commences and the wrapping is applied firmly and continuously. Once applied, the wrapping is immediately removed by pulling on the free end of the loop (Davies, 1985). The reduction of swelling allows greater facilitation of active movement. This is a treatment that can be applied easily by carers prior to, and in between, episodes of physiotherapy. It has very specific, local effects and may prove very useful when swelling is restricting functional improvement in the hand.

CONCLUSION

A variety of techniques used by physiotherapists working in neurology have been discussed. It is not possible to give detailed descriptions of their exact application but brief outlines have been given and references provided for further information. Many of the techniques used require further research either to validate their use and/or to establish appropriate guidelines for their application.

REFERENCES

Adler SJ, Beckers D, Buck M. *PNF in Practice*. Berlin & Heidelberg: Springer Verlag; 1993.

Ageranioti S, Hayes K. Effects of vibration in hypertonia and hyperreflexia in the wrist joint of patients with spastic hemiparesis. *Physiother Can* 1990, **42**:24-33.

Baker L. Clinical uses of neuromuscular electrical stimulation. In: Nelson R Currier D, eds. *Clinical electrotherapy*, Connecticut: Appleton and Lange; 1991:143-170.

Barton L, Wolf S. Use of EMG feedback in stroke rehabilitation. In: Gordan W, ed. *Advances in Stroke Rehabilitation*. Boston: Andover Medical Publishers; 1993.

Bishop B. Neurophysiology of motor responses evoked by vibratory stimulation. *Phys Ther* 1974, **54**(12): 1273-1282.

Bobath B. *Adult Hemiplegia: evaluation and treatment*. Oxford: Heinemann; 1990.

Bohannon RW. Tilt table standing for reducing spasticity after spinal cord injury. *Arch Phys Med Rehab* 1993a, **74**:1121-1122.

Bohannon RW. Muscle strength in patients with brain lesions: measurement and implications. In: Harms-Ringdahl K, ed. *Muscle strength*. Edinburgh: Churchill Livingstone; 1993b:187-225.

Bromley I. *Tetraplegia and Paraplegia. A guide for physiotherapists*. Edinburgh: Churchill Livingstone; 1985.

Brouwer B, Sousa de Andrade. The effects of slow stroking on spasticity in patients with multiple sclerosis: A pilot study. *Physiother Theory Pract* 1995, **11**:13-21.

Butler P, Nene A. The biomechanics of fixed ankle foot orthoses and their potential in the management of cerebral palsied children. *Physiother* 1991, **77**:81-88.

Carr EK, Kenney FD. Positioning of the stroke patient: a review of the literature. *Int J Nurs Stud* 1992, **29**:355-36.

Carriere B. *The Swiss ball: when, why and how to use it in patient treatment*. Berlin: Springer Verlag; 1997.

Caudrey D, Seeger B. Biofeedback devices as an adjunct to physiotherapy. *Physiother* 1981, **67**:371-376.

Davies PM. *Steps to Follow. A guide to the treatment of adult hemiplegia*. Berlin Heidelberg: Springer-Verlag; 1985.

Davies PM. *Right in the middle. Selective trunk activity in the treatment of adult hemiplegia*. Berlin Heidelberg: Springer-Verlag; 1990.

Davis BC, Harrison RA. *Hydrotherapy in Practice*. Edinburgh: Churchill Livingstone; 1988.

De Weerdt W, Harrison M. The use of biofeedback in physiotherapy. *Physiother* 1985, **71**: 9-12.

Dickstein R, Hocherman S, Pillar T, *et al*. Stroke rehabilitation three exercise therapy approaches. *Phys Ther* 1986, **66**:1233-1237.

Edelstein J. Prosthetic assessment and management. In: Sullivan S, Schmitz T, eds. *Physical rehabilitation assessment and treatment*. Philadelphia: FA Davis Co.; 1988.

Edwards S, Charlton P. Splinting and the use of orthoses in the management of patients with neurological disorders. In: Edwards S, ed. *Neurological Physiotherapy: a problem-solving approach*. Edinburgh: Churchill Livingstone; 1996:161-188.

Edwards RG, Lippold OCJ. The relation between force and integrated electrical activity in fatigued muscle. *J Physiol* 1956, **312**: 677-681.

Engardt M, Knutsson E, Jonsson M, *et al*. Dynamic muscle strength training in stroke patients: effects on knee extension torque, electromyographic activity, and motor function. *Arch Phys Med Rehabil* 1995, **76**:419-425.

Era P, Lahtinen U, Harri-Lehtonen, *et al*. The effect of conventional movement training and trampoline training on balance and gait in chronic hemiplegic patients. *Physio Theory Pract* 1991, **7**:223-230.

Faghri PD, Rodgers MM, Glaser RM, *et al*. The effects of functional electrical stimulation on shoulder subluxation, arm function recovery and shoulder pain in hemiplegic stroke patients. *Arch Phys Med Rehabil* 1994, **75**:73-79.

Farber S. A multisensory approach to neurorehabilitation. In: Farber S, ed. *Neurorehabilitation: a multisensory approach*. Philadelphia: WB Saunders Co.; 1982:115-177.

Firoozbakhsh K, Kunkel C, Scremin A, *et al*. Isokinetic dynamometric technique for spasticity assessment. *Am J Phys Med Rehabil* 1993, **72**: 379-385.

Flowers K. String wrapping versus massage for reducing digital volume. *Phys Ther* 1988, **68**:57-59.

Garland SJ, Hayes KC. Effects of brushing on electromyographic activity and ankle dorsiflexion in hemiplegic subjects with foot drop. *Physiother Can* 1987, **39**:239-247.

Gibb G. Acupuncture: a medical viewpoint. *NZ J Physiother* 1981, **9**: 11-14.

Glanz M, Klawansky S, Stason W, *et al*. Biofeedback therapy in poststroke rehabilitation: a meta-analysis of the randomised controlled trials. *Arch Phys Med Rehabil* 1995, **76**:508-515.

Glasser L. Effects of isokinetic training on the rate of movement during ambulation in hemiparetic patients. *Phys Ther* 1986, **66**:673-676.

Goldberg J, Sullivan SJ, Seaborne DE. The effect of two intensities of massage on H-reflex amplitude. *Phys Ther* 1992, **72**:449-457.

Goldspink G, Williams PE. Muscle fibre and connective tissue changes associated with use and disuse. In: Ada L, Canning C, eds. *Key issues in neurological physiotherapy*. Oxford: Butterworth-Heinemann; 1990:197-218.

Goulet C, Arsenault AB, Levin MF, *et al*. Absence of consistent effects of repetitive transcutaneous electrical stimulation on soleus H-reflex in normal subjects. *Arch Phys Med Rehabil* 1994, **75**:1132-1136.

Hale LA, Fritz VU, Goodman M. Prolonged static muscle stretch reduces spasticity - but for how long should it be held? *SA J of Physio* 1995, **51**:3-6.

Hochreiter NW, Jewell M, Barber L, *et al*. Effect of vibration on tactile sensitivity. *Phys Ther* 1983, **6**:934-937.

Hollis M. *Massage for physiotherapists*. Oxford: Blackwell Scientific Publications; 1987.

Johansson B. Has sensory stimulation a role in stroke rehabilitation? *Scand J Rehabil Med* 1993, **29**:87-96.

Johnstone M. *Restoration of normal movement after stroke*. Edinburgh: Churchill Livingstone; 1995.

Kerrigan DC, Sheffler LR. Spastic paretic gait: an approach to evaluation and treatment. *Crit Rev Rehab Med* 1995, **7**:253-268.

Kisner C, Colby LA. *Therapeutic exercise: foundations and techniques*. Philadelphia: FA Davis Co.; 1990.

Klingenstierna U, Gosman-Hedström G, Claesson L, *et al*. Can acupuncture improve the functional outcome in stroke patients? *Proceedings of 12th International Confederation for Physical Therapy*. Washington DC; 1995:748.

Kukulka C, Haberichter PA, Mueksch AE *et al*. Muscle pressure effects on motoneuron excitability: A special communication. *Phys Ther* 1987, **67**:1720-1722.

Leandri M, Parodi CI, Corrieri N, *et al*. Comparison of TENS treatments in hemiplegic shoulder pain. *Scand J Rehabil Med* 1990, **22**:69-72.

Leddy M. Sling for hemiplegic patients. *Br J Occup Ther* 1981, **44**:158-160.

Lee JM, Warren MP, Mason AM. Effects of ice on nerve conduction velocity. *Physiother* 1978, **64**:2-6.

Lehmann J, De Lateur B. Application of heat and cold in the clinical setting. In: Lehmann J, ed. *Therapeutic heat and cold*. Baltimore: Williams and Wilkins; 1990:633-644.

Leonard JA, Hicks JE, Nelson VS, *et al*. Prosthetics, Orthotics, and assisitive devices. 1. General concepts. *Arch Phys Med Rehabil* 1989, **70**:S195-S201.

Leone J, Kukulka C. Effects of tendon pressure on alpha motoneuron excitability in patients with stroke. *Phys Ther* 1988, **68**:475-480.

Lovgreen B, Cody FWJ, Schady W. Muscle vibration alters the trajectories of voluntary movements in cerebellar disorders - a method of counteracting impaired movement accuracy? *Clin Rehab* 1993, **7**:327-336.

Low J, Reed A. *Electrotherapy explained, principles and practice*. Oxford: Butterworth-Heinemann Ltd; 1990.

MacPhail HE, Kramer JF. Effect of isokinetic strength-training on functional ability and walking efficiency in adolescents with cerebral palsy. *Dev Med Child Neurol* 1995, **37**:763-775.

Martin J. The Halliwick method. *Physiotherapy* 1981, **67**:288-291.

Mason C. One method for assessing the effectiveness of fast brushing. *Phys Ther* 1985, **65**:1197-1202.

McCormack G. The Rood approach to the treatment of neuromuscular dysfunction. In: Pedretti L, Zoltan B, eds. *Occupational Therapy Practice skills for physical dysfunction*. St Louis: Mosby Co.; 1990:311-333.

Melis EH, Torres-Moreno R, Chilco L, *et al*. Application of ambulatory assistive devices and functional electrical stimulation to facilitate the locomotion of spinal cord injured subjects. *Proceedings of 12th International Congress of World Confederation for Physical Therapy*. Washington DC: 1995:772.

Mills V. Electromyographic results of inhibitory splinting. *Phys Ther* 1986, **64**:190-193.

Moore M, Kukulka C. Depression of Hoffmann reflexes following voluntary contraction and implications for proprioceptive neuromuscular facilitation therapy. *Phys Ther* 1991, **71**:321-333.

Moreland J, Thomson MA. Efficacy of electromyographic biofeedback compared with conventional physical therapy for upper-extremity function in patients following stroke: a research overview and meta-analysis. *Phys Ther* 1994, **74**:534-545.

Morris SL, Sharpe M. PNF revisited. *Physio Theory Prac* 1993, **9**:43-51.

Murphy C. Massage – The roots of the profession. *Physio* 1993, **79**:546.

O'Daniel B, Krapfl B. Spinal cord injury. In: Payton O, ed. *Manual of Physical Therapy*. New York: Churchill Livingstone; 1989.

Oldham JA, Howe TE, Peterson T, *et al*. Electrotherapeutic rehabilitation of the quadriceps in elderly osteoarthritic patients: a double blind assessment of patterned neuromuscular stimulation. *Clin Rehab* 1995, **9**:10-20.

Payton O. *Manual of physical therapy*. New York: Churchill Livingstone; 1989.

Petrofsky J. Functional electrical stimulation and its application in the rehabilitation of neurologically injured adults. In: Finger S, *et al.*, eds. *Brain Injury and Recovery: theoretical and controversial issues*. New York: Plenum Press; 1988.

Pette D. Skeletal muscle adaptation in response to chronic stimulation. In: Nix WA, Vrbová G, eds. *Electrical stimulation and neuromuscular disorders*. Berlin: Springer-Verlag; 1986: 12-20.

Pope PM. Postural management and special seating. In: Edwards S, ed. *Neurological physiotherapy: a problem-solving approach*. Edinburgh: Churchill Livingstone; 1996: 135-160.

Reid Campion M. *Adult Hydrotherapy*. Oxford: Heinemann; 1990.

Richardson DLA. The use of the tilt table to effect passive tendo-Achilles stretch in a patient with head injury. *Physio Theory Prac* 1991, **7**:45-50.

Robichaud J, Agostinucci J, Vander Linden D. Affect of air-splint application on soleus muscle motoneuron reflex excitabilty in nondisabled subjects and subjects with cerebrovascular accidents. *Phys Ther* 1992, **72**(3):176-185.

Rutherford OM, Jones DA. Contractile properties and fatiguability of the human adductor pollicis and first dorsal interosseus: a comparison of the effect of two chronic stimulation patterns. *J Neurol Sci* 1988, **85**:319-331.

Scott OM, Vrbová G, Hyde SA, *et al*. Effects of electrical stimulation on normal and diseased human muscle. In: Nix WA, Vrbová G, eds. *Electrical stimulation and neuromuscular disorders*. Berlin: Springer-Verlag; 1986: 125-131.

Seib T, Price R, Reyes MR, *et al*. The quanitative measurement of spasticity: effect of cutaneous electrical stimulation. *Arch Phys Med Rehabil* 1994, **75**:746-750.

Skinner AT, Thomson AM. *Duffield's exercise in water*. London: Ballière Tindall; 1983.

Smith K. Hydrotherapy in neurological rehabilitation. In: Reid Campion, ed. *Adult Hydrotherapy*. Oxford: Heinemann; 1990:70-103.

Stokes M, Cooper R. Muscle fatigue as a limiting factor in functional electrical stimulation; a review. *Physiother Prac* 1989, **5**:93-90.

Sullivan SB. Strategies to improve motor control. In: Sullivan S, Schmitz T, eds. *Physical rehabilitation assessment and treatment*. Philadelphia: FA Davis Co.; 1988.

Sullivan SJ, Williams LRT, Seaborne DE, *et al*. Effects of massage on alpha motorneurone excitability. *Phys Ther* 1991, **71**:555-560.

Suzuki T, Fujiwara T, Yase Y, *et al*. Electrophysiological study of spinal motor neurone function in patients with cerebrovascular diseases – characteristic appearances of the H-reflex and F-wave. *Proceedings of 12th International Congress of World Confederation for Physical Therapy*. Washington DC: 1995:798.

Tardieu C, Lespargot A, Tabary C, *et al*. For how long must the soleus muscle be stretched each day to prevent contracture? *Dev Med Child Neur* 1988, **30**:3-10.

Twist D. Effects of a wrapping technique on passive range of motion in a spastic upper extremity. *Phys Ther* 1985, **65**:299-304.

Umphred DA, McCormack GL. Classification of common facilitatory and inhibitory techniques. In: Umphred DA, ed. *Neurological Rehabilitation*. St Louis: Mosby Co.; 1990:111-161.

Vang MM, Coleman KA, Gardner MP, *et al*. Effects of functional electrical stimulation on spasticity. *Proceedings of 12th International Congress of World Confederation for Physical Therapy*. Washington DC: 1995:574.

Voss DE, Ionta M, Meyers B. *Proprioceptive neuromuscular facilitation: patterns and techniques*. New York: Harper and Row; 1985.

Wallen M, O'Flaherty S. The use of the soft splint in the management of spasticity of the upper limb. *Aust Occup Ther J* 1991, **38**:227-231.

Wallen M, Mackay S. An evaluation of the soft splint in the acute management of elbow hypertonicity. *Occup Ther J Res* 1995, **15**(1):3-16.

Wang R. Effect of proprioceptive neuromuscular facilitation on the gait of patients with hemiplegia of long and short duration. *Phys Ther* 1994, **74**:1108-1115.

Whalley Hammell K. S*pinal cord injury rehabilitation*. London: Chapman and Hall; 1995.

Wells P. Introduction. In: Wells P, Frampton V, Bowsher D. *Pain Management*. Oxford: Butterworth-Heinemann Ltd; 1994:1-2.

Wells P, Frampton V, Bowsher D. *Pain Management*. Oxford: Butterworth-Heinemann Ltd; 1994.

Williams PE, Catanese T, Lucey EG, *et al*. The importance of stretch and contractile activity in the prevention of connective tissue accumulation in muscle. *J Anat* 1988, **158**:109-114.

Williams PE. Use of intermittent stretch in the prevention of serial sarcomere loss in immobilised muscle. *Annals Rheu Dis* 1990, **49**:316-317.

Zachazewski JE, Eberle ED, Jefferies M. Effect of tone-inhibiting casts and orthoses on gait: A case report. *Phys Ther* 1982, **62**:453-455.

Zoltan B, Ryckman D. Head injury in adults. In: Pedretti L, Zoltan B, eds. *Occupational Therapy Practice skills for physical dysfunction*. St Louis: Mosby Co; 1990:623-647.

Zorowitz RD, Idank D, Ikai T, *et al*. Shoulder subluxation after stroke: a comparison of four supports. *Arch Phys Med Rehabil* 1995, **76**:763-761.

Zupan, Gregoric M. Long-lasting effects of electrical stimulation upon muscles of patients suffering from progressive muscular dystrophy. *Clin Rehab* 1995, **9**:102-109.

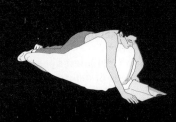

25 H Thornton & C Kilbride

PHYSICAL MANAGEMENT OF ABNORMAL TONE AND MOVEMENT

CHAPTER OUTLINE

- Physical managment of spasticity
- Other abnormalities of muscle tone
- Factors influencing decision making in management of muscle tone

- Measurement of effectiveness of tone management
- Movement abnormalities
- Case histories

INTRODUCTION

Movement dysfunction is a complicated area in itself but with the additional problem of tonal disorders it becomes extremely challenging to the physiotherapist. Appropriate management of movement dysfunction, irrespective of underlying cause, requires a broad knowledge of different areas, which include:

- Normal motor control.
- Biomechanics.
- Kinesiology.
- Neuroplasticity.
- Learning theory.
- Anatomy.

This chapter describes the physical management of spasticity and other abnormalities of muscle tone and movement. As evaluation of practice increases and new theoretical frameworks emerge, new developments are being made in this exciting area of physiotherapy.

Spasticity is a velocity-dependent increase in resistance to passive movement (Katz & Rymer, 1989). It is taken in the context of peripheral and central components, reflecting the current theory that spasticity is a manifestation of both disordered motor control and adaptive changes in the

periphery (Dietz & Berger, 1983; Hufschmidt & Mauritz, 1985). In the clinical setting, signs of spasticity commonly observed by the physiotherapist include positive support reaction, flexor withdrawal, grasp reaction, extensor thrust and recognised synergies (Bobath, 1990). The pathophysiology of spasticity other tone and movement abnormalities are discussed in Chapter 5.

Spasticity occurs in many neurological conditions and its association with those conditions is discussed in the relevant chapters of this book.

PHYSICAL MANAGEMENT OF SPASTICITY

Spasticity not only limits function but can lead to the development of contractures, causing permanent changes in joint alignment. Means of management include general handling, specific treatment techniques and education of the patient and carer.

MOVEMENT AND HANDLING

The use of manual handling techniques is one of the principal means available to the neurological physiotherapist in the physical management of spasticity. The importance of afferent input and its effects on muscle tone have been described by Musa (1986). To achieve functional gains, treatment is aimed at the maintenance of soft tissue length, the modulation of tone and the re-education of movement.

Maintenance of Soft Tissue Length
The need for prevention of adaptive changes, in addition to contractures, is gaining wider clinical recognition. The changes that occur in a muscle when it has been maintained in a shortened or lengthened position have been discussed in Chapter 24. Without the full range of motion, peripheral changes cause muscle imbalance (see Chapter 23) and this compounds any central motor dysfunction (Ada & Canning, 1990; Carr & Shepherd, 1995). It has been suggested that the development of disability is less severe if soft tissue adaptation is minimised (Perry, 1980). To achieve this the therapist can use the following modalities.

Stretching, Assisted and Passive Movements
When handling a patient, the therapist must perceive and adapt to any changes in muscle tone that are a direct response to the movement. The patient should be as fully involved in movement as the current status allows.

The importance of carrying out assisted or passive movements of the limbs, head, neck and trunk through their full range is paramount. Trunk stretches, for instance, should be carried out in the semiconscious or unconscious patient in a supine position by taking both legs through flexion to the chest and rotating them to alternate sides. Attention should be paid to muscles that cross two or more joints. During the movement the patient should be taken out of his or her preferred posture. There are no established guidelines on how often this should be carried out. The relevant literature suggests intervals from 30 minutes to 6 hours (Tardieu et al., 1988; Williams, 1990).

Rotation is important to modulate any excess of flexion or extension. All movements should be performed with care, confidence and variety. Guiding the patient's own movement is preferable to purely passive stretches. Movement should not be too vigorous, with limbs manifesting high tone, and should never be forced. It has been argued that overvigorous movement could be a causative factor in heterotopic ossification (Ada & Canning, 1990), although the subject is still under debate (Davies, 1994).

Caution also needs to be exercised when moving limbs that are flaccid or of mixed tone. This is due to the risk of overstretching and subsequent joint damage. Continuous passive movement (CPM) machines are used in the orthopaedic field to mobilise joints. In neurological physiotherapy, CPM can be beneficial in gaining range following orthopaedic intervention to remove heterotopic ossification, and in late-stage head injuries. Stretching techniques are discussed in detail in Chapter 24.

Positioning
Positioning, whether in bed or seated in a chair, is very important and is considered in a separate section of this chapter and also in Chapters 7 & 8.

Soft Tissue and Joint Alignment
Soft tissue shortening can hinder the recovery of movement or reinforce the presence of abnormal movement. The alignment of muscles, tendons and joints should be observed carefully to ensure that shortening is not being masked by compensatory movements.

As an example of this, Ryerson (1988) described the foot progressing through three stages of deformity as a form of compensation. Kilbride (1993) evaluated some treatment modalities to ameliorate these problems. These are essentially a form of soft tissue massage that aim to elongate the structures and realign the joints to improve sensorimotor feedback. This is significant as malalignment precludes normal muscle activity. Grillner (1981) demonstrated that the position of the hip is vitally important in the facilitation of correct muscular activity for gait in the cat. To improve the quality and recruitment of muscle activity, correct alignment of the limbs is essential.

Weight Bearing
Standing is an excellent way of maintaining length in soft tissues. It is thought to be effective in altering tone via the vestibular system, which is a major source of excitatory influence to extensor muscles, whilst reciprocally inhibiting flexor muscles (Markham, 1987; Brown, 1994). Standing can be carried out whilst the patient is still unconscious, if medically stable, using a tilt table.

The use of tilt tables is an effective method for stretching the Achilles tendon (Richardson, 1991). However, to ensure the functional mobility of the foot, additional mobilisation of the individual joints is needed if it is to perform its specific roles of shock absorber and rigid lever for push off.

Alternatively, backslabs (Davies, 1994) or standing frames may be used to assist effective standing. The patient can be stood between two therapists and movements such as righting reactions incorporated to make the activity more demanding on the nervous system. Bearing weight through the upper limbs may be used to maintain length and influence muscle tone but must be carried out with extreme care. Normal biomechanical alignment of the upper limb must be maintained by external rotation at the shoulder (Ryerson & Levit, 1991) and the wrist joint should not be overstretched.

Modulation of Muscle Tone
Movement and alteration of the alignment of particular parts of the body can influence muscle tone in other areas indirectly. For example, mobilisation of the trunk and shoulder girdle can lead to a decrease in tone throughout the arm (Davies, 1985; Bobath, 1990). The trunk, head and shoulder and pelvic girdles have been found to be particularly influential in altering muscle tone (Bobath, 1990), although this is largely based on anecdotal evidence.

The alteration of muscle tone may be augmented by presynaptic inhibition from the periphery, leading to neuroplastic adaptation (Lumberg, 1979; Musa, 1986). The rotational element here is extremely important and is emphasised in the approaches of propnoceptive neuromuscular faciliation (PNF); (Voss *et al.*, 1985) and of Bobath (1990).

Although each patient should be assessed for the best response to movement and handling, Table 25.1 illustrates a few basic guidelines for dealing with patients who demonstrate 'spasticity' or other motor dysfunction.

Re-education of Movement

Most re-education of movement is based on one of two theoretical models. These are the neurophysiological model and the motor control model, and are discussed in Chapters 22 & 24.

POSITIONING AND SEATING

Good positioning and seating are essential to:
- Maximise function.
- Reduce sustained postures.
- Prevent pressure sores (Settle, 1987).
- Maintain soft tissue length.
- Reduce discomfort and noxious stimuli.

Sufficient support should be provided to allow the patient to cope with the force of gravity, without using excessive abnormal activity which could otherwise lead to deformity. The reader is referred to Pope (1996) for a detailed review of posture and seating.

Although the importance of positioning is generally accepted (Carr & Kenney, 1992), evaluation is at an early stage (Carr & Kenney, 1994). Liaison with occupational therapists, nurses and rehabilitation technicians is essential to ensure optimal provision of equipment.

Positioning in Bed

Lying supine with one pillow under the head is generally thought to encourage extensor spasticity (Davies, 1994). Where this position cannot be avoided, e.g. in a patient with head injury and unstable intracranial pressure (ICP), the physiotherapist must try to minimise its undesirable effects. This may be achieved by breaking up the position, using wedges to prevent mass extension and by increasing the regularity of stretches and limb movement.

The prone position can be very helpful for the patient with head injury and mass extension. It can be achieved on a bed but commercially produced bean bags can be extremely useful for gaining good shoulder protraction and for work on head extension (Figure 25.1). However, patients with tracheotomies or severe contractures may be unable to achieve the prone position.

In general, lying on the side is good as it breaks up the classic flexion and extension synergies, and relieves pressure. The use of pillows, wedges and 'T' rolls can greatly assist in providing adaptable support and allowing change of position (Figure 25.2). Positioning charts that illustrate these postures are useful to ensure consistency and for education of staff.

Mattresses

Each patient should have a mattress that matches his or her needs. Mattresses are selected by the nursing staff and so adequate liaison is essential. Although a bed with an air-filled mattress, designed to relieve pressure, may seem most appropriate, these beds can result in flexion contractures unless careful attention is paid to stretches and standing. Getting the patient out of such a bed can also be extremely difficult unless an overhead hoist is available. As overhead hoists are rare in most district hospitals the patient risks spending too much time in a highly flexed static position. In general, it is preferable to select a mattress that offers adequate pressure relief whilst allowing

Handling techniques used in the treatment of abnormal muscle tone						
Disorder	Speed	Range	Repetition	Voice	Base of support	Other
↑ Tone	Slow	Large	Yes	Quiet, minimal	Large	Longitudinal traction
↓ Tone	Moderate to fast	Small	Yes	Brisk, loud	Small	Graded resistance, quick stretch, compression
Dystonia	Varied	Varied	No	Cognitive, verbal cues or automatic	Use of distal key points ie: hands and feet	Compression
Rigidity	Slow	Large	Yes	Quiet with verbal cues	Large	Longitudinal traction

Table 25.1 Handling techniques used in the treatment of abnormal muscle tone.
(Adapted with permission from Mary Lynch.)

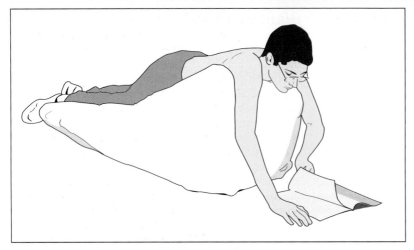

Figure 25.1 The use of a bean bag to induce a comfortable prone position.

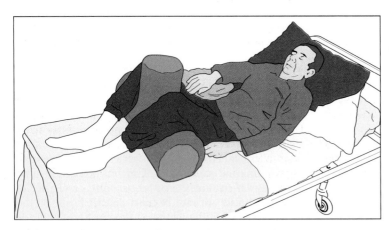

Figure 25.2 The use of a 'T' roll to prevent lower limb extension and adduction.

ease of transfer, and to encourage regular turning and change of position.

For acute head injuries where ICP is a problem, the use of the latest electronic pressure beds should be considered. These constantly turn the patient, providing changing weight distribution and thereby positive effects on respiratory function.

For patients with uncontrolled movements, reduced sensation, or cognitive or perceptual deficits, the use of cot sides, or placing the mattress on the floor, should be considered to prevent injury from the patient falling out of bed.

Sitting

A correct sitting position in a patient with severe disability may best be achieved through the provision of a wheelchair with a suitable seating system. This also allows the patient to maintain a good posture while being moved.

For seating to be effective it must be matched to the needs of the patient. In the early stages of rehabilitation, when a patient's condition reduces mobility, adapting a standard chair to the individual patient may be appropriate. Support needs to be proximal and should be sufficient to allow the patient to sustain good posture. This can improve carry-over of treatment (Chiu, 1995).

For patients with a marked neurological deficit the assessment for custom-made seating systems must be made by a specialist.

Hospitals and rehabilitation units should have a range of wheelchairs and seating systems available for short-term loan. This is particularly useful for patients in the acute stage where needs may change rapidly. For example, a patient may initially require a very supportive system but eventually require only a basic wheelchair. Patients in the acute stage of injury must be prevented from developing abnormal postures and compensatory strategies (Mulcahy *et al.*, 1993). Head supports, arm supports, trays for supporting an affected shoulder and the positioning of the arm where the patient can easily see it should all be considered. Special seating systems for the neurological patient were reviewed by Pope (1996).

SPLINTING

The best approach to contractures remains prevention but this is not always possible. Despite splinting, positioning and regular assisted or passive movements, some patients still develop some soft tissue adaptation. Whilst it is not easy to identify patients at risk, the following factors may be useful indicators:

- Evidence of adaptation occurring with current intervention.
- Inability to stand a patient up for medical reasons.
- The presence of a lower limb fracture.
- Low Glasgow coma scale (GCS) score (i.e. <9) and decerebrate rigidity.
- Low staffing levels (if staffing levels are low, splinting may be a necessary adjunct to physiotherapy).

In general, unconscious immobile patients with altered muscle tone are at most risk from contractures.

If high muscle tone is evident before plastering, a good casting position may be difficult to achieve. Subject to consultation with the medical and nursing staff, muscle tone can be temporarily reduced with a muscle relaxant (see Chapter 28) or a paralysing agent if the patient is still being ventilated. This allows a good casting position to be achieved more easily.

For lower limb fractures the foot should be encased within the cast. A platform should be built under the toes to prevent clawing and shortening of the toe flexors.

If a patient has contractures when first assessed for rehabilitation, a choice has to be made between surgical intervention and non-invasive means. A conservative approach should be considered if handling alters muscle tone, if movement is felt or observed, or if there is a soft end-feel. A preliminary cast should be applied if there is any doubt about the approach. If casting is going to be successful, a gain in range of motion is usually evident after the removal of the first plaster. A radiograph should be taken to exclude heterotopic ossification.

Contractures can be considered in two categories: connective tissue adaptation; and sarcomere changes in muscle (see Chapter 24). Connective tissue loses its extensibility due to a possible loss of fluid and proliferation of collagen (Akeson et al., 1977). Development of contractures can have a varied time scale, depending on the underlying pathology (e.g. there is a more insidious onset with stroke than with incomplete spinal or head injury).

The most likely sites for contractures are:

- Shoulders.
- Elbows.
- Wrist and fingers.
- Hips.
- Knees.
- Ankle (Achilles tendon).
- Spine.

Other joints may also be affected and consideration should be given to the pelvis, trunk (including ribcage), neck and jaw. Attention to the jaw can avoid the unfortunate situation where the patient is prevented from feeding only because he or she is unable to open the mouth fully.

Plastering may be precluded if the condition of the patient's skin or vascular system is poor. Aggressive behavioural changes can also preclude plastering if the cast would present a danger to the patient or others.

Main Forms of Splinting

Different types of splint were described and reviewed by Edwards & Charlton (1996).

Prophylactic Splinting

Prophylactic (i.e. preventive) splinting may be necessary for patients with brain injury who have a low GCS or marked spasticity. It may also be appropriate for patients who need more than positioning and assisted movements to maintain joint range (Conine et al., 1990). Prophylactic splinting can take the form of plaster boots for the Achilles tendon and plaster cylinders or backslabs for the limbs. Barnard et al. (1984) reported a significant reduction in the overall level of spasticity after using plaster boots. However, in the absence of independent movement, any gains achieved may be difficult to maintain, particularly in the presence of persistent muscle tone.

Pressure splints (Johnstone, 1995), used for periods during the day, can be an alternative in some cases and, in the presence of mildly increased tone, strapping may suffice.

Corrective Splinting or Serial Casting

Corrective splinting is used to increase range of movement (ROM) in the presence of contracture. Two common methods are serial casting in the form of cylinders or drop-out casts (Booth et al., 1983). The advantage of the drop-out cast is that active movement can still be encouraged and function is not so compromised. Cast braces are useful for slowly correcting contracted joints, especially at the elbow when the contracture is >90°. A risk factor may be swelling, which can occur around the elbow or knee.

Cones and resting splints can be used to address tightness in the wrist and fingers. The wrist position must be corrected before the fingers. The cone splint can also be used to inhibit tone, although it is important to have the wide end of the cone on the ulnar side to inhibit power grip.

Dynamic Splinting

Dynamic splinting aims to facilitate recovery and assist stability for improved function. Examples are ankle-training braces (Burdett et al., 1988), the Walk-easy (Kelly, 1993), and hinged ankle-foot orthoses (AFOs). Orthoses are discussed in Chapter 24 and by Edwards & Charlton (1996).

Strapping is an alternative short-term method and can be applied to virtually any joint. It can be extremely useful for the ankle and shoulder complexes. Strapping is gaining in popularity in conjunction with increased knowledge of 'musculoskeletal' muscle imbalance treatment approaches (Sahrmann, 1987; see Chapter 23).

Orthotic Insoles

The use of orthotic insoles should be explored with the podiatry department if available. A primary goal of foot orthoses is to aid the maintenance and redistribution of weight-bearing patterns (Lockard, 1988). In cases where the alignment is good and there is minimal contracture, orthotic insoles may be preferable to other means, in 'walking out' contracture.

EQUIPMENT
Equipment to aid independence in mobility and standing includes various types of wheelchairs and standing aids.

Electric and Patient-propelled Wheelchairs
Wheelchair mobility allows independence and arguments for chairs propelled by patients emphasise the independence this gives (Blower, 1988). However, for stroke patients, self-propelling a wheelchair is a unilateral activity involving only the sound side, often with substantial effort. Over time this can result in poor posture, asymmetry, back pain and contractures (Ashburn & Lynch, 1988). It has also been shown to increase spasticity (Cornall, 1991). An alternative within the rehabilitation unit is to loan such patients electric wheelchairs so that they can be independent without increasing their spasticity. An electric wheelchair may also need to be considered for long-term use by some stroke patients where self-propelling could increase their spasticity to the point where it interferes with functional abilities. Cognitive and perceptual difficulties can, however, limit a patient's ability to use an electric wheelchair and each patient must be carefully assessed for suitability.

Other patients requiring electric wheelchairs include those with progressive neurological disorders such as multiple sclerosis (MS) and motor neurone disease. Correct positioning may need to be aided by seating support systems (see above and Chapter 8).

Aids to Standing
There are a number of devices available on the market that aid standing. The use of a standing frame or tilt table has the benefit of enabling a patient to maintain a standing position for a reasonable length of time, often without the assistance of a carer or therapist. Many patients who are wheelchair-bound can develop flexor tone due to the constant posture of sitting. Daily standing can be effective in maintaining tone at a manageable level whilst maintaining joint range. It could be argued that provision of aids is essential to patients who are unable to stand unaided, so that they may maintain their condition and thus prevent costly complications. Evidence to justify this is sparse.

Gymnastic Balls
The use of gymnastic balls to provide mobile support can encourage mobility, stability and postural reactions. As with all equipment, the effectiveness of the gymnastic ball depends on the skill of the physiotherapist in ensuring its appropriate and effective use (see Chapter 24).

OTHER SPECIFIC TECHNIQUES
The techniques mentioned below in relation to spasticity are discussed in more detail in Chapter 24.

Thermal Treatments
Ice has a temporary effect in reducing muscle tone and can be used as an adjunct to other treatment methods or as a means of controlling tone in a specific area. It has been shown to be effective in the treatment of a painful shoulder in hemiplegia (Calliet, 1980; Partridge et al., 1990). The application of heat packs can assist in achieving a range of movement (Sapega et al., 1981).

Electrical Stimulation
This treatment is not widely used in neurology in the UK. Recent research suggests that it may have a place in the control of muscle tone in certain patient groups (see Chapter 24). Also, surgical procedures to implant electrical stimulators have been reported to be effective for reducing spasticity (Sindou et al., 1991).

Hydrotherapy
During hydrotherapy the water has a dual role, providing both support and warmth. The support facilitates stretching of the large muscle groups and helps achieve movement in the trunk. The warmth has a relaxing effect. Conversely, isolating individual small joint movements can be difficult. Hydrotherapy can be used to alter muscle tone and joint ROM prior to a treatment on dry land.

The use of hydrotherapy for patients with spinal injury is widespread, although there is a great diversity of provision (Mahony et al., 1993). There is some evidence that hydrotherapy may be beneficial for patients after strokes (Taylor et al., 1993); its limited use may reflect lack of availability and high demand on staff time. Considerable care should be taken in using hydrotherapy for patients with MS as they are often adversely affected by the heat (although this can be addressed by reducing the pool temperature; see Chapter 11).

Biofeedback
The effectiveness of electromyographic (EMG) biofeedback machines in the treatment of increased muscle tone is as yet unproven (Moreland & Thomson, 1994). It can provide the patient with useful feedback between therapy sessions, but only where the patient has the ability to assimilate this information. Balance monitors that provide feedback on weight distribution (Sackley, 1990) for patients in standing and sitting require investigation.

EDUCATION OF THE PATIENT
Although it is important to educate the patient about his or her condition, this needs to be specifically tailored to the patient's abilities and desire to know. Different individuals react and cope differently to disability. The physiotherapist must judge what information to provide and when to provide it, but it is the patient who decides when or if to use this information. A review system to monitor the patient can be useful where information needs to be given in stages. It is important to collaborate with the patient when setting goals to ensure management is both appropriate and feasible.

Patients need to know how to deal with their spasticity and, if possible, identify any triggers to muscle spasms. Particular attention should be given to identifying nociceptive stimuli such as those from skin, bladder and bowel (and even tight clothing and wrinkled seat cushions). If a spasm occurs the patient may be able to learn to 'breathe through it' (i.e. exhale fully whilst the spasm is occurring). This may help to prevent the patient tensing and thus increasing the spasm. Some patients will be able to gain some further cognitive control over their spasms, but this is not always possible. For example, patients with clonus can be taught to push down through the long axis of the lower leg via the knee. This gives a prolonged stretch and so inhibits the over activity in the muscles concerned.

A home programme may be part of the overall management of muscle tone. Even if the patient is unable to carry out all the specified exercises or stretches independently, he or she should be able to direct a carer and thus retain responsibility. In some cases the spouse or partner may not see this as part of his or her role and this view should be respected. Patient compliance with a home programme sometimes increases if the exercises are incorporated into everyday life (e.g. linking them with the washing up). There may be an additional need to explain any medical or pharmaceutical interventions and how these can be combined with physical methods to optimise the effect.

EDUCATION OF THE CARER

From the outset of any education programme the carer should be as fully involved as is appropriate. In particular, he or she should be included in the goal-setting process, particularly for the long-term goals. Although direct liaison with carers can be difficult, every endeavour should be made, even if this means telephoning or writing to them. The carer must be fully instructed in methods of moving or assisting the patient that are appropriate to the level of disability. It is also necessary to confirm the carer's competence in these skills. This may be an ongoing process, involving sessions in the home environment, but needs to be well established prior to discharge. The carer should also be given relevant information about support groups or networks (see 'Associations and Support Groups').

OTHER ABNORMALITIES OF MUSCLE TONE

The clinical features and medical management of hypotonia, rigidity and dystonia are discussed in Chapter 5.

HYPOTONIA

When dealing with persistent low muscle tone, care must be taken to avoid damage to joints or overstretching of muscles. If muscles are elongated this can present difficulty in recruitment due to alteration in the length–tension curve (Ada & Canning, 1990; and Chapter 23). If the patient is mobile, great care must be paid to the knee joint which may be in constant hyperextension, and orthoses may need to be considered. Correct alignment is essential when patients with low tone are stood up in order to avoid undue pressure on the joints and surrounding structures.

The flaccid shoulder sometimes seen following damage to the central nervous system (CNS) can lead to traction of the brachial plexus and soft tissues. This causes pain; various support devices for the arm are available that may be useful in alleviating this pain (see Chapter 24).

RIGIDITY

The physiotherapist will see two main types of rigidity. These are the rigidity of Parkinson's disease and decerebrate rigidity in head injury (see Chapter 5). In Parkinson's disease, the physiotherapist must understand the pharmacological management, and therapy must be timed accordingly. Treatment is especially aimed at maintenance of posture through regular exercise. Rigidity in the patient with head injury will rapidly result in contractures, and preventive physical measures are usually required. Some of the rarer conditions that may present with rigidity are 'stiff-man syndrome', atypical spinal cord lesions, and Schwartz–Jampel syndrome (Thompson, 1993).

DYSTONIA

This has been described as mobile rigidity or 'sustained involuntary muscle contractions' (Pentland, 1993). Clinically, treatment should aim to increase proprioceptive input by compression or stretch. In this condition there is a tendency to adopt static postures; mobile weight bearing through hands and feet will allow the patient to feel postural adaptation.

FACTORS INFLUENCING DECISION MAKING IN MANAGEMENT OF MUSCLE TONE

These factors include: the type of neurological condition; physical and cognitive abilities of the patient; carry-over of treatment effects into everyday activities; severity of the tonal abnormality; current and previous function; and other medical interventions.

DIAGNOSIS AND PROGNOSIS

The importance of, and the approach to, the management of muscle tone will depend on the patient's diagnosis. For the patient with a terminal primary tumour of the brain and a life expectancy of a few months, the priorities must be to get the patient as functional as possible quickly, to help him or her to be comfortable and to address rapidly changing needs. Emphasis would be on provision of equipment, and advice to carers regarding transfers and positioning for comfort. It would be inappropriate to carry out long physically oriented treatments where no improvement was anticipated. It would also be a waste of resources.

For the patient with a rapidly deteriorating condition, such as motor neurone disease, a stronger emphasis on monitoring and management would be most appropriate.

Factors such as fatigue in MS patients and ICP in patients with acute head injuries influence physical management. In acute head injury where the prognosis is unknown, a high level of treatment and work towards optimal recovery is required. Although the patient is at particular risk of developing contractures in the acute stage, emphasis is often placed on respiratory problems. In such cases insufficient attention can be given to the long-term physical problems. This is where the use of prophylactic splints might be indicated.

Where the patient does not have a diagnosis on which to base a prognostic assessment, the physiotherapist must treat those symptoms that present. However, prediction of change is difficult and regular reviews are essential. For conditions that can follow a relapsing and remitting course, such as MS, access to therapy at an appropriate time in the course of the disease is again essential.

THE ABILITY TO LEARN

The ability to change physically is inextricably linked to the cognitive capacity to learn and to take on new information (Turnbull, 1982; Riddoch et al., 1995). It is therefore important for the physiotherapist to realise that the response to physical rehabilitation cannot be seen in isolation from cognition, motivation, premorbid ability, behavioural difficulties, and perceptual and communication dysfunction. This area is covered in more detail in Chapter 27 on psychological management.

POTENTIAL FOR PHYSICAL CHANGE

When handling a patient, certain signs indicate a potentially favourable outcome for prolonged physical change. These include:

- A change in tone in response to handling or positioning.
- The ability to follow a movement.
- The presence of any movement, however small.
- The presence of some muscle tone (as opposed to flaccidity).

CARRY-OVER AND TEAMWORK

Carry-over can be defined as the extent to which treatment gains are maintained and used functionally between treatment sessions.

The management of spasticity requires a 24-hour approach for maximum effectiveness. It is essential that the whole rehabilitation team works towards common goals and has the knowledge and skills necessary to provide a co-ordinated approach. Interdisciplinary working practices can help such co-ordination, but these require commitment (Davis et al., 1992). For example, the speech and language therapist could undertake treatment while the patient is in a standing frame, or a perching stool could be used to encourage a more extended posture during activities in other therapies. Similar consideration should be given to modifying physiotherapy treatments on the advice of other therapists and, when conflicts arise, all disciplines should be ready to compromise in the interests of the patient. Regular communication between staff in the form of joint goals, joint treatment sessions, meetings, multidisciplinary notes, and training may increase effectiveness.

The physiotherapist has an important role in teaching not only the patient and relatives, but also the other team members, how to manage the physical aspects of the patient's care. The importance of teamwork was emphasised in the Kings Fund Forum conference (1988) entitled *The Treatment Of Stroke.*

SEVERITY

The severity of increased muscle tone is difficult to quantify, either objectively or subjectively (see below). It can cause problems in seating, positioning and transfers, and the pain and discomfort suffered by the patient can lead to disturbed sleep. The therapist needs to be aware that some patients actually require a high level of extensor activity in their legs to be able to walk functionally. Altering tone should be considered only when it is of benefit to the patient. When reducing tone, care should be taken to ensure that by the end of the treatment session the patient has achieved some normal activity that improves his or her function or assists in nursing care.

Abnormal tone may not be constant and hence the wider picture should always be sought by a full assessment. In the patient with high muscle tone, splinting and medical measures may be required. Severity may also influence the frequency of treatment and the emphasis placed on management as opposed to physical handling. For example, a customised seating system in conjunction with a precise positioning programme would be crucial in an immobile patient but less important in an independent walker.

CURRENT AND PREVIOUS FUNCTION

It is vital to take a holistic view of the patient when making decisions about the management of tonal difficulties. Details of the patient's previous lifestyle should be considered, as well as his or her aspirations for the future. Quality of life is both personal and subjective: the individual must be consulted and goals must be set jointly. The views of the patient's family and friends should be sought if it is not possible to converse fully with the patient.

OTHER MEDICAL INTERVENTIONS

It is important for the physiotherapist to understand both the capabilities and the limitations of each available treatment. Resources should not be wasted carrying out treatments that are not effective, or where other means would be more appropriate. The therapist needs a basic understanding of the medical means of controlling spasticity (see Chapter 28 and chapters on specific neurological conditions). Drugs may be appropriate where physical means alone prove inadequate but, due to the potential side effects, careful consideration needs to be given to their use. Pain increases spasticity and so the use of analgesia should be considered. It should be remembered that not all patients are able to communicate and request painkillers. The physiotherapist's skills in assessing tone can also play a valid role in evaluating the effectiveness of drug therapy.

Injections of botulinum toxin may be a useful adjunct to therapy, especially where a particularly localised problem with spasticity is identified (Park, 1995). This will result in inactivity in the muscle for a few months. Local nerve blocks may reduce muscle activity or pain, and so give the patient the opportunity to achieve movement (Skeil & Barnes, 1994). Where there are marked contractures it may be appropriate to consider orthopaedic surgery such as tendon lengthening or soft tissue releases. In some patients intrathecal baclofen may be used, especially where spasticity is a major problem and there is virtually no function in the affected limbs (Campbell *et al.*, 1995). There are also neurosurgical procedures that can be beneficial for suitable patients (Sindou *et al.*, 1991).

MEASUREMENT OF EFFECTIVENESS OF TONE MANAGEMENT

Assessment scales are discussed in Chapter 4; those used specifically to assess muscle tone are discussed here and were also reviewed by Haas & Crow (1995).

SPECIFIC SCALES FOR SPASTICITY AND TONE

The subjective assessment of muscle tone is carried out routinely by both doctors and physiotherapists by passively moving the limbs. Increase in muscle tone may be recorded as mild, moderate or severe but there is no agreement on how these categories are defined (DeSouza, 1987). Spasticity can be variable and depend on position, mood, base of support, temperature, stress, pain or time. Standardisation of as many of these factors as possible is necessary if attempting to measure this difficult clinical manifestation.

The Ashworth Scale is a well known measure of tonal changes. It has two forms, the standard test and a modified version (Bohannon & Smith, 1987). The reliability of this scale has been established only for the elbow and this should be considered prior to its adoption (Wade, 1992).

The Motor Assessment Scale (Carr *et al.*, 1985) includes a measure of tone and disability items. The Oswestry Scale is based on clinical observations and is graded from 0 to 5, i.e. no spasticity, mild spasticity, moderate spasticity, severe spasticity, very severe spasticity, and solely spastic (Goff, 1976).

FUNCTIONAL SCALES

Disability or handicap scales have a limited role in the assessment of spasticity. They can assess the effects of spasticity on disability but, because spasticity is an impairment not a disability, they cannot measure spasticity directly. The more sensitive the scale, the more clinically useful it is likely to be, although this may mean it is less statistically reliable (Kidd *et al.*, 1995). The Barthel Index has been used widely but is not very sensitive. More recently the Functional Independence Measure (FIM) and the Functional Assessment Measure (FAM) have been developed. With seven levels, these have greater sensitivity (Hall, 1992). The Barthel and FIM are generally accepted but further research is required to establish the most valid and reliabile scales, and these may differ for different disorders. No gold standard for assessing disability exists at present (see Chapter 4).

MOTOR SCALES

There are a number of scales that concentrate on the motor abilities. These may be more sensitive to changes achieved through physical therapy. Partridge *et al.* (1987) described a milestone assessment for strokes that is based on the achievement of movements. Other motor assessments include the Rivermead Motor Assessment, the Motor Club Assessment Scale (Ashburn, 1982) and the Motor Assessment Scale (Carr *et al.*, 1985).

OTHER MEASURES

None of the measures described below assesses muscle tone directly but they are used to assess aspects of function that may be influenced by abnormal tone and thus be altered by management of tone.

Range of Movement

The most common instrument used is a goniometer, which measures changes in joint ROM as an indirect measure of tonal changes. Electrogoniometers can also be used but these are not widely available in the clinical setting. A micrometer can also be used to measure linear changes, such as the height of the heel from the floor, and is more accurate than a simple ruler. Spinal motion can be measured with a flexible ruler.

Walking Tests

A test based on timed 10-metre walks during which steps are counted has been shown to be of use (Holden *et al.*, 1986; Collen *et al.*, 1990). Longer distances or times can also be used if the procedure is standardised. This test is simple and quick to administer and measure. A paper walkway gives much useful information in the absence of a gait laboratory (i.e. stride length, step width and length).

Painted Footprints

This allows changes in weight distribution to be recorded and is a useful way of documenting the realignment of the foot complex.

Photography

Periodic photographs allow comparison over time. The procedure needs to be standardised to ensure that the same perspective and distance are used each time.

Video Recording

The use of video recordings is an excellent means of documenting change in posture and movement (Stillman, 1991).

Goal Setting

Goal setting is widely used and can be meaningful to both the therapist and the patient. It has, however, been criticised for subjectivity. If correctly used in the context of an integrated care pathway, it fosters a critical analysis of achievement (Baldry & Rossiter, 1995). A stated goal should contain the elements of who, what, when, and how (Davies & Crisp, 1980).

Adverse Occurrences

It is possible to use undesirable signs such as pain (Dvir & Panturin, 1993) and frequency of spasms to assess the outcome of intervention.

MOVEMENT ABNORMALITIES

Neurological disease can present in many ways and can often exhibit a mixed picture. An important role for the physiotherapist can be to provide information regarding physical impairments. Often it may be the experienced neurophysiotherapist who identifies that a patient has a tremor or specific focal abnormality. Any physical findings that are not apposite to the diagnosis of the patient should be discussed with the medical staff.

Movement abnormalities can severely limit mobility, e.g. ataxia or functional activities involving the upper limbs, e.g. tremor and athetosis. Severely disabled patients who are unable to talk may be further limited in their ability to communicate if movement abnormalities preclude the use of computers and other communication aids.

The approach to movement abnormalities involves careful assessment and knowledge of the diagnosis. The following are some specific points for particular movement disorders which have also been reviewed by Edwards (1996).

ATAXIA

Ataxia is associated with a disturbance in the sensory or vestibular system, or a lesion in the cerebellum, and occurs in conditions such as MS and Friedreich's ataxia (see Chapter 11). In cerebellar ataxia the patient generally presents with low muscle tone (Diener & Dichgans, 1992). This may be masked by increased tone in certain muscle groups if the patient has used a spastic synergy to gain some stability. Treatment should concentrate on creating stability around proximal joints and in the trunk to give the patient a background on which to move. Where the patient uses compensatory activity, the physiotherapist needs to consider how this may best be achieved to prevent over-dominance of one movement or posture.

Measures available to give the patient stability include supportive seating (Figure 25.3), weighted frames and damping devices such as the 'neater eater'. The use of weights is discussed in the literature (Morgan, 1975) but in practice may be inappropriate if the ataxia is too generalised. In MS patients, fatigue may make the use of weights impractical. Case History B, below, describes a patient with ataxia.

TREMOR

Tremors may occur in many neurological conditions including Parkinson's disease, brain injury and MS. Cleeves *et al.* (1994) described less common tremors. Drug therapy is usually effective to some extent and the provision of adaptive equipment should be considered. Clinicians treating head injuries should be aware of a tremor that can develop long after the actual head injury (Cleeves *et al.*, 1994).

ATHETOSIS

Management and the provision of equipment is very important (see Chapter 19). Clinicians may see this

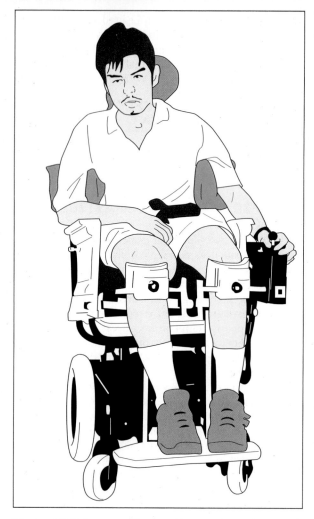

Figure 25.3 A supportive seating system allows this very ataxic young man to be able to drive an electric wheelchair.

condition more frequently in adults in the future, as the life expectancy of children with cerebral palsy rises.

BRADYKINESIA

This disorder, in which movements are slowed, is most commonly seen in conjunction with Parkinson's disease (see Chapter 12). Treatment should be concentrated at the time when drug therapy has been maximised. Exercise programmes that teach compensatory strategies may be beneficial (Kamsa *et al.*, 1995).

OTHER MOVEMENT DISORDERS

There has been little evaluation of therapy in the rarer movement abnormalities. Choreiform movements are discussed in Chapter 13 on Huntington's disease. The therapist should carry out a detailed assessment and consider each individual case on the basis of the clinical presentation.

CASE HISTORIES

For each case history a certain point in the patient's rehabilitation has been described. The aim of these presentations is to give an overview, not provide detailed descriptions of treatment.

CASE A – SPASTICITY
The Patient
Steve, a 24-year-old man, suffered a head injury from a climbing accident. Initially he was admitted to a neurosurgical unit where he underwent a craniotomy and removal of a haematoma from the frontoparietal region. Scanning revealed widespread contusions. He was intubated and ventilated for a week and bilateral prophylactic plaster boots were applied as he had extensor tone in both lower limbs. He developed a flexion contracture of his right arm, which could not be splinted due to a large abrasion. Four weeks after the accident he was transferred back to a general surgical ward in his local general hospital and assessed.

Problems Identified
Steve was fed nasogastrically because he was at risk of aspiration. He had marked extensor tone in the lower limbs but could use his left arm functionally. His right arm had no functional movement and had flexor tone with contracture. He was unable to sit independently and had attention-seeking behaviour. His family were very supportive.

Decision Making
Regular team meetings were arranged and the family were invited to therapy sessions and to a case conference. At the case conference the team identified a requirement for long-term rehabilitation to maximise Steve's functional recovery; he was referred to a specialist rehabilitation centre.

Action Taken
It was decided to give Steve a percutaneous endoscopic gastrostomy (PEG) in liaison with the speech and language therapist, dietitian and surgeon. A joint session with the occupational therapist provided him with a temporary supportive seating package. As part of the treatment the plaster boots were removed and ROM was maintained by daily standing. Serial drop-out casts were applied to his right arm and led to increased range. All staff tried to ignore inappropriate behaviour and socially rewarded good behaviour. Nursing staff and family were advised on positioning and methods of transfer. He was transferred to the rehabilitation unit after 2 months.

Evaluation of Outcome
Steve's range of flexion at the elbow and ankles was measured. Baseline charts were kept to monitor periods of attention-seeking behaviour. Functional and behavioural goals were set jointly by the team, Steve and his family. He achieved the functional goals of independent sitting and dressing his upper body.

CASE B – ATAXIA
The Patient
Jenny, a 26-year-old single mother, had been previously diagnosed as having partial paraplegia due to MS. She was referred for outpatient physiotherapy by a neurologist, following a relapse. Jenny had been confined to a wheelchair for 3 years and presented in low mood and with social isolation. She had fears about losing her 4-year-old daughter if she approached social services for any help. Her wheelchair was small, the canvas sagged, and she found it difficult to propel for long distances.

Problems Identified
On examination, Jenny was found to have low muscle tone in her trunk, with overactivity of the hip flexors and some contracture in the adductors. She compensated by using her arms for support in a flexed internally rotated position. She was unable to stand and spent all day sitting. Her flexor spasms were getting worse, and she had only flickers of activity in her lower limbs. She was very emotional on assessment and cried when asked about how she managed with daily tasks.

Decision Making
The worsening spasms were of great concern as this suggested increasing spasticity. Prompt action was needed to prevent this interfering with her transfers. There was also reduced range in the hips and knees. On examination she had more activity in her trunk than she was currently using. It appeared that she had developed habitual postures resulting from her relapse. Her psychological state needed support.

Action Taken
Active treatment included teaching Jenny to relax through spasms, and to be much more aware of what triggered them. She kept a diary detailing when she got a spasm and why it happened. The therapist made backslabs to enable her to stand therapeutically, enabling alignment of trunk on pelvis and active work around her trunk through activities with the upper limbs. After a trial period with a standing frame, Jenny was provided with a frame for use at home and began to stand daily. She was also given a perching stool which she could manage to transfer onto for use in the kitchen. She was referred for assessment for a lightweight wheelchair and for advice about a 'buggy' for outdoor mobility. Once the relationship between Jenny and her physiotherapist was established she agreed to visit her GP's counsellor and to attend the local MS support group.

Evaluation of Outcome
By the time of discharge Jenny was getting spasms only rarely. This factor had been used for evaluation. She was going out regularly and subjective assessment suggested that her mood had improved substantially. Her daughter attended a nursery in the morning, giving Jenny some free time to manage the household tasks. Most importantly, she had incorporated into her daily life activities such as standing and adopting different postures that would maintain her abilities.

REFERENCES

Ada L, Canning C. Anticipating and avoiding muscle shortening, In: Ada L, Canning C, eds. *Key issues in neurological physiotherapy: foundations for practice*. Oxford: Butterworth Heinemann; 1990:219-237.

Akeson WH, Amiel D, Mechanic GL, *et al*. Collagen cross-linking alterations in joint contractures: changes in the reducible cross-links in periarticular connective tissue collagen after nine weeks of immobilisation. *Connect Tiss Res* 1977, **5**:15-19.

Ashburn A. A physical assessment for stroke patients. *Physiother* 1982, **68**:109-113.

Ashburn A, Lynch. Disadvantages of the early use of electric wheelchairs in the treatment of hemiplegia. *Clin Rehab* 1988, **2**:327-331.

Baldry JA, Rossiter D. Introduction of integrated care pathways to a neuro-rehabilitation unit. *Physiother* 1995, **81**:432-434.

Barnard P, Dill H, Eldredge P, *et al*. Reduction of hypertonicity by early casting in a comatose head-injured individual. A case report. *Phys Ther* 1984, **64**:1540-1542.

Blower P. The advantages of the early use of wheelchairs in the treatment of hemiplegia. *Clin Rehab* 1988, **2**:323-325.

Bobath B. *Adult hemiplegia: evaluation and treatment,3rd edition*. Oxford: Butterworth-Heinnemann; 1990.

Bohannon RW, Smith MB. Interrater reliability of a modified Ashworth Scale of muscle spasticity. *Phys Ther* 1987, **67**:206-207.

Booth BJ, Doyle M, Montgomery J. Serial casting for the management of spasticity in the head-injured adult. *Phys Ther* 1983, **63**:1960-1966.

Brown P. Pathophysiology of spasticity – editorial. *J Neurol Neurosurg Psychiat* 1994, **57**:773-777.

Burdett RG, Borello-France D, Blatchly C, *et al*. Gait comparison of subjects with hemiplegia walking unbraced with ankle foot orthosis and with an Air Stirrup ® Brace. *Phys Ther* 1988, **68**:1197-1203.

Calliet R. *The shoulder in hemiplegia*. Philidelphia, FA Davis; 1980.

Campbell SK, Almeida GL, Penn RD, *et al*. The effects of intrathecally administered baclofen on function in patients with spasticity. *Phys Ther* 1995, **75**:352-362.

Carr EK, Kenney FD. Positioning of the stroke patient: a review of the literature. *Int J Nurs Stud* 1992, **29**:355-369.

Carr EK, Kenney FD. Observing seated posture after stroke: a reliability study. *Clin Rehab* 1994, **8**:329-333.

Carr JH, Shepherd RB, Ada L. Spasticity: research findings and implications for intervention. *Physiother* 1995,**81**:421-429.

Carr JH, Shepherd RB, Nordholm L, *et al*. Investigation of a new motor assessment scale for stroke patients. *Phys Ther* 1985, **65**:175-176.

Chui ML. Wheelchair seating and positioning. In: Montgomery J, ed. *Physical therapy for traumatic brain injury*. New York: Churchill Livingstone; 1995:117-136.

Cleeves L, Findley LJ, Marsden CD. Odd tremors. In: Marsden CD, Fahn S, eds. *Movement disorders*. Oxford: Butterworth-Heinemann; 1994:434-458.

Collen FM, Wade DT, Bradshaw CM. Mobility after stroke: reliability of measures of impairment and disability. *Int Disability Stud 1990,* **12**:6-9.

Conine TA, Sullivan T, Machie T, *et al*. Effect of serial casting for the prevention of equinus in patients with acute head injury. *Arch Phys Med Rehab* 1990, **70**:310-312.

Cornall C. Self-propelling wheelchairs: The effects on spasticity in hemiplegic patients. *Physio Theory Practice* 1991, **7**:13-21.

Davies ADM, Crisp AG. Setting performance goals in geriatric nursing. *J Adv Nurs* 1980, **5**:381-388.

Davies PM. *Steps to follow. A guide to the treatment of adult hemiplegia*. Berlin Heidelberg: Springer-Verlag; 1985.

Davies PM. *Starting again. Early rehabilitation after traumatic brain injury or other severe brain lesion*. Berlin Heidelberg: Springer-Verlag; 1994.

Davis A. Davis S, Moss N, *et al*. First steps towards an interdisciplinary approach to rehabilitation. *Clin Rehab* 1992, **6**:237-244.

De Souza LH. The measurement and assessment of spasticity. *Clin Rehab* 1987, **1**:89-96.

Diener HC, Dichgans J. Pathophysiology of cerebellar ataxia. *Mov Disord* 1992, **7**:95-109.

Dietz V, Berger W. Normal and impaired regulation of muscle stiffness in gait: a new hypothesis about muscle hypertonia. *Exp Neurol* 1983, **79**:680-687.

Dvir Z, Panturin E. Measurement of spasticity and associated reactions in stroke patients before and after physiotherapeutic intervention. *Clin Rehab* 1993, **7**:15-19.

Edwards S. Abnormal tone and movement as a result of neurological impairment - considerations for treatmen. In: Edwards S, ed. *Neurological physiotherapy: a problem-solving approach*. London: Churchill Livingstone; 1996:63-86.

Edwards S, Charlton P. Splinting and the use of orthoses in the management of patients with neurological disorder. In: Edwards S, ed. *Neurological physiotherapy: a problem-solving approach*. London: Churchill Livingstone; 1996:161-188.

Goff B. Grading of spasticity and its effect on voluntary movement. *Physiother* 1976, **62**:358-361.

Grillner S. Control of locomotion in bipeds, tetrapodes and fish. In: Brooks, V, ed. *The Handbook of Physiology* Volume *III Section 3. The nervous system II Motor Control*. Baltimore: American Physiological Society; Waverley Press; 1981:1179-1236.

Haas BM & Crow JL. Towards a clinical measurement of spasticity. *Physiother* 1995, **81**:474-479.

Hall KM. Overview of functional assessment scales in brain injury rehabilitation. *Neuro Rehab* 1992, **2**:98-113.

Holden MK, Gill KM, Magliozzi MR. Gait assessment for neurologically impaired patients: standards for outcome. *Phys Ther* 1986, **10**:1530-1539.

Hufschmidt A, Mauritz KH. Chronic transformation of muscle in spasticity: a contribution to increased tone. *J Neurol Neurosurg Psych* 1985, **48**:676-685.

Johnstone M. *Restoration of normal movement after stroke*. Edinburgh: Churchill Livingstone; 1995.

Kamsa YPT, Browner W, Johannes PWF, *et al*. Training of compensational strategies for impaired gross motor skills in Parkinson's disease. *Physio Theory Pract* 1995, **11**:209-229.

Katz RT, Rymer WZ. Spastic hypertonia: mechanisms and measurement. *Arch Phys Med Rehabil* 1989, **70**:144-155.

Kelly V. The walk-easy dorsiflexion assistor. *Physiother* 1993, **79**:254-256.

Kidd D, Stewart G, Baldney J, *et al*. The functional independence measure: a comparative validity and reliability study. *Disabil Rehab* 1995, **17**:10-14.

Kilbride CB. *Positive supporting reaction: the evaluation of physiotherapy intervention* [*unpublished MSc thesis*]. London: University of East London; 1993.

Kings Fund Forum. The treatment of stroke. *BMJ* 1988, **297**:126-128.

Lockard MA. Foot othoses. *Phys Ther* 1988, **68**:1866-1873.

Lumberg A. A multisensory control of spinal reflex pathways. *Progress Brain Res* 1979, **50**:11-28.

Mahony M, McGraw-Non K, McNamara N, *et al*. Aquatic intervention for patients with spinal cord injury. Aquatic physical therapy. *J Aquatic Sect Am Phys Ther Assoc* 1993, **1**:10-16 & 20.

Markham CH. Vestibular control of muscular tone and posture. *J Can Sci Neurol* 1987, **14**:493-496.

Moreland J, Thomson MA. Efficacy of electromyographic biofeedback compared with conventional physical therapy for upper-extremity function in patients following stroke: a research overview and meta-analysis. *Phys Ther* 1994, **74**:23-32.

Morgan MH. Ataxia and weights. *Physiother* 1975, **61**:332-334.

Mulcahy CM, Pountney TE, Nelham RL, *et al*. Adaptive seating for the motor handicap: problems, a solution, assessment and perscription. *Physiother* 1988, **74**:347-352.

Musa I. The role of afferent input in the reduction of spasticity. *Physiother* 1986, **72**:179-182.

Park DM. Spasticity in adults. In: Moore P, ed. *Handbook of botulinum toxin treatment*. London: Blackwell Science; 1995:209-221.

Partridge CJ, Edwards S, Johnston M. Recovery from physical disability after stroke: normal patterns as a basis for evaluation. *Lancet* 1987, Feb 14:373-375.

Partridge CJ, Edwards SM, Mee R, *et al*. Hemiplegic shoulder pain: a study of two methods of physiotherapy treatment. *Clin Rehab* 1990, **4**:43-49.

Pentland B. Parkinsonism in dystonia. In: Greenwood R *et al*., eds. *Neurological rehabilitation*. Edinburgh: Churchill Livingstone; 1993:475-484.

Perry J. Rehabilitation of spasticity. In: Feldman RG, Young RR, Koella W, eds. *Spasticity: disordered motor control*. Chicago: Year Book Medical Publishers; 1980:87-100.

Pope PM. Postural management and special seating. In: Edwards S, ed. *Neurological physiotherapy - a problem-solving approach*. London: Churchill Livingstone; 1996:135-160.

Richardson DLA. The use of the tilt table to effect passive tendo-achilles stretch in a patient with head injury. *Physio Theory Pract* 1991, **7**:45-50.

Riddoch MJ, Humphreys GW, Bateman A. Cognitive deficits following stroke. *Physiother* 1995, **81**:465-493.

Ryerson SD. The foot in hemiplegia. In: Hunt G, ed. *Physical therapy of the foot and ankle*. New York: Churchill Livingstone; 1988:109-131.

Ryerson S, Levit K. The shoulder in hemiplegia. In: Donatelli R, ed. *Physical therapy of the shoulder, 2nd edition*. New York: Churchill Livingstone; 1991:117-149.

Sackley CM. The relationship between weight bearing, asymmetry after stroke, motor function and activities of daily living. *Physio Theory Pract* 1990, **6**:179-185.

Sahrmann S. Muscle imbalances in orthopaedic/neurologic patients. In: *Proceedings of 10th International Congress of World Confederation for Physical Therapy*. Sydney: International Congress for Physical Therapy; 1987:836-841.

Sapega AA, Quendenfield TC, Moyer RA, *et al*. Biophysical factors in range of motion exercises. *Physician Sportsmed* 1981, **9**:57-65.

Settle CM. Seating and pressure sores. *Physiother* 1987, **73**:455-457.

Sindou M, Abbott R, Keravel Y, eds. *Neurosurgery for spasticity, a multidisciplinary approach*. Wien: Springer-Verlag; 1991.

Skeil DA, Barnes MP. The local treatment of spasticity. *Clin Rehab* 1994, **8**:240-246.

Stillman B. Computer-based video analysis of movement. *Aust J Physiother* 1991, **37**:219-227.

Tardieu C, Lespargot A, Tabary C, *et al*. How long must the soleus muscle be stretched each day to prevent contracture? *Devel Med Child Neurol* 1988, **30**:3-10.

Taylor EW, Morris D, Shaddeau S, *et al*. Effects of water walking on hemiplegic gait. Aquatic physical therapy. *J Aquatic Sect Am Phys Ther Assoc* 1993, **1**:10-13.

Thompson PD. Stiff muscles. *J Neurol Neurosurg Psychiat* 1993, **56**:121-124.

Turnbull GI. Some learning theory implications in neurological physiotherapy. *Physiother* 1982, **68**:38-41.

Voss DE, Ionta MK, Myers BJ. *Proprioceptive neuromuscular facilitation patterns and techniques, 3rd edition*. Philadelphia: Harper & Row; 1985.

Wade DT. *Measurement in neurological rehabilitation*. New York: Oxford University; 1992.

Williams PE. Use of intermittent stretch in the prevention of serial sarcomere loss in immobilised muscle. *Ann Rheumat Dis* 1990, **49**:3-16.

PAIN MANAGEMENT IN NEUROLOGICAL REHABILITATION

CHAPTER OUTLINE

- **Neurophysiology of pain**
- **Chronic pain**

- **Pain management in practice**

INTRODUCTION

Chronic pain syndromes pose a particular challenge to the physiotherapist in neurological practice because, whilst the psychology of a patient may be a stronger influence on outcome than is his or her physical status, instigating and maintaining change in physical activity is crucial to rehabilitation. Indeed, the role of psychology in the physiotherapy of chronic conditions has merited an editorial in a physiotherapy journal (Harding & Williams, 1995a). The same authors have argued elsewhere (1995b) that the physiotherapist working with chronic pain has the same aims as in any other specialty; i.e. to improve fitness and mobility and to educate the patient about the condition. However, the achievement of these aims for the patient in chronic pain often requires different means, based on psychological principles. Why should the patient's psychology affect the treatment of a physical pain syndrome?

The importance of psychological aspects to the understanding and recovery of the person with persistent pain stems from the primary experience of pain being wholly subjective. Pain cannot be observed directly. The International Association for the Study of Pain (IASP) has defined pain as 'an unpleasant and emotional experience associated with actual or potential tissue damage or described in terms of such damage'. Science has not yet made the measurement of experience a straightforward matter. Turk (1989), in a classic discussion of this dilemma, likened the investigator who was trying to measure pain to a hunter who goes into the woods to catch an animal no-one has ever seen but whose damaging effects are clear to all. The only way the hunter can decide which tracks to follow is by adopting assumptions about the nature of the quarry. Similarly, clinicians and scientists attempting to investigate and treat pain know the effects of pain from their daily work, yet no precise definition for measurement exists to date.

Clinicians must rely on secondary sources from which to infer the magnitude and quality of the pain experience. Broadly, these are either physiological (e.g. autonomic response), motor activity (e.g. guarding, moaning, facial expressions), self-report (e.g. visual-analogue scales, numerical ratings, descriptive adjectives, questionnaires), or other indicators such as health-care use and medication levels. Part of the complexity of pain phenomena is that self-reports of pain vary greatly in the extent to which they coincide with either psychophysiology or motor activity. It seems that we are interrogating at least three response systems that may correlate at times but are at best loosely coupled.

Melzack & Wall (1965) suggested that sensory, affective and cognitive factors combine to create an individual's pain experience. Melzack (1975) designed the McGill Pain Questionnaire to assess each of these three components, by analysing the patient's selection of adjectives which best describe the pain. It is by no means certain, however, that verbal labels can accurately represent the pain experience. The complexities of the experience of pain in both the laboratory and clinic are discussed by Melzack & Wall (1984), in a text that can be helpful to both professionals and patients. The shortcomings of measurements for pain led clinicians to move towards assessing the patient, in terms of physical pathology, psychosocial and behavioural variables, rather than the pain as an isolated phenomenon (Turk & Rudy, 1987).

NEUROPHYSIOLOGY OF PAIN

Recent advances of functional imaging techniques have increased our understanding of the central processing that affects sensation, emotion and cognition. For example, a positron emission tomography (PET) study of patients with mononeuropathies revealed activation of bilateral anterior insular, posterior parietal, lateral inferior prefrontal and posterior cingulate cortices, compared to a pain-free state created by regional nerve blocks. In addition, both the right anterior cingulate cortex (ACC) and Brodmann area were also activated, regardless of the laterality of the neuropathy (Hsieh et al,. 1995). The ACC may be important in chronic pain syndromes: it has involvement in avoidance learning, it is rich in opioid receptors and it may process the affective component of pain experience. There are two neuronal clusters in the ACC that have links with 'attention' and 'motor control and motor intention'; these two functions could be implicated in psychological pain-management techniques that target cognition and behaviour. The basic anatomy and physiology of pain have been outlined in Chapter 1 and will not be repeated here. A brief reference to basic aspects of acute and chronic pain is Coniam & Diamond (1994).

PEOPLE WITH CHRONIC PAIN

A person with chronic pain is likely to be inactive and unable to fulfil normal social roles, such as family member, employee or leisure partner. Behavioural theory has offered a conceptual framework for understanding and treating this disability that has received considerable empirical support. It suggests that the behaviour of patients with chronic pain is influenced by social and environmental stimuli and consequences. The reinforcement schedules for well and illness behaviour are entirely controlled by the immediate social group. Pain complaints often bear little relationship to organic pathology (Fordyce, 1976). Limping, grimacing or verbal complaints signal pain and elicit attention and consideration from others. Some consequences of pain behaviour, such as extra care-giving by friends and relatives, or the avoidance of aversive situations such as a stressful workplace, serve to reinforce and maintain pain behaviour.

Because of his or her frequent interactions with the patient, a spouse is able to be very influential in shaping the patient's behaviour. Significant associations have been found between the responses of a spouse and the activity of the patient. Flor et al. (1987) reported that patients who viewed their spouses as highly solicitous responders to pain behaviours, were more likely both to report their pain as more severe and to have low activity levels. Using a methodology that has been developed and validated to observe directly the behaviour between spouse and patient (Romano et al., 1991), Romano et al. (1995) demonstrated that solicitous responses from the spouse to the patient's pain behaviours were associated with greater pain behaviour and disability amongst patients with chronic pain.

Many programmes for pain management explicitly address this issue, involving spouses and teaching them to respond positively to increased patient activity and other well behaviours and, conversely, to respond less solicitously to pain behaviours. Negative exchanges with care-givers or criticism from family members may have adverse consequences for both physical and psychological well-being that exceed the beneficial effects of positive support (Kerns et al., 1991). Prospective studies are few, but they suggest that patient hostility may precede increases in criticism by the spouse (Lane & Hobfell, 1992).

PAIN AND DEPRESSION

Depressed patients often report pain and depression, and depressive symptoms are frequently found in patients with chronic pain. A large population survey of middle-aged people (Rajala et al., 1994) demonstrated that pain was more common amongst the depressed than the non-depressed population, and many of the depressed subjects reported pain in multiple anatomical sites. Assessed according to the International Classification of Diseases (ICD-9; WHO, 1989), the prevalence of depressive neurosis was reported to be 21% in a British pain clinic population (Tyrer et al., 1989). Depression may be a consequence of pain and the limitations it imposes on the patient's life, or it may be a sign of an underlying distress, which renders a person more vulnerable to the causation and maintenance of a chronic pain syndrome. In a 10-year follow-up sample of a general population, depressive symptoms predicted future musculoskeletal pain episodes, but not vice versa (Leino & Magni, 1993).

There is evidence from correlational analyses that it is the perceived impact that the pain has on the patient's life that predicts depression, rather than the absolute level of pain experienced. A path analysis of the self-report cognitive and emotional scores of 10 chronic pain patients was conducted by Turk et al. (1995). Pain Intensity significantly influenced perceptions of Interference and Life Control, which in turn affected depression scores. However, pain intensity was not directly related to depression.

Although less well studied than depression, anger is another prominent negative emotion in chronic pain (Wade et al., 1990; Hatch et al., 1991). Fernandez & Turk (1995) have suggested a list of objects and reasons for anger (Table 26.1). If the expression of anger is inhibited, then the patient runs the risk of experiencing more pain and depression. However, unchecked expression of anger may disrupt interpersonal relations and affect treatment outcome. This analysis led Fernandez & Turk (1995) to postulate an optimal regulation of anger that represents a better adjustment by the patient to the condition.

The beliefs and expectations of patients with chronic pain have been shown to be critical facilitators of, or impediments to, their recovery. For example, DeGood & Kiernan (1996) asked out-patients with chronic pain, 'Who do you think is at fault for your pain?'. The responses were grouped according to whether a patient identified his or her employer, another person, or no-one. Only half those

Attributions about objects of anger and appraisals about reasons for anger amongst people with chronic pain	
Agent (object of anger)	**Action (reason for anger)**
Causal agent of injury/illness	Chronic pain
Medical health care providers	Diagnostic ambiguity; treatment failure
Mental health professionals	Implications of psychogenicity or psychopathology
Attorneys and legal system	Adversarial dispute, scrutiny and arbitration
Insurance companies; social security system	Inadequate monetary coverage or compensation
Employer	Cessation of employment; job transfer; job retraining
Significant others	Lack of interpersonal support
God	'Predetermined' injury and consequences; ill fate
Self	Disablement, disfigurement
The whole world	Alienation

Table 26.1 Attributions about objects of anger and appraisals about reasons for anger amongst people with chronic pain. (Redrawn from Fernandez & Turk, 1995, with permission.)

patients who had experienced a work-related injury blamed their employers. The patients who faulted their employers were more likely to feel unfairly treated by the employers before and after the injury. This was despite there being no difference amongst the three groups in terms of current pain intensity or activity limitation. However, those patients who blamed their employers or another person, reported greater mood and behavioural disturbance, poorer response to past treatments and lesser expectations of future benefit. It may be that the sense of suffering is increased when pain is seen as the result of others' lack of caution or concern.

COPING WITH CHRONIC PAIN

Differences in the use of coping strategies for pain may be significant in adjusting to chronic pain. Active coping by patients with chronic pain is related to psychological well-being. In contrast, passive coping is strongly related to psychological distress and depression (Snow-Turek et al., 1996). Cross-sectional studies show that active strategies such as positive self-statements, the use of coping self-statements and increasing activities are associated with better physical and psychological functioning in patients with chronic pain. In contrast, the use of rest to cope with pain, and other passive strategies, appears to be associated with worse physical functioning. Measures of coping with pain have been developed; e.g. the Chronic Pain Coping Inventory (Jensen et al., 1995) includes positive items (such as 'imagined a calming or distracting image to help me relax') and negative items (such as 'walked with a limp to decrease the pain').

PAIN MANAGEMENT IN PRACTICE

Management of pain includes: initial assessment of the problem; planning treatment and setting goals; treatment strategies; and monitoring progress.

ASSESSMENT

Some measurement of a patient's physical function and everyday activity is an essential prerequisite to starting treatment. It provides a quantitative description of the patient's current situation, which can then be used to monitor treatment progress and maintenance. Many useful tools for measuring pain and its effects have been developed, with good reliability and validity. Provided that they are selected and used with an appreciation of their limitations, some of which were outlined in the first part of this chapter, they can be of great benefit to both the clinician and the researcher. Harding et al. (1994) have described a battery for assessing the physical functioning of patients with chronic pain, which reportedly took only 45 minutes to complete prior to treatment. The reliability, validity and acceptability of seven tests of speed and endurance are recorded. Some measures of pain for specific anatomical sites have been developed, which have high face validity and therefore facilitate patient co-operation. For example, the Pain Index for the Knee (Lewis et al., 1995a) offers a clinical procedure for assessing knee pain, with some basic transportable equipment, and takes only 5–10 minutes for each knee. It involves 10 standardised knee movements (four active, six passive), which are then scored by the assessor, largely in terms of the subject's pain behaviour. The Curtin Back Screening Questionnaire has been demonstrated to discriminate between people with different degrees of disability resulting from occupational low-back pain (Harper *et al.*, 1995) and has good psychometric properties. It is reportedly self-administered in 30 minutes and scored in 3 minutes, and is designed for a range of settings from primary care to the specialist clinic.

RECORDS

Because of the many emotional and cognitive variables that can influence a patient's understanding of his or her condition, self-report is only one facet of information gathering. For instance, patients with pain tend to under-report their activity levels, as compared to objective measures of activity (Turk *et al.*, 1992). Any report or rating of pain over time necessarily depends on memory for pain, which in itself is complex and problematic (Erskine *et al.*, 1990). A structured system of record keeping and diaries is therefore essential. For research purposes, electronic data-logging devices have been developed (Lewis *et al.*, 1995b) and these could be adapted for clinical use.

STRATEGIES FOR PAIN MANAGEMENT

Medication for pain is outlined in Chapter 28 and will not be considered here, except in passing. A fairly detailed and accessible account of psychological pain-management strategies can be found in chapters 8 to 13 of Turk *et al.* (1983). It can often be a great surprise to the patient that pain levels and painful body parts are not to be the focus of treatment, but rather general fitness and activity levels, physical confidence and attitude. However, some patients with chronic pain are resigned to the persistence of their condition and may not require a great deal of persuasion, but rather welcome an approach offering constructive help and real hope, and which has only minimal risks.

Relaxation

Relaxation is often an essential part of most pain-management programmes, especially in the early stages. The classical Jacobsen exercises, involving the clenching and relaxing of various muscle groups, are not usually the technique of choice for neuropathic pain because they tend to increase muscle tension. Patients with chronic pain who receive relaxation training report greater decrease in pain, decrease in psychological distress and decrease in functional disability, compared to patients on a waiting list or in attention-placebo control conditions (Turk *et al.*, 1983). Applied relaxation training (ART) has been demonstrated to be more effective at treating upper extremity pain associated with repetitive workplace tasks than either electromyography (EMG) biofeedback alone, or EMG biofeedback combined with ART (Spence *et al.*, 1995). The authors suggest that, whereas ART creates feelings of control over pain by influencing muscle tension levels, any involvement of machinery reduces feelings of control and reinforces conceptions of pain as a primarily physical and mechanical phenomenon. It is certainly true that ART teaches a more flexible and portable skill, which can be employed in a variety of situations.

Setting Goals

The setting of goals serves a number of purposes: (1) there is an explicit contract describing what is expected of the patient in terms of physical progress over the next few weeks; (2) the patient and his or her family have a clear account of a realistic rate of progress; and (3) the patient's progress can be monitored against the agreed goals, and success or failure noted. Initially, the therapist may need to offer extensive guidance in setting goals, but it is always essential to take careful and detailed account of the patient's preferences and current situation.

Pacing

Pacing involves the gradual increase of activity, in a structured, graded way, in line with the patient's increasing stamina and pain-management skills. Most patients are surprised at how little activity they are required to perform at the outset and this can lead them to view their treatment as a step backwards; this requires careful explanation and education. The ideal baseline is far below the personal maximum level of effort. Any sign of exhaustion or pain, suggesting that a person is approaching his or her activity limit, is evidence that the baseline has been set too high. The baseline level of activity or exercise should be performed by the patient relatively easily and should be achievable on any day, not just 'good days'. Sometimes the baseline levels of activity can appear trivial to an outsider. For example, a severely disabled, bed-bound woman with chronic pain started with a baseline that amounted to little more than five slight shifts of each foot on the bed, three times a day, but that was the level at which the team could engage her and from which she could start to build her confidence.

Cognitive Therapy

People with chronic pain will have a different outlook on life from that of healthy people. They will tend to fasten on negative events, predict the future negatively, denigrate themselves, experience a great deal of guilt, discount positive events and successes, and 'catastrophise', i.e. follow trains of thoughts that lead to a disastrous potential outcome from a relatively minor setback. This skewing of their perception of themselves and their lives can be overcome and normalised, by a technique known as cognitive therapy. This identifies, records and challenges mistakenly negative thoughts and attitudes; challenges them by exploring or gathering evidence related to them; and systematically and routinely counters them with replacement 'healthy' thoughts.

Self-help Books

It can be extremely useful for a person with chronic pain to read about pain and its management. There are pitfalls though: the book may offend or anger the patient by being irrelevant to, or inaccurate about, his or her condition; the patient may become obsessed with the details of the condition and never move beyond diagnosis and terminology; or the patient may think that he or she could have written a more expert and insightful book, either before or after reading the one that you recommend. However, judicious timing and matching of patients to books can bring dividends. These books can extend the time each week a person thinks constructively about his or her pain; they can serve as a memo, to remind the patient and extend the contents of treatment sessions; they can introduce new topics, such as the role of the family, in a less threatening way than a face-to-face discussion might be able to do; and family members, who may not be able to attend sessions, can become acquainted with some basic principles of pain management. For physiology and anatomy, Coniam & Diamond (1994) is good. Three self-help books which have proved useful in clinical work are Shone (1992), Sternbach (1987) and White (1990).

OVERVIEW OF PAIN STRATEGIES

It is not known which individual components or combinations of strategies are the most effective, or even necessary, within a pain-management programme. No two programmes are alike, even within the same hospital and when run by the same staff, because the patients' individual personalities and experiences on the programme affect the content and emphasis. It may be that different aspects are helpful to particular patient profiles, or at particular stages of rehabilitation and maintenance. It is sometimes argued that strategies in themselves do not represent the core process in pain management and rehabilitation, but rather serve as agents that contribute to the primary process, which is one of establishing feelings of control.

There is an experimental study which provides evidence for the importance of control in the experience of pain (Holroyd et al., 1984). College students suffering from recurrent tension headache were recruited and assigned to one of four EMG biofeedback training groups. All were told that they were learning to decrease frontal EMG. All subjects were shown two graphs on a VDU, one graph showing dramatic improvement, the other showing modest improvement. Half of the subjects were told that the dramatically improving line represented their progress and the modestly improving line was an average performance (the 'high-success group'). The other half of the subjects were told that the dramatically improving line was the average performance and the modestly improving line was their own performance (the 'low-success group'). Although all subjects were led to believe that they were learning to decrease EMG activity, the high- and low-success groups were further split into two separate feedback schedules, with half the subjects in each group receiving feedback for decreasing EMG activity, but the other half receiving feedback for increasing EMG activity. Regardless of whether their experimental feedback led them to increase or decrease their actual EMG activity, the high-success group reported greater reduction in tension headache (53%) than the low-success group (26%).

Performance feedback was also related to cognitive changes, including feelings of control over pain and beliefs about being able to perform everyday activities despite pain. The authors concluded that the effectiveness of EMG training in tension headache may be mediated by cognitive changes induced by performance feedback and not primarily by reductions in EMG activity.

CLINICAL ASPECTS OF NEUROPATHIC PAIN

It is likely to be the case that your first contact with a person with chronic pain will be an uncomfortable experience. The patient may be firmly entrenched in the view that nothing can help the pain. Patients with chronic pain are often extremely bitter and distrustful of healthcare professionals. They may produce lengthy and colourful accounts of their pain and previous operations and treatments. They may have had, or report, previous unsuccessful or painful experiences of physiotherapy. The task of the physiotherapist in the first session is to engage them. You must somehow convince them that it is worth coming back for the next session, that changes are possible, that their lives can get better. Strategies to effect this include: emphasising your expertise; not reinforcing exclamations of pain and other pain behaviour, whilst remaining respectful and interested; examining range of movement (as far as is possible); and offering some immediate education about joint care, sitting posture or environmental aids.

It is a great privilege if a person with chronic pain agrees to enter a treatment programme with you; the patient will almost certainly have suffered many therapeutic disappointments previously and will be risking another by daring to start hoping again. A good way of encouraging people with chronic pain to continue with pain-management programmes is to induce positive change early. Relaxation will often do this, offering some modulation of pain experience and therefore evidence that the problem is not completely intractable, as the patient may have professed or believed at initial assessment.

The intractability and persistence of some neuropathic pain syndromes should not be underestimated. People experiencing neuropathic pain can be driven to extreme and even bizarre behaviours. The clinician must be aware of all possibilities and alert to them. For example, Mailis (1996) reported four cases of self-injurious behaviour in people with painful dysaesthesiae. Whilst these are the exception rather than the rule, they serve as a reminder of the range of behavioural disturbances that pain can induce.

THE PAIN MANAGEMENT TEAM

A team approach to chronic pain goes some way to addressing the many interrelated factors that serve to influence and maintain a chronic pain syndrome. It also should ensure a continuity of approach. It allows a greater number of patients to receive the attention of several specialists within a short period of time, leading to savings in time and costs. However, teams are not a panacea. The individual characteristics of team members exert great influence over the team's character and effectiveness. Time must be allocated for meetings and other team functions. 'Participatory democracy tends to be a cumbersome and slow-moving process' (Segraves, 1989).

The role of the various professionals in the team is in line with each particular discipline's skills and expertise. The neurologist will be involved in the initial examination and investigations of the patient and the diagnosis. A neurosurgical opinion may be sought. Medication may be prescribed. Most pain clinics involve a pain anaesthetist, who will examine the patient, may request further investigations and may perform some procedures and adjust medication. A psychiatrist may be involved if there are reasons to consider psychotropic medication, although as a general rule most pain-management programmes seek to reduce medication. A psychologist will usually be involved once pain management, as opposed to more active treatments, is under consideration. The psychologist will be involved in the psychosocial assessment of the patient and planning the cognitive aspects of treatment.

The physiotherapist will be involved in assessment and the planning of physical treatment (the role of the physiotherapist in the pain-management team is discussed in detail by Harding & Williams, 1995b). In some centres, a nurse may oversee the reduction of medication and an occupational therapist may assist patients with household and work activities. Once a pain-management programme is instigated, all staff must be able to discuss and reinforce the basic principles of increasing activity and well behaviour, pacing, using relaxation strategies, maintaining the exercise programme, at least rudimentary cognitive therapy, and goal setting.

The organisation of teams has been described in sports terms by Segraves (1989), not entirely for reasons of humour. Three models are identified:

1. Baseball teams, in which individuals function and are evaluated independently, hardly interacting; the team manager's concern is 'batting order'.
2. Football teams, which require more interaction but are basically a co-ordinated hierarchical service; this is best suited to large organisations, or many independent units.
3. Basketball teams, which require continuous team member awareness, co-operation, adjustment and spontaneous reaction; the coach is an enabler rather than a director; this flexible and dynamic system tends to work where numbers are small.

OUTCOMES

There is a growing body of evidence that psychological pain-management programmes, delivered by a multidisciplinary team, result in significant benefit for a substantial proportion of recruited patients and that this improvement is generally maintained over a number of years. In a large study, Maruta et al. (1990) reported a 70% success rate at discharge from an in-patient pain-management programme, which was maintained by very nearly half of those successfully treated at 3-year follow-up. These figures are similar to those reported in a previous study from the same institution. These outcomes are particularly encouraging when one considers the severe disability, emotional distress and excessive medication use that is typical of the patients who are admitted to these programmes.

REFERENCES

Coniam SW, Diamond AW. *Practical pain management.* Oxford: Oxford University Press; 1994.

DeGood DE, Kiernan B. Perception of fault in patients with chronic pain. *Pain* 1996, **64**:153-160.

Erskine A, Morley S, Pearce S. Memory for pain: a review. *Pain* 1990, **41**:255-266.

Fernandez E, Turk DC. The scope and significance of anger in the experience of chronic pain. *Pain* 1995, **61**:165-175.

Flor H, Kerns RD, Turk DC. The role of spouse reinforcement, perceived pain, and activity levels of chronic pain patients. *J Psychosom Res 1987,* **31**:251-259.

Fordyce, WE. *Behavioural methods for chronic pain and illness.* St Louis: Mosby; 1976.

Harding V, Williams ACdeC. Applying psychology to enhance physiotherapy outcomes. *Physiother Theory Prac* 1995, **11**:129-132.

Harding V, Williams ACdeC. Extending physiotherapy skills using a psychological approach: cognitive-behavioural management of chronic pain. *Physiother* 1995, **81**:681-688.

Harding V, Williams A CdeC, Richardson PH *et al.* The development of a battery of measures for assessing physical functioning of chronic pain patients. *Pain* 1994, **58**:367-375.

Harper AC, Harper DA, Lambert LJ, *et al.* Development and validation of the Curtin Back Screening Questionnaire (CBSQ) - a discriminative disability measure. *Pain* 1995, **60**:73-81.

Hatch JP, Schoenfeld LS, Boutros NN, *et al.* Anger and hostility in tension-type headache. *Headache* 1991, **31**:302-304.

Hsieh JC, Belfrage M, Stone-Elander S, *et al.* Central representation of chronic ongoing neuropathic pain studied by positron emission tomography. *Pain* 1995, **63**:225-236.

Holroyd KA, Penzien DB, Hursey KG, *et al.* Change mechanisms in EMG biofeedback training: cognitive changes underlying improvement in tension headache. *J Con Clin Psychol* 1984, **52**:1039-1053.

Jensen MP, Turner JA, Romano JM, *et al.* The chronic pain coping inventory: development and preliminary validation. *Pain* 1995, **60**:203-216.

Kerns RD, Southwick S, Giller EL, *et al.* The relationship between reports of pain related social interactions and expressions of pain and affective distress. *Behav Ther* 1991, **22**:101-111.

Lane C, Hobfell SE. How loss affects anger and alienates potential supporters. *J Con Clin Psychol* 1992, **60**:935-942.

Leino P, Magni G. Depressive and distress symptoms as predictors of low back pain, neck-shoulder pain, and other musculoskeletal morbidity: a 10-year follow-up of metal industry employees. *Pain* 1993, **53**:89-94.

Lewis B, Bellamo R, Lewis D, *et al.* A clinical procedure for assessment of severity of knee pain. *Pain* 1995, **63**:361-364.

Lewis B, Lewis D, Cumming G. Frequent measurement of chronic pain: an electronic diary and empirical findings. *Pain* 1995, **60**:341-347.

Mailis A. Compulsive targeted self-injurious behaviour in humans with neuropathic pain: a counterpart of animal autotomy? Four case reports and a review of the literature. *Pain* 1996, **64**:569-578.

Maruta T, Swanson DW, McHardy MJ, *et al.* Three year follow-up of patients with chronic pain who were treated in a multidisciplinary pain management centre. *Pain* 1990, **41**:47-53.

Melzack R. The McGill pain questionnaire: major properties and scoring methods. *Pain* 1975, **1**:277-299.

Melzack R, Wall PD. Pain mechanisms: a new theory. *Sci* 1965, **150**:971-979.

Melzack R, Wall PD. *The challenge of pain.* London: Penguin; 1984.

Rajala U, Uusimaki A, Keinanen-Kiukaanniemi S, *et al.* Prevalance of depression in a 55 year old Finnish population. *Soc Phychiatry Psychiat Epidemiol* 1994, **29**:126-130.

Romano JM, Turner JA, Friedman LS, *et al.* Observational assessment of chronic pain patient-spouse behavioural interactions. *Behav Ther* 1991, **22**:549-567.

Romano JM, Turner JA, Jensen MP, *et al.* Chronic pain patient-spouse behavioral interactions predict patient disability. *Pain* 1995, **63**:353-360.

Segraves KB. Bringing it all together: developing the clinical team. In: Camic PM, Brown FD, eds. *Assessing chronic pain: a multidisciplinary handbook.* New York: Springer-Verlag; 1989:229-248.

Shone N. *Coping successfully with pain.* London: Sheldon Press; 1992.

Snow-Turek AL, Norris MP, Tan G. Active and passive coping strategies in chronic pain patients. *Pain* 1996, **64**:455-462.

Spence SH, Sharpe L, Newton-John T, *et al.* Effect of EMG biofeedback compared to applied relaxation training with chronic, upper extremity cumulative trauma disorders. *Pain* 1995, **63**:199-206.

Sternbach R. *Mastering pain.* London: Arlington Press; 1987.

Turk DC. Assessment of pain: the elusiveness of a latent construct. In: Chapman CR, Loeser J, eds. *Advances in pain research and therapy, Vol 12: Issues in pain measurement.* New York: Raven; 1989:267-280.

Turk DC, Kerns RD, Rosenberg R. Effects of marital interaction on chronic pain and disability: examining the down side of social support. *Rehabil Psychol* 1992, **37**:259-274.

Turk DC, Meichenbaum D, Genest M. *Pain and behavioural medicine: a cognitive behavioral approach.* New York: Guilford Press; 1983.

Turk DC, Okifuji A, Scharff L. Chronic pain and depression: role of perceived impact and perceived control in different age cohorts. *Pain* 1995, **61**:93-101.

Turk DC, Rudy TE. Assessment of chronic pain patients. *Behav Res Ther* 1987, **25**:237-249.

Tyrer SP, Capon M, Peterson DM *et al.* The detection of psychiatric illness and psychological handicaps in a British pain clinic population. *Pain* 1989, **36**:63-74.

Wade JB, Price DD, Hamer RM, *et al.* An emotional component analysis of chronic pain. *Pain* 1990, **40**:303-310.

White AA. *Your aching back.* New York: Simon and Schuster; 1990.

World Health Organization. *Mental disorders, glossary and guide to their classification in accordance with the 9th revision of the international classification of diseases.* Geneva: WHO; 1989.

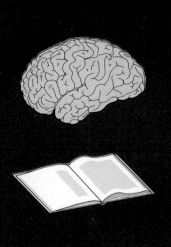

27 JG Beaumont

CLINICAL PSYCHOLOGY IN NEUROLOGICAL REHABILITATION

CHAPTER OUTLINE

- **Approaches in clinical neuropsychology**

- **Neuropsychological consequences of neurological disorders**

INTRODUCTION

The field of clinical psychology that is concerned with neurological disorders has now become known as clinical neuropsychology. Although in the UK there is no formal definition of a clinical neuropsychologist, developments are currently under way which may soon result in the establishment of professional qualifications in neuropsychology. In practice, clinical neuropsychologists are Chartered Clinical Psychologists with specialist experience and expertise in the field of neuropsychology, and often title themselves 'Neuropsychologist'.

Whilst clinical neuropsychology is only now emerging as an independent area of professional psychology, it has a history as long as the history of modern scientific psychology. From the end of the last century, psychologists have investigated the behavioural effects of lesions to the brain, not only for the light this study could shed on the operation of normal brain processes but also from a genuine concern to alleviate the distress and disability resulting from neurological injury and disease.

Clinical neuropsychology was given an inevitable stimulus by the two World Wars, the study of missile wounds proving a fertile ground for the association of specific psychological deficits with defined regions of the brain. This research carried significant implications for a debate, inherited from nineteenth-century neurology, which occupied at least the first half of this century, about the nature of the representation of psychological functions in the brain. Put rather crudely, the opposite poles of the debate argued either for the highly localised and specific representation of functions, or for a mass action view whereby psychological functions are distributed across the entire cerebral cortex. This debate has never been finally resolved, but the position that most clinical neuropsychologists now adopt is one of relative localisation: that many functions are localised to regions of the cortex but cannot be more finely localised. This is often qualified by a tertiary model of cortical function in that the primary cortex, subserving sensation and discrete motor control is quite highly localised; the secondary cortex, subserving perception and the control of movements is rather less localised; and the tertiary or association cortex, supporting all higher-level functions, is much less clearly localised. Current developments in connectionist theory, which suggest radical models for neuropsychological processes are, however, starting to modify these views. For a fuller discussion, see Beaumont (1996) and for illustrations see Code *et al.* (1996).

Only within the last two decades has rehabilitation become an active focus of interest for clinical neuropsychology. Before that time clinicians saw their role as primarily one of assessment, either in the context of diagnosis or of vocational adjustment. The widespread introduction of modern neuroimaging greatly diminished the contribution of neuropsychology to diagnosis and as a result the embarrassing period of neglect of rehabilitation, both in terms of research and of practical interventions, came to an end. Rehabilitation is now the central focus of neuropsychology and assessment is understood, quite properly, as only a significant stage towards the planning of rehabilitation and management.

APPROACHES IN CLINICAL NEUROPSYCHOLOGY

Clinical psychological management involves detailed assessment, which is discussed prior to reviewing interventions.

NEUROPSYCHOLOGICAL ASSESSMENT

Neuropsychological assessment should be understood as the essential precursor to the planning and implementation of rehabilitation. It is not an end in itself, but is designed to provide a description in psychological terms of the client's current state with respect to the clinical problems being addressed. Such a description should provide an insight into the processes which are no longer functioning normally in that individual, and so provide the rationale upon which the intervention is based. Subsequent reassessments allow progress to be monitored and interventions to be adjusted, according to the client's current state. Rehabilitation should never proceed without an adequate assessment having been undertaken.

The Three Traditions

There are historically three traditions in clinical neuropsychology. The first, most eloquently expressed in the work of Luria (see Christensen, 1974), is based upon behavioural neurology, although it is a much more sophisticated extension of it. The approach is based upon the presentation of simple tasks, selected in a coherent way from a wide variety of tests available, which any normal individual can be expected successfully to complete without difficulty. Any failure on the task is a pathological sign and the pattern of these signs, in skilled hands, allows a psychological description to be built up.

The second tradition, associated with work in North America, is a psychometric battery-based approach, most notably expressed in the Halstead–Reitan and Luria Nebraska Neuropsychological Test Batteries (any apparent theoretical link with the approach of Luria is quite illusory). In this approach a standard, and often large, battery of tests is administered to all clients and the resulting descriptions arise out of a psychometric analysis of the pattern of test scores.

The third approach, the normative individual-centred approach, has been dominant in Europe, particularly in the UK. It relies upon the use of specific tests, associated wherever possible with adequate normative standardisation, which are selected to investigate hypotheses about the client's deficits; testing these hypotheses permits the psychological description to be built up. Whilst requiring a high level of expertise, this neuropsychological detective work can be more efficient and provide a finer degree of analysis, when applied intelligently. In practice, many neuropsychologists employ a mixture of these approaches, although the normative individual-centred approach is generally becoming more dominant.

Cognitive Functions

The greater part of neuropsychological assessment concentrates upon cognitive functions at present: perception, learning, memory, language, thinking and reasoning. This is a reflection of the principal interests of contemporary psychology. There is a bewildering variety of test procedures available to the clinical neuropsychologist, but most involve the presentation of standardised test materials in a controlled way; this can yield reliable scores which are then interpreted with respect to appropriate normative data. These norms may be more or less adequate for the clinical population under consideration, and there are certainly some excellent, some very good, and some rather inadequate tests.

Even a partial description of the most popular tests is outside the scope of this chapter, but a good introduction may be found in Harding & Beech (1996), and a more thorough account in Crawford et al. (1992) and in Lezak (1995).

Behavioural Assessment

Assessment of behaviour (as distinct from specifically cognitive performance), usually in relation to undesirable behaviours or defective interpersonal or social skills, relies more directly upon observational recording. Here the object is to identify the antecedents of the behaviour under investigation, and then to analyse the consequences of the behaviour for the individual. In this way an understanding can be gained of what 'causes' the behaviour, and what maintains the behaviour in the individual's repertoire. This information can be used to construct a programme designed to modify the behaviour (see below) or simply be used to provide feedback to the client to assist him or her to gain the insight to modify his or her own behaviour.

Behavioural sampling—the regular observation and recording of relevant aspects of behaviour for fixed samples of time—is frequently employed, and carers may also be requested to maintain records or diaries of specific events. Video recording, sometimes with detailed analysis, may also be employed.

Affective States

Clinical neuropsychologists are also commonly asked to evaluate other aspects of behaviour: affective states, motivation, insight, adjustment to disability, pain and, often most difficult of all, the possible psychological basis of apparently organic neurological states. It is for this reason, amongst others, that a thorough training in clinical psychology is considered essential for neuropsychological practice. A certain number of standard questionnaires and rating scales are available to assist in this assessment, but the neuropsychologist must commonly rely upon clinical experience and expertise in forming a judgement.

Outcome Measures and the Quality of Life

The political climate of health service changes in the UK has forced healthcare providers to consider the outcome of their interventions, and this can only be to the advantage of clients. Psychologists, because of their expertise in the measurement of behaviour, have been prominent in the development of outcome measures. Within neuropsychological rehabilitation there is a variety of measures, of which the Barthel Index (Wade, 1992) is widely used, and FIM–FAM (Functional Independence Measure–Functional Assessment Measure; Ditunno, 1992; Cook *et al.*, 1994) is growing in popularity as it can be linked to problem-oriented and client-centred rehabilitation planning. However, none of the available scales is adequate to assess the status of severely disabled clients (see Chapter 4), and there is also a lack of good measures of the specific outcome of psychological interventions. Research is actively being undertaken to fill these gaps.

Allied to the need to assess outcomes has been a growing interest in 'quality of life' (QoL), recognising that not only functional and physical status should be considered but also the individual's personal feelings and life experience. A central problem is that QoL is not a unitary concept and encompasses a range of ideas, from the spiritual and metaphysical to cognitions about health and happiness. What is clear is that QoL relates not in a direct, but in a very complex, way to health status, physical disability and handicap, and that the precise nature of this relationship has yet to be clarified.

Cognitive Neuropsychology

Cognitive neuropsychology should be understood as a distinct, and currently very fashionable, approach within neuropsychology. Of growing importance over the past decade, cognitive neuropsychology concentrates upon the single case and seeks to explain psychological deficits in terms of the components of cognitive information-processing models. Such models, which are now quite detailed in respect of functions such as reading, spelling and face recognition, are based upon experimental data derived from normal individuals and from clinical investigations. These models are modular, and dysfunction can be understood in terms of the faulty performance of either the modules or the connections between them.

Cognitive neuropsychological analysis has been of enormous importance in developing our understanding of both normal and abnormal cognitive psychological functions within the brain but, partly because of the resources required to analyse a problem fully using this approach in the individual case, it has not made such a great impact upon the clinical practice of neuropsychologists.

NEUROPSYCHOLOGICAL INTERVENTIONS

Management strategies include cognitive and behavioural interventions as well as psychotherapy.

Cognitive Interventions

Cognitive interventions aim to reduce the impact of deficits in the areas of memory, learning, perception, language, and thinking and reasoning. How this is achieved depends in part upon the model of recovery that is adopted but, in general, requires either new learning or the development of strategies which bypass the abnormal components in the system. There are often a variety of routes by which an end result may be achieved. Perhaps trivially, consider how many ways 9 may be multiplied by 9 to achieve 81. There

are in fact at least 9 ways. If you learnt the solution by rote learning, you may well find that your children have been taught a different method: 9 x 10 – 9, or the fact that the first digit of the solution is 9 – 1 and that the two digits of the answer sum to 9. These are different 'strategies' of finding the solution. If the previously available strategy has been lost, it may be more successful to teach a new strategy that relies upon different brain mechanisms.

Besides the explicit teaching of new strategies, appropriately structured training may be employed; this is often based upon 'error-free learning', which has been shown to be most effective following head injury. Aids to performance, which may be either external (such as diaries to aid memory) or internal (mnemonics), may also be successfully employed. These interventions are more fully developed in some areas than others, and have been used most extensively in the rehabilitation of memory (Wilson & Moffat, 1992; Kapur, 1994), but the basic principles can be applied in any area of cognitive function (see also Riddoch & Humphreys, 1994).

Behavioural Interventions

Behavioural interventions are less widely employed but may be appropriate to address the remediation of undesirable behaviours and in situations where the residual cognitive function of the individual is severely limited. These interventions are based upon psychological learning theory which, put rather simply, states that behaviour is determined by its consequences. Behaviour which leads to a 'good' outcome for the individual will increase in frequency; that which has an undesirable outcome for the individual will decrease in frequency. Behaviours that are desirable (from the perspective of the rehabilitation goals) can therefore be increased by ensuring that they are positively reinforced (given a good outcome for the individual), whilst undesirable behaviours do not receive such reinforcement. In laboratory situations, negative reinforcement (punishment) might be used to reduce the frequency of a behaviour, but in a clinical situation its use would be extremely exceptional (perhaps only in relation to a significant life-threatening behaviour and then only with informed consent); in practice, the lack of positive reinforcement is sufficient for the undesired behaviour to reduce in frequency.

The range of behavioural techniques is both wider and more sophisticated than this brief account might suggest, and in certain selected contexts these approaches may be highly effective (Wood, 1990). However, the demands on resources and staff skills are high, given that a behavioural programme must be applied consistently, contingently and continuously, often over a very protracted period. For this reason, behavioural approaches are less commonly employed outside specialist facilities, although they are perhaps unreasonably neglected within other rehabilitation contexts.

Psychotherapy; Staff, Team and Organisational Support; Research

Psychologists in neuropsychological practice are also involved in a variety of more general clinical psychological issues. Amongst these is the provision of psychotherapy or counselling, which may follow one of a large variety of models and is often eclectic in nature, addressing issues of personal loss, life changes, and adjustment to disability. Psychotherapeutic techniques appropriate to neuropsychological disability are relatively underdeveloped, and are associated with a number of specific problems such as cognitive limitations and impairment of memory.

Because of their specialist knowledge of human and social relations, and of organisational processes, psychologists will advise and provide practical support to the construction and functioning of clinical teams, besides giving staff support at an individual level. Staff stress is often high in neurological care settings, and the health and welfare of staff is important not only as an end in itself, but also because it has consequences for the care of patients.

Psychologists, who have been trained in methods of research design and analysis, are also commonly active in research relating to neurodisability and in supporting the research of others, and regard it as an important aspect of their role.

NEUROPSYCHOLOGICAL CONSEQUENCES OF NEUROLOGICAL DISORDERS

The consequences and management of neuropsychological problems cannot be discussed in any detail in this chapter but several useful texts exist (e.g. Riddoch & Humphreys, 1994; Beaumont *et al.*, 1996; Kolb & Whishaw, 1996).

GENERAL CONSIDERATIONS

The neuropsychological consequences of neurological disease depend upon a number of factors, not all of which are determined by the neurological aetiology.

Focal versus Diffuse

Focal, relatively localised, lesions result in quite different effects from lesions which diffusely affect the cerebral cortex. Most specific neuropsychological deficits of cognitive function are associated with relatively focal lesions (following trauma, tumours, or surgical intervention), and these have generally been the area of study of neuropsychologists. By contrast, diffuse lesions (following infections, generalised degeneration or widespread closed head injury) tend to affect level of consciousness, attention, motivation and initiation and affect, rather than specific psychological functions.

Acute versus Chronic

Acute lesions have greater effects than chronic lesions. In the acute period following the acquisition of a lesion there may be widespread disruption of psychological functions, together with changes in the level of consciousness, confusion and loss of orientation. Amnesia is common in the acute period, and the duration of post-traumatic amnesia, before continuous memory and full orientation return, is the best indicator of the severity of the lesion (see Chapter 8). Neuropsychological consequences diminish over time, most of the recovery occurring within the first 6–12 months, but with further improvements occurring over the next year or a little longer.

Progressive versus Static; Speed of Development

Lesions that continue to develop, such as tumours and degenerative conditions, have a greater impact than lesions that are essentially static after the initial acute period, such as trauma, cerebrovascular accidents and surgical interventions. The assumption is that the brain accommodates more readily the presence of a static lesion, but must continue to adapt to a developing lesion.

Within progressive lesions, those that develop more rapidly will cause greater psychological disruption than those which develop more slowly. This effect is seen most clearly in the case of tumours, where slow-growing tumours such as meningiomas have much less effect than more rapidly growing tumours such as gliomas. Indeed, meningiomas may grow to a very considerable size before they cause sufficient interference with psychological function to come to medical attention; this is most unlikely to happen in the case of the more aggressive tumours, where a much smaller lesion will have dramatic behavioural consequences.

Site and Lateralisation

The site is obviously of relevance in the case of a focal lesion, and will determine the neuropsychological consequences within the principle of relative localisation (see above). Lateralisation, whether the lesion is primarily located in the left or right hemisphere of the cerebral cortex, is also of relevance as the psychological functions assumed by the two hemispheres are known to differ. There is an enormous literature on cerebral lateralisation, which was the most prominent research topic of neuropsychology for the two decades from about 1960, and most functions show some degree of differential lateralisation. The clearest case is speech, which is exclusively located in the left hemisphere of about 95% of right-handed individuals (Beaumont *et al.*, 1996; Kolb & Whishaw, 1996).

Age of Acquisition

The age at which a lesion is acquired may also be of relevance, as the effects are less in the younger patient and throughout the childhood years (the Kennard principle). This was previously attributed to an increased 'plasticity' of the developing brain, in that alternative regions could subsume the functions previously destined to be located in the area containing the lesion. However, there is now some doubt over this hypothesis, partly due to accumulating evidence for the continuing neural adaptability of the brain in adult life (see Chapter 6). The explanation may lie at least as much in the cognitive flexibility of the developing psychological systems and the greater opportunities for alternative forms of learning in the pre-adult period.

SPECIFIC AETIOLOGIES

As stated above, it is not possible to describe the management of neuropsychological problems in the conditions mentioned in this section. As well as the psychology texts cited in this chapter, the reader is referred to a book on neurological rehabilitation which devotes sections to cognitive and behavioural problems (Greenwood *et al.*, 1993).

Head Injury

Head injury is the most common cause of neurodisability for which rehabilitation is undertaken (see Chapter 8). It affects young males more than any other group and effective intervention can result in a very favourable outcome. Head injuries range from very mild to very severe and profound, with dramatic differences in the behavioural consequences up to and including prolonged coma and vegetative states. The lesions associated with head injury are generally focal or multifocal, and static, although acceleration–deceleration closed head injuries may result in widespread and diffuse lesions across the cortex. An important consideration is that even apparently very mild head injuries associated with a brief period of concussion may sometimes have significant behavioural consequences in terms of anxiety, depression, changes in personality and subtle disorders of memory, with consequent effects upon occupational performance, social activity and personal relationships.

Stroke

Stroke, perhaps because it tends to occur in the more elderly, has received less attention than head injury. The effects of strokes and other cerebrovascular accidents will depend upon the area and proportion of the arterial distribution which is lost, ranging from the whole territory of one of the main cerebral arteries, which is a substantial proportion of the cortex, down to relatively discrete focal lesions associated with a distal portion of one of these arteries (see Chapter 7). Although the neuropsychological consequences depend primarily on the area of cortex affected, the picture is often complicated by the occurrence of further, perhaps minor, strokes that prevent the psychological condition being stable, and by associated arterial disease, which may result in more general and perhaps fluctuating insufficiency of the blood supply to the entire cortex.

Degenerative Conditions

Interest in the degenerative conditions from a neuropsychological perspective has grown in recent years. Other than the dementias of later life, principally dementia of the Alzheimer type, which are clearly associated with deficits of cognitive function of a progressive nature, there are a number of other degenerative conditions which occur in adult life, but of which the neuropsychological consequences are only beginning to be understood. Multiple sclerosis, the most common neurological disease of the population, Parkinson's disease, Huntington's disease and motor neurone disease, sometimes referred to collectively as the subcortical dementias, are all associated with cognitive, affective and behavioural deficits in a significant proportion of those with the disease, and almost all those whose disease progresses to an advanced stage suffer psychological sequelae (see Chapters 11–14). Disorders of memory, attention and affect are common as primary consequences of the disease in this group, and there are naturally significant psychological disturbances associated with being a sufferer from one of these diseases.

Spinal Injuries

Spinal cord injury clearly differs from other neurological conditions in that the patient has suffered a disabling condition, but all neural systems supporting psychological functions are intact (see Chapter 9). The main issue is therefore one of adjustment to the disability, both in terms of the primary impairment dependent upon the spinal cord lesion, and the secondary consequences of handicap that follow from the disability. Amongst the primary disabilities are loss of mobility and other functional capacities (especially if the upper limbs are affected), together with loss of bladder and bowel control and, most importantly for psychological health, sexual function may also be affected. Depression is very common following spinal injury, and the facilitation of insight and adjustment to the disability is a primary task for the neuropsychologist.

CONCLUDING ISSUES

Factors that influence psychological management and that need to be considered include the cognitive ability and psychological adjustment of the patient, and a collaborative team approach.

COGNITIVE ABILITY

An important determinant of the psychological effects of neurological injury or disease is the cognitive status of the individual. Besides specific cognitive deficits, which may limit both psychological and functional adjustment to the disease, more general factors such as attentional capacity, motivation, and the capacity for learning and the acquisition of skills will all contribute to the eventual outcome.

Pre-morbid intellectual capacity will also be a factor; it is known that the best protective factor against dementia in advanced age is to be as an adult more intelligent, and the same principle applies to all neuropsychological deficits. The more you have, the less you will be affected by a given loss, and the more you have left with which to compensate. Nevertheless, those who functioned at a high intellectual level with a mentally demanding occupation before illness may also be more acutely aware of relatively subtle deficits in their ability and this may have a disproportionate effect upon their capacity to pursue a previous occupation.

Relatively intact cognitive abilities may contribute to the ability to benefit from rehabilitation interventions, and to gain insight and consequent adjustment to the disability, although in some severely affected individuals the lack of insight and memory for what has been lost may result in an unawareness which is in some respects protective, even if it cannot be regarded as psychologically healthy.

PSYCHOLOGICAL ADJUSTMENT

Good psychological adjustment depends upon: satisfactory insight into the events and psychological changes that have occurred and a personal acceptance of these changes; an appropriate adjustment of the perception of self; a modification of beliefs and personal goals; and the acquisition of appropriate strategies to compensate as far as is possible for any residual handicap. It implies not only psychological adjustment, but also the re-establishment of personal, family and social relationships, both intimate and more distant. It may also involve occupational adjustment and redefinition of personal roles in all these contexts. This the psychologist must understand and have the skills to facilitate.

It should also be recognised that not all those who acquire neurological diseases had perfect psychological adjustment before the problem occurred; occasionally, the personality of a patient, as perceived by those close to him or her, has actually been improved by the condition. Not everyone who is neurologically intact is in good psychological health, and the goal of returning the client to this state may be confounded by circumstances quite unrelated to the neurological problem.

THE PROCESS OF CARE

Neuropsychologists generally work within a team, particularly in rehabilitation settings. They must contribute to the team not only by their support, but also by effectively playing the appropriate multidisciplinary role within the team. A psychologist who is privileged to work within an expert and committed team will respect the particular contributions made by other team members. They will come to realise that it is only by the collaborative efforts of the disciplines within the team that the optimal outcome will be achieved for the patient, and that the patient will have the best chance of a good psychological adjustment to his or her condition and obtain the best quality of life that is possible.

REFERENCES

Beaumont JG. Neuropsychology. In: Beaumont JG, Kenealy PM, Rogers MJC, eds. *Blackwell dictionary of neuropsychology*. Oxford: Blackwell Publishers; 1996;523-531.

Beaumont JG, Kenealy PM, Rogers MJC, eds. *Blackwell dictionary of neuropsychology*. Oxford: Blackwell Publishers; 1996.

Christensen A-L. *Luria's neuropsychological investigation*. Copenhagen: Munksgaard; 1974.

Code C, Wallesch C-W, Lecours A-R, Joanette Y. *Classic cases in neuropsychology*. Hove: Psychology Press; 1996.

Cook L, Smith DS, Truman G. Using Functional Independence Measure profiles as an index of outcome in the rehabilitation of brain-injured patients. *Arch Phys Med Rehabil* 1994, **75**:390-393.

Crawford JR, Parker DM, McKinlay WW. *A handbook of neuropsychological assessment*. Hove: Lawrence Erlbaum Associates; 1992.

Ditunno JF Jr. Functional assessment measures in CNS trauma. *J Neurotrauma* 1992, **9**(Suppl 1): S301-305.

Greenwood R, Barnes MP, McMillan TM, *et al. Neurological rehabilitation*. London: Churchill Livingstone; 1993.

Harding L, Beech JR. *Assessment in neuropsychology*. London: Routledge; 1996.

Kapur N. *Memory disorders in clinical practice*. Hove: Lawrence Erlbaum Associates; 1994.

Kolb B, Whishaw IQ. *Fundamentals of human neuropsychology, 4th edition*. New York: WH Freeman and Co.; 1996.

Lezak M. *Neuropsychological assessment, 3rd edition*. New York: Oxford University Press; 1995.

Riddoch MJ, Humphreys GW. *Cognitive neuropsychology and cognitive rehabilitation*. Hove: Lawrence Erlbaum Assoc.; 1994.

Wade DT. The Barthel ADL index: guidelines. In: Wade DT, ed. *Measurement in neurological rehabilitation*. Oxford: Oxford University Press; 1992:177-178.

Wilson BA, Moffat N. *Clinical management of memory problems, 2nd edition*. London: Chapman & Hall; 1992.

Wood RL. *Neurobehavioural sequelae of traumatic brain injury*. London: Taylor & Francis; 1990.

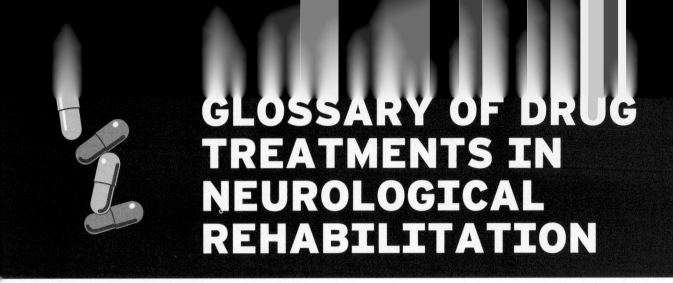

GLOSSARY OF DRUG TREATMENTS IN NEUROLOGICAL REHABILITATION

CHAPTER OUTLINE

Drugs used in the control and treatment of:

- Epilepsy and seizures
- Spasticity
- Parkinson's disease
- Movement abnormalities
- Multiple sclerosis
- Stroke
- Head and spinal cord injury

- Inflammation
- Pain
- Trigeminal neuralgia
- Migraine
- Depression
- Bowel disorders
- Diarrhoea/faecal incontinence
- Bladder disorders

Drug therapy in patients with neurological disorders is aimed mainly at treating and controlling symptoms of conditions for which there is usually no cure. The majority of these disorders are chronic and require multiple drug therapy. The way in which individual patients handle and respond to drugs may vary. Furthermore, the actions and side effects of many drugs are dose-dependent and may mask or exaggerate the underlying neurological condition. The reader is thus encouraged to take account of the combined effects of all drugs prescribed when planning, administering and assessing care for a patient.

The aim of this glossary is to provide the physiotherapist with information on how drugs may influence or interfere with the management of a patient; it thus focuses only on the uses and side effects that are considered of interest to a physiotherapist. It is not possible to provide an exhaustive guide or to discuss drugs in the context of pathology

and the reader should refer to relevant chapters for the latter. Those requiring comprehensive information about a particular drug are referred to the *British National Formulary* (Joint Formulary Committee, 1997), the *ABPI Compendium of Data Sheets* (Association of the British Pharmaceutical Industry, 1996–1997) and *Martindale: The Extra Pharmacopoeia* (The Royal Pharmaceutical Society, 1996). Generic names for drugs tend to be fairly standard internationally. For trade names used outside the UK, readers should refer to their national book. A pharmacist may also prove a valuable resource for advice on issues relating to multiple drug therapy.

Table 28.1, at the end of this glossary, lists generic (non-proprietary) names, widely known proprietary names, and drug use in neurological conditions. Non-proprietary drug names are listed in bold type and proprietary drug names are listed in italics in the following glossary.

1. DRUGS USED TO CONTROL EPILEPSY AND SEIZURES

Carbamazepine (Tegretol)
Use: All forms of simple and complex partial seizures and tonic, clonic seizures. Also used in trigeminal neuralgia and, recently, as prophylaxis in manic depression. Has little or no use in absent seizures. May be used alone or with other anticonvulsants.
Side effects: Ataxia, diplopia, drowsiness, dizziness, vertigo, tremor, headache, nausea, diarrhoea, dry mouth, itching, behavioural disturbance and agitation.

Clonazepam (Rivotril)
Use: Status epilepticus, myoclonus and all forms of epilepsy.
Side effects: Drowsiness, fatigue, dizziness, muscle hypotonia, co-ordination disturbances, paradoxical aggression, irritability and mental changes.

Ethosuximide (Zarontin)
Use: Absent seizures (periods of lack of awareness or response but without convulsions).
Side effects: Drowsiness, dizziness, ataxia, dyskinesia, headache, extrapyramidal side effects, lethargy and fatigue, gastrointestinal disturbances, weight loss, psychotic states, irritability, hyperactivity, sleep disturbances, night terrors, inability to concentrate and aggressiveness.

Gabapentin (Neurontin)
Use: As an adjunct in the treatment of partial seizures with or without secondary generalisation that are not satisfactorily controlled with other antiepileptics.
Side effects: Drowsiness, dizziness, ataxia, fatigue, nystagmus, headache, tremor, diplopia, nausea and vomiting, and dysarthia.

Lamotrigine (Lamictal)
Use: May be used alone or as an adjunct in partial seizures, primary and secondary generalised tonic–clonic seizures.
Side effects: Drowsiness, diplopia, blurred vision, dizziness, insomnia, headache, ataxia, tiredness, gastrointestinal disturbances, aggression, tremor, agitation and confusion.

Phenobarbitone
Use: Status epilepticus and all forms of epilepsy except absent seizures.
Side effects: Drowsiness, lethargy, depression, ataxia, paradoxical excitement, restlessness, and confusion in elderly.

Phenytoin (Epanutin)
Use: Effective in tonic–clonic and partial seizures. Has a narrow therapeutic index and the relationship between dose and plasma concentrations is not linear, thus a small increase in dosage may lead to a large rise in plasma concentration with acute toxic side effects.
Side effects: Nystagmus, blurred vision, ataxia, slurred speech, decreased co-ordination, mental confusion, paraesthesia, drowsiness, vertigo, dizziness, insomnia, motor twitching, headache, nausea, vomiting, constipation, tremor, rarely dyskinesias, peripheral neuropathy and lymphadenopathy.

Primidone (Mysoline)
Use: Essential tremor and all forms of epilepsy except absent seizures.
Side effects: Drowsiness, ataxia, headache, dizziness, nausea and vomiting, and visual disturbances.

Sodium Valproate (Epilim)
Use: All forms of epilepsy.
Side effects: Ataxia, tremor, sedation, gastric irritation, nausea, oedema, hyperactivity and behavioural disturbances.

Topiramate (Topamax)
Use: As an adjunct in the treatment of partial seizures with or without secondary generalisation, not satisfactorily controlled with other antiepileptics.
Side effects: Ataxia, confusion, dizziness, fatigue, paraesthesia, emotional lability, aphasia, diplopia, nausea, nystagmus and speech disorder.

Vigabatrin (Sabril)
Use: Chronic epilepsy not satisfactorily controlled by other antiepileptics.
Side effects: Drowsiness, fatigue, dizziness, nervousness, irritability, headache, aggression, psychosis, excitation and agitation, occasional increase in seizure frequency, diplopia and gastrointestinal disturbances.

2. DRUGS USED TO CONTROL SPASTICITY

The effectiveness of drugs in reducing spasticity varies with the mode of application and the condition of the patient. For example, baclofen given intrathecally may be more effective than when given orally in some patients.

Baclofen (Lioresal)
Use: Chronic and severe spasticity resulting from multiple sclerosis, spinal cord lesions, cerebral palsy and brain injury.
Side effects: Sedation, light-headedness, dizziness, ataxia, headache, tremor, nystagmus, paraesthesias, convulsions, muscular pain and weakness, gastrointestinal and urinary disturbances, increased sweating, and paradoxical increase in spasticity.

Botulinum toxin (Dysport)
Use: Under investigation for treatment of chronic and

severe spasticity in multiple sclerosis and brain injury; injected into muscle, e.g. to relieve hip adductor or elbow flexor spasticity.
Side effects: Muscle weakness.

Dantrolene (Dantrium)
Use: Chronic severe spasticity.
Side effects: Drowsiness, dizziness, weakness, malaise, fatigue, nervousness, diarrhoea, nausea, headache, less frequently constipation, dysphagia, speech and visual disturbances, seizures, dyspnoea, and urinary incontinence or retention.

Diazepam (Valium), Methocarbamol (Robaxin), Orphenadrine (Disipal)
Use: For short-term symptomatic relief of muscle spasms of varied aetiology with the exception of muscle spasm resulting from coma, pre-coma, brain damage, epilepsy or myasthenia gravis.
Side effects: Light-headedness, fatigue, dizziness, drowsiness, nausea and paradoxical restlessness.

Phenol
Use: Intrathecal block to reduce lower limb spasticity and help control pain.
Side effects: Non-specific damage to other neural structures.

3. DRUGS USED IN PARKINSON'S DISEASE

There are two groups of anti-parkinsonian drugs, the dopaminergic and the antimuscarinic drugs.

DOPAMINERGIC ANTI-PARKINSONIAN DRUGS

Amantadine (Symmetrel)
Use: Parkinson's disease, with the exception of drug-induced extrapyramidal symptoms.
Side effects: Nervousness, dizziness, convulsions, blurred vision, gastrointestinal disturbances and peripheral oedema.

Apomorphine (Britaject)
Use: Patients with frequent 'on–off' fluctuations in motor performance which are inadequately controlled by conventional antiparkinsonian medication.
Side effects: Dyskinesia during the 'on' periods, postural instability and falls, increase in cognitive impairment, nausea, vomiting, sedation, postural hypotension, euphoria, light-headedness, restlessness and tremors.

Bromocriptine (Parlodel)
Use: Idiopathic Parkinson's disease, both alone or in combination with levodopa.
Side effects: Nausea, vomiting, constipation, headache, dizziness, postural hypotension, drowsiness, vasospasm of the fingers and toes particularly in patients with poor peripheral circulation, confusion, psychomotor excitation, dyskinesia and leg cramps.

Levodopa (Brocadopa, Larodopa) used with a dopa-decarboxylase inhibitor, e.g. Benserazide (Co-beneldopa, Madopar) or Carbidopa (Co-careldopa, Sinemet)
Use: Idiopathic parkinsonism, with the exception of drug-induced extrapyramidal symptoms.
Side effects: Ataxia, gait abnormalities, numbness, agitation, postural hypotension, dizziness, psychiatric symptoms which include hypomania and psychosis, drowsiness, headache, flushing, sweating, nausea, vomiting, dysphagia, peripheral neuropathy, diplopia, blurred vision, urinary retention and incontinence, and fatigue.

Lysuride Melate (Revanil)
Use: Treatment of Parkinson's disease, both alone or in combination with levodopa.
Side effects: Nausea, vomiting, sudden severe fall in blood pressure in early stages of treatment, dizziness, headache, lethargy, malaise and drowsiness.

Pergolide (Celance)
Use: As an adjunct to levodopa in the treatment of Parkinson's disease.
Side effects: Body pain, abdominal pain, nausea, dyspepsia, dyskinesia, somnolence, diplopia, dyspnoea, insomnia, constipation or diarrhoea, and hypotension.

Ropinirole (Requip)
Use: Parkinson's disease, more useful as an adjunct to levodopa.
Side effects: Nausea, abdominal pain, vomiting, oedema, somnolence, dyskinesia, confusion and occasionally severe hypotension.

Selegiline (Eldepryl)
Use: Idiopathic parkinsonism, with the exception of drug-induced extrapyramidal symptoms, alone or in combination with levodopa.
Side effects: Hypotension, nausea and vomiting, andagitation.

ANTIMUSCARINIC ANTI-PARKINSONIAN DRUGS

Benzhexol Hydrochloride (Artane), Benztropine Mesylate (Cogentin), Biperiden (Akineton), Orphenadrine Hydrochloride (Disipal), Procyclidine Hydrochloride (Kemadrin).
Use: Parkinson's disease and drug-induced extrapyramidal symptoms.
Side effects: Dry mouth, gastrointestinal disturbances, dizziness, blurred vision, urinary retention, nervousness, and in high doses in susceptible patients, mental confusion, excitement, sedation (with Benztropine and Biperiden), and psychiatric disturbances which may necessitate discontinuation of treatment.

4. DRUGS USED TO CONTROL MOVEMENT ABNORMALITIES

Movement disorders covered here include essential tremor, chorea (e.g. in Huntington's disease), tics and related disorders.

Benzhexol Hydrochloride (Artane)
Use: In some movement disorders at high doses.
Side effects: Previously described in section on anti-parkinsonian drugs.

Botulinium toxin (Dysport)
Use: Blepharospasm, hemifacial spasm and spasmodic torticollis.
Side effects: Ptosis, lacrimation, eye irritation, diplopia, increased electorphysiologic jitter in some distant muscles, bruising, weakness of neck muscles, dysphagia and dryness of mouth. Excessive doses may produce distant and profound neuromuscular paralysis, reversed with time.

Chlorpromazine (Largactil), Haloperidol (Serenace, Haldol), Pimozide (Orap), Clonidine (Dixarit), Sulpiride (Dolmatil)
Use: Motor tics, adjunctive treatment in choreas and Gilles de la Tourette syndrome.
Side effects: Extrapyramidal symptoms such as dystonic reactions and akathisia, Parkinsonism, tremor, tardive dyskinesia, drowsiness, in more rare instances, agitation, convulsions, antimuscarinic symptoms such as dry mouth, nasal congestion, constipation, difficulty in micturition and blurred vision.

Piracetam (Nootropil)
Use: Myoclonus of cortical origin.
Side effects: Hyperkinesia, drowsiness and nervousness.

Primidone (Mysoline)
Use: Benign essential tremor.
Side effects: Drowsiness, nystagmus, ataxia, nausea, vomiting, headache and dizziness.

Propranolol (Inderal)
Use: Treatment of essential tremor or tremor associated with anxiety or thyroytoxicosis.
Side effects: Postural hypotension, peripheral vasoconstriction, paraesthesia, dizziness, mood changes, psychoses, gastrointestinal disturbances and fatigue.

Tetrabenazine (Nitoman)
Use: Movement disorders due to Huntington's chorea, senile chorea and related neurological conditions.
Side effects: Drowsiness, gastrointestinal disturbances, extrapyramidal dysfunction and hypotension.

5. DRUGS USED IN MULTIPLE SCLEROSIS (MS)

Corticosteroids: Methylprednisolone (Depo-Medrone)
Use: To hasten recovery following a relapse.
Side effects: Cushing's syndrome, hypotension, mental disturbances and muscle wasting.

Dopaminergic drugs: Amantadine (Symmetrel) or Pemoline (Volital)
Use: To treat fatigue associated with MS.
Side effects: Nervousness, restlessness, tremor, dizziness, convulsions, headache, blurred vision, gastrointestinal disturbances, peripheral oedema, dry mouth, sweating, tics and Gilles de la Tourette's syndrome.

Beta-1a-Interferon (Avonex) Beta-1b-Interferon (Betaferon)
Use: To reduce the frequency and severity of relapses in patients with relapsing–remitting MS.
Side effects: Injection site reactions, anxiety, convulsions and confusion.

Isoniazid/Pyridoxine
Use: To treat tremor associated with MS. Does not affect progression or remission of disease.
Side effects: Nausea, vomiting, peripheral neuritis, convulsions and psychotic episodes.

Cannabis, Tetrahydrocannabinol (Dranabinol)
Use: Under investigation for the treatment of tremor, spasticity, ataxia and muscle pain associated with MS; currently classed as Schedule I Controlled Drug and a licence from the Home Office is needed for investigational use.
Side effects: Weakness, dry mouth, dizziness, impairment of posture and balance.

6. DRUGS USED IN STROKE

Sequelae seen in stroke can vary depending on the site of lesion and the type of haemorrhage, thrombosis or embolism (see Chapter 7). Drug treatment is aimed at controlling the symptoms and treating the predisposing risk factors such as hypertension, diabetes, hyperlipidaemia, obesity, smoking and alcohol excess. In addition, the following may be prescribed depending upon need: anticonvulsants, antiplatelet drugs such as aspirin, anti-spasticity drugs such as baclofen, anticoagulant drugs such as warfarin (contraindicated following cerebral haemorrhage) and nimodipine, a calcium channel blocker to prevent vascular spasm following subarachnoid haemorrhage (SAH).

7. DRUGS USED IN HEAD AND SPINAL CORD INJURY

A prolonged or incomplete recovery may follow injury, and drug treatment is aimed at treating the sequelae such as post-traumatic epilepsy (1), spasticity (2), pain (9), depression (12) and loss of autonomic functions such as bladder and bowel control (13–15). Excessive bronchial and salivary secretions are treated with oral or transdermal administration of hyoscine.

8. DRUGS USED TO TREAT INFLAMMATION

STEROIDAL ANTI-INFLAMMATORY DRUGS

Dexamethasone *(Decadron)*, Hydrocortisone *(Hydrocortistab)*, Methylprednisolone *(Depo-Medrone)*, Prednisolone *(Deltastab)*, Triamcinolone *(Adcortyl, Kenalog, Lederspan)*
Use: Injected locally into soft tissue or joints for anti-inflammatory effect to relieve pain, increase mobility and reduce deformity.
Side effects: Occasionally, reaction at the site of injection.

NON-STEROIDAL ANTI-INFLAMMATORY DRUGS

Aspirin, Azapropazone *(Rheumox)*, Diclofenac *(Voltarol)*, Diflunisal *(Dolobid)*, Ibuprofen *(Brufen)*, Indomethacin *(Indocid)*, Ketoprofen *(Alrheumet, Orudis, Oruvail)*, Mefenamic Acid *(Ponstan)*, Naproxen *(Naprosyn, Synflex)*, Phenylbutazone *(Butacote)*, Piroxicam *(Feldene)*
Use: To treat pain and inflammation.
Side effects: Headache, dizziness, fatigue, vertigo, drowsiness, convulsions, peripheral neuropathy, muscle weakness, involuntary muscle movements, aggravation of epilepsy and parkinsonism, gastrointestinal side effects such as nausea, dyspepsia, abdominal pain, oedema, hypotension and diplopia.

9. DRUGS USED TO CONTROL PAIN

NON-OPIOID ANALGESICS
Nefopam *(Acupan)*
Side effects: Nausea, vomiting, dry mouth, nervousness, lightheadedness, drowsiness, confusion, urinary retention, blurred vision and sweating.

Paracetamol (Panadol)
Side effects: Rash.

NON-STEROIDAL ANTI-INFLAMMATORY DRUGS TO CONTROL PAIN
Use: Previously described under the section on Drugs Used to treat Inflammation.
Side effects: Listed above under the Anti-inflammatory section.

OPIOID ANALGESICS
Buprenorphine *(Temgesic)*, Codeine, Dextropropoxyphene in combination with Paracetamol as Co-proxamol, Diamorphine, Dihydrocodeine *(DF118)*, Dipipanone *(Diconal)*, Fentanyl *(Sublimaze)*, Meptazinol *(Meptid)*, Morphine *(Oramorph, MST Continus)*, Pethidine, Tramadol *(Zydol)*
Side effects: Nausea, vomiting, constipation, drowsiness, hypotension, difficulty with micturition, dry mouth, sweating, headache, facial flushing and vertigo.

10. DRUGS USED TO TREAT TRIGEMINAL NEURALGIA

Carbamazepine (Tegretol)
Side effects: Listed under section on Drugs Used to control Epilepsy and Seizures (1).

Phenytoin (Epanutin)
Side effects: Listed under section on Drugs Used to cotrol Epilepsy and Seizures (1).

Tricyclic antidepressants: Amitriptyline *(Tryptizol)*, Clomipramine *(Anafranil)*, Dothiepin *(Prothiaden)*, Imipramine *(Tofranil)*, Lofepramine *(Gamanil)*, Trimipramine *(Surmontil)*
Side effects: Dry mouth, nausea, constipation, sedation, blurred vision, difficulty with micturition, syncope, postural hypotension, sweating, tremor, rashes, hypersensitivity reactions, behavioural disturbances, movement disorders and dyskinesias, convulsions, numbness, paraesthesia of extremities, peripheral neuropathy, inco-ordination, extrapyramidal symptoms, dizziness, weakness, fatigue and headache.

11. DRUGS USED TO TREAT MIGRAINE

Clonidine *(Dixarit)*
Use: Prophylaxis of recurrent migraine.
Side effects: Dry mouth, sedation, dizziness and nausea.

Methysergide *(Deseril)*
Use: Prevention of recurrent migraine and cluster headache.
Side effects: Nausea, vomiting, heartburn, drowsiness, dizziness, postural hypotension, mental and behavioural disturbances, oedema, rashes, leg cramps and paraesthesias of extremities.

Pizotifen *(Sanomigran)*
Use: Prophylaxis of vascular headache, cluster headache and migraine.
Side effects: Dry mouth, nausea, constipation, drowsiness and dizziness.

Propranolol (*Inderal*)
Use: Migraine prophylaxis.
Side effects: See section 4.

Ergotamine (*Cafergot, Migril*)
Use: Treatment of migraine.
Side effects: Nausea, vomiting, abdominal pain, paraesthesia, peripheral vasoconstriction, pain and weakness in the extremities, numbness, muscle cramps and occasionally increased headache.

Paracetamol with an antiemetic such as Metoclopramide (*Paramax*)
Use: Treatment of migraine.
Side effects: Metoclopramide can cause extrapyramidal symptoms of dystonic type, tardive dyskinesia, neuroleptic syndrome, drowsiness, restlessness and diarrhoea.

Sumatriptan (*Imigran*)
Use: Treatment of migraine.
Side effects: Chest pain and tightness, sensations of tingling, heat, heaviness, pressure or tightness in any part of the body, flushing, dizziness, weakness, paraesthesia, seizures, hypotension, nausea, vomiting, fatigue and drowsiness.

12. DRUGS USED TO TREAT DEPRESSION

TRICYCLIC ANTIDEPRESSANTS

Amitriptyline (*Tryptizol*), **Clomipramine** (*Anafranil*), **Dothiepin** (*Prothiaden*), **Imipramine** (*Tofranil*), **Lofepramine** (*Gamanil*), **Trimipramine** (*Surmontil*)
Side effects: See section 10.

OTHER ANTIDEPRESSANTS RELATED TO THE TRICYCLICS
Maprotiline (*Ludiomil*), **Mianserin** (*Bolvidon*), **Trazodone** (*Molipaxin*)
Side effects: As for the tricyclic antidepressants but with milder antimuscarinic side effects.

MONOAMINE OXIDASE INHIBITORS
Phenelzine (*Nardil*), **Isocarboxazid** (*Marplan*), **Tranylcypromine** (*Parnate*)
Side effects: Postural hypotension, dizziness, drowsiness, headache, weakness, fatigue, dry mouth, constipation, other gastrointestinal disturbances, oedema, agitation, tremors, nervousness, blurred vision, difficulty in micturition, sweating, convulsions, and psychotic episodes with hypomanic behaviour.

REVERSIBLE MONOAMINE OXIDASE INHIBITORS
Moclobemide (*Manerix*)
Side effects: Dizziness, nausea, headache, restlessness and agitation.

SELECTIVE SEROTONIN REUPTAKE INHIBITORS (SSRI)
Citalopram (*Cipramil*), **Fluoxetine** (*Prozac*), **Fluvoxamine** (*Faverin*), **Paroxetine** (*Seroxat*), **Sertaline** (*Lustral*)
Side effects: Nausea, vomiting, diarrhoea, dry mouth, dyspepsia, headache, agitation, drowsiness, tremor, dizziness, fatigue, seizures, dyskinesia, movement disorders and sweating.

13. DRUGS USED IN BOWEL DISORDERS

Bulk-forming laxatives: Bran, Ispaghula husk, Methylcellulose, Sterculia (*Celevac, Fybogel, Isogel, Normacol, Trifyba, Regulan*)
Side effects: Flatulence, abdominal distension, and gastrointestinal obstruction or impaction.

Faecal softeners: Arachis oil (rectally), Docusate (orally)
Side effects: Abdominal cramps.

Osmotic laxatives: Lactilol, Lactulose, Magnesium salts (*Epsom salts*), **Phosphates** (*Fletcher's enemas*), **Sodium Citrate** (*Microlette*).
Side effects: Flatulence, cramps and abdominal discomfort.

Stimulant laxatives: Bisacodyl (*Dulcolax*), **Danthron** (*Co-danthramer, Co-danthrusate*), **Docusate Sodium** (*Dioctyl*), **Glycerol, Senna** (*Senokot*), **Sodium Picosulphate** (*Picolax*)
Side effects: Increased intestinal motility and abdominal cramps; prolonged use can precipitate atonic colon and hypokalaemia.

14. DRUGS USED TO TREAT DIARRHOEA/FAECAL INCONTINENCE

Codeine Phosphate
Side effects: Nausea, vomiting, difficulty with micturition and dry mouth.

Loperamide (*Imodium*)
Side effects: Abdominal cramps and abdominal bloating.

Diphenoxylate/Atropine combination (*Lomotil*)
Side effects: As for codeine.

15. DRUGS USED IN BLADDER DISORDERS

URINARY RETENTION
Alpha Blockers: Alfuzosin (*Xatral*), **Doxazosin** (*Cardura*), **Indoramin** (*Doralese*), **Prazosin** (*Hypovase*), **Terazosin** (*Hytrin*)
Side effects: Sedation, dizziness, postural hypotension,

weakness, lack of energy, headache, dry mouth, nausea, urinary frequency and incontinence.

Parasympathomimetic agents: Bethanechol (Myotonin), Distigmine (Ubretid)
Side effects: Nausea, vomiting, sweating and blurred vision.

URINARY FREQUENCY, ENURESIS, INCONTINENCE
Flavoxate (Urispas), Oxybutynin (Cystrin, Ditropan), Propantheline (Probanthine)
Side effects: Dry mouth, constipation, diarrhoea, blurred vision, nausea, abdominal discomfort, facial flushing, difficulty in micturition, headache, dizziness and drowsiness.

Cross reference of generic and proprietary drug names and their use in neurological disorders

Drug name	Drug name	Drug use (Glossary reference)
Acupan*	Nefopam	Pain (9)
Adcortyl*	Triamcinolone	Inflammation (8)
Akineton	Biperiden*	Parkinson's (3)
Alfuzosin	Xatral*	Urinary retention (15)
Alrheumet*	Ketoprofen	Pain, Inflammation (8,9)
Amantadine	Symmetrel*	Parkinson's (3), Fatigue in MS (5)
Amitriptyline	Tryptizol*	Trigeminal neuralgia (10), Depression (12)
Anafranil*	Clomipramine	Trigeminal neuralgia (10), Depression (12)
Apomorphine	Britaject*	Parkinson's (3)
Arachis oil		Laxative (13)
Artane*	Benzhexol	Parkinson's (3), Tremor (4), Chorea (4), Tics (4)
Aspirin		Pain, Inflammation (8,9)
Avonex*	Beta-1a Interferon	MS (5)
Azapropazone	Rheumox*	Pain, Inflammation (8,9)
Baclofen	Lioresal*	Spasticity (2)
Benzhexol	Artane*	Parkinson's (3), Tremor (4), Chorea (4), Tics (4)
Benztropine	Cogentin*	Parkinson's (3)
Beta 1a Interferon	Avonex*	MS (5)
Beta-1b Interferon	Betaferon*	MS (5)
Betaferon*	Beta-1b Interferon	MS (5)
Bethanechol	Myotonin*	Urinary retention (15)
Biperiden	Akineton*	Parkinson's (3)
Bisacodyl	Dulcolax*	Laxative (13)
Bolvidon*	Mianserin	Depression (12)
Botulinium toxin	Dysport*	Torticollis, Blepharospasm (4), Spasticity (2)
Britaject*	Apomorphine	Parkinson's (3)
Brocadopa*	Levodopa	Parkinson's (3)
Bromocriptine	Parlodel*	Parkinson's (3)
Brufen*	Ibuprofen	Pain, Inflammation (8,9)
Buprenorphine	Temgesic*	Pain (9)
Butacote*	Phenylbutazone	Pain, Inflammation (8,9)

Table 28.1 Cross reference of generic and proprietary drug names and their use in neurological disorders.
*Proprietary drug names

Drug name	Drug name	Drug use (Glossary reference)
Cafergot*	Ergotamine	Migraine (11)
Cannabis		MS (5)
Carbamazepine	Tegretol*	Seizures (1), Trigeminal neuralgia (10)
Cardura*	Doxazosin	Urinary retention (15)
Celance*	Pergolide	Parkinson's (3)
Chlorpromazine	Largactil*	Motor tics, Chorea (4)
Cipramil*	Citalopram	Depression (12)
Citalopram	Cipramil*	Depression (12)
Clomipramine	Anafranil*	Trigeminal neuralgia (10), Depression (12)
Clonazepam	Rivotril*	Seizures (1)
Clonidine	Dixarit*	Motor tics, Chorea (4),Migraine (11)
Co-beneldopa	Madopar*	Parkinson's (3)
Co-careldopa	Sinemet*	Parkinson's (3)
Co-proxamol	Dextropropoxyphene/ Paracetamol	Pain (9)
Codeine		Pain (9), diarrhoea (14)
Cogentin*	Benztropine	Parkinson's (3)
Cystrin*	Oxybutynin	Urinary frequency (15)
Dantrium*	Dantrolene	Spasticity (2)
Dantrolene	Dantrium*	Spasticity (2)
Decadron*	Dexamethasone	Inflammation (8)
Deltastab*	Prednisolone	Inflammation (8)
Depo-Medrone*	Methylprednisolone	Inflammation (8)
Deseril*	Methysergide	Migraine (11)
Dexamethasone	Decadron*	Inflammation (8)
Dextropropoxyphene/ Paracetamol	Co-proxamol	Pain (9)
DF118*	Dihydrocodeine	Pain (9)
Diamorphine		Pain (9)
Diazepam	Valium*	Status epilepticus (1), Spasticity (2)
Diclofenac*	Voltarol*	Pain, Inflammation (8,9)
Diconal*	Dipipanone	Pain (9)
Diflunisal	Dolobid*	Pain, Inflammation (8,9)
Dihydrocodeine	DF118*	Pain (9)
Dioctyl*	Docusate sodium	Laxative (13)
Diphenoxylate/Atropine	Lomotil*	Diarrhoea (14)
Dipipanone	Diconal*	Pain (9)
Disipal*	Orphenadrine	Parkinson's (3), Spasticity (2)
Distigmine	Ubretid*	Urinary retention (15)
Ditropan*	Oxybutynin	Urinary frequency (15)
Dixarit*	Clonidine	Motor tics, Chorea (4), Migraine (11)
Docusate sodium	Dioctyl*	Laxative (13)
Dolmatil*	Sulpiride	Motor tics, Chorea (4)
Dolobid*	Diflunisal	Pain, Inflammation (8,9)
Doralese*	Indoramin	Urinary retention (15)
Dothiepin	Prothiaden*	Trigeminal neuralgia (10), Depression (12)
Doxazosin	Cardura*	Urinary retention (16)
Dulcolax*	Bisacodyl	Laxative (13)
Dysport*	Botulinium toxin	Torticollis, Blepharospasm (4)
Eldepryl*	Selegiline	Parkinson's (3)
Epanutin*	Phenytoin	Seizures, Status epilepticus (1)

Drug name	Drug name	Drug use (Glossary reference)
Epilim*	Sodium valproate	Seizures (1)
Epsom salts*	Magnesium sulphate	Laxative (13)
Ergotamine	Cafergot*, Migril*	Migraine (11)
Ethosuximide	Zarontin*	Seizures (1)
Faverin*	Fluvoxamine	Depression (12)
Feldene*	Piroxicam	Pain, Inflammation (8,9)
Fentanyl	Sublimaze*	Pain (9)
Fibre	Isogel*,Fybogel*,Normacol*, Trifyba*, Regulan*	Laxative (13)
Flavoxate	Urispas*	Urinary frequency (15)
Fletcher's enemas*	Phosphate enemas	Laxative (13)
Fluoxetine	Prozac*	Depression (12)
Fluvoxamine	Faverin*	Depression (12)
Gabapentin	Neurontin*	Seizures (1)
Gamanil*	Lofepramine	Trigeminal neuralgia (10), Depression (12)
Glycerol		Laxative (13)
Haldol*	Haloperidol	Motor tics, Chorea (4)
Haloperidol	Haldol*, Serenace*	Motor tics, Chorea (4)
Hydrocortisone	Hydrocortistab*	Inflammation (8)
Hydrocortistab*	Hydrocortisone	Inflammation (8)
Hyoscine	Kwells*, Scopaderm*	Reduce secretions (7)
Hypovase*	Prazosin	Urinary retention (15)
Hytrin*	Terazosin	Urinary retention (15)
Ibuprofen	Brufen*	Pain, Inflammation (8,9)
Imigran*	Sumatriptan	Migraine (11)
Imipramine	Tofranil*	Trigeminal neuralgia (10), Depression (12)
Imodium*	Loperamide	Diarrhoea (14)
Inderal*	Propranolol	Essential tremor (4), Migraine (11)
Indocid*	Indomethacin	Pain, Inflammation (8,9)
Indomethacin	Indocid*	Pain, Inflammation (8,9)
Indoramin	Doralese*	Urinary retention (15)
Isocarboxazid	Marplan*	Depression (12)
Isogel*,Fybogel*, Normacol*, Trifyba*, Regulan*	Fibre	Laxative (13)
Isoniazid/Pyridoxine		MS (5)
Kemadrin*	Procyclidine	Parkinson's (3)
Kenalog*	Triamcinolone	Inflammation (8)
Ketoprofen	Alrheumet*,Orudis*,Oruvail*	Pain, Inflammation (8,9)
Kwells*	Hyoscine	Reduce secretions (7)
Lactitol		Laxative (13)
Lactulose		Laxative (13)
Lamictal*	Lamotrigine	Seizures (1)
Lamotrigine	Lamictal*	Seizures (1)
Largactil*	Chlorpromazine	Motor tics, Chorea (4)
Larodopa*	Levodopa	Parkinson's (3)
Lederspan*	Triamcinolone	Inflammation (8)
Levodopa	Brocadopa*, Larodopa*	Parkinson's (3)
Lioresal*	Baclofen	Spasticity (2)
Lofepramine	Gamanil*	Trigeminal neuralgia (10), Depression (12)
Lomotil*	Diphenoxylate/Atropine	Diarrhoea (14)
Loperamide	Imodium*	Diarrhoea (14)

Drug name	Drug name	Drug use (Glossary reference)
Ludiomil*	Maprotiline	Depression (12)
Lustral*	Sertraline	Depression (12)
Lysuride	Revanil*	Parkinson's (3)
Madopar*	Co-beneldopa	Parkinson's (3)
Magnesium sulphate	Epsom salts*	Laxative (13)
Manerix*	Moclobemide	Depression (12)
Maprotiline	Ludiomil*	Depression (12)
Marplan*	Isocarboxazid	Depression (12)
Mefenamic Acid	Ponstan*	Pain, Inflammation (8,9)
Meptazinol	Meptid*	Pain (9)
Meptid*	Meptazinol	Pain (9)
Methocarbamol	Robaxin*	Spasticity (2)
Methylprednisolone	Depo-Medrone*	Inflammation (8)
Methysergide	Deseril*	Migraine (11)
Mianserin	Bolvidon*	Depression (12)
Microlette*	Sodium citrate solution	Laxative (13)
Migril*	Ergotamine	Migraine (11)
Moclobemide	Manerix*	Depression (12)
Molipaxin*	Trazodone	Depression (12)
Morphine	MST Continus*, Oramorph*	Pain (9)
MST Continus*	Morphine	Pain (9)
Myotonin*	Bethanechol	Urinary retention (15)
Mysoline*	Primidone	Essential tremor (4), Seizures (1)
Naprosyn*	Naproxen	Pain, Inflammation (8,9)
Naproxen	Naprosyn*, Synflex*	Pain, Inflammation (8,9)
Nardil*	Phenelzine	Depression (12)
Nefopam	Acupan*	Pain (9)
Neurontin*	Gabapentin	Seizures (1)
Nimodipine	Nimotop*	SAH (6)
Nimotop*	Nimodipine	SAH (6)
Nitoman*	Tetrabenazine	Chorea (4)
Nootropil*	Piracetam	Myoclonus (4)
Oramorph*	Morphine	Pain (9)
Orap*	Pimozide	Motor tics, Chorea (4)
Orphenadrine	Disipal*	Parkinson's (3), Spasticity (2)
Orudis*	Ketoprofen	Pain, Inflammation (8,9)
Oruvail*	Ketoprofen	Pain, Inflammation (8,9)
Oxybutynin	Cystrin*, Ditropan*	Urinary frequency (15)
Panadol*	Paracetamol	Pain (9)
Paracetamol	Panadol*	Pain (9)
Paracetamol/Metoclopramide	Paramax*	Migraine (11)
Paramax*	Paracetamol/Metoclopramide	Migraine (11)
Parlodel*	Bromocriptine	Parkinson's (3)
Parnate*	Tranylcypromine	Depression (12)
Paroxetine	Seroxat*	Depression (12)
Pemoline	Volital*	Fatigue in MS (5)
Pergolide	Celance*	Parkinson's (3)
Pethidine		Pain (9)
Phenelzine	Nardil*	Depression (12)
Phenobarbitone		Seizures (1)
Phenol		Spasticity (2)

Drug name	Drug name	Drug use (Glossary reference)
Phenylbutazone	Butacote*	Pain, Inflammation (8,9)
Phenytoin	Epanutin*	Status epilepticus (1), Seizures (1)
Phosphate enemas	Fletcher's enemas*	Laxative (13)
Picolax*	Sodium Picosulphate	Laxative (13)
Pimozide	Orap*	Motor tics, Chorea (4)
Piracetam	Nootropil*	Myoclonus (4)
Piroxicam	Feldene*	Pain, Inflammation (8,9)
Pizotifen	Sanomigran*	Migraine (11)
Ponstan*	Mefenamic Acid	Pain, Inflammation (8,9)
Prazosin	Hypovase*	Urinary retention (15)
Prednisolone	Deltastab*	Inflammation (8)
Primidone	Mysoline*	Essential tremor (4), Seizures (1)
Probanthine*	Propantheline	Urinary frequency (15)
Procyclidine	Kemadrin*	Parkinson's (3)
Propantheline	Probanthine*	Urinary frequency (15)
Propranolol	Inderal*	Essential tremor (4), Migraine (11)
Prothiaden*	Dothiepin	Trigeminal neuralgia (10), Depression (12)
Prozac*	Fluoxetine	Depression (12)
Requip*	Ropinirole	Parkinson's (3)
Revanil*	Lysuride	Parkinson's (3)
Rheumox*	Azapropazone	Pain, Inflammation (8,9)
Rivotril*	Clonazepam	Seizures (1)
Robaxin*	Methocarbamol	Spasticity (2)
Ropinirole	Requip*	Parkinson's (3)
Sabril*	Vigabatrin	Seizures (1)
Sanomigran*	Pizotifen	Migraine (11)
Scopaderm*	Hyoscine	Reduce secretions (7)
Selegiline	Eldepryl*	Parkinson's (3)
Senna	Senokot*	Laxative (13)
Senokot*	Senna	Laxative (13)
Serenace*	Haloperidol	Motor tics, Chorea (4)
Seroxat*	Paroxetine	Depression (12)
Sertaline	Lustral*	Depression (12)
Sinemet*	Co-careldopa	Parkinson's (3)
Sodium citrate solution	Microlette*	Laxative (13)
Sodium Picosulphate	Picolax*	Laxative (13)
Sodium valproate	Epilim*	Seizures (1)
Sublimaze	Fentanyl*	Pain (9)
Sulpiride	Dolmatil*	Motor tics, Chorea (4)
Sumatriptan	Imigran*	Migraine (11)
Surmontil*	Trimipramine	Trigeminal neuralgia (10), Depression (12)
Symmetrel*	Amantadine	Parkinson's (3), Fatigue in MS (5)
Synflex*	Naproxen	Pain, Inflammation (8,9)
Tegretol*	Carbamazepine	Seizures (1), Trigeminal neuralgia (10)
Temgesic*	Buprenorphine	Pain (9)
Terazosin	Hytrin*	Urinary retention (15)
Tetrabenazine	Nitoman*	Chorea (4)
Tofranil*	Imipramine	Trigeminal neuralgia (10), Depression (12)
Topamax*	Topiramate	Seizures (1)
Topiramate	Topamax*	Seizures (1)
Tramadol	Zydol*	Pain (9)

Drug name	Drug name	Drug use (Glossary Reference)
Tranylcypromine	Parnate*	Depression (12)
Trazodone	Molipaxin*	Depression (12)
Triamcinolone	Adcortyl*,Kenalog*,Lederspan	Inflammation (28,8)
Trimipramine	Surmontil*	Trigeminal neuralgia (10), Depression (12)
Tryptizol*	Amitriptyline	Trigeminal neuralgia (10), Depression (12)
Ubretid*	Distigmine	Urinary retention (15)
Urispas*	Flavoxate	Urinary retention (15)
Valium*	Diazepam	Status epilepticus (1), Spasticity (2)
Vigabatrin	Sabril*	Seizures (1)
Volital*	Pemoline	Fatigue in MS (5)
Voltarol*	Diclofenac*	Pain, Inflammation (8,9)
Xatral*	Alfuzosin	Urinary retention (15)
Zarontin*	Ethosuximide	Seizures (1)
Zydol*	Tramadol	Pain (9)

REFERENCES

Association of the British Pharmaceutical Industry. *ABPI Compendium of Data Sheets*. London: Datapharm Publications Ltd; 1996-1997.

Joint Formulary Committee. *British National Formulary, Number 34*. London: British Medical Association & Royal Pharmaceutical Society of Great Britain; 1997.

The Royal Pharmaceutical Society. *Martindale: The Extra Pharmacopoeia, 31st edition*. London: The Pharmaceutical Press; 1996.